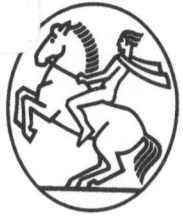

William E. Stewart II

The Interferon System

Second, enlarged edition

Springer-Verlag Wien GmbH

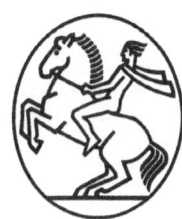

William E. Stewart II
Interferon Laboratories
Sloan-Kettering Institute for Cancer Resarch
New York, N. Y., U. S. A.

With 23 Figures

Library of Congress Cataloging in Publication Data. Stewart, William E. 1940–   . The interferon system.
Bibliography: p. Includes index. 1. Interferons. I. Title. [DNLM: 1. Interferon. QW 800 S852i.]
QR 187.5.S73. 1981.599.02'95.81–1775

ISBN 978-3-7091-8617-6   ISBN 978-3-7091-8615-2 (eBook)
DOI 10.1007/978-3-7091-8615-2

Preface to the First Edition

This book is an update of *Interferon*, published in 1969 by Dr. Jan Vilček. The field of interferon research has since expanded from its former narrow treatment of interferon strictly as an antiviral substance, such that *The Interferon System* now encompasses cellular modulations ranging from immune alterations to cell proliferative restrictions to antitumor activities. The steadily increasing number of these *non-antiviral* functions of interferons emphasizes the need for a comprehensive – and critical – review of the entire literature of interferon studies.

The text, with its supporting bibliography, provides complete coverage of interferon research. A newcomer to the area should find here all the information necessary to understand why interferon, which has been studied for more than twenty years and which originally stirred excitement over its clinical prospects, is still inspiring speculation about this potential. For those already familiar with the seemingly perpetual clinical promise of interferon, this volume should serve as a valuable reference source, the largest bibliography on the subject ever to appear under one cover.

Clearly, this book should be considered only as an introduction to the topic and as a reference source; most questions about the interferon system are still unanswered – even unasked. Hopefully this summation and critical evaluation of work done to date will stimulate and facilitate further progress.

New York, N. Y., February 1979   **William E. Stewart II**

Preface to the Second Edition

This second edition of *The Interferon System* includes an Appendix to the References to incorporate most of the papers that have been published on interferon between mid-1978 and the end of 1980. I have also included references to several of the older papers that were not referred to in the original text, to provide as complete a reference source on interferon as possible. The text, however, remains unchanged.

The format for the Second Edition derives from the fact that the publishers exhausted their supply of the First Edition in less than two years, and I felt it was premature to attempt a revision of the text at this stage. Data collection in the field of interferon research is presently proceeding at a rapid rate, both in basic molecular biology and in clinical evaluations. Hence, it will likely be some time before I shall undertake to revise the text for the Third Edition. However, be assured that when I do so, I shall again interject critical evaluations (personal animus?) against anyone publishing erroneous information on The Interferon System.

New York, N. Y., February 1981 **William E. Stewart II**

Contents

I. Introduction

In preparing this volume, I have attempted to cover each of the various aspects of what has become collectively known as *The Interferon System*. I have tried to include as much of the entire literature on this topic as possible, both from an historical perspective and an up-to-date account, so that this work will serve both as an introduction to the subject and as a comprehensive reference source for the field. Where it has not been feasible to include in depth discussion on each topic, I have attempted to reference ample literature; next to knowing is knowing where to find-out!

I have been aided enormously in this effort by my many colleagues who sent me their manuscripts over the past months, often even before they were accepted for publication. This cooperation has allowed this review to have even more emphasis on recent works than would otherwise have been possible at this date.

As this study is written, interferon has been known for 21 years (yet another decade since Jan Vilček [1969] phrased this sentence in the introduction to his monograph). The elegantly straight-forward studies reported by the late Alick Isaacs and by Jean Lindenmann (Isaacs and Lindenmann, 1957) immediately clarified vast accumulations of mysterious effects of how one virus, in either a cell culture or in an animal, could interfere with the ability of another virus to replicate or to cause disease.

From their original observations have come all the vast literature that has accumulated over the past 20 years and which is condensed here into this volume. These studies have shown that the significance of interferon by far exceeds the original expectations of its discoverers. Indeed, the nature of the numerous effects of interferons on virus infections, on cell replication, on immune responses, and on cell functions which are described in this text make it tempting to speculate that we have not yet realized the full significance of the interferon system.

The clinical potential of interferons, natural, non-toxic, cellular products with broad spectrum antiviral activity, was immediately recognized. However, many years of research in numerous laboratories have been necessary to reduce obstacles that initially seemed insurmountable for this potential to eventually be realized. The studies distilled in this review demonstrate how advances in the basic knowledge of interferon regulatory mechanisms have allowed large scale production of interferons for both preliminary clinical trials and partial purification and characterization. The early data from these limited clinical trials have shown the promise of interferons both as antiviral agents in prophylaxis and treatment of viral infections and in the treatment of human tumors. Such initial successes have greatly increased the demand for large-scale production and extensive purification and characterization of interferons. In view of the accelerated progress in interferon studies it was recently stated in one manuscript that there are still gaps in our knowledge of the interferon system; it appears more likely that our knowledge is but a small gap in our ignorance of the interferon system.

A. An Historical Perspective

1. The Phenomenon of Viral Interference

About 4 decades have passed since the phenomenon of viral interference was first described as the protective action of a neutrotropic yellow fever virus against a viscerotropic strain of the same virus in monkeys (Hoskins, 1935) and with antigenically unrelated viruses (Findlay and MacCullum, 1937). Thus, the quest was underway for the mediator of viral interference for some 2 decades before Isaacs and Lindenmann (1957) assigned a name to it. Interim demonstrations of virus-virus inhibitions, both in animals and in cell cultures were numerous and were reviewed extensively by Schlesinger (1959). It seems likely that many workers were dealing with "interferons" (Lennette and Koprowski, 1946; Burnet and Fraser, 1952; Nagano and Kojima, 1954); indeed, "facteur inhibitor" (Nagano, 1967; Nagano, 1975) seems to qualify as an interferon (or should it be the other way around?).

Viral interference is characterized as the ability of one virus to interfere with the replication of another (challenge) virus; some viruses are able to induce interference even when they are unable themselves to replicate; and the interference is often not due to failure of the challenge virus to attach to the refractory cell or to enter it.

2. Discovery of Interferon

The exquisitely simple original experiment demonstrating interferon is illustrated in Fig. 1: Isaacs and Lindenmann added heat-inactivated influenza virus to pieces of chicken egg chorioallantoic membranes. These membranes were then washed to remove unadsorbed virus and were incubated at 37° C for serveral hours. Membrane fragments were removed from the culture fluid and fresh membrane fragments were incubated in this medium for 18–24 hrs at 37° C. Live influenza virus was then added and its replication was inhibited. Thus, the tissues exposed to inactivated virus had released a factor that transferred interference (virus resistance) to fresh tissues, the factor was called *interferon*.

It was shortly demonstrated that interferon was stable on dialysis against buffers ranging from pH 1–10, was destroyed by trypsin but not by ribonuclease or deoxyribonuclease, was not sedimented by centrifugation at 100,000 Xg but was precipitated by ammonium sulfate, and it did not inactivate virus directly but rendered cells resistant to virus (Isaacs, Lindenmann, and Valentine, 1957; Lindenmann, Burke, and Isaacs, 1957). Induction of interferon was also demonstrated with U. V.-inactivated influenza virus (Burke and Isaacs, 1958a) and other myxoviruses (Burke and Isaacs, 1958b). Tyrrell (1959) found an interferon in cultures of calf kidney cells infected with live influenza virus; this interferon had no detectable activity in chick cells and vice versa, thus giving rise to the concept of "species specificity" of interferons. Henle *et al.* (1959) demonstrated an interferon in a stable line of mouse cells, and Ho and Enders (1959a, b) found a human interferon induced by live poliovirus in primary human cell cultures.

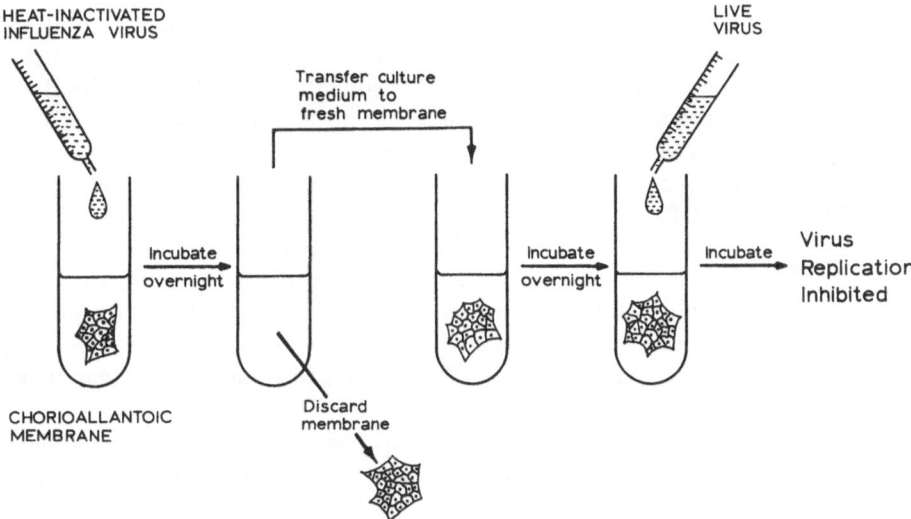

Fig. 1. The discovery of interferon. A schematic representation of the original experiment of Isaacs and Lindenmann (1957)

It is now known that virtually all types of viruses can induce interferon in most types of vertebrate animal cells, either in cell cultures or in the whole organism (see Section III. A). Also, interferons can inhibit virtually all types of viruses (see Part IX).

3. Interference Mediated by Other Mechanisms

Interferon has been shown to be responsible for the vast majority of viral interferences studied (Henle *et al.* 1959; Isaacs, 1959a, b, c; Burke and Isaacs, 1960; Wagner, 1960; Vilcek, 1960; Henderson and Taylor, 1961; Strandstrom, Sandelin, and Oker-Blom, 1962; Neva and Weller, 1964; Friedman, 1964; Parkman *et al.*, 1964; Vilcek, 1964a). However, other methods of interference between viruses have been described. Henle and Henle (1943) and Zeigler, Lavin, and Horsfall (1944) found that chick allantoic cells exposed to U. V.-inactivated influenza virus became resistant to live influenza virus; this was attributed to destruction of cellular receptors for the virus. Similarly, U. V.-inactivated Newcastle disease virus induced resistance to live Newcastle disease challenge virus (Baluda, 1957). The inactivated virus rapidly destroyed the homologous viral receptors on the cell surface (Baluda, 1959). The cells returned to full susceptibility to virus challenge in about 1–3 days when virus receptors had been regenerated. A similar mechanism of non-interferon-mediated interference was described by Crowell and Syverton (1961) with Coxsackie viruses in persistently infected HeLa cells. Coxsackie B 1 virus could not attach to cells infected with Coxsackie B 3 virus, while herpes, vaccinia and polioviruses were not prevented from infecting and destroying the cells.

Huang and Wagner (1966) demonstrated that defective T particles of vesicular stomatitis virus could interfere with replication of infectious B particles of this virus. Inhibition was accomplished if T particles were added as late as 2 hours after B particles, indicating that interference was not due to inhibition of adsorption. The short RNA segments obtained from the T particles were reported to compete with the longer RNA segments obtained from the B particles for synthetic sites (Stampfer, Baltimore, and Huang, 1969). Defective interfering particles have now been demonstrated in a vast number of virus-cell systems, and may play a role in the natural recovery process from viral diseases (Huang and Baltimore, 1970; Stewart II, 1973; Huang, 1977).

Marcus and Carver (1965) described that African green monkey kidney cell cultures infected with rubella virus became resistant to Newcastle disease virus, but did not become resistant to a number of other viruses. This "intrinsic interference" was not due to destruction of receptors for Newcastle disease virus and could also be induced by Sindbis, West Nile and polioviruses (Marcus and Carver, 1967).

Thus, the studies of the viral interference phenomenon have elucidated at least four distinguishable mechanisms whereby one virus particle can restrict the replication of another:
1. destruction of receptors
2. defective interfering particles
3. intrinsic interference
4. interferon induction

B. An Overview of the Interferon System

In order to introduce the interferon system, I have attempted to schematically represent the components of the system in Fig. 2. Reading from left to right in this scheme will reveal the different aspects of the interferon system that will be described in detail in this text, in the diagrammed sequence.

The interferon-related chain of events is initiated by the interaction of any of a variety of *interferon inducers* with an animal cell. This inducer molecule triggers *induction mechanisms* which activate the transcription of normally silent *genetic information for interferon production* which transcribes *interferon messenger RNA(s)*. *Interferon production* results when this message is translated into proteins which are modified and secreted as *interferons*. *Interferon-binding* to susceptible cells then initiates a number of alterations in cells that could best be described as "pleiotypic alterations" (Stewart II *et al.*, 1973a). It appears that certain of these changes are direct surface alterations whereas others require activation of another set of normally silent *genetic information for interferon action(s),* which function through their respective messenger RNA(s) and protein mediator(s). These various *cellular alterations induced by interferons* are measurable as virus resistance, cell multiplication inhibition, effects on cell surfaces, regulation of interferon synthesis (enhancing and inhibiting), and immunomodulations.

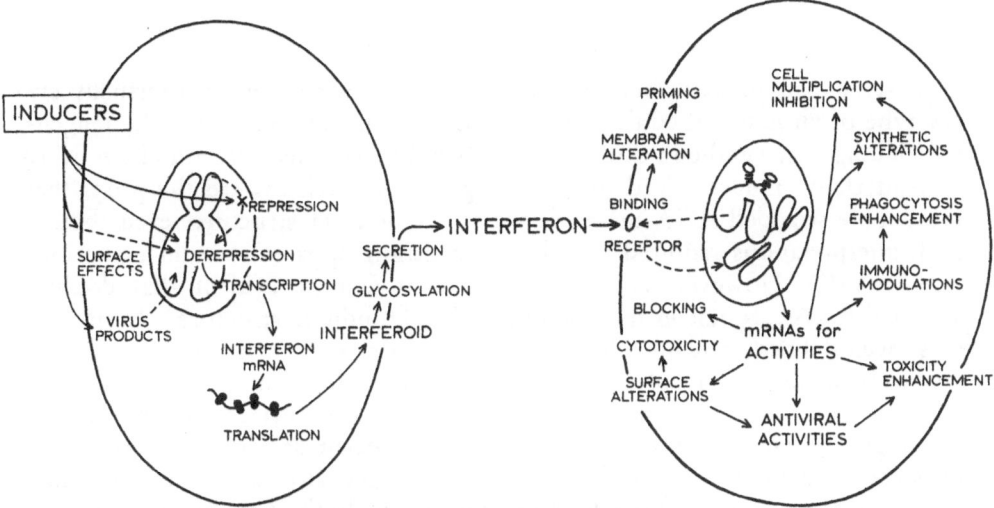

Fig. 2. The interferon system. This schematic representation of events at the cellular level leading to production of interferon and alteration of cells by the interferon produced is illustrated in two adjacent cells; it could also be diagrammed for the induced interferon to act upon the producing cell

1. Interferon Inducers

The number of interferon-inducing substances has increased steadily over the years until it is now perhaps easier to list those substances which are not known to induce interferons than to enumerate those which do so (see Part III). The inducers include numerous representatives of all the major virus groups, microorganisms, bacterial and fungal products, natural and synthetic nucleic acids, complex and simple polymers, various low molecular weight substances, mitogens, and immune recognition responses. Some of these inducers are able to induce interferons in a wide variety of cells either in the animal or in tissue cultures, while others are able to induce interferons only in specific cell populations *in vivo.* Several schemes have been proffered which classify inducers according to structures, amounts of interferon induced, types of cells induced, or physico-chemical properties of the interferon induced. However, the enormity of substances that have been found to induce interferon in virtually every vertebrate animal system investigated and the amazing similarity of activity spectra of all these interferons indicates the fundamental role of interferons in a number of biological processes.

It has often been argued that, as interferons are induced by viruses and inhibit virus replication, this inducer-action relationship shows that this antiviral activity is their true "significance". However, as mitogens have also been found to induce interferons, and as interferons inhibit cell multiplication, it could as well be interpreted that interferons are fundamentally related to restriction of growth. Further, the finding that interferons are induced by immune recognition responses and are able to suppress immune reactions suggests interferons' significance is immunomodulatory in this inducer-action relationship.

2. Induction Mechanisms

Several years of work in a number of laboratories revealed that virtually every type of virus tested could induce interferons in some systems. The tangential finding that synthetic double-stranded polyribonucleotide complexes were also interferon inducers lead to great surges of research toward the proof that the double-stranded RNA molecule was "the" inducer structure, even though such interpretations required ignoring or belittling apparently valid exceptions (see Part III). However, as truth will out, it is now evident that double-stranded RNAs are not in fact the one-and-only inducer structures. Even with these well-defined, potent inducers, it is still, after some ten years of work in several labs, not even resolved whether the inducer must enter the cells to trigger interferon production or can do so from the cell surface. It becomes increasingly evident that interferon induction may occur as a rather non-specific response to a variety of insults to cells. Apologetically, some authors must even admit to having poured literally fortunes in both time and money into seemingly endless searches for a better interferon inducing double-stranded RNA than the one first serendipitously tested, polyriboinosinic-polyribocytidylic acid (poly I. poly C) (Field et al., 1967a). Such searches, while enormously expanding bibliographies, all show that these efforts have been in vain (DeClercq, 1974; Torrence and DeClercq, 1977). These screenings have also failed to define why poly I. poly C is the best of the double-stranded RNA class of inducers.

It is possible that some classes of inducers may act directly on the cell membranes to trigger the induction of interferon. Other inducers may act by inactivation of regulatory mechanisms responsible for preventing constitutive production of interferon, and others may act directly to derepress interferon genetic information. Some inducing agents, such as single-stranded RNA viruses or DNA viruses may of course have to form double-stranded replicative products to act as interferon inducers.

It is ironic that the most promising lead on the possible mechanism of interferon induction has not come from any of the studies on defining the molecular structure of polyribonucleotide complexes but rather has come from recent studies on purification and characterization of interferons themselves. DeMaeyer-Guignard, Thang, and DeMaeyer (1977) described that interferons bind very selectively to single-stranded synthetic polyribonucleotides and posed the interesting possibility that low levels of spontaneously (constitutively) produced endogenous interferon in cells might be bound by certain structures such as viral or non-viral polyribonucleotides (and possibly other structural classes of inducers); it might be this depletion of basal-level endogenous interferon that serves as the interferon induction mechanism.

3. Genetic Information for Interferon Production

The genetic analysis of interferon production has allowed chromosomal assignments of structural and regulatory genes for certain interferons (see Part V). The genetic locus for human fibroblast interferon has been assigned to chromosome 5 (Tan, 1977) and has been localized further to the long arm of this chromosome, with regulatory information apparently located on the short arm of the same chromosome. Gene dosage studies measuring the amounts of this interferon produced from various human aneuploid cells, mono-, di- or polysomic for chromosome 5 or with translocations of its arms confirmed these assignments. However, it is still not known whether human leukocyte interferon is translated from messages transcribed from this chromosome.

Studies *in vivo* have shown that mouse interferon is produced from loci which segregate independently for different inducing viruses. These studies suggest there is more than one structural gene for interferon in mice.

4. Interferon Messenger RNA

From the first demonstrations that interferon production was inhibited by inhibitors of RNA and protein synthesis, it was assumed there were messenger RNAs specific for this molecule, and such was demonstrated by DeMaeyer-Guignard, DeMaeyer and Montagnier (1972) who extracted messenger RNA from mouse cells induced to synthesize interferon with polyr I. polyrC (see Part VI). This message preparation was applied to cultures of chick embryo fibroblasts which then produced mouse interferon, which could be identified by its lack of antiviral activity on chicken cells and activity on mouse cells. Thus this experiment showed that mouse interferon messenger RNA could be isolated from induced cells (but not from uninduced cells) and that this message could be taken up as an apparently intact molecule by heterologous cells and translated into a protein foreign to the host cells, which was then released into the culture medium. This observation has been confirmed by a number of investigators who have successfully translated mouse interferon messenger RNA, human fibroblast interferon messenger RNA and human lymphoblastoid cell interferon messenger RNA in heterologous cells, in various cell-free protein translating systems and in *Xenopus laevis* oocytes microinjected with these messages.

This technique is presently being used to quantitate the interferon messenger RNA during the induction and production phases of the interferon production curve as a means to investigate the regulation mechanisms on interferon synthesis. Also, many laboratories are presently undertaking to obtain purified interferon messenger RNAs which can then be retro-copied into a DNA segment for gene-splicing into a prokaryotic cell. Such applications of the rapidly developing techniques of recombinant DNA research would appear to hold hope for the large amounts of interferon that will be demanded for its wide clinical exploitation.

5. Interferon Production

Once interferon messenger RNA arrives in the cytoplasm of the induced cell it is translated into interferon(s) which are glycosylated and excreted from the cell. It appears, however, that another messenger RNA is induced concomitantly with the interferon messenger RNA, and that this message translates into a protein involved in termination of interferon message translation (see Part VI. A). Normally termination of interferon production, both in animals and in cell cultures is followed by a period of refractoriness to repeated interferon inductions. It is not clear whether this hyporesponsiveness is an interferon-mediated regulatory mechanism or whether the factor(s) responsible for termination of interferon message transcription and/or translation mediate this refractoriness.

It has been possible by discriminant applications of antimetabolites shortly after induction of interferon messenger RNAs to prevent the normally rapid termination of interferon production in cell cultures and thus to greatly accentuate interferon production. Application of this "superinduction" ("superproduction?") technique has allowed greatly increased production of human fibroblast interferons (Havell and Vilček, 1972).

6. Interferons

Once liberated from cells interferons can be concentrated and purified by a variety of physicochemical techniques. All native interferons seem to be relatively small glycoproteins occuring as single-chain polypeptides (see Part VI). Interferons have in common that they are all apparently proteins and that they all induce antiviral activity in cells by a process requiring cellular RNA- and protein-synthetic processes. However, they differ remarkably in terms of stabilities to denaturing agents: some interferons are completely stable when boiled in a mixture of urea, sodium dodecyl sulfate and 2-mercaptoethanol, while others are completely destroyed by this treatment; some are completely stable to treatment at pH2 while others are completely inactivated by acid pH. Even interferon produced from different cells in the same animal can differ in these respects. "Species specificity" of interferons, a property often felt useful for defining interferons, is now considered a hollow term, for even interferons from the same animal induced by the same inducer can differ drastically in this respect: human leukocyte interferons are significantly active on cells from a wide range of animals, whereas human fibroblast interferons are devoid of activity in many of these same animal cells.

Several interferons have been purified to very high specific activities (greater than 10^8 units[1]/per milligram of protein) and at least one (human leukocyte interferon) has recently been purified to homogeneity, with a specific activity of about 10^9 units per milligram of protein (Lin and Stewart II, 1978).

The carbohydrate components of some interferons have been enzymatically and chemically cleaved, and carbohydrate moieties have been prevented from being added in vivo by glycosylation inhibitors. Such studies have revealed that carbohydrate moieties of these interferon proteins are not involved in antigenicity, activity, or hydrophobicity. While the carbohydrate components of

---

[1] A unit of interferon is often defined as the reciprocal of the dilution of an interferon preparation which can reduce replication of a sensitive virus by a given percent; a meaningful unit must always be equated to international reference interferons (see Part II. F).

certain interferons account for their size and charge heterogeneities (for example the various components of human leukocyte interferon and of mouse L cell interferons) it does not account for heterogeneities exhibited between human leukocyte and human fibroblast interferons. These latter heterogeneities thus likely reflect differences in primary structures resulting from their being different gene products.

The finding that interferon proteins can retain activity in their deglycosylated forms increases hopes for obtaining a proteolytically-derived small active fragment of interferon ("interferoid") which could be chemically synthesized.

Recently it has been demonstrated that in addition to what – for lack of a better term – we shall call "classical" interferons, which are acid stable, there is another class of interferons which are acid labile. These latter interferons have been called "immune" interferons, "mitogen-type" interferon, and type II interferons. It appears that these interferons are also different from each of the classical (type I) interferons in antigenicity and heterospecific antiviral activities. It will hopefully someday be resolved what these differences mean to the molecules, the cells and the animals.

7. Interferon Binding

The ability of interferons to exert activities in cells apparently is dependent on the presence of receptors for the interferons on the cell which is able to recognize the interferon (see Part V. III. C). The amount of interferon binding to cells has often been shown to correlate with their sensitivity to the interferon, and in human cells this binding has been found to correlate with the same chromosome responsible for sensitivity to action of interferon, suggesting that this chromosome codes for the interferon receptor (Wiranowska–Stewart, and Stewart II, 1977). Once interferon binds to the cell it becomes resistant to proteolytic digestion, but it is not resolved whether it is actually taken up by the cells to exert its activity.

8. Genetic Information for Interferon Actions

Interferon does not induce antiviral activity in cells whose RNA and protein synthesizing systems are arrested, and it does not induce virus resistance in enucleated cells. Thus, cellular genetic functions are needed for interferon to exert its antiviral activities. In the human system it has been demonstrated that chromosome 21 must be present for human cells to respond to interferons, but it seems likely that this chromosome codes for interferon receptor rather than the antiviral factors per se.

9. Cellular Alterations Induced by Interferons

a) Antiviral States

Interferons transform cells into the antiviral state through a process involving synthesis of new cellular messenger RNA and protein. This has lead to many searches for the presumed antiviral protein, which has eluded workers for more than a decade. The antiviral mechanism of interferon interrupts the replication of at least most viruses at the level of synthesis of viral macromolecules. It does not usually appear to inhibit attachment of viruses, their entry into cells or their uncoating, but blocks transcription and/or translation of viral genetic information. An exception appears to be certain tumor-virus systems where interferon treatment may inhibit release and/or maturation of the virions even though the syntheses of the major viral components are not inhibited (see Part IX. B 4). The key word here may be *major* viral components, for inhibition of translation of message for production of an essential *minor* viral component may be responsible for the final inhibition observed, even though it might at first appear to be prevention by a "novel" antiviral mechanism. This seems a likely possibility as it is clear that the interferon translation inhibitory activity exerts discriminatory inhibiton of translation of messages of different viruses, some being exquisitely sensitive, others being quite resistant, and cellular messages (as a whole, at least) being apparently less sensitive than viral messages.

b) Priming and Blocking

Almost as soon as interferons were discovered it was observed that they exerted alterations in cells not related to induction of antiviral activity: Burke and Isaacs (1958 b) found that cells treated with interferon prior to addition of an interferon inducing virus were able to make more interferon than cells not previously treated with interferon; they referred to this phenomenon as *priming*. However, it was several years before this was clearly recognized as the first non-antiviral function of interferon (Stewart II, Gosser and Lockart, 1971 a). Additionally this effect may be a direct alteration of cells, as cells do not seem to require newly induced cell protein synthesis to become primed.

Another effect of interferon on its own production is that seen when cells are treated for several hours with relatively large doses of interferons. Such cells when subsequently induced to make interferon produce less than cells not previously treated with interferon. This phenomenon referred to as *blocking* (Stewart II, Gosser and Lockart, 1971 b), unlike priming, requires new cellular protein synthesis during interferon treatment for its development.

Interferon treatment has also been shown to augment the levels of certain cellular products other than interferons.

c) Enhanced Susceptibility to Toxicity of Double-Stranded RNA

Interferon-treated cells are often more sensitive than untreated cells to the cytotoxicity of double-stranded RNAs and vaccinia virus, provided the latter is able to synthesize new products (Stewart II *et al.*, 1972), possibly double-stranded RNA molecules themselves. It is not clear what mechanisms are involved in this effect but it may reflect an interferon-induced alteration of cell membranes and/or a double-stranded RNA-dependent nuclease and/or protein inhibitor.

d) Effects on Cell Surfaces

Not that the above alterations are not themselves cell surface alterations, but additionally, interferon has been shown to change the electrophoretic mobility of cells, and to enhance the expression of certain surface antigens.

e) Effects on Cell Multiplication

The cell-multiplication-inhibitory activity of interferons has been a contested issue since it was first described about 15 years ago, and it has only recently been convincingly demonstrated to the satisfaction of most critics that this is indeed a phenomenon attributable to interferon (Stewart II *et al.*, 1976). Interferons can decrease cell growth rates, and lower the saturation density to which cells will grow. It can inhibit the ability of tumor cells to form colonies in soft-agar, and it can inhibit the blastogenic responses of cells to mitogens. *In vivo*, interferon can inhibit the regeneration of liver tissue, and its antitumor activities in animals and in man may be partially attributable to its cell-multiplication-inhibitory activity. Additionally the death of newborn mice treated with interferon preparations may represent an adverse consequence of interferon inhibiting tissue development during a critical growth phase (Gresser *et al.*, 1975).

f) Immunomodulations

On the one hand interferon preparations have been shown to enhance the phagocytic activity of macrophages and to enhance the specific cytotoxicity of lymphocytes for target cells. Certain doses of interferons have been reported to enhance primary antibody responses, and to enhance tumor cell rejection.

On the other hand, interferon preparations have been reported to inhibit blastogenesis induced by allogeneic cells, to inhibit primary antibody responses, to inhibit graft-versus-host reactions and prolong allograft survivals, to inhibit delayed-type hypersensitivity reactions, and to inhibit tumor cell rejection.

Thus the immunomodulatory actions of interferon may depend on timing of interferon treatment and the dose of interferon.

C. The Interferon System *in vivo*

1. Interferons as Prophylactic and Therapeutic Agents in Animals

The literature on interferons in the natural recovery process from acute viral diseases is enormous, and most of these were equivocal in the assignment of a crucial role for interferon (see Stewart II, 1973, for review). Recent studies, however, have convincingly demonstrated that interferon is in fact one of the most important early determinants of recovery or non-recovery from a number of viral diseases. Gresser *et al.* (1976c) showed that mice treated with antiserum active against mouse interferon were killed by amounts of herpes simplex virus several hundred times less than an LD50 for a mouse not receiving anti-interferon.

An exogenous dosage of interferon or an interferon inducer can also protect an animal against certain viral diseases (see Part XII). Generally this treatment is much more effective if interferon or inducer is given prophylactically rather than therapeutically.

Similarly, interferons can inhibit the growth of a number of tumors in animals whether these are spontaneous, transplanted or induced by RNA or DNA tumor viruses.

2. Interferons in the Clinic

Interferon has been demonstrated to exert a mildly protective effect in man against the "common cold", but the amount of interferon required for this modest effect was enormous. On the other hand recent trials of interferons in chronic active hepatitis patients have provided rather impressive results with relatively low interferon investment (Greenberg *et al.*, 1976). Thus it may prove possible to clinically evaluate interferons even with the presently limited supplies of interferons if the proper disease model is tested. The recent results with herpes keratitis show a clear clinical application (Sundmacher, Neumann-Haefelin, and Cantell, 1976a, b; Sundmacher *et al.*, 1976), and a number of trials are presently underway with preliminary results building hopes for more successes.

Meanwhile the trials of human leukocyte interferons in osteogenic sarcomas are continuing with the data increasing in significance with each passing day (Strander *et al.*, 1974, 1977; Strander and Cantell, 1974; Cantell, 1977; Adamson *et al.*, 1977; Strander, 1977a, b, c).

It is presently only the limited availability of interferon that prevents its testing in a great variety of human viral diseases and cancers. Likely it will take a dramatic demonstration of clinical efficacy of interferon before the investments for research and scale-up production will be forthcoming.

Meanwhile, the study of the interferon system as a model for cell regulatory mechanisms pushes efforts toward its purification and characterization, its genetic mappings and studies on its action mechanisms. Since the interferon system involves both interferon producing and interferon responding cells it provides a unique model for intercellular communications whose main components can be isolated and quantitated.

II. Interferon Assays

It seems desirable to cover interferon assays as a preliminary section to detailed description of the various components of the interferon system, because it is necessary that the reader understand what "an interferon unit" means and how it is derived to intelligably follow discussions of the relative merits of interferon inducers, the significance of specific activities of interferon preparations, or the relative interferon sensitivities of cells or viruses.

A. General Considerations

Perhaps the most often encountered question while lecturing on the interferon system is "what is an interferon unit"? This can only be answered by describing how interferons are quantitated. To date the only way to assay interferon is to indirectly measure the activities that it exerts on cells. Generally, this is accomplished by measuring any of a vast number of parameters of virus replication in the interferon-treated cells, but it is also possible to quantitate interferons by measuring their abilities to exert various other alterations such as priming, double-stranded RNA toxicity enhancement, or cell-multiplication-inhibition. Whichever indirect effect of interferon on cells one chooses to measure as an indirect quantitation of interferon activity, one must always ascertain that the effect is attributable to interferon by characterization of the active component; criteria for acceptance of a substance as an interferon were first delineated by Lockart (1966) and will be described in Part VII. A.

Considering only the methods for assaying interferons based on measuring antiviral activities, there are as many ways to quantitate interferons as there are ways of measuring virus replication, and virtually all of these have been employed. All interferon assays require living tissue cultures and these can be selected from an enormous variety, both primary and stable, homologous or sometimes heterologous. Then there is the choice of the challenge virus to be used. In the following sections the rational basis for such decisions will be discussed.

Assays are often picked for different reasons. If one wishes to assay hundreds or thousands of samples with suspected high levels of interferon, one would willingly sacrifice sensitivity and precision and select a simple method involving least manipulations, while if one had one or only a few samples to assay which were suspected of low levels of interferon, one would choose an assay perhaps more laborious but with high sensitivity and precision. Considerations such as available supplies, speed (time required to get the answer), and reproducibility often influence choice of assays, and a safety factor is sometimes a determinant of the challenge virus selected; few people chose to use rabies virus as their assay challenge, though it is highly sensitive to many interferons, and some laboratories are prevented by government restrictions from using the convenient and interferon-sensitive vesicular stomatitis virus.

"Units" of interferon are reciprocals of endpoint dilutions of an interferon preparation. Thus a unit of interferon could vary enormously with the same interferon preparation depending on sensitivity of the cells to the interferon, sensitivity of the virus, or the numerous factors influencing the assays, as will be described below. For this reason several international reference interferon preparations have been made available to investigators, so that units for interferons can be equated to these reagents, which are described in Section II. F.

B. Dose-Response Relationships

An interferon preparation is diluted serially in culture medium and each dilution is incubated, usually overnight, with the test cells, which are then infected with the selected challenge virus. When one is trying to characterize an inhibitor as an interferon, it is necessary to remove the preparations and wash the cultures before adding the challenge virus to remove any non-specific extracellular virus inhibitors that might be present. In each assay it is necessary to include cultures treated with diluent alone, for cell controls, left uninfected, and for virus controls. After appropriate intervals the virus growth parameter is measured in each of the culture series. Endpoints are usually derived by plotting dilutions of the test interferon preparation against percent of function measured in cell controls. This plot normally produces linear slopes near the ranges corresponding to about 25–75% virus growth (Lindenmann and Gifford, 1963a, b; Cantell and Paucker, 1963a; Finter, 1968; Stewart II, Scott, and Sulkin, 1969). These sigmoidal relationships are found with each of the interferon assay methods described below (Finter, 1973a), whether the assayed inhibition is a viral function, cell multiplication, or any of the several nonantiviral functions detectable (Gresser et al., 1971; Hilfenhaus et al., 1976; Stewart II et al., 1973a; 1976). Virus-induced cytopathology can be reliably and conveniently measured as a 50% inhibition endpoint, while virus yield-inhibition assays provide more reliable data when $\log_{10}$ reductions are plotted, using 0.5 $\log_{10}$ or greater inhibition as endpoint.

To compare the potency of a particular interferon preparation with that of another, the slopes of the dose-response curves must be parallel (Finter, 1973 a) However, such parallel lines are not always found in practice. Interferon preparations may be contaminated with different substances that influence the slopes (Finter, 1966 b); also, Havell, Berman and Vilček (1975) found that human leukocyte interferon and human fibroblast interferon preparations, regardless of their degrees of purity, showed different dose-response curves when both were assayed in human diploid fibroblast cultures by inhibition of vesicular stomatitis virus yields. Similar observations have been made by Edy, Billiau, and Desomer (1976a) and Hilfenhaus (1977) using human leukocyte interferon and human fibroblast interferon assayed by inhibition of virus cytopathology. These results emphasize the problem of comparing titers of interferon preparations even of the same animal species, even when a reference interferon has been included (Vilček, Havell, and Yamazaki, 1977; Schwartz and Villani-Price, 1977). These observations have necessitated production of interferon reference preparations for both human leukocyte and human fibroblast interferons (Section II. F).

If one examines dose-response data, it is apparent that, even with low dilution steps (2-fold) and these dilutions plotted against any measurable biological function, the significance of assays of less than 2-fold difference is negligible, and significant figures on interferon titers disappear almost after the first digit (Jordan, 1972a, b). Nonetheless, some authors persistently report that their assays vary less than 10%, and present titers with four or five figures (Carter *et al.*, 1975a; Chadha *et al.*, 1974). Thus it must be repeatedly emphasized that, regardless of the assay employed, *two-fold differences in interferon titers are of marginal significance; less than that is insignificant.*

C. Assay Methods

1. Plaque-Reduction Assays

The ability of viruses to form plaques affords a convenient method for quantitation of virus and, hence, to detect its inhibition. Wagner (1961) first employed this measure for interferon assays, which has become one of the most widely used interferon assays. Usually, the interferon preparations are serially diluted in 2-fold or 3-fold steps in maintenance medium and added to confluent monolayer cultures of cells in plate cultures. After overnight incubation at 37° C the cultures are drained and washed and inoculated with a convenient number of plaque-forming particles of the challenge virus. After an adsorption period of about 1 hour at 37° C, inocula are removed and cell sheets are overlaid with a semisolid nutrient mixture, usually containing agar. After solidification of overlays, plates are inverted and incubated at 37° C until plaques have developed (usually 1 to 3 days, depending on the virus-cell combination). The reciprocal of the dilution of the interferon preparation reducing the plaque-count to 50% of that in virus control plates is the titer, often referred to as a plaque-depressing-dose-50% (PDD50) endpoint unit (Stewart II, Scott, and Sulkin, 1969).

The plaque-reduction assay is a laborious method, involving previous preparation of large numbers of monolayer cultures for each sample to be assayed; it requires relatively large sample volumes and numerous manipulations of cultures and is extremely expensive in terms of consumable supplies. Reproducibility is poor as cells may vary from time to time in their responses to the interferon or to the virus so that endpoints may not fall within the dilution series, or the plaque numbers may be too many or too few for optimal counts (Sellers and Fitzpatrick, 1962; Finter, 1966b; Stewart and Gandhi, 1967; Aboud, Weiss, and Salzberg, 1976). This assay is in wide use and may have merits in assays of particular types of interferons (Epstein, 1976a) and the aesthetic gratification of having accomplished it, but as a second for previous warnings offered by Finter (1973a), I caution that if one contemplates assaying more than a few interferon samples, one cannot afford this assay.

2. Yield-Reduction Assays

The direct measurement of virus yields from interferon treated cells is a technique that has several advantages over the plaque-reduction assay. First, this assay can be used in various modifications with all challenge viruses, whereas plaque-reduction assays can only be performed with the relatively limited numbers of viruses that form plaques in a particular cell. Yield-reductions can be measured as infectious virus or viral products (haemagglutinins, haemadsorption, or neuraminidase). This method usually excels in sensitivity and accuracy (Sellers and Fitzpatrick, 1962; Sreevalsan and Lockart, 1962; Baron and Buckler, 1963; Finter, 1967a; Hallum and Youngner, 1966). The assay can be successfully accomplished over a wide range of infectious multiplicities of challenge virus, so that effects on either single or multiple cycles of virus replication can be investigated, and thus can be used to determine resistance of cells at various times after treatment with interferon (Baron, Buckler and Dianzani, 1968).

a) Reduction of Infectious Virus Yields

The direct quantitation of virus yields by infectivity has been used in many laboratories. Usually the amount of virus is measured after a single cycle of replication (Finter, 1967a; Stewart II and Lockart, 1970; Gallagher and Khoobyarian, 1971; Ito and Montagnier, 1977). Measuring virus yields as infectious units is, of course, a laborious and expensive process, in time and consumable supplies and cannot be contemplated for handling of large numbers of interferon assays.

b) Reduction of Haemagglutinin Yields

This measure of virus replication was the one first used to demonstrate that virus replication was inhibited by the substance later to be named interferon (Isaacs and Lindenmann, 1957). The original method was laborious and imprecise and did not prove satisfactory in some laboratories (Finter, 1967a; Stanton and May, 1973). However, Oie et al. (1972a) developed a sensitive variation of this type of assay in cells infected with Sindbis virus. This assay can also be performed with encephalomyocarditis virus (Jordan, 1972c) with high sensitivity and precision. Haemagglutinin yield-reduction assays with encephalomyocarditis virus or GD-VII virus have recently been shown to be sensitive and precise for measuring human and mouse interferons in a variety of homologous and heterologous cell species (Lvovsky and Levy, 1976; Jameson, Dixon and Grossberg, 1977)

c) Reduction of Haemadsorption

The quantitative haemadsorption assay for interferon, described by Finter (1967a), involves infection of interferon-treated cells with Sendai virus or influenza virus (Finter, 1967a, 1968), and replacing medium with suspensions of erythrocytes which adsorb to infected cells. After washing monolayers, red cells are lysed by hypotonic solution and liberated haemoglobin is quantitated by optical density measurement. A modification of this method has been described using ^{51}Cr-labelled erythrocytes to quantitate haemadsorption (Emodi et al., 1975a).

d) Reduction of Neuraminidase Yields

Reduction of the neuraminidase produced by influenza virus has been used to assay chicken interferon (Sedmak and Grossberg, 1973), human interferons, monkey, rabbit, hamster and mouse interferons (Sedmak, Grossberg, and Jameson, 1975). This method is reported to be reproducible, rapid, sensitive and convenient, provided the cell system used is a good producer of neuraminidase.

3. Cytopathic Effect (CPE)-Inhibition Assays

A number of viruses cause cell damage that can be visualized in the light microscope, and any of these cytopathic effects can be used to quantitate protection of cells by interferon. Two major methods of this assay are in wide usage, one based on microscopic reading of cell damage and one based on an indirect measure of the cell damage by amounts of a vital dye taken up by cells.

a) CPE-Reading Method

This method was first used by Ho and Enders (1959a), and has been used to assay nearly every type of interferon that has been described, against a great number of viruses (Sellers and Fitzpatrick, 1962; Fantes, O'Neill and Mason, 1964; Wheelock and Sibley, 1965; Kono and Ho, 1965; Bucknall, 1967; Billiau and Buckler, 1970; Bucknall, 1970; Ahl and Rump, 1976; Viehauser, 1977). The main advantages of this method are simplicity, speed and economy of samples and supplies, with introduction of semimicro-titration trays (Tilles and Finland, 1968; Dahl and Degre, 1972; Dahl, 1973).

I shall describe the semimicroassay system used in this laboratory that allows two workers to assay thousands of samples of human and murine interferons each week with nearly 100% success-rate.

Growth medium is introduced into each well of 96 well plastic microtiter trays, 50 μl/well. The interferon sample (25 μl) is introduced into the first well of the row and the solution is mixed with a fresh micropipette tip. An aliquot (25 μl) is transferred to the next well and mixed with a fresh micropipette tip[2], etc. After dilutions are made, including on each tray a standardized interferon preparation assay series and wells for virus controls and cell controls, trays are exposed to sterilizing ultraviolet-irradiation (Stewart II and Sulkin, 1966). Freshly trypsinized cell suspensions are then introduced into each well (0.1 ml containing about 2 × 10^4 cells) and trays are incubated at 37° C overnight. A

---

[2] If serial dilutions are made with the same tip throughout, artifactually high titers can be produced (T. Chudzio, 1977, personal communication).

suspension of vesicular stomatitis virus containing about 10^4 plaque-forming units in 50 μl of serum-free medium is introduced into each well, except cell controls, and trays are incubated about 24 hours at 37° C, at which time virus controls show 100% CPE. Endpoints are read as 50% protection, and as illustrated in Figure 3, are reliable within 0.5 log$_{10}$ dilutions and end-point can be interpolated reproducibly to 0.3 log$_{10}$ differences. However, at this level, the least satisfactory aspect of this assay method imposes itself, for subjectivity must decide differences of less than 2-fold.

b) Dye-Uptake Method

This modification of the CPE-inhibition assay, introduced by Finter (1969), relieves the imagination of the worker from visually reading the CPE. When the virus-induced damage has developed, a vital dye, neutral red (about 10^{-5} gm%), is added to all cultures which are incubated for 2 hours. Cultures are then washed and dye which was taken up by living cells is eluted into acid-alcohol and quantitated colorimetrically. This method requires considerably more manipulations than the CPE-reading method but has the same sensitivity and is more precise (Finter, 1969; McLaren, 1970).

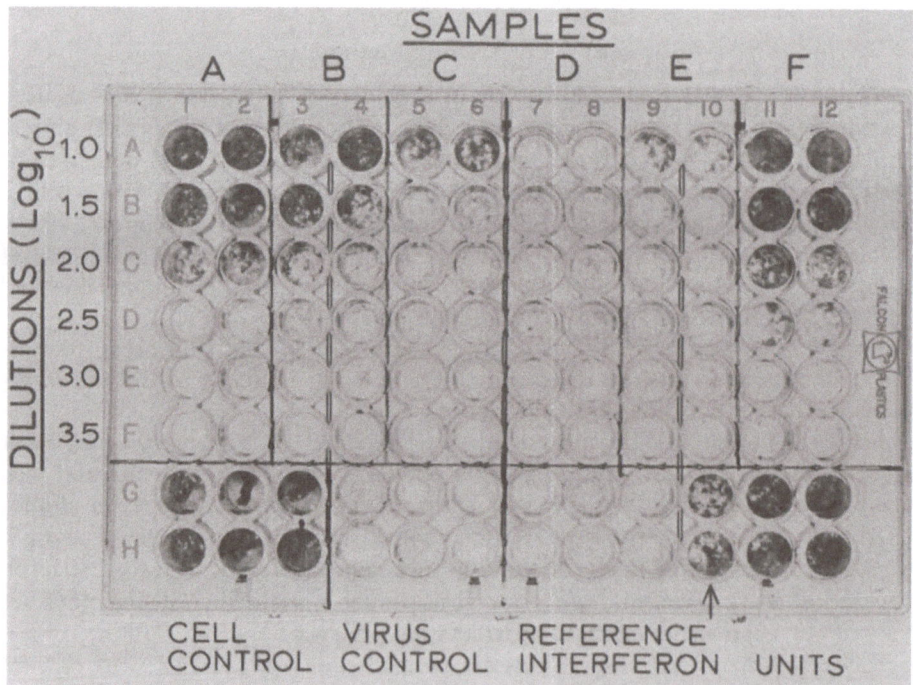

Fig. 3. Microtiter tray assay by CPE-reading method. The titers of the samples estimated from visual microscopic readings were: A, 100 units/ml; B, 60 units/ml; C, 20 units/ml; D, <10 units/ml; E, ~10 units/ml; F, 200 units/ml. Reference interferon assay 1 unit at arrow

This dye-binding CPE-inhibition assay was adapted to a semimicroassay method for rabbit interferon by Armstrong 1971), and several similar systems are currently in use for numerous interferons (Pidot, 1971; Havell and Vilcek, 1972; McManus, 1976; Borden and Leonhardt, 1977).

4. Radiochemical Assays

As it is possible to label viral RNA by incorporating radiolabelled RNA-precursors into the culture medium; it is possible to detect interferon-induced virus inhibition by inhibition of this incorporation of radiolabel. Allen and Giron (1970) assayed mouse interferons by incorporating tritiated uridine into media of MM virus-challenged cultures treated with Actinomycin D. After several hours cells were scraped into cold buffer and acid-insoluble material was precipitated with 5% trichloroacetic acid (TCA) and radioactivity counted. The endpoint was referred to in inhibition of Nucleic Acid Synthesis – 50% (INAS50) units. This method was sensitive and precise and gave reproducible results (McWilliam et al., 1971), and various modifications have been used satisfactorily in a number of laboratories to assay other interferons (Koblet, Kohler, and Wyler, 1972; Atkins et al., 1974; Ito et al., 1975). One modification of this method has been to grow the cells directly in scintillation vials (Suzuki, Akaboshi, and Kobayash, 1974).

A similar method has been described using reovirus as the challenge and determining the amount of label incorporated into ribonuclease-resistant double-stranded RNA (Vassef et al., 1973); this method did not require treating cells with Actinomycin D, and was quick and easy.

5. Other Antiviral Assays

Numerous other methods of antiviral assays of interferons have been developed and most of them are in limited use, though most have specific utilities.

a) Reverse Transcriptase Inhibition Assay

The ability of interferon to inhibit replication of certain oncornaviruses can be measured in terms of elaboration of reverse transcriptase from the interferon-treated cells. This was recently developed into an assay referred to as the reverse-transcriptase-reduction-dose 50% (RTRD50) assay (Aboud, Weiss, and Salzberg, 1976). Cultures of chronically oncornavirus-producing NIH/3T3 cells infected with Moloney murine leukemia virus were incubated overnight with interferon and incubated with fresh medium for 3 to 4 hours; medium was then assayed for reverse transcriptase activity (by incorporation of ^{3}H-thymidine). This method was reported to offer about the same sensitivity as the PDD50-VSV method (Stewart II, Declercq and Desomer, 1972a) with better reproducibility and had the advantage of being accomplished within a 24 hour period. Presumably such an assay could be devised for other species of interferons.

2*

b) Immunofluorescence Assay

An immunofluorescence assay based on counting of infected cells was first employed by Boxaca and Paucker (1967) for L cells infected with vesicular stomatitis virus. It was later used by Kozikowski and Hahon (1969) and reportedly gave reproducible results. It has been used to assay human interferons, and the unit of measure, an $ICDD_{50}$ (50% infected cell-depressing dilution) was similar to one international reference human interferon unit (Hahon, 1974).

While this method might have applications for determining interferon sensitivities of certain non-cytocidal viruses (e. g. rabiesvirus), it would seem to have limited utility for routine assays.

c) EB Virus-Expression Assay

An assay of interferon by its ability to inhibit numbers of Daudi line of lymphoblastoid cells expressing early antigen of EB virus was developed by Adams et al. (1975) and has understandably yet not been used outside that laboratory (Liden and Adams, 1975). Supposedly this assay is relatively reliable to detect one unit of human leukocyte interferon, but reading the procedure hardly impresses one with any of its merits. It is by far the most laborious method encountered in the interferon literature.

d) Cytochemical Assays

The first demonstration of the effect of interferon on a non-viral agent (the psittacosis agent) was described by Sueltenfuss and Pollard (1963) as an assay for chick interferon. Infected cells were stained with acridine orange and inhibited psittacosis agents could be enumerated at the non-infectious "red ball" stage under fluorescence microscopy.

A variation of this method was developed to show that replication of non-cytocidal rabiesviruses were sensitive to interferons (Stewart II and Sulkin, 1968). This method employed either acridine orange staining or the May-Gruenwald-Giemsa staining and counting of cells containing cytoplasmic inclusion bodies.

e) Agar Diffusion Assays

Diffusion of interferon through agar overlays of cell cultures was used by Porterfield (1959, 1964) to quantitate interferon, the area of protection against challenge virus being proportional to the concentration of interferon in the diffusion well. This technique has since been used in various modifications by other laboratories (Bradish and Allner, 1970; Yoshino and Morishima, 1970).

f) pH Indicator Assay

A method was described for assaying interferon protection of cells against virus by color change of a pH indicator dye, the protected cultures changing color as the cells metabolize the media (Paucker, 1965). Its enormity of pitfalls prevented its wide acceptance.

6. Non-Antiviral Assays

Interferons have been shown to induce a number of alterations in cells that can be measured without using virus growth parameters. Certain of these non-antiviral alterations have been used to quantitate interferons, but are not yet in wide use for this purpose *per se* because it is yet not resolved whether all interferons are identical in ability to induce these alterations (see Section X), and antiviral assays are generally so much more precise and easily accomplished. Therefore, these assays are covered in the specific section relating to the non-antiviral alterations induced (priming, toxicity enhancement, cell-multiplication-inhibition; see Section X).

D. Factors Influencing Interferon Assays

Interferon assays involve an enormous number of variable which can significantly influence the apparent titers obtained. Multiple choices in assay systems can be made for the type of cells used, the challenge virus, each of the many assay methods described above, and the specific conditions affecting assay results as described below can each be manipulated to influence assay outcomes within any of the above cell-virus-assay method sets. Obviously a large number of these factors must be chosen arbitrarily by the investigator. The following partial listings are indications to assist in making the choices somewhat more rational and pointing out potential variables that can be encountered once the cell-virus-assay method set has been selected. Many of these variables will be discussed in greater detail in relation to their effects on the antiviral mechanism of action of interferons (Section VIII. D).

1. Non-Interferon Contaminants

Virtually all interferon assays are performed with interferon preparations where interferon is practically the *least* component in the preparation.

Some of the non-interferon material in these preparations may derive from the substances used to stimulate interferon. These residual inducers must be eliminated or destroyed to avoid induction of interferon during the assay. Residual viral inducers can be removed by ultracentrifugation; many viruses can be destroyed by acid treatment (however, many interferons are also destroyed by pH2; see Section VII. A. 3), or heating at 65° C for 1 hour (Cantell *et al.*, 1965), but many interferons are unstable at this temperature. A convenient method for inactivation of inducing viruses is exposure to sterilizing UV-irradiation. This has been used with many interferons: chick interferon (Isaacs and Burke, 1959; Zemla and Vilček, 1961), human interferons (Mayer, 1962; Stewart II, Scott and Sulkin, 1969) and mouse interferon (Lockart, 1963). This method of inactivation has the added advantage of destroying bacterial contaminants in the interferon preparations. Residual virus can also be eliminated by neutralizing antiserum (Burke and Buchan, 1965). Non-viral inducers such as double-stranded RNA can be eliminated by digestion with ribonuclease (Lockart, 1973).

Interferon preparations may contain non-specific viral inhibitors which can be eliminated by washing the cell cultures after interferon treatment before applying the challenge virus (Finter, 1965; Gifford, 1963a; Buckler and Baron, 1966).

Interferon preparations may also be contaminated with substances that mask interferon action. A number of factors have been reported in interferon preparations or sera which antagonize the action of interferons (Chany and Brailovsky, 1967; Truden, Sigel, and Dietrich, 1967; Lidin and Adams, 1975; Cembrzynska–Nowak, 1977; Rytel, 1975; Epstein and Salmon, 1974; Fournier et al., 1974; Galliot et al., 1973; Sheaff and Stewart, 1969; Broudeur, Legar, and Brailovsky, 1973; Rossman and Vilček, 1970). These inhibitors of interferon action will be described in detail as they relate to the antiviral action of interferons (Section VIII. D. 4).

Some contaminants in interferon preparations may be toxic in the assay cells and thus inhibit the ability of the cell to replicate the challenge virus, or it may directly inactivate the challenge virus. Thus it is always important to ascertain that the inhibition observed results form an inhibitory activity fulfilling the criteria for interferons (see Section VII. A. 7).

2. Period of Interferon Exposure

Cells treated with interferon require several hours to develop maximum antiviral activity. It is usually convenient to incubate cultures overnight with the interferons before challenge virus is added, but shorter intervals are sometimes used to speed results (Wagner, 1961; Lindenmann and Gifford, 1963b; Finter 1967a). However, many assay systems require significantly longer interferon treatment than others: Jordan (1972a) found that chick cells developed full antiviral activity by 6 hrs of interferon treatment while mouse cells required 24 hr period of exposure. The advantage of rapid results must be weighed against lower assay sensitivity.

3. Challenge Multiplicity

In most assay systems, the higher the virus challenge ratio of infectious virus per cell, the lower the titers (Lindenmann and Gifford, 1963a, b; Finter, 1967a; Ke et al., 1970; Stewart II, unpublished data). With CPE-reading assay method it is important to use just sufficient virus to ensure complete cell kill within the desired time, as more virus appreciably lowers the sensitivity of the assay. Using low multiplicities of infection with interferon inducing and sensitive viruses can give increased assay sensitivity, apparently as the first virus cycles induced interferon which then acts additively.

4. Assay Duration

Interferon titers obtained at earliest times after virus control cultures are distinguishable from cell controls will be higher than the titers of the same samples determined at a later time (Sellers and Fitzpatrick, 1962; Gifford, Toy and Lindenmann, 1963). This likely results from virus growing more slowly in interferon-treated cells and from decay of the antiviral state induced by interferon (see Section XI. A. 1).

5. Concentration vs. Volume

Interferon effects are dependent on the interaction of interferons with the sensitive cells, and this interaction has been shown to follow the law of mass action (Stewart II, 1975a), so that cells with greater sensitivity bind more interferon than less sensitive cells when the interferon concentration is constant (Stewart II, Declercq and Desomer, 1972b); on the other hand, the total amount of interferon bound by cells is independent of the volume of interferon sample to which they are exposed (see Section VIII. C. 1). Similarly, numerous studies have shown that while the total mass units of interferon applied (i. e., volume X concentration) has no effect on level of antiviral activity, antiviral levels are determined by the concentration of the interferon solution (Wagner, 1961; Stewart and Sheaff, 1972; Burke, 1970; Gifford and Toy, 1970; Lieberman et al., 1974; Borden and Leonhardt, 1977). Thus interferon titers obtained in assays should be referred to in units per ml. Some authors have used terms such as interferon units/4 ml because they applied 4 ml samples to their assay cultures (Bausek and Merigan, 1970a, b). Others using microtiter assays have reported units/0.05 ml, and have extrapolated their titers in units/ml by multiplying by a factor of 20. Indeed, the same endpoint dilution is obtained with the 4 ml-volume assay and the 0.05 ml volume assay. Some authors have quoted interferon used in μliters, unexplainably (Radke et al., 1974).

Similarly, if an animal is inoculated with 0.1 ml of an interferon whose endpoint dilution is 1/10,000, the animal receives 1,000 units of interferon; some authors have stealthily avoided this issue with cautious phrases, such as: each animal was inoculated with 0.1 ml of a sample whose activity was 10^4 when 0.05 ml was applied to microtiter cultures.

6. Aging Effect

The "age" of cells has been reported to effect interferon sensitivity of assays in two ways: one type of "age" effect has referred to age of the embryo whose tissues were used to make the assay culture and another type of "age" effect has been the prolonged cultivation of cell cultures. Both "aging" effects increase sensitivities of the interferon assays.

Isaacs and Baron (1960) found that chorioallantoic tissue or minced whole embryo tissue of very young (6-day old) chicken embryos differed from that from older (11 to 13 day old) embryos in being much less sensitive to the antiviral action of interferon; similar differences were found in mouse embryo tissue. Similarly, Cantell et al. (1965) reported that the sensitivity of chick embryo cell monolayers to the antiviral action of interferon increased with age of the embryos; an interferon titrating 32 units per ml in cultures from 6-day old embryos titrated 1024 units per ml in cultures from 13-day embryos (Cantell and Valle, 1965). Cells from human embryos were reported to show age-correlated increase, with cells from the least mature embryos being least interferon sensitive and those from oldest embryos being most sensitive (Siewers, John and Medearis, 1970). Grossberg and Morahan (1971) offered a possible explanation for this in vivo age-related increase. They found that cells from 6-day chick embryos were considerably less sensitive to interferon than those from 13-day embryos (greater than 30-fold difference); however, addition of a small percentage of young embryo cells to cultures from older embryos greatly decreased the interferon sensitivity (more than ten-fold) of the mixed cultures. They, therefore, postulated that young embryo cells elaborate a repressor of interferon action. They reported that medium from cultures of young embryo cells contained a factor antagonistic to interferon action which if added before, during, or even after interferon exposure of 13-day embryo cultures eliminated their interferon sensitivity. It has not been determined whether embryonic age of cells relates to sensitivity to the non-antiviral cell-multiplication inhibitory-action of interferon; if so, this anti-interferon activity might be related to pro-liferative potential.

Cantell and Paucker (1963b) found that cultures of HeLa cells incubated for 1 to 2 days before interferon treatment were much less sensitive to the interferon than cultures of the HeLa cells "aged" 6 to 10 days before interferon exposure. They showed that this was not due to recovery from toxicity of dispersion. Carver and Marcus (1967) found that chick embryo cells aged in vitro for 7 days were 2 to 8-fold more sensitive than 1 to 2-day old cultures (from embryos of the same age). Similar findings were reported by Lockart (1967), Rossman and Vilček (1969), and May and Stanton (1974). Billiau and Buckler (1970) found that rat embryo cells kept for about 2 weeks were about six-fold more interferon sensitive than fresh cultures, and McLaren (1970) found that mouse L cell cultures aged several days were more interferon sensitive. Practically no information is available to explain this in vitro aging effect, but Korsantiya, Smorodintsev and Gwozdilova (1967) have reported that fresh chick embryo cells possess greater interferon-destructive activity than cultures aged 6 to 10 days. Unfortunately, translation of this article does not allow determining whether this "destruction" of interferon activity might be elaboration by the younger cultures of an antagonist of interferon action.

Lvovsky and Levy (1975) have recently made use of the in vitro aging phenomenon to develop highly sensitive assays for human and mouse interferons. Cultures of human fibroblasts or mouse L cells aged 5 days at 30° C and then 1 day at 37° C before treatment with interferon were 16–30 fold and 10-fold, respectively, more sensitive to the interferons. This assay is good for testing samples for minimal interferon levels, but the lack of foresight required to predict assay needs makes overnight cultures more convenient for routine assays, though perhaps less sensitive.

E. Choice of an Assay System

The assay system consists of a cell, and challenge agent and the method to measure the effect.

1. Assay Method of Choice

The choice of assay method can depend on the number of samples to be assayed, as a laboratory generating several thousands of chromatographic fractions each week must consider expense of consumables whereas a laboratory assaying few samples need not be overly concerned with this factor. For other than economic considerations, assays are usually chosen for personal prejudice of the investigator.

2. Cells of Choice

The first determinant of which cell to use is the animal species of the interferons to be assayed. Owing to the host-range limitations of many interferons it is almost always best to select cells from the homologous species (though the several exceptions to this will be discussed; Section VII A 2).

For convenience sake it is usually best to choose continuous cell lines over primary cultures, if these are otherwise comparable. Some investigators have found that primary cells are more sensitive than continuous cell lines (Stewart II, Declercq and Desomer, 1972b; DeMaeyer-Guignard, DeMaeyer and Montagnier, 1972), but this may be compensated by in vitro "aging" described above and must be balanced against the problem of variations in challenge virus sensitivities of different batches of primary cultures (Finter, 1968; Ke et al., 1970; Stewart II, unpublished data). Also, even different clones of continuous cell lines can vary significantly in interferon sensitivity (P. T. Allen, personal communication, 1970; Stewart II, Declercq and Desomer, 1972b).

Aneuploid cells have provided tools for genetic studies of the interferon system and use of human cells with genetic components determining sensitivity to human interferons has provided cells trisomic for human chromosome 21 with increased interferon sensitivity for assay purposes (Tan, Tischfield, and Ruddle, 1973).

3. Virus of Choice

The virus most often used for interferon assays is vesicular stomatitis virus (Finter, 1973a). This virus has a broad host range, willproduce cytopatology and plaques in most cell types, is relatively sensitive to interferon in cells of most animal species, and is not a particular safety hazard. However, its use is restricted in some countries (e. g., England).

It is important to note that the relative sensitivity of viruses to interferon is determined by the species of the cells used in the assay (Stewart II, Scott, and Sulkin, 1969). Thus, while a given virus may be more sensitive than another virus to the resistance induced in one species of cells by interferon, it may be less sensitive than this same virus in another species of cells (Stewart II and Lockart, 1970; Ahl and Rump, 1976; Ito and Montagnier, 1977). Therefore, in choosing a challenge virus for assays of an interferon that has not been previously described it is impossible to generalize interferon sensitivities of particular viruses or even classes of viruses. The relative interferon sensitivities of a number of viruses in a number of animal cell systems are presented in Section IX. A. 2 and Table 14.

F. Reference Interferons and Standard Interferons

Whatever assay method is chosen, owing to the myriad variables that can be anticipated (and often some that cannot), it is usually observed that the apparent potency of a given interferon preparation can vary significantly at different assays. To adjust assay results to take into consideration such fluctuations, a laboratory standard interferon preparation must be included in each assay series. Such adjustments against a laboratory standard interferon will allow results within that laboratory to be quantitatively evaluated. To relate the results of one laboratory to those of other laboratories, each laboratory standard interferon must be calibrated against an international research reference interferon preparation. Without such internal and interlaboratory standardization of "units" it would be impossible to equate results in different laboratories (Finter, 1968; 1973a).

Thus, several international reference interferons have been made available by the National Institute for Medical Research, London, and the National Institutes of Health, Bethesda[3]. Chick interferon reference preparation (62/4) was prepared in 1961 by the British Medical Research Council, and a human leukocyte reference interferon (69/19) was established in 1971. Mouse reference interferon (G002-902-026) and rabbit reference interferon (G019-901-028) were prepared by the Research Resources Branch of the National Institutes of Allergy and Infectious Disease (U. S. A.). Recently, a new human fibroblast reference interferon has been prepared by the NIAID; this reagent should be used to calibrate human fibroblast interferons instead of the human leukocyte reference interferon, as these two types of interferons have been found to give dissimilar dose-response curves (Section VII. C. 1). A reference human leukocyte interferon preparation has also been produced by the N. F. Gamaleya Institute of Epidemiology and Microbiology, U. S. S. R. Academy of Medical Sciences, U. S. S. R. (Polezhaev, Makariev, and Aleksandrova, 1974).

It is likely that other reference interferon preparations will be forthcoming, particularly as more information becomes available on the Type II interferons and regarding the heterogeneity of interferons. By incorporation of a laboratory standard that is regularly calibrated against an appropriate reference interferon in each set of assays (Fig. 3) it is possible to make appropriate adjustments for assay sensitivity fluctuations so that results can be expressed in *international reference units*.

---

[3] These interferon reference reagents can be obtained by qualified investigators from the Division of Biological Standards, National Institute for Medical Research, Mill Hill, London, England, or from Research Resources Branch, NIAID, NIH, Bethesda, MD 20014, U.S.A.

III. Interferon Inducers

The first inducer of interferon to be discovered was a virus, influenza (Isaacs and Lindenmann, 1957). In the several years following this discovery, it became apparent that practically each cell-virus interaction attempted was capable of elaborating an interferon. In fact virologists were so diligently mixing viruses and cells to determine if the particular virus of their interest induced interferon, it was several years before anyone found out that substances other than viruses were capable of inducing interferons. In 1963, Isaacs and his associates demonstrated that "foreign" nonviral nucleic acids, either heterologous cell RNA or chemically-modified homologous cell RNA, could induce interferon production (Rotem, Cox and Isaacs, 1963; Isaacs, Cox and Rotem, 1963). In 1964, bacteria and bacterial endotoxins were found to induce interferons in chickens (Ho, 1964a; Youngner and Stinebring, 1964; Stinebring and Youngner, 1964) and the mold product statolon, from *Penicillium stoloniferum* (Kleinschmidt, Cline, and Murphy, 1964), was found to induce interferon in mice. It was later found that several intracellular microorganisms, such as TRIC agents (Hanna, Merigan, and Jawetz, 1967) and *Toxoplasma gondii* (Rytel and Jones, 1966) induced interferon in cell culture and in vivo. Then synthetic polyanions such as pyran copolymer (Regelson, 1967) and the double-stranded polyribonucleotides, polyriboinosinic acid-polyribocytidylic acid (poly rI·poly rC) (Field *et al.*, 1967a) were added to the list, followed by immune recognition reactions (Green, Cooperband, and Kibrick, 1969) and the synthetic low molecular weight compound tilorone hydrochloride, which was able to induce serum interferon in mice after oral administration (Krueger and Mayer, 1970; Mayer and Krueger, 1970). The recent years have seen publication of numerous reports of low molecular weight synthetic interferon inducers with such exciting names as BL-20803 (Siminoff *et al.*, 1973), N, N-dioctadecyl-N', N'-Bis (2-hydroxyethyl) propanediamine (Hoffman *et al.*, 1973), MA-56 (Soehner, Grambardella, and Hou, 1974), and U-25,166 (Nichol, Weed, and Underwood, 1976). It has also been recently recognized that certain antibiotics (e. g., 9-methylstreptimidone; Saito *et al.*, 1974, 1976), radioprotective chemicals (Khaitovich and Lvovsky, 1975; Lvovsky *et al.*, 1977) and basic dyes (Diederich, Lodemann, and Wacker, 1973) can induce interferons.

Clearly any classification of these inducers is tentative (Ho and Armstrong, 1975). Each of these classes of inducers shows differences in intensities of interferon responses induced, cell types effected *in vivo* or *in vitro*, the time of appearance of the interferon (reflecting either the types of cells induced or dif-

Table 1. *Animal viruses reported to induce interferons* [a]

Virus	in vivo	in vitro	References
1. Human Interferons			
Influenza-A	+	+	Gresser and Dull (1964); Andrews (1961)
Influenza-B	+		Smorodintsev et al. (1970)
Parainfluenza-1 (Sendai)		+	Gresser (1961 a)
Parainfluenza-3		+	Chany (1960)
Newcastle disease		+	Baron and Isaacs (1962)
Measles	+	+	Petralli, Merigan, and Wilbur (1965a); DeMaeyer and Enders (1961)
Mumps	+	+	Cantell (1961); Waddell, Wilbur, and Merigan (1968)
Rubella		+	Neva and Weller (1964)
Respiratory syncytial	+	+	Ray, Gravelle, and Chin (1967); Moehring and Forsyth (1971)
Rabiesvirus		+	Wiktor et al. (1972)
Vesicular stomatitis		+	Marcus and Sekellick (1977); Vilcek, Yamazaki and Havell (1977)
Chikungunya		+	Zimmermann et al. (1972)
Sindbis		+	Gresser and Enders (1962)
Western equine encephalitits		+	Luby, Sanders, and Sulkin (1971)
St. Louis encephalitits	+		Luby et al. (1969)
Yellow fever	+	+	Wheelock and Sibley (1965); Wheelock and Edelman (1969)
Poliovirus-Type 1		+	Gresser, Chany, and Enders (1965)
Poliovirus-Type 2	+	+	Smorodintsev et al. (1970); Ho and Enders (1959 a, b)
Encephalomyocarditis		+	Stewart II, Gosser, and Lockart (1971 a)
Rhinovirus-2	+	+	Smorodintsev et al. (1971 a); Fiala (1972)
Rhinovirus-12	+	+	Gatmaitan, Stanley, and Jackson (1973)
Rhinovirus-15	+		Cate, Douglas, and Couch (1968)
Coxsackie-A 21	+		Cate, Douglas, and Couch (1968)
Reovirus-2		+	Oie, Loh, and Ratnayake (1973)
Blue tongue		+	Jameson and Grossberg (1977)
Adenoviruses		+	Lysov et al. (1971)
Varicella-zoster	+	+	Vaczi, Horvath, and Hadhazy (1965)
Human cytomegalovirus		+	Vaczi, Horvath, and Hadhazy (1965); Glasgow (1974)

[a] Strain differences, active or inactivated conditions not designated.

Table 1 (continued)   Interferon Inducers   29

Virus	*in vivo*	*in vitro*	References
Herpes simplex		+	Rasmussen *et al.* (1974)
Vaccinia	+	+	Wheelock (1964); Epstein, Stevens, and Merigan (1972)

2. Monkey Interferons

Influenza-A		+	Burke and Isaacs (1958 a)
Parainfluenza-1 (Sendai)		+	Burke and Isaacs (1958 b)
Parainfluenza-5		+	Hsiung (1962)
Newcastle disease		+	Barahona and Melendez (1971)
Measles		+	McKimm and Rapp (1977 a)
Rubella		+	Parkman, Buescher, and Artenstein (1962)
Rabies	+		Wiktor *et al.* (1976)
Chikungunya	+	+	Barbosa *et al.* (1974); Uhlendorf, Zimmerman, and Baron (1973)
Sindbis		+	Stewart II and Lockart (1970)
Dengue		+	Russell *et al.* (1966)
Poliovirus-type 2		+	Stewart II, Gosser, and Lockart (1971 a)
Encephalomyocarditis		+	Stewart II, Gosser, and Lockart (1971 a)
Rice dwarf virus		+	Takehara and Suzuki (1973)
Simian Virus-40		+	Diderholm (1963)

3. Mouse Interferons

Influenza-A	+	+	Isaacs and Hitchcock (1960); Finter (1965)
Parainfluenza-1 (Sendai)	+	+	Baron and Buckler (1963); Henle *et al.* (1959)
Parainfluenza-3	+		Craighead (1966)
Newcastle disease	+	+	Baron and Buckler (1963); Henle *et al.* (1959)
Mumps		+	Henle *et al.* (1959); Holmes, Gilson, and Dienhardt (1964)
Rabies	+		Wiktor, Koprowski, and Rorke (1972)
Vesicular stomatitis	+	+	Wagner *et al.* (1963); Younger and Wertz (1968)
Sindbis	+		Baron and Buckler (1963)
Chikungunya	+	+	Baron *et al.* (1966 a); Glasgow and Habel (1963)
Western equine encephalitis		+	Lockart (1963)
Eastern equine encephalitis		+	Wagner (1963 b)
Semliki forest	+	+	Finter (1965)

Table 1 (continued)

Virus	*in vivo*	*in vitro*	References
O'Nyong-Nyong	+		Hitchcock and Porterfield (1961)
Bunyamwera	+		Baron *et al.* (1966 a)
Rift valley fever	+		Higashihara (1971)
West Nile	+		Vainio, Gwatkin, and Koprowski (1961)
Tahyna	+		Bardos and Sejcovicova (1966)
St. Louis encephalitis	+		Monath and Borden (1971)
Encephalomyocarditis	+	+	Baron, Barban, and Buckler (1964); Giron (1969)
Coxsackie B1	+		Heineberg, Gold, and Robbins (1964)
Coxsackie B3	+		Rytel (1969)
Rhinovirus-2		+	Stewart II, Gosser and Lockart (1971 a)
Lactic dehydrogenase	+	+	Lagwinska *et al.* (1975)
Junin	+		Boxaca, Guerreo, and Savy (1973)
Mouse hepatitis	+.		Malluci (1964)
Reovirus-3	+	+	Jameson, Schoenherr, and Grossberg (1977); Gauntt (1973); Lai and Joklik (1973)
Rice dwarf		+	Takehara and Suzuki (1973)
Blue tongue	+		Huismans (1969); Jameson, Schoenherr, and Grossberg (1977)
Colorado tick fever		+	Dubovi and Akers (1972)
Lymphocytic choriomeningitis	+		Riviere and Bandu (1977); Merigan, Oldstone, and Welsh (1977)
Friend leukemia	+		Gresser *et al.* (1967 b, d)
Moloney leukemia	+		Sinkovics and Howe (1964)
Rauscher leukemia	+		Glasgow and Friedman (1970); Toth, Vaczi, and Berencsi (1971 a)
Mouse mammary tumor	+		DeMaeyer *et al.* (1974)
Murine cytomegalovirus	+	+	Henson and Smith (1964); Henson, Smith, and Gherke (1966)
Minute virus of mice	+		Harris, Coleman, and Morahan (1974)
Polyoma	+	+	Friedman and Rabson (1964); Allison (1961)
Herpes Simplex	+	+	Sydiskis and Schultz (1966); Glasgow and Habel (1963)
Vaccinia	+	+	Verlinde and Dret (1963); Baron and Buckler (1963); Glasgow and Habel (1962 a, b)

4. Bovine Interferons

Influenza-A		+	Tyrrell (1959)

Table 1 (continued)   Interferon Inducers   31

Virus	*in vivo*	*in vitro*	References
Parainfluenza-1 (Sendai)		+	Smorodintsev (1968)
Parainfluenza-3		+	Hermodsson (1964)
Newcastle disease		+	Hermodsson (1963)
Foot and mouth disease	+	+	Straub and Ahl (1976); Dinter (1960)
Semliki forest		+	Finter (1964 a)
Bovine rhinovirus		+	Smorodintsev (1968)
Bovine viral diarrhea	+		Rinaldo *et al.* (1976)
Infectious bovine rhinotracheitis	+	+	Todd, Volenec, and Paton (1972); Fulton and Rosenquist (1976 b)

5. Rabbit Interferons

Virus	*in vivo*	*in vitro*	References
Influenza-A	+	+	Isaacs and Westwood (1959 a); Andrews (1961)
Parainfluenza-3		+	Acton and Myrvik (1966)
Newcastle disease	+	+	Postic *et al.* (1966); Levy-Koenig, Golgher, and Paucker (1970 a, b)
Mumps		+	Cantell and Tommila (1960)
Rabies		+	Wiktor, Postic, and Koprowski (1972)
Eastern equine encephalitis	+	+	Ho (1973)
Sindbis	+	+	Ho and Breinig (1965); Schleupner *et al.* (1969)
Reovirus-3	+		Tytell *et al.* (1967)
Rice dwarf		+	Takehara and Suzuki (1973)
Blue tongue	+		Jameson, Schoenherr, and Grossberg (1977)
Shope papilloma	+		Langston and Sobin (1967)
Herpes simplex	+	+	Force, Stewart, and Haff (1965); Fujibayashi, Hooks, and Notkins (1975)
Vaccinia		+	Nagano and Kojima (1958)

6. Hamster interferons

Virus	*in vivo*	*in vitro*	References
Influenza-A	+	+	Wiktor, Postic, Ho, and Koprowski (1972); Pollikoff *et al.* (1962)
Parainfluenza-1 (Sendai)		+	Menezes (1972)
Newcastle disease	+	+	Baron *et al.* (1966 a); Henle and Henle (1963)
Rabies	+		Stewart II and Sulkin (1966)
Venezuela equine encephalitis	+		Jahrling (1975); Jahrling, Navarro, and Scherer (1976)
Polyoma	+	+	Porwit-Bobr and Ptak (1966); Talas, Weisfeiler, and Batkai (1968)

Table 1 (continued)

Virus	in vivo	in vitro	References
7. Bat interferon			
Japanese encephalitis	+	+	Stewart II, Allen, and Sulkin (1969)
8. Rat interferon			
Parainfluenza-1 (sendai)		+	Zimmerman et al. (1972)
Newcastle disease	+	+	VanRossum and Desomer (1966); Biernacka and Lobodzinska (1973)
Sindbis	+	+	Desomer and Billiau (1966); Cocito, DeMaeyer and Desomer (1962 a, b)
Chikungunya	+	+	Mendelson, Kapusta, and Dick (1970)
Semliki forest		+	DeMaeyer and DeMaeyer-Guignard (1967)
Respiratory syncytial	+		Grodnitskaya and Dreizen (1975)
Kilham rat virus		+	Kilham et al. (1968)
Vaccinia		+	DeMaeyer and DeMaeyer-Guignard (1963)
9. Sheep interferons			
Chikungunya	+	+	Rinaldo, Overall, and Glasgow (1975)
Blue tongue		+	Rinaldo, Overall, and Glasgow (1975)
Herpes simplex		+	Rinaldo, Overall, and Glasgow (1975)
10. Pig interferons			
Newcastle disease		+	Gresser et al. (1974)
Hog Cholera	+	+	Torlone, Titoli, and Gialetti (1965)
11. Guinea-pig interferons			
Newcastle disease		+	Kaplan et al. (1962)
Chikungunya		+	Friedman et al. (1962)
Herpes simplex	+		Tokumaru (1967)
12. Cat interferon			
Newcastle disease	+	+	McCullough (1972); Rodgers et al. (1972)
13. Dog interferons			
Influenza-A		+	Depoux (1965)
Newcastle disease		+	Desmyter and Stewart II (1976)
Herpes simplex		+	Aurelian and Roizman (1965)
14. Chicken interferons			
Influenza-A	+	+	Isaacs and Lindenmann (1957)
Influenza-B	+	+	Hahnemann and Reinicke (1965); Smorodintsev et al. (1970)
Influenza-C	+	+	Cantell et al. (1965)

Table 1 (continued)　　　　　　　　Interferon Inducers　　　　　　　　33

Virus	*in vivo*	*in vitro*	References
Parainfluenza-1 (Sendai)	+		Cantell *et al.* (1965)
Parainfluenza-5	+	+	Hsiung and VandeWater (1966)
Newcastle disease	+	+	Isaacs (1962); Levine (1962); Burke and Isaacs (1958 a, b)
Vesicular stomatitis	+	+	Isaacs (1962); Cooper and Bellett (1959)
Chikungunya	+	+	Isaacs (1962); Ruiz-Gomez and Isaacs (1963 a, b)
Sindbis		+	Ho (1961)
Western equine encephalitis		+	Lockart (1964)
Eastern equine encephalitis		+	Wagner (1963 b)
Mayoro		+	Henderson and Taylor (1961)
O'Nyong-Nyong	+		Isaacs (1962)
Bunyamwera	+		Isaacs (1962)
Kumba	+	+	Isaacs (1962); Gifford, Mussett, and Heller (1964)
Rio Bravo		+	Jordan (1972 a)
Japanese encephalitis		+	Grossberg and Scherer (1964)
Powassan	+		Larke (1965)
Yellow fever	+		Isaacs (1962)
West Nile	+		Isaacs (1962)
Tick-Borne encephalitis		+	Vilcek (1960)
Dengue		+	Sather and Hammon (1963)
Reovirus-3		+	Long and Burke (1971)
Fowl plague	+	+	Isaacs (1962); Burke and Isaacs (1958b)
Duck hepatitis	+		Sueltenfuss and Pollard (1963)
Molluscum contagiosum		+	Friedman-Kien and Vilcek (1967)
Rous sarcoma	+	+	Force and Stewart (1966); Bader (1962)
Polyoma		+	Ustacelebi and Williams (1973)
Human adenoviruses	+	+	Beladi and Pusztai (1967); Ho and Kohler (1967); Pusztai *et al.* (1969)
Celo-Avian adenovirus		+	Markovits and Coppey (1971)
Gal-Adenovirus of chickens		+	Bakay (1969)
Pseudorabies		+	Lomniczi (1974 a, b)
Marek's disease	+	+	Hong and Sevoian (1971); Kaleta and Bankowski (1972 a, b)
Herpes simplex		+	Fruitstone, Waddell, and Sigel (1964)
Fowlpox		+	Asch and Gifford (1970)
Vaccinia	+	+	Isaacs (1962); Asch and Gifford (1970)

Table 1 (continued)

Virus	in vivo	in vitro	References
15. Reptile interferons (tortoise)			
Parainfluenza-1 (Sendai)		+	Falcoff and Fauconnier (1965)
Newcastle disease		+	Galabov (1973); Vassileva and Galabov (1975); Galabov and Velichkova (1975)
Sindbis		+	Galabov, Savov, and Vassileva (1973)
Semliki forest		+	Galabov, Petrinova, and Savov (1973)
West nile		+	Galabov, Petrinova, and Savov (1973)
16. Fish interferons			
a) Fathead minnow interferon			
Reovirus-2		+	Oie and Loh (1971)
Infectious pancreatic necrosis		+	Gravelle and Malsberger (1965)
b) Red swordtail interferon			
Reovirus		+	Kelly and Loh (1973)
c) Blue striped grunt interferon			
Grunt fin agent		+	Beasley, Sigel, and Clem (1966)
d) Rainbow trout interferon			
Egtved rhadbo virus		+	Kinkelin and Dorson (1973)
Infectious pancreatic necrosis	+	+	Kinkelin and LeBerre (1974); DeSena and Rio (1975)

ferent induction-production mechanisms), and the types of interferons induced. In the discussion in this Section, I shall describe the inducers with examples of the systems in which they induce interferons. Mechanisms of induction and origins (cell types) will be described in Section IV, and the physicochemical characterizations of the heterogeneity of the interferons produced will be covered in Section VII. C.

A. Animal Viral Inducers

The number of viruses that have been shown to induce interferons has grown to include every major virus group. Table 1 shows a listing of some of these viruses arranged by the animal cells induced; this arrangement is for convenience as reference source for interferons of the different species. It is apparent that inducer viruses can be either single-stranded RNA viruses, double-stranded RNA viruses, or DNA viruses. The majority of viruses that have been tested can induce interferon in the intact animal or in cell cultures. Interferon-like substances have also been reported to be produced by mosquito cells infected with arbovirus (Enzmann, 1973); however, this report could not be confirmed by others (Takehara, 1975a, b; Murray and Morahan, 1973). To date, interferon production seems to be reliably demonstrated only in vertebrates and their cells.

Several viruses have earned reputations as "good" inducers, as they have consistently induced relatively high levels of interferons in a variety of systems. A "good" inducer in this regard would be Newcastle disease virus after either intravenous injection into animals (Henle *et al.*, 1959; Baron and Buckler, 1963; Ho *et al.*, 1970) or cell cultures (Ho *et al.*, 1970; Stewart II, Gosser, and Lockart, 1971b, 1972).

Some viruses are regarded as "poor inducers" because several investigators have reported failures to induce interferons with these agents in their particular system. Adenoviruses have failed to induce detectable interferon in several animals and cell cultures (Ray, Gravelle, and Chin, 1967; Ho, 1973), although they do induce interferons in others (Beladi and Pusztai, 1967; Ho, 1973; Pusztai *et al.*, 1969). Cytomegaloviruses failed to induce interferons in some human or mouse cells (Glasgow *et al.*, 1967; Osborn and Medearis, 1966) but did so in others (Vaczi, Horvath, and Hadhazy, 1965; Henson and Smith, 1964; Oie *et al.*, 1975).

However, the classification of viral inducers as "good" or "poor" is not particularly meaningful or enlightening. Even "good" viral inducers can differ significantly; some strains of Newcastle disease virus induce significantly less than other strains (Ho *et al.*, 1970; W. E. Stewart II, unpublished data). Also, rabiesvirus which has been repeatedly reported to be a poor inducer, or non-inducer in cell cultures (Fernandes, Wiktor, and Koprowski, 1964; Wiktor, Fernandes, and Koprowski, 1964) is a "good" inducer of interferon in hamster brain tissue (Stewart II and Sulkin, 1966). Lymphocytic choriomeningitis virus, which causes persistent infections in mice, was reported to not induce interferon in this system (Wagner and Snyder, 1962). However, Riviere *et al.* (1977) found that administration of antibodies specific for mouse interferon to mice infected with lymphocytic choriomeningitis virus greatly increased the levels of this virus in their sera, suggesting that endogenous interferon induced by this virus was responsible for the restricted replication of the virus. Also, polioviruses that did not induce detectable interferon in several cell cultures (Isaacs, 1963a; Stewart II, Gosser and Lockart, 1971a) were able to induce interferons in these cells after the cultures were primed with interferon (Section X. C.).

A number of other factors can affect the ability of viruses to induce interferons. Several of these variables relate to the metabolic effects of viruses on the cells, such that slightly inactivated (heat, ultraviolet radiation, etc.) "poor" inducer virus may become a "good" inducer (Ho and Breinig, 1965; Goorha and Gifford, 1970a; Gandhi Burke, and Scholtessek, 1970). The implications of these studies to the mechanisms of interferon induction will be discussed (Section IV). At present it suffices to state that most, if not all, viruses are able to induce interferons.

A few viruses deserve special mention as their interferon inducing property adds more to our knowledge of the interferon system than just another virus on the list.

1. Adenoviruses

It has been observed that adenovirus type 12 failed to induce interferon in several mouse, monkey, human or hamster cell cultures, but induced interferon in hamsters after intravenous inoculation (Ho, 1973). Beladi and Pusztai (1967) induced interferon in chick embryo cells with adenovirus 9. Adenovirus type 12 induced interferon in chicks (Pusztai *et al.*, 1969) and in chick embryo fibroblasts (Pusztai *et al.*, 1976) but not in human, monkey, rabbit, hamster or mouse cells. A curious effect of trypsin on adenoviruses was observed (Beladi and Pusztai, 1967; Ho and Kohler, 1967; Pusztai *et al.*, 1974): it destroyed the interferon inducing ability of the viruses without affecting their infectivity. However, heating at 56° C destroyed both interferon inducing activity and infectivity of adenoviruses (Pusztai *et al.*, 1969). Roszotoczy (1976a) showed that the amount of interferon induced by human adenoviruses was increased by about 10-fold by priming the cells before induction. To my knowledge, adenoviruses have not been shown to induce interferons in other than human and chick cell systems.

2. Myxo-Paramyxo Inducers

The first inducer of interferon was influenza-A virus, and this inducer has been the most widely used of all the viral inducers, inducing interferon in man and human cell cultures, monkey cell cultures, mice and mouse cell cultures, calf cells, rabbits and rabbit cells, hamsters and hamster cells, dog cells, chickens and in chicken cells. Sendai virus was found by Gresser (1961a) to induce interferon in human leukocyte cultures, and is presently used for induction of the entire worlds's supply of human leukocyte interferon for clinical use (Mogensen and Cantell, 1977). Sendai virus has been used to induce interferons of several animal species. Newcastle disease virus is among the best inducers of interferons *in vivo* and *in vitro* in human cells, in mouse cells and in mice, in rabbit cells and in rabbits, rats, pig, guinea-pig, cat, dog, chicken and fish cells (see Table 1), making it a dependable agent for trials of interferon induction in a previously untested system.

3. Rhabdoviruses

Rabiesvirus was long thought defective in interferon inducing ability (Wiktor, Fernandes, and Koprowski, 1964; Fernandes, Wiktor, and Koprowski, 1964), as no interferon was found in human or rabbit cell cultures infected with rabiesvirus. However, when inoculated into hamsters, its replication in the brain induced high levels of interferon, with lower levels of interferon in several other tissues (Stewart II and Sulkin, 1966). Several vaccine strains of rabiesviruses have been found to induce interferons in human and rabbit cells (Wiktor *et al.*, 1972) and in monkeys (Wiktor *et al.*, 1976) and mice (Wiktor, Koprowski, and Rorke, 1972), their inducing potential correlating with their prophylactic potentials as antirabies vaccines.

Vesicular stomatitis virus induces interferon in mouse cells and chicken cells, but has earned a reputation as a poor inducer as it does so very modestly, likely attributable to its propensity for rapidly terminating cellular protein synthesis. Marcus and Sekellick (1977) recently described a defective interfering particle of vesicular stomatitis virus with covalently linked (±) RNA of message and antimessage which was an efficient inducer in chicken and human cells.

Another rhabdovirus, Egtved virus, was found to induce interferon in rainbow trout cells (Kinkelin and Dorson, 1973).

4. "Arbovirus" Inducers

The conglomerate of viruses that, during interferon's infancy and adolescence, were called "arboviruses" have been used extensively in cell cultures and animals to induce serum interferons, brain interferons and tissue culture interferons. Many of these agents induce high titers of circulating interferons in animals that coincide with viremias (Baron et al., 1966a), and Wheelock and Sibley (1965) found that the 17-D vaccine strain of Yellow Fever virus induced circulating interferon in man.

An interesting recent finding with Venezuelan equine encephalitis virus was reported by Jahrling, Navarro and Scherer (1976). They found that this virus induced extremely high titers of interferon (about 70,000 units/ml of serum) in the hamster, an animal that some workers have considered to be defective in interferon production (Grossberg, Smith, and Sedmak, 1975), even though it was known to produce interferon when infected with rabiesvirus (Stewart II and Sulkin, 1966).

5. Diplorna Viruses

The double-stranded RNA-containing reoviruses were tested for interferon inducing activity soon after it was found that synthetic double-stranded RNA induced interferon (Lampson et al., 1967), and reovirus-3 was found to induce interferon in rabbits (Tytell et al., 1967), but not impressively. Reoviruses were found to induce modest levels of interferon in human cells (Oie, Loh, and Ratnayake, 1973), mice and mouse cells (Gauntt, 1973; Lai and Joklik, 1973), in chicken cells (Long and Burke, 1971), and in fish cells (Oie and Loh, 1971). Rice dwarf virus induced interferon in monkey, mouse and rabbit cells (Takehara and Suzuki, 1973), and Colorado tick fever induced interferon in mouse cells (Dubovi and Akers, 1972).

Bluetongue virus, an arbovirus, was found to induce interferon in sheep cells (Rinaldo, Overall, and Glasgow, 1975) and in mice (Huisman, 1969), again at relatively unremarkable levels. However, Jameson, and Grossberg (1977) found this virus to induce large amounts of interferon in human cell cultures (10,000 to 60,000 units/ml), being slightly better than Sendai virus in human buffy-coat suspensions, and levels of over 100,000 units/ml of plasma in mice and rabbits (Jameson, Schoenherr and Grossberg, 1977). These data clearly re-emphasize the naivety of generalizing groups of viruses as "good" or "poor" inducers.

6. Lymphocytic Choriomeningitis Virus

To harp further on this point, I point to the recent studies of interferon inducing potential of lymphocytic choriomeningitis virus. This virus, both in vivo and in vitro, appeared to have solid credentials as a non-inducer (Traub, 1961; Wagner and Snyder, 1962; Volker, Larsen, and Pfau, 1964; Youn and

Barski, 1966), though the related M-P virus had been reported to induce low levels of interferon in mice (Padnos, Shimonaski and Came et al., 1971). Then Merigan, Oldstone, and Walsh (1977) found that this virus induced high levels of interferon in normal mice and even higher levels in nude mice. Also, Riviere and Bandu (1977) found significant levels of circulating interferon in lymphocytic choriomeningitis virus-infected mice. So much for the concept of classifying viruses as "good" and "poor" inducers!

Most investigators have used viruses that had been previously shown to induce interferons. The listings in Table 1, showing the relatively limited number of agents tested, and the recent findings of more efficient viral inducers in some of the animal cell systems, emphasize the need to continue looking for a better viral interferon inducer.

B. Non-Viral Inducers of Interferons

This section should actually be entitled non-*animal* viral inducers of interferons as many of the agents initially regarded as non-viral agents that could induce interferons have been found to owe their interferon-inducing activity to plant or bacterial virus particles in them, as we shall see.

1. "Foreign" Nucleic Acids

Isaacs (1961, 1963b) proposed that interferon production might be a defensive response of cells to intrusion of "foreign" nucleic acids. He and his associates reported that crude RNA preparations from heterologous cells or homologous preparations modified by chemical treatment would induce interferons in cell cultures (Rotem, Cox, and Isaacs, 1963; Isaacs, Cox, and Rotem, 1963). This observation proved difficult to confirm and subsequently fell into disrepute. However, other reports of interferon induction by RNA preparations extracted from uninfected cells (DeMaeyer, DeMaeyer–Guignard, and Montagnier, 1971; Kimball and Duesberg, 1971) suggest an explanation for this induction by crude preparations extracted from cells.

2. Fungal Extracts

A listing of fungal products reported to induce interferons is given in Table 2. Statolon, a product of fermentation of *Penicillium stoloniferum* was found to induce interferon in animals and in cell cultures (Kleinschmidt, Cline, and Murphy, 1964; Kleinschmidt and Murphy, 1965, 1967). The active component of statolon was originally believed to be an anionic polysaccharide, but it was later found that its interferon-inducing potential resided in virus particles from the *Penicillium* mycelia (Kleinschmidt and Ellis, 1967; Ellis and Kleinschmidt, 1967). This virus was subsequently found to contain double-stranded RNA (Kleinschmidt et al., 1968).

Helenine, a product from *Penicillium funiculosum*, was also found to induce interferon (Rytel, Shope, and Kilbourne, 1966) and again the active component was found to be a double-stranded RNA component present in polyhedral virions in the preparation (Lampson et al., 1967; Banks et al., 1968). *Aspergillus foetidus*, *P. chrysogenium* and *P. cyaneofulvum* were also

Table 2. *Microorganisms and their products reported to induce interferons*

Inducer	in vivo	in vitro	References
I. Fungi			
A. Mycophage from			
Aspergillus foetidus	+	+	Banks *et al.* (1970)
Cortinelluf shiitake	+	+	Suzuki, Suganuma, and Ishida (1974)
Lentinus edodes	+	+	Tsunonada and Ishida (1970)
Penicillium cyaneofulvum	+	+	Banks *et al.* (1969)
Penicillium funiculosum	+	+	Lampson *et al.* (1967); Rytel, Shope and Kilbourne (1966)
Penicillium stoloniferum	+	+	Kleinschmidt, Cline, and Murphy (1964); Kleinschmidt and Murphy (1965)
B. Fungal extracts			
Alternaria tenvis	+		Youngner (1970)
Candida albicans – Mannan	+		Borecky *et al.* (1967)
Streptomyces kanamyceticus – Kanamycin	+		Lukas and Hruskova (1968)
Streptomyces griseus – cycloheximide	+	+	Youngner, Stinebring, and Taube (1965); Tan and Berthold (1977)
Streptomyces sp. – Lymphomycin	+		Suzuki, Suganuma, and Ishida (1974)
Streptomyces sp.	+		Suzuki, Saito, and Ishida (1977)
II. Bacteria			
A. Intact bacteria			
Aerobacter sp.	+		Youngner (1970)
Bordetella pertussis	+		Borecky and Lackovic (1967)
Brucella abortus	+		Youngner and Stinebring (1964)
Brucella melitensis	+		Bousquet *et al.* (1973)
Corynebacterium parvum	+		Kirchner *et al.* (1977)
Escherichia coli	+		Ho (1964 a)
Francisella tularensis	+		Lukas and Hruskova (1967)
Haemophilus influenzae	+		Degre and Dahl (1974)
Klebsiella aerogenes	+		Degre and Dahl (1974)
Listeria monocytogenes	+		Lukas and Hruskova (1967)
Salmonella typhimurium	+		Stinebring and Youngner (1964)
Serratia marcescens	+		Stinebring and Youngner (1964)
Staphylococcus aureus	+		Degre and Dahl (1974)
Salmonella typhi	+		Kandefer-Szerszen (1973)

Table 2 (continued)

Inducer	in vivo	in vitro	References
B. Bacterial products			
Aerobacter sp.			
– Endotoxin	+		Smith and Wagner (1967 a, b)
Bordetella pertussis			
– components	+		Kojima, Yoshida, and Nakase (1973)
Brucella abortus			
– Spheroplasts	+		Ramuz *et al.* (1974)
– Endotoxin	+		Kono (1967)
– Lipopolysaccharide	+		Youngner, Feingold, and Chen (1973)
– Lipid A	+		Youngner, Keleti, and Feingold (1974)
Corynebacterium diphtheriae			
– Toxoid			Green *et al.* (1970)
Escherichia coli			
– Endotoxin	+		Stinebring and Youngner (1964)
– Protein	+		Grossberg *et al.* (1972)
Hemophilus influenzae			
– Extract	+	+	DeClercq and Merigan (1969 a)
Klebsiella pneumoniae			
– Capsular Polysaccharide	+		Kato, Nakashima, and Ohta (1975)
Mycobacterium tuberculosis			
– Cell Wall	+		Nagano *et al.* (1971)
– PPD			Stinebring and Absher (1970)
Pseudomonas aeruginosa			
– Endotoxin	+		Kojima, Homma, and Abe (1971)
Salmonella minnesota			
– Lipid A	+		Schiller *et al.* (1976)
Salmonella enteridis			
– Endotoxin	+	+	DeClercq and Merigan (1969 a)
Salmonella typhi			
– Endotoxin			Oh and Gill (1966)
O-Antigen	+		Galabov and Galabov (1972);
– Detoxicated			
O-Antigen	+		Galabov and Galabov (1973)
Salmonella typhimurium			
– Lipopolysaccharide	+		Keleti, Feingold, and Youngner (1974)
– Lipid A	+		Youngner, Feingold, and Chen (1973)
Staphylococcus aureus			
– Enterotoxin A	+		Johnson, Stanton, and Baron (1977)
C. Bacteriophage			
Escherichia coli-Phage T4	+		Kleinschmidt, Douthart, and Murphy (1970)
– dsRNA from phage f2	+	+	Doskocil *et al.* (1971)
– dsRNA from phage MU9	+	+	Field *et al.* (1967 b)
Pseudomonas phageolica			
– dsRNA from phage Ø6	+		Kleinschmidt, Van Etton, and Vidaver (1973)

Table 2 (continued)

Inducer	in vivo	in vitro	References
III. Chlamydia			
Trachoma-inclusion Conjunctivitis Agents	+	+	Merigan and Hanna (1966); Jekin and Lu (1967)
Psittacosis	+	+	Kozikowska and Hahon (1970)
IV. Rickettsiae			
Coxiella burneti	+	+	Kazar (1966); Hahon and Kozikowska (1968)
Rickettsia mooseri		+	Kohno *et al.* (1970)
Rickettsia prowazeki	+		Kazar (1966)
Rickettsia tsutsugamushi		+	Hopps *et al.* (1964)
V. Mycoplasma			
Acholeplasma laidlawii	+		Rinaldo *et al.* (1973)
Acholeplasma sp. ØG1	+		Fauconnier and Wroblowski (1974)
Mycoplasma arthritidis	+		Rinaldo *et al.* (1974 a, b)
Mycoplasma pulmonis	+		Cole *et al.* (1975, 1976)
Mycoplasma pneumoniae	+	+	Rinaldo (1976); Sokhey, Soloviev and Vasilieva (1977)
VI. Protozoa			
Bensonita jellisona	+		Remington and Merigan (1969)
Encephalitozoon cuniculi		+	Armstrong *et al.* (1973)
Eperythrozoon coccoides	+		Suntharasami and Rytel (1973)
Plasmodium berghei	+		Huang, Schultz, and Gordon (1968)
Toxoplasma gondii	+		Rytel and Jones (1966); Freshman *et al.* (1966)
Trypanosoma cruzi	+		Rytel and Marsden (1970)

found to contain an interferon inducing virus (Banks *et al.*, 1968, 1970; Buck, Chain and Himmelweit, 1971).

Interferon induction has also been reported with extracts of the edible mushrooms *Lentinus edodes* and *Cortinelluf shiitake;* again the active component was found to be a double-stranded RNA (Tsunonada and Ishida, 1970; F. Suzuki *et al.*, 1974).

The yeast *Candida albicans* produces a polysaccharide, mannon, which induces interferon in mice (Borecky *et al.*, 1967), and the *Streptomyces* elaborate kanamycine and cycloheximide, both of which induce interferon production *in vivo* (Lukas and Hruskova, 1968; Youngner, Stinebring, and Taube, 1965). The *Streptomyces* have been reported to elaborate the antibiotics lymphomycin and 9-methylstreptimidone, both of which induce interferons in rabbits and mice, respectively (Suzuki, Suganuma, and Ishida, 1974; Saito *et al.*, 1976; Suzuki, Saito, and Ishida, 1977).

3. Bacteria and Bacterial Products

A listing of bacterial products reported to induce interferons is given in Table 2. The first report of bacteria being able to induce interferon was probably by Gledhill (1959), who showed that mice inoculated with bacterial endotoxin contained a factor in their sera which exerted a "sparing effect" against virus diseases. Youngner and Stinebring (1964) reported that chickens and mice inoculated with live *Brucella abortus, Serratia marcescens* or *Salmonella typhimurium* or *E. coli* endotoxin produced interferon. Ho (1964) found interferon in rabbits injected with live *E. coli* or endotoxin. It is important to note that while Youngner and Stinebring reported this interferon to be acid stable (to pH 3), Ho found the *E. coli* and endotoxin-induced interferons were labile at pH 2. Interferon was also induced in mice by *Brucella* (Hallum, Youngner, and Stinebring, 1965), and rats made interferon when inoculated with *E. coli* (Desomer and Billiau, 1966). Interferon was found in the aqueous humor, urine and cerebrospinal fluids of rabbits inoculated with *Salmonella typhosa* endotoxin (Oh, 1966; Oh and Gill, 1966).

Ke and Ho (1967) found that while rabbit interferons induced by endotoxin and virus were similar in stabilities at pH 4, virus-induced interferons were stable at pH 2 while endotoxin-induced interferon was destroyed, suggesting their origins from different cells. In this regard, it is important to emphasize that none of the many endotoxins tested have been able to induce interferon in cell cultures (Kono, 1967; Matisova *et al.*, 1970) with the exception of the unconfirmed claim that both *Hemophilus influenza* extract and *Salmonella enteritidis* endotoxin induced "significant" interferon levels in cultures of human skin fibroblasts (DeClercq and Merigan, 1969a).

Interferon has been induced by cell wall components of *Bordetella pertusis* (Kojima, Yoshida and Nakase, 1973), *Mycobacterium tuberculosis* (Nagano *et al.*, 1971), by *Salmonella sp.* (Keleti, Feingold and Youngner, 1974) and O-antigen (Galabov and Galabov, 1972, 1973). The lipid A component of the lipopolysaccharide was the more active portion (Youngner, Feingold, and Chen, 1973; Schiller *et al.*, 1976).

Brucella abortus spheroplasts were active (Ramuz *et al.*, 1974), as was an aqueous-ether extractable component called BRU-PEL (Youngner, Keleti, and Feingold, 1974; Feingold, Keleti, and Youngner, 1976).

Standard mixed bacterial vaccines (*Klebsiella aerogenes, Haemophillus influenza* and *Staphylococcus aureus*) and each of these individually induced interferon in mice (Degre and Dahl, 1971, 1974) but not in man (Rytel *et al.*, 1974). *Klebsiella pneumoniae* capsular polysaccharide was an inducer in mice (Kato, Nakashima, and Ohta, 1975).

In addition to these assorted components of bacteria that induce interferons, bacteria have been found to contain phage which also induce interferon (see Table 2). The coliphage T4 induced interferon in mice (Kleinschmidt, Douthart, and Murphy, 1970) as did *Pseudomonas phaseolica* phage ∅ 6

(Kleinschmidt *et al.*, 1973; Kleinschmidt, Van Etten, and Vidaver, 1974). The *E. coli* f₂ phage replicative form double-stranded RNA (Doskocil *et al.*, 1971; Fuchsberger *et al.*, 1972) was able to induce both *in vivo* and *in vitro*.

4. Other Microorganisms Inducing Interferons

A list of the microorganisms inducing interferons is presented in Table 2. These include representatives from most of the major groups of microorganisms. Many of these agents have been shown to induce interferons in animals and in tissue cultures.

a) Chlamydia

The TRIC (trachoma-inclusion conjunctivitis) agents induce interferons in mice and mouse L cells (Merigan and Hanna, 1966; Hanna, Merigan, and Jawetz, 1967) and in human cell cultures (Jenkin and Lu, 1967). The psittacosis agent was found to induce interferon in leukocyte cultures (Kozikowska & Hahon, 1970).

b) Rickettsiae

R. tsutsugamushi was found to induce interferon in chick embryo cells (Hopps *et al.*, 1964) and a number of other *Rickettsiae* were found to induce interferons in mice (Kazar, 1966; Brezina, Kazar and Schramek, 1968; Hahon and Kozikowska, 1968).

c) Mycoplasmas

The mycoplasmas were reported by several investigators to not induce interferons (Armstrong and Paucker, 1966; Singer, Barile, and Kirschstein, 1969; Smirnova and Kagan, 1971; Yershov and Zhadanov, 1965). However, Rinaldo and his associates (Rinaldo *et al.*, 1973) found that *Acholeplasma laidlawii*, an isolate contaminating fetal lamb kidney cultures, was able to induce interferon in ovine leukocyte cultures. Interferon was not induced by heat-killed mycoplasmas or cell-free filtrates of mycoplasma 1 cultures. A mycoplasma obtained from a plant, *Acholeplasma sp.* Ø G 1, was found to induce interferon in mice (Fauconnier and Wroblowski, 1974). Several animal mycoplasmas were found to induce interferon (up to about 10,000 units/ml serum) in mice, but not in mouse cell cultures (Rinaldo *et al.*, 1974a; Cole *et al.*, 1975). The induction of interferon by the mycoplasmas was apparently not attributable to their contamination with interferon-inducing virus, as at least one mycoplasmal virus isolate failed to induce interferon (Rinaldo *et al.*, 1974b). This should be confirmed with other mycoplasmal virions before this is generalized. These microorganisms were also found to induce interferons in sheep and human lymphocyte cultures (Cole *et al.*, 1976; Rinaldo, 1976).

d) Protozoa

Interferons have been induced by various protozoa in cell cultures and in animals.

Toxoplasma gondii was found to induce a later interferon response in mice, beginning at 8 hours and persisting for about 72 hours (Rytel and Jones, 1966; Freshman *et al.*, 1966). It did not induce interferon in mouse cell cultures.

Mice inoculated with *Trypanosoma cruzi* (Rytel and Marsden, 1970) or *Plasmodium berghei* (Huang, Schultz, and Gordon, 1968) produced interferons. However, interferon was not detected in sera of human beings during acute illness with malaria or with subclinical *T. cruzi* infections (Rytel, Rose and Stewart, 1973).

Interferon was induced in mice by *Besnoitia jellisoni* (Remington and Merigan, 1969) and by *Eperythrozoon coccoides* (Suntharasamai and Rytel, 1973). Another protozoan, *Encephalitozoon cuniculi*, a contaminant of rabbit cell cultures, was found to make these cultures resistant to virus infections and to induce interferon in them (Armstrong *et al.*, 1973).

Thus, with all the microorganisms and their products found to induce interferons, either in animals or in cell cultures or both, it is impossible to identify a common inducing entity. Many of the crude fungal and bacterial products described owe their inducing potencies to contaminating virions, many of which contain double-stranded RNAs. However, many of the inducers are free of nucleic acids.

The likelihood that these stimuli act on different cell types is suggested both by the inability of most of the non-viral inducers to induce in cell cultures and by the different properties of the interferons induced (Section VII. C. 1).

5. Mitogens and Immune Recognition Induction

A number of substances which stimulate lymphocyte blastogenesis and proliferation also induce interferons. These stimuli include both mitogens and immune recognition reactions associated with lymphocyte transformation.

a) Mitogens

Wheelock (1965a) found that phytohemagglutinin, an extract of red kidney beans *Phaseolus vulgaris*, induced interferon production in suspensions of human leukocytes. He attributed this to stimulation of mitotic activity in lymphocytes, as phytohemagglutinin was unable to induce interferon in other cell cultures (Edelman and Wheelock, 1966). Pokeweed mitogen, from *Phytolacca americana*, and another mitogen streptolysin-O were also able to induce interferon in human leukocyte suspensions (Friedman and Cooper, 1967). Antilymphocytic sera (Falcoff, E., *et al.*, 1972a; Falcoff, Oriol, and Iscaki, 1972) and Concanavalin A (Wallen, Dean and Lucas, 1973), as well as the other mitogenic interferon inducers, usually induce interferon before increased DNA synthesis (Falcoff, Oriol, and Iscaki, 1972; Green, Cooperband and Kibrick, 1969; Stobo *et al.*, 1974).

It has been shown that these different mitogens do not all induce the same cell populations, as they induce interferons at different times (Wheelock, 1965a; Richmond, 1969; Epstein, Kreth and Herzenberg, 1974a, b) having different properties (Wietzerbin *et al.*, 1977a, b). Evidence for distinct cellular origins of interferons induced by different mitogens will be discussed (Section VI. B. 1). Generally, these can be classified as those induced by B cell mitogens and T cell mitogens. Several studies have shown that addition of macrophages to mitogen-stimulated lymphocyte cultures increases interferon production significantly (Epstein, Cline and Merigan, 1970, 1971a; Wietzerbin et al., 1977a, b).

b) Immune Recognition Induction

Peritoneal macrophages of animals immune to certain specific inducers were found to produce more interferon than such cells from non-immune animals when exposed to the immunogen (Glasgow, 1966). Green, Cooperband, and Kibrick (1969) reported that lymphocytes from patients sensitized to PPD, diphtheria toxoid or tetanus toxoid produced interferon when exposed to these specific antigens, whereas lymphocytes from non-sensitized patients failed to produce interferons in response to such stimuli.

This immune recognition induction was demonstrated in mice infected with *Mycobacterium tuberculosis* BCG and subsequently inoculated with the mycobacterial antigen PDD (Stinebring and Absher, 1970), often producing several thousand units of interferon per ml of serum (Salvin, Youngner, and Lederer, 1973). The instability properties of such interferons at pH 2 were so markedly different from "classical" interferons that they were termed "Type II" to distinguish them from classical acid-stable, "Type I" interferons (Section VII. A. 3.).

Epstein, Cline, and Merigan (1971a) found that the production of interferon in sensitized lymphocytes by PPD was, like PHA-stimulated interferon in nonsensitized lymphocytes (Epstein, Cline, and Merigan, 1972), enhanced by addition of macrophages. She and her associates have also shown that vaccinia viral antigen stimulated interferon production in sensitized human lymphocytes; again, macrophages significantly augmented interferon production (Epstein, Stevens, and Merigan, 1972). Significantly, there was no correlation between the extent of lymphocyte transformation and interferon production. Macrophage-lymphocyte interaction was also required for optimum interferon production in white cell suspensions from patients with herpes simplex infections induced with herpes virus antigen (Rasmussen et al., 1974). Similar findings were reported by Valle et al. (1975a, b) using human T cell-enriched lymphocyte suspensions, who showed that the "memory" for immune-recognition interferon response was carried by the T cells, not the macrophages. Fujibayashi, Hooks, and Notkins (1975) showed that splenic leukocytes from rabbits immunized with herpes simplex virus could produce interferon when exposed to antigen-antibody complexes of herpes antigen and anti-herpesvirus antibody.

Svet-Moldavsky, and his coworkers (1974) were able to induce interferons in mice by injection of allogeneic spleen cells, whereas syngeneic cells did not induce interferon. These interesting studies also showed that trysinized syngeneic cells acquired ability to induce interferon.

Several of these mitogenic and immune-recognition sets are recognizable as those known to induce various other lymphokines.

c) Induction by Tumor Cells

A recent report has described human interferon induction by human tumor cells mixed with lymphocytes (Trinchieri, Santoli, and Knowles, 1977). It is not yet clear whether this induction results from "tumor" antigens present on the surface of the cells, but the interferon is produced with the same production kinetics as virus-induced interferons (see below). Previously, Svet-Moldavsky and his associates (Svet-Moldavsky, Nemirovskaya, and Osipova, 1974; Svet-Moldavsky *et al.*, 1974) found interferon induction in response to syngeneic tumor cells in mice. Interferon was produced in response to methylcholanthrene-induced sarcoma, spontaneous hemangiopericytoma, Lewis lung adenocarcinoma and leukemia L_{1220} cells, interferon (about 100 units/ml) appearing about 15 to 20 hours after inoculation of the cells.

6. Synthetic Inducers

A great variety of synthetic compounds have been found which are able to induce interferons (Table 3). These range from the high molecular weight double-stranded polyribonucleotides, polyriboinosinic acid·polyribocytidylic acid, to the low molecular weight propanediamine and radioprotective mercaptoalkylamines. It would be romantic to believe that from basic knowledge derived from experiments on different inducer structure-function relationships these synthetic compounds have been produced from specific blueprints for interferon-inducing structures. In fact, quite the opposite has been the case: each of the synthetic inducer classes has been found accidentally or through trial-and-error screenings. Many hypotheses have been proposed for structural requirements for better polynucleotide inducers, and after exhaustive testing of such compounds, the one originally, accidentally, found is still the best inducer. A number of structural features of high molecular weight inducers have been proposed that should enhance interferon inducing potency (DeClercq, 1974); unfortunately, such supposed structure-function requirements have not held up under further experimentation (Thang *et al.*, 1977).

The different classes of synthetic interferon inducers, like the different classes of natural inducers, differ in the populations of cells induced, in the kinetics of appearance of interferons induced, in being able to induce interferon *in vitro* or *in vivo* and in the range of animal species in which they are active. The polyribonucleotides are the most widely active inducers in terms of action *in vivo* and *in vitro* and in range of animal species in which they induce interferon, while the low molecular weight inducers are generally active only *in vivo* and in only certain species.

a) Anionic Polymers

1. Polycarboxylates, Sulfates and Phosphates

Early attempts to correlate interferon inducing activity with structure of the inducer were unsuccessful. Kleinschmidt and Ellis (1967), acting on the assumption that statolon owed its interferon-inducing activity to its polyanionic nature, investigated synthetic polyanions as inducers, without success. Others,

Table 3. *Synthetic inducers of interferons*

Inducer	in vivo	in vitro	References
A. Anionic polymers			
1. Polycarboxylates			
– Pyran (maleic anhydride divinyl ether)	+		Regelson (1967)
– Polyacrylic acid	+		Merigan and Finkelstein (1968)
– Polymethacrylic acid	+		Desomer, Billiau, and Declercq (1968)
– Polyacetal carboxylic acid (chlorite-oxidized oxymylose; COAM)	+		Claes et al. (1970)
– Polyacrylic acid-poly-allylsucrose (carbopol)	+		Declercq and Luczak (1977)
2. Polysulfates			
– Polyvinylsulfate	+		Came et al. (1969)
3. Polyphosphates			
– Dextran-Phosphate	+		Suzuki, Suzuki, and Imaya (1971)
B. Polynucleotides			
1. Polyribonucleotides			
– Homopolymers e. g., single-stranded	+	+	Baron et al. (1969)
poly rI	+	+	Thang et al. (1977)
– Homopolymer pairs e. g., poly rI·poly rC	+	+	Field et al. (1967 a)
poly rA·poly rU	+	+	Vilcek et al. (1968)
– Alternating Copolymers e. g., poly rI-rC·poly rA-rU	+	+	Colby and Chamberlin (1969)
– Homopolymer·Copolymer e. g., poly rI·poly rC-rG	+	+	Matsuda et al. (1971)
2. Polydeoxyribonucleotides			
– Homopolymer pairs e. g., poly dA·poly dT		+	Vilcek et al. (1968)
3. Polyribonucleotide Analogues			
– Thiophosphate for phosphate e. g., poly sI·poly sC	+	+	Black et al. (1972)
– Halogen for 2'-hydroxyl e. g., poly rA·poly 2'-FU		+	Declercq and Janik (1973)
– Vinyl for sugar-phosphate e. g., poly rI·poly vinyl C		+	Pitha and Pitha (1971)
4. Polyribonucleotide Pair·Aggregates			
– poly rI·poly rC+ DEAE-Dextran	+	+	Dianzani et al. (1968)
– poly rI·poly rC·poly·L·Lysine	+	+	Levy et al. (1974)

Table 3 (continued)

Inducer	in vivo	in vitro	References
C. Low molecular weight inducers			
1. Tilorone			
Bis-diethylaminoethyl-fluorenone	+		Krueger and Mayer (1970)
		+	Degre and Glaz (1977)
2. Cationic Dyes			
Acridine	+		Diederich, Lodemann, and Wacker (1972)
Quinacrine	+		Glaz et al. (1973)
3. Propanediamine			
N, N-dioctadecyl-N', N'-bis (2-hydroxyethyl) propanediamine	+		Hoffmann et al. (1973)
4. BL-20803 4(3-dimethylaminopropyl-amino)-1, 3-dimethyl-1H-pyrazolo- 3, 4–5 quinoline dihydrochloride	+		Siminoff et al. (1973)
5. MA-56 Bis-ω-piperidinylacetyl-dibenzofuran hydrochloride	+		Soehner, Gambardella, and Hou (1974)
6. AET 5,2-aminoethyl-isothiouronium	+	+	Lvovsky et al. (1977)
7. U-25, 166 2-amino-5-bromo-6-methyl-4-pyrimidinol	+		Nichols, Weed, and Underwood (1976)

however, working under the same presumption, were able to induce interferon in animals and in man with the polyanionic complex maleic anhydride-divinyl ether copolymer, Pyran (Regelson, 1967; Merigan, 1967a; Merigan and Regelson, 1967). Other such copolymers of maleic anhydride (Merigan, 1967a; Declercq and Merigan, 1969b), polyacrylic acids and polymethacrylic acids (Merigan and Finkelstein, 1968; Desomer, Billiau and Declercq, 1968), and a variety of chlorite-oxidized polysaccharides, such as chlorite-oxidized oxyamylose, COAM (Claes et al., 1970) induced interferons in mice after intravenous or intraperitoneal injections.

The interferon-inducing capacity of polycarboxylates correlates with increasing molecular weight (Declercq, 1971; Niblack and McCreary, 1971; Mohr, Brown and Coffey, 1972). Another structural feature required for interferon induction by polycarboxylates is apparent from a two-dimensional representation of its structure (Fig. 4): the regular and dense distribution of negative charges. This requisite for induction is confirmed by the inactivity of uncharged polymers such as dextrans, polyacrylamide and other charge-deficient polymers (Desomer, Billiau, and Declercq, 1968; Merigan and Finekstein,

1968; Claes *et al.*, 1970; Remington and Merigan, 1970). There is also a distinct correlation between toxicity of the polycarboxylates and their interferon-inducing ability which seems in turn to relate to their structural stability (Merigan and Regelson, 1967; Billiau, Desmyter, and Desomer, 1970). Carbopol, a polymer of acrylic acid cross-linked with allylsucrose was recently also reported to be an interferon-inducer, albeit weakly so (Declercq and Luczak, 1977).

Polyvinyl sulfate (Came *et al.*, 1969) and dextran phosphate (Suzuki, Suzuki, and Imaya, 1971; Suzuki *et al.*, 1972, 1975) were also found to induce interferon in mice, presumably for the same structure-function arguments put forth for the polycarboxylates.

2. *Polynucleotides*

As it was known that double-stranded polyribonucleotides were adjuvants for production of antibodies, it seemed reasonable to test these polymeric complexes for their abilities to augment interferon induction. In fact, it was found that the double-stranded polyribonucleotide complex of polyriboinosinic acid·polyribocytidylic acid (poly rI· poly rC) was itself an efficient interferon inducer in rabbits, in microgram amounts (Field *et al.*, 1967a). Poly rI·poly rC also induced interferon in cell cultures, as did polyribouridylic acid·polyriboadenylic acid, though the latter was less effective. Single-stranded homopolyribonucleotides apparently were ineffective (Field *et al.*, 1968). In the decade since this initial discovery of poly rI·poly rC as an interferon inducer, a vast literature has accumulated testifying to the exhaustive efforts to find a better double-stranded RNA inducer in terms of ability to induce as much interferon with less toxicity or more interferon for the same amount of toxicity. These extensive and expensive searches for inducers with improved therapeutic indexes have been entirely fruitless (for extensive listings see Colby, 1971; Declercq, 1974; Pitha and Hutchinson, 1977, Declercq and Torrence, 1977). In a number of articles a number of supposed structural requirements for interferon induction by synthetic polyribonucleotides are put forth (Colby *et al.*, 1971; Colby and Morgan, 1971; Colby, 1971; Declercq and Merigan, 1969c; Colby and Chamberlin, 1969; Johnston *et al.*, 1975; Bobst *et al.*, 1976; Carter and Pitha, 1971; Carter *et al.*, 1972; Hutchinson, Johnston and Eaton, 1974; Kleinschmidt, 1972). In the following discussion, I shall present each of these criteria and present evidence supporting or contradicting them. Such evaluations emphasize that even with the enormous amount of resources put into this research area, we still have no better double-stranded polynucleotide-type inducer than the first one tested. Not only that, we now know less about the structural requirements of these inducers than we "knew" before (Declercq, Wells, and Merigan, 1970; Declercq and Merigan, 1971c; Declercq *et al.*, 1971).

The following apparent structural requirements have been propounded for interferon-inducing activity of polynucleotides:

i) *High Molecular Weight.* Reduction of the molecular weight of poly rI·poly rC by sonication resulted in loss of activity (Lampson *et al.*, 1970).

However, others reported just the opposite effect of sonic disruption (Shiokawa and Yaoi, 1972). Some workers have found that the activity of poly rI·poly rC depends more upon the size of poly rI than poly rC (Tytell et al., 1968; Mohr et al., 1972; Carter et al., 1972; Declercq, Stewart II, and Desomer, 1973b; Stewart II and Declercq, 1974). Others have, however, suggested that both polynucleotides are equal in size-function effect (Wacker et al., 1969; Niblack and McCreary, 1971; Morahan et al., 1972; Arimura, 1975). These data can be interpreted that there is a size-range from about 5 S to about 10 S within which the polynucleotides are optimally active, losing activity on each side of this size-range (Declercq, 1974; Pitha and Hutchinson, 1977). Similar results have been reported for complexes of poly rG and poly rC, with the size of the poly rG being more crucial for activity (Timowsky et al., 1973; Vilner et al., 1974, 1976).

ii) 2'-Hydroxyl Group. The presence of ribose is apparently essential for interferon induction by synthetic polynucleotides. Several studies reported that deoxyribose-containing polynucleotides were inactive (Vilček et al., 1968; Colby and Chamberlin, 1969; Hutchinson, Johnston, and Eaton, 1974). Also numerous substitution at the C-2' position caused loss of activities (Black et al., 1972; Declercq, Zmudska, and Shugar, 1972; Declercq and Janik, 1973; Declercq, Rothman, and Shugar, 1974; Torrence et al., 1973a; Merigan and Rothman, 1974; Tso et al., 1976). Many of these modifications might be expected to increase the interferon inducing activity of the polymers, as they resulted in increased resistance to degradation by pancreatic ribonuclease (Declercq, 1974). Most of the polynucleotides with C-2' substitutions also fulfilled the structural requirements for inducers in size and thermal stability. Thus, loss of the 2'-OH was apparently directly responsible for activity losses.

It was reported that with partial substitutions of 2'-hydroxyl groups with 2'-O-methyl groups, polynucleotide complexes formed which were still active, and the 2'-O-methylation in poly rI strands was less detrimental on activity than insertions of these groups into the poly rC strands (Merigan and Rothman, 1974; Tso et al., 1976). Replacements of ribosyl residues by deoxyribosyl residues in either the purine strand or the pyrimidine strand eliminated interferon-inducing activity (Pitha and Pitha, 1974).

It was also reported that substitutions in the 2'-hydroxyl group that resulted in loss of interferon-inducing activity also resulted in loss of reactivity with anti-double-stranded RNA-antibodies (Johnston et al., 1975).

iii) Nucleolytic Resistance. The resistance of polynucleotide complexes to nucleolytic degradation has been associated in many studies with their interferon-inducing capabilities. Certain polynucleotides with thiophosphate substituions of the phosphate group were more resistant to nuclease activity and were more efficient inducers (Declercq, Eckstein and Merigan, 1969; Declercq et al., 1969, 1970).

Addition of the polycation DEAE-dextran increased the stability of double-stranded RNA to ribonuclease degradation and increased its interferon inducing activity in numerous systems (Dianzani et al., 1968; Dianzani, Gagnoni, and Cantagalli, 1970; Tilles, 1970; Billiau et al., 1970; Stewart II and Lockart, 1970; Pitha and Carter, 1971a; Richmond, 1971; Dianzani, Baron,

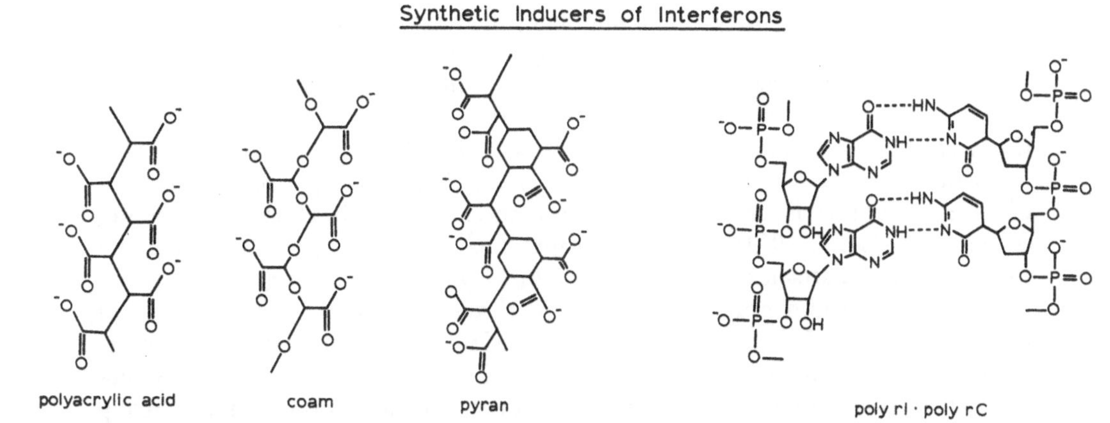

Synthetic Inducers of Interferons

polyacrylic acid   coam   pyran   poly rI · poly rC

tilorone

acridine   quinacrine   BL-20803   BL-3849A

U-25166   propanediamine   AET

Fig. 4. Structural features of synthetic interferon inducers

and Buckler, 1971; Mecs and Rosztoczy, 1971; Rosztoczy, 1971; Vilček, Barmak, and Havell, 1972; Wacker et al., 1972). In many of the in vitro systems, the requirement for the DEAE-dextran is absolute: in mouse cell cultures no interferon is induced by poly rI·poly rC alone, at any concentration, but high levels of interferon are induced by poly rI·poly rC in the presence of DEAE-dextran (Rosztoczy, 1971; Stewart II, Gosser, and Lockart, 1971a).

Polylysine has also been reported to facilitate interferon induction by polyribonucleotide complexes. Poly-D-lysine was originally used (Rice et al., 1970, 1971), but later studies have used poly-L-lysine, as the former polymer formed precipitates with poly rI·poly rC (Levy et al., 1974). The complex of poly rI·poly rC·poly-L-lysine prepared in a solution of carboxymethyl cellulose is referred to as poly ICLC. Poly ICLC also exhibited increased ribonuclease resistance. In this regard it should be noted that poly rI·poly rC alone has been found to induce disappointingly low levels of interferons in primates, including man (DeVita et al., 1970; Young, 1971; Hill et al., 1972).

Serum from certain animals, including man, have been reported to contain high levels of double-stranded ribonucleases (Nordlund, Wolff, and Levy, 1970). Poly ICLC has, however, been shown to be a more efficient inducer of interferons than poly rI·poly rC in animals (Olsen *et al.*, 1976) and in primates (Levy *et al.*, 1974, 1975, 1976; Stephen *et al.*, 1977; Sammons *et al.*, 1977).

It has also been shown that poly rI·poly rC enclosed in phospholipid particles is a better interferon inducer *in vivo* than is naked poly rI·poly rC (Straub, Garry, and Magee, 1974), possibly because such liposomes protect the inducer from nucleolytic attack (Magee *et al.*, 1976; Mayhew *et al.*, 1977).

However, certain poly rI·poly rC complexes have been modified in ways that have decreased their resistance to nucleases without decreasing their interferon-inducing activities (Carter *et al.*, 1972; Tso *et al.*, 1976). Also, polynucleotides whose 2'-OH groups were substituted with a methyl or azido group or halogen were more resistant to nuclease but were not active (Black *et al.*, 1972; Declercq and Janik, 1973; Torrence *et al.*, 1973a, b).

iv) Ordered Secondary Structure. The presence of a stable, highly-ordered base-paired structure, i. e., double-stranded, is usually found to be essential for polyribonucleotides to induce interferons (Merigan, 1970; Colby, 1971; Declercq, 1974; Pitha and Hutchinson, 1977). The stability of polynucleotide base-pairings can be measured from the temperature at which 50% of double-stranded structure is dissociated into the single-stranded structures (Tm). The polyribonucleotide complexes having Tm higher than 60° C have usually been found to have higher interferon-inducing activity than those with lower Tm values (Declercq and Merigan, 1970a; Morahan *et al.*, 1972).

Other experiments have suggested that while both component strands are necessary for interferon induction, secondary structure of the complex was not critical (Carter *et al.*, 1972; Pitha and Carter, 1971b). Poly rI·poly rC complexes with strand interruptions in poly rI strands were less effective inducers than complexes with strand interruptions in poly rC, but the differences were not correlated with Tm value changes (Pitha and Pitha, 1973), nor was it correlated with sensitivities to nuclease hydrolysis.

These studies have thus condensed the structural "requirements" of polynucleotides for interferon induction to: 1. Presence of 2'-hydroxyl group; 2. High molecular weight; 3. Nucleolytic resistance; 4. Double-strandedness. Unfortunately these criteria have such flagrant violators to these rules that chaos begins to erode the prettiness of the picture painted by ten years of interferon inducer-structure dogma. For example:

i. Certain polynucleotide complexes have been prepared which fulfill *all* of the previously "recognized requirements" for being effective interferon inducers (high molecular weight, double-strandedness, high Tm, adequate resistance to nuclease and presence of 2'-OH groups), but such complexes were, inexplicably, completely inactive (Torrence *et al.*, 1975).

ii. Certain polynucleotides which clearly do not fulfill these "requirements" are effective inducers. The clearest example of such an inducing polynucleotide was recently reported by Thang *et al.* (1977), who found that certain preparations of single-stranded poly rI were efficient interferon inducers both *in vivo* and *in vitro*. No satisfactory rationalization for this has been offered, but this report certainly gives credence to the several earlier reports of interferon induction by single-stranded RNAs, both synthetic (Baron *et al.*, 1969; Pitha and Pitha, 1974; Billiau *et al.*, 1969) and single-stranded, non-replicating viruses (Dianzani *et al.*, 1970; Gandhi, Burke, and Scholtissek, 1970; Meager and Burke, 1972; Dianzani, Pugliese, and Baron, 1974, 1975).

b) Low Molecular Weight Inducers

1. Tilorone

A number of small synthetic molecules have been discovered to induce interferon (Fig. 4). The first of these, identified by Krueger and Mayer (1970), was bis-diethylaminoethylfluorenone, an orange, water-soluble compound (molecular weight of 412) known as tilorone hydrochloride. This compound, given orally, intraperitoneally or subcutaneously to mice, induced high levels of circulating interferon between 12 and 48 hours (Mayer and Krueger, 1970; Krueger *et al.*, 1971; Declercq and Merigan, 1971a). Several analogues of this structure have also been reported to be active (Meindl, Bodo, and Huppy, 1976). In most studies, tilorone did not induce interferon in cell cultures (Declercq and Merigan, 1971a; Stringfellow and Glasgow, 1972b), but did so in human leukocyte suspensions (Dennis *et al.*, 1972), though Degre and Glaz (1977) have recently reported tilorone to induce interferon in human fibroblast cultures. Tilorone has been found to be toxic in doses near those required for interferon induction in mice (Glaz and Talas, 1973; Gibson *et al.*, 1976). Unfortunately, tilorone is a poor inducer in man (Kaufman *et al.*, 1971).

2. Cationic Dyes

Several basic dyes were found to induce interferon in mice following intraperitoneal injection (Diederich, Lodemann, and Wacker, 1972). Toluidine blue, methylene blue, trypaflavine and acridine orange were each active *in vivo* but not *in vitro* (Diederich, Lodemann, and Wacker, 1973). Acridine was more active than the structurally similar quinacrine (Glaz *et al.*, 1973; Glaz and Talas, 1975).

3. Propanediamine

N, N-d-octadecyl-N', N'- bis (2-hydroxyethyl) propanediamine was found to induce interferon in mice (Hoffman *et al.*, 1973) when inoculated intraperitoneally, and in man it induced nasal interferon when applied topically in nose drops (Gatmaitan, Stanley, and Jackson, 1973; Panusarn *et al.*, 1974) but not in cats, dogs, pigs, monkeys or rabbits. Its apparent high therapeutic index has raised hopes for its clinical application (Douglas and Betts, 1974; Stanley *et al.*, 1976).

4. BL-20803

4 (3-dimethylaminopropylamino) − 1, 3-dimethyl-1 H-pyrazolo [3, 4-b] quinoline dihydrochloride induced interferon in mice, either parenterally or

orally (Siminoff *et al.*, 1973). It was not active in cell cultures (Siminoff, 1975, 1976). A variety of analogues of BL-20803 have also been found to induce interferon in mice and in mouse spleen leukocytes (Siminoff and Crenshaw, 1977; Crenshaw, Luke, and Siminoff, 1976). One of these, a 7-methyl derivative called BL-3849 A, induces high levels of interferon in mice (Kern *et al.*, 1976).

5. MA-56

Bis-ω-piperidinylacetyl-dibenzofuran·HCl was reported to induce low levels of interferon in mice when administered orally (Soehner, Gambardella and Hou, 1974).

6. AET

5, 2-aminoethylisothiouronium, a radioprotective mercaptoalkylamine, and several related compounds, have recently been found to induce interferons in mice and in both mouse and human non-lymphoid cell cultures (Khaitovich and Lvovsky, 1975; Lvovsky *et al.*, 1977). Thus these compounds become the first low molecular weight synthetic inducers that are active both *in vivo* and *in vitro*. Studies are underway to determine the effectiveness of these inducers in primates.

7. U-25, 166

A substituted pyrimidine, 2-amino-5-bromo-6-methyl-4-pyrimidinol was found to induce high levels of interferon in cats, mice and rats when administered orally or parenterally (Nichol, Weed, and Underwood, 1976). Though inactive in fibroblast cultures, it was active in mouse thymus and spleen organ cultures, whereas tilorone was not (Stringfellow, 1977a; Stringfellow and Weed, 1977). U-25, 166 is relatively non-toxic for cats at doses inducing high levels of interferon and was effective when administered orally as a suspension or in capsules. No reports have appeared of its effectiveness in primates.

Thus the search goes on for a better interferon inducer, having shifted from inducing viruses to ten years of seemingly endless explorations of polynucleotide modifications, to the synthetic low molecular weight inducers. Early evidence suggests that these small molecules will fall into several distinct classes of inducers, dependent on which cell populations are effected. Possibly within each of these classes structural requirements will be recognized as have been proposed for the polynucleotides, and perhaps subsequent reviews will deal with these. Clearly, when confronted with the diversity of natural and synthetic inducers of interferons listed in Tables 1, 2 and 3, it is difficult to rationalize a single inducer structure.

C. Interferon (?) Inducers

An aspect of interferon inducers that has received very little attention in interferon literature is that many *interferon* inducers (as they are called by interferonologists) are called other types of inducers by immunologists and assorted cell biologists. Indeed, as I hope to emphasize in Fig. 5, these same substances have been reported to induce a variety of substances ("lymphokines") which exert a variety of effects on cells. Many of these other factors are present in interferon preparations (or from another point of view, interferons are present in preparations of many of these factors). This realization must be kept in mind when attributing various activities to the interferons in such broths (Section X). Also, it should be of interest to determine the ability of each of the various classes of inducers for their abilities to induce several of these other lymphokines. Perhaps the inducing abilities of certain of these compounds is less specific for interferon than has been supposed.

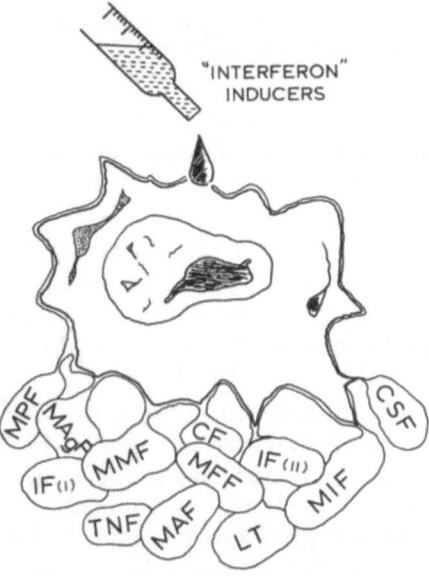

Fig. 5. Inducers of Interferons and other lymphokines

When cells are exposed to various substances that have often been thought of as interferon inducers, they usually produce a number of other lymphokines which can be assayed by a wide variety of methods, and usually derive their names from the activity measured: TNF, tumor necrosis factor; MAF, macrophage activation factor; LT, lymphotoxin; MIF, migration inhibitory factor; IF(I), interferon-type I; IF(II), interferon-type II; CSF, colony-stimulating factor; MFF, macrophage fusion factor; MMF, macrophage mitogenic factor; MAgF, macrophage aggregation factor; to name only a few. The evidence separating these is often conflicting; some may be identical, but measured for different effects. Many are in some crude "interferon" preparations and some are in many crude preparations: Hoffmann et al. (1976); Klimpel et al. (1975; 1977); Block et al. (1977); Lai, Alpers, and Mackay-Scollay (1977); O'Reilly et al. (1977); Trudgett (1976); Havredaki and McNeill (1975); Imanishi (1975); Salvin et al. (1975a, b); Archer and Young (1974); Goguel and Nauciel (1974); Salvin, Nishio, and Shonnard (1974); McNeill (1973); McNeill and Gresser (1973); Salvin, Youngner and Lederer (1973); Youngner and Salvin (1973); Haber, Rosenau, and Goldberg (1972)

D. Uninduced (Spontaneous) Interferons

The following examples of interferon production are perhaps attributable to *unrecognized* inducers.

A number of instances of spontaneous production of interferon in apparently uninduced cultures have been reported. Clearly, in view of all the possible types of inducers it seems likely that some cells might inadvertantly be induced, especially during preparation of cultures of lymphoid cells, as such cells can be stimulated by so many of the different classes of inducers. On the other hand, some constitutive production of interferons might represent apparently defective regulation mechanisms.

Henle and Henle (1965) found that Burkitt's lymphoma cell cultures spontaneously produced interferon, and interpreted this as evidence for persistent viral infection of these cells. However, several others reported that leukocytes from peripheral blood and bone marrow cells obtained from healthy individuals can produce interferons without apparent stimulus (Deinhardt and Burnside, 1967; Northrup and Deinhardt, 1967; Hasse et al., 1970; Minnefor et al., 1970).

Smith and Wagner (1967a) found that cultures of rabbit leukocytes (macrophages) produced interferon in the absence of known viral infection. Uninfected polymorphonuclear leukocytes, rabbit kidney or spleen cells did not produce interferon under similar culture conditions. Yields of interferon from uninfected macrophages were about 1 percent or less of yields from virus-induced macrophages. Protein synthesis inhibitors and actinomycin D treatment inhibited production of the spontaneous interferon. Interestingly, the spontaneously produced interferon was less stable to acid or heat than the virus-induced interferon (Smith and Wagner, 1967b).

Uninduced interferon production has been reported from hamster peritoneal exudates (Talas, Weiszfeiler, and Batkai, 1968; Talas, 1969; Talas, Szolgay, and Rozsa, 1972). A spontaneous production of interferon by mouse peritoneal macrophages was attributed to contamination with endotoxin or bacteria, as no interferon was produced by similar cells obtained from germ-free mice (DeMaeyer, Fauve and DeMayer-Guignard, 1971). Similar findings with conventional and germ-free mouse peritoneal macrophages were reported by Ito et al. (1976a).

Spontaneous interferon production was also found in cultures of bone marrow cells of patients with multiple myeloma (Epstein and Salmon, 1974), but none was found in cultures from normal individuals. Archer and Young (1974) reported that Burkitt's lymphoma-derived cell lines spontaneously produced both interferon and macrophage migration inhibitory factor. Lidin and Adams (1975), and Adams et al. (1975) found that some lines of EB virus-carrying lymphoid cells produced interferon while others did not. Recently, Tovey et al. (1977b), in agreement with the findings of Haase et al. (1970), found no correlation between expression of EB virus early antigen and spontaneous interferon production by human lymphoblastoid cells. When these cells were induced with 5-bromodeoxyuridine, spontaneous interferon production was markedly enhanced (Tovey et al., 1977b). Also, it was reported that 5-iododeoxyuridine potentiated production of interferon in these cells when induced by measles virus (Volckaert-Vervliet and Billiau, 1977).

Spontaneous producers of interferon which could represent regulatory mutants in the interferon system would offer tools for probing the regulation of interferon production. One candidate for such a mutation has been reported which is apparently a virus-resistant cell line because of this regulation defect (Morgan, Colby, and Hulse, 1973; Jarvis and Colby, 1978).

It seems possible that certain cells, perhaps all cells, constitutively produce low levels of interferon, some producing enough to be detectable. The maintenance-role of this endogenous interferon in the interferon induction mechanism has recently been suggested (DeMayer-Guignard, Thang, and DeMayer, 1977; Thang, DeMayer-Guignard, and DeMayer, 1977), as will be discussed in detail elsewhere (Section IV. C. 3.).

IV. Induction Mechanisms

The diversity of agents able to stimulate the synthesis of interferons defies all attempts to recognize common inducer structure. Indeed, the finding of several distinct classes of interferon inducing substances suggests there might be several different interferon induction mechanisms. The following discussions will review the data showing that all interferon appearing after stimulation by each of the inducers are synthesized *de novo* and that different inducers can induce interferons in different cell populations. I shall evaluate the data for or against the unifying hypothesis that all viruses, RNA or DNA-containing, trigger interferon production by forming "the inducing structure" double-stranded RNA, and shall describe alternative induction mechanisms that have been proposed.

A. The Interferon Induction-Production Curve

The interaction of any of the inducers (viral or non-viral, natural or synthetic) with any of the sensitive cell systems (either *in vivo* or *in vitro*) results in an induction-production curve similar to that illustrated in Fig. 6, though the kinetics of each of the phases can vary in different cellinducer combinations. After addition of the inducing substance there is always a period of time when no interferon is detectable. This period, which is designated the *Interferon Induction Phase*, is usually from about 1 to 8 hours long. In the system illustrated (mouse L-cells induced with either Newcastle disease virus or poly rI·poly rC) this period usually lasts about 6 or 8 hours (Lancz and Johnson, 1969; Stewart II, Gosser, and Lockart, 1971a, b; Youngner and Hallum, 1969). The induction phase is followed by a first appearance of interferon and its rapid rise within an hour or so to its maximum level. Production is normally maintained at this level for only a few hours, then rapidly declines to undetectable levels. The time from onset of interferon synthesis (the end of the Induction phase) to termination of its synthesis will be referred to as the *Interferon Production Phase;* the events occurring in this phase will be described in Section VI.

Clearly, distinct events occur in each of these phases between the initial interaction of the inducer with the cells and the onset and termination of interferon production. It is only when these components are analyzed independently that they reveal several important aspects of the mechanisms involved in the regulation of interferon synthesis.

1. The Induction Phase

The first event leading to appearance of interferon in an animal or a cell culture is the interaction of the interferon inducer with a cell sensitive to it. This interaction can, at least in some cases, lead to uptake of the inducer and its processing within the cell to "trigger" the derepression of genetic information coding for interferon production. Therefore, the induction phase incorporates all the events from interaction of the inducer and cell to beginning of transcription of the cellular genetic information for interferon. Thus, at any time during the induction phase the interferon response to the inducer can be aborted by inhibitors of DNA-dependent RNA synthesis.

On the other hand, the production phase incorporates transcription of interferon messenger RNA, its translation and posttranslational modification processes and its transport out of the cell. During this period, interferon synthesis can be averted by inhibitors of protein synthesis.

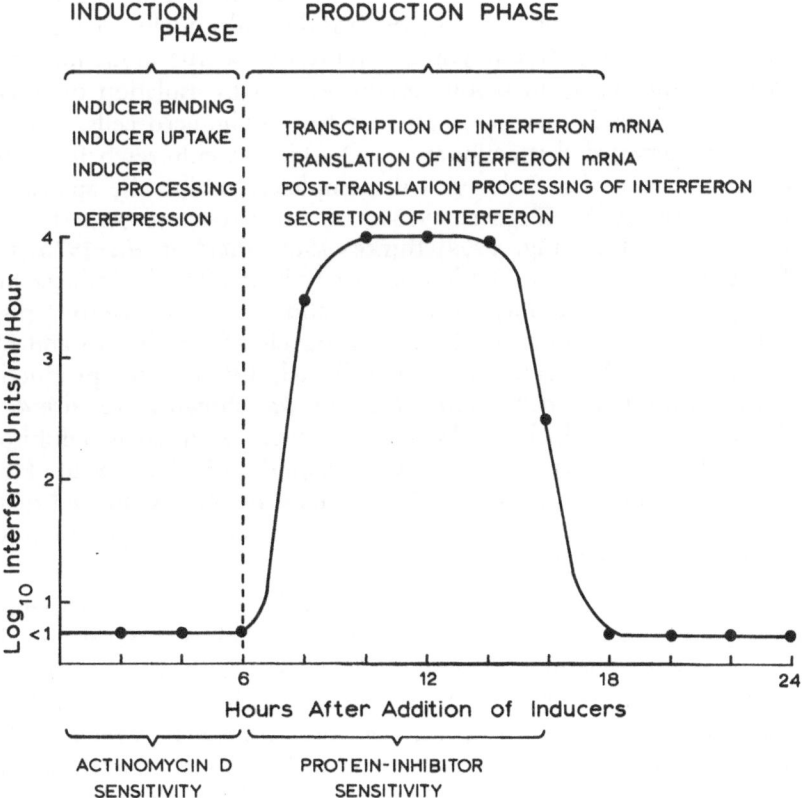

Fig. 6. The Interferon Induction-Production curve. The system diagrammed is typical for mouse L929 cells induced with Newcastle disease virus (Stewart II, Gosser, and Lockart, 1971a)

a) True Induction?

Nearly every type of cell tested, either *in vivo* or *in vitro,* primary cultures or established cell lines, has been found to be able to produce interferon in response to some types of inducers. The exceptions are so rare that they are usually referred to as "VERO-like", to identify with the monkey cell line first characterized by Desmyter, Rawls and Melnick (1968) as apparently being defective in ability to produce interferon (Cantell and Paucker, 1963b; Schafer and Lockart, 1970; Stewart II, Scott, and Sulkin, 1969; Stewart, Lutkus, and Sulkin, 1970; Morgan, 1967a, b; Blach-Olszenska and Cembrzynska-Nowak, 1977). In nearly all these interferon-competent cells the interferon potential is latent; that is, not expressed (the few exceptions of "spontaneous" interferon production were discussed previously; Section III. D.), and it is therefore assumed that interferon production is regulated by a repressor mechanism and that interferon induction represents a derepression mechanism (Burke, 1965; Vilček, 1969). Alternatively, induction could result from the cell producing a derepressor in response to the inducer, or production could result from inactivation of a cell mechanism responsible for destroying interferon or its message, thus not representing a true induction mechanism at all, but rather a *production* regulation. It has become evident that *both* induction and production regulations of interferon exist (Havell, 1977; Pitha and Hutchinson, 1977).

The evidence that interferon synthesis represents a true induction has been provided by studies using metabolic inhibitors and by isolation of interferon messenger RNA from induced cells but not from uninduced cells. It has been repeatedly demonstrated that actinomycin D added to cultures before addition of either viral or non-viral inducers will completely inhibit the appearance of interferon (Heller, 1963; Wagner, 1963a, b; Anderson and Atherton, 1964; Ho, 1964b; Ho and Breinig, 1965; Burke, 1965; Field *et al.,* 1970; Colby, 1971). Similarly, actinomycin D addition at any time after the inducer but before first appearance of interferon also aborts the interferon response (Stewart II, Gosser, and Lockart, 1971a, b; Havell, 1977; Gifford and Heller, 1963; Wagner, 1964; Walters, Burke, and Skehel, 1967). Also, production of interferon from the induced interferon message was shown to require *de novo* synthesis of protein, which could be prevented with such inhibitors as puromycin, fluorophenylalanine or cycloheximide (Burke, 1965; Ho and Breinig, 1965; Wagner and Huang, 1965). Some experiments showed that production of interferon in animals also required newly expressed genetic information (Ho and Kono, 1965).

The ability of cells to express new genetic information was also shown to be necessary, as ultraviolet irradiated cells lost their interferon producing capacity if irradiated before induction (DeMaeyer-Guignard and DeMayer, 1965b; Burke and Morrison, 1965; Cogniaux-LeClerc, Levy and Wagner, 1966). Recently it has also been shown that the cell nucleus is required for interferon production, as enucleated cells were unable to make interferon (Burke and Veomett, 1977), and specific chromosomes have been shown to be responsible for interferon production (Cassingena *et al.,* 1971; Tan, Creagan, and Ruddle, 1974a, b; see Section V).

This evidence suggests that, at least in some inducer-cell combinations, the appearance of interferon represents true induction.

b) Preformed Interferons?

Early reports on induction of interferons *in vivo* or in leukocyte suspensions by several of the non-viral inducers (e. g., endotoxins, etc.) showed that many of these substances lead to appearance of interferons much more rapidly than do viruses (Youngner and Stinebring, 1964; Ho, 1964 a). This, combined with apparently different cellular origins of the interferons appearing in response to some of the different inducers (i. e., endotoxins not being active in cultured cells), suggested that different induction mechanisms were involved for induction of interferons by the non-viral inducers. Ho and Kono (1965) and Youngner, Stinebring and Taube (1965) found that the appearance of interferon in mice and rabbits injected with endotoxin was not inhibited by a dose of actinomycin D that inhibited liver RNA synthesis by more than 95 percent; also, cycloheximide at protein inhibitory levels was unable to prevent interferon appearance induced with endotoxin, but did inhibit appearance of interferon induced by virus (or *Brucella abortus*) (Ke *et al.*, 1966; Youngner, Stinebring, and Taube, 1965). These authors thus concluded that the endotoxin-in-interferon response was merely a release of a "preformed" interferon, whereas virus-induced interferon (and *Brucella*-induced) was newly synthesized, thereby requiring longer to appear and being sensitive to inhibitors (Youngner, Stinebring, and Taube, 1965).

Numerous supporting papers subsequently appeared on "preformed" interferons, but the picture soon became obscure. It was found that statolon-induced interferon was not inhibited in mice by cycloheximide (Youngner and Stinebring, 1966), at least not circulating interferon. However, spleen levels of interferon induced by statolon were inhibited by this treatment (Merigan, 1967 b). Actinomycin D inhibited interferon synthesis in rabbits injected with virus, but did not inhibit interferon response to endotoxin (Ho and Kono, 1965).

It has been hypothesized that endotoxins caused release of interferon from cells containing it by damaging them so that they "leak" interferon (Vilček, 1969). In this regard Sauter and Gifford (1966) had found release of both interferon and lysosomal enzymes in mice injected with endotoxin. It was often concluded that endotoxins were not "true" inducers (Vilček, 1969).

It was then also observed that appearance of interferon in rabbits injected with poly rI·poly rC was also resistant to inhibition by cycloheximide, and it was concluded that synthetic double-stranded RNA stimulated release of "preformed" interferon (Youngner and Hallum, 1968). To the contrary, induction of interferon in cultured cells by poly rI·poly rC was inhibited by actinomycin D (Field *et al.*, 1968; Vilček *et al.*, 1968).

It was, however, observed that the poly rI·poly rC-induced interferon appeared in human fibroblast cultures more rapidly than did virus-induced interferon in the same cultures and the response to the former inducer was less sensitive to metabolic inhibitors than the latter (Finkelstein, Bausek, and Merigan,

1968; Bausek and Merigan, 1970a, b). This correlation between time of interferon synthesis (length of induction phase) and sensitivity to metabolic inhibitors is frequent, and will be discussed below (Tan et al., 1970; Stewart II,
Gosser, and Lockart, 1971b).

The appearance of interferon in peritoneal macrophage or spleen cell cultures inoculated with endotoxin was sensitive to inhibition by actinomycin D
or puromycin (Kobayashi, Yasin, and Masuzumi, 1969; Smith and Wagner,
1967a, b; Smith et al., 1973). Studies using slices of tissues from animals injected with poly rI·poly rC showed that the interferon response to this inducer
was inhibited by actinomycin D (Ho and Ke, 1970).

Similar studies revealed that while the induction of interferon in rabbits by
endotoxin was somewhat more resistant to inhibitors than was virus-induced
interferon, it was inhibited by higher levels (Ho, Ke, and Armstrong, 1973).
Thus, it now appears that all the inducers are "true" inducers, that none cause
release of "preformed" interferon, and reports claiming "release of previously
cleared interferon" by inducers should be disregarded (Chester, Declercq, and
Merigan, 1972). Though not all inducer classes have been tested, it now seems
likely that all interferon is produced *de novo*.

2. *The Interaction of Inducer and Cell*

The initial interaction of inducers with cells would appear to be different
for each inducer class, and it is not possible to look for a common "trigger" at
this stage of the induction process. The initial interaction of viruses with cells
is apparently insufficient to stimulate the derepression event; rather, some ev-
ent(s) subsequent to adsorption, penetration and uncoating is usually required
(Burke, 1973; Lockart et al., 1968). Also, interferon can be induced with infectious viral RNA, so it is not the adsorption, penetration or uncoating processes *per se* that "trigger" interferon (Stewart II, Gosser, and Lockart, 1971a).

On the other hand, the trigger for interferon induction by the mitogens,
immune recognition reactions, or endotoxins might result from direct cell surface alterations. It should be possible to test this by using mitogens immobilized on agarose beads as inducers.

The initial interaction of polynucleotides with cells has been repeatedly
studied, and so far it is still not known whether these substances induce interferon from the cell surface or from inside the cells. Poly rI·poly rC was found
to adsorb rapidly to cells but biological activity induction did not correlate
with the rapid binding (Black et al., 1972; Declercq, Wells, and Mergan, 1972;
Field et al., 1972a; Kelly and Levy, 1973; Pitha and Pitha, 1973; Pitha, Marshall, and Carter, 1972). It was postulated by Colby and Chamberlain (1969)
that specific cell receptors could recognize the inducing polynucelotide configuration. However, to date not quantitative differences in polynucelotide bindings to cells have correlated with inducing activity (Declercq and Desomer,
1973a; Declercq, 1974). In some studies it was reported that cell-bound poly
rI·poly rC was more accessible to ribonucelase on cells in which it was the
most effective inducer (Declercq and Desomer, 1973a; Declercq and
Stewart II, 1974a); however, this claim could not be substantiated in other
studies (Stewart II, unpublished data).

A large number of attempts over several years have been made to determine whether poly rI·poly rC attached to solid matrices was able to induce antiviral activity without entering the cells (Declercq and Desomer, 1972 a, 1974; Taylor-Papidimitrious, and Kallos, 1973; Bachner et al., 1975; Hutchison and Merigan, 1975; Wagner, Bugianesi, and Shen, 1971; Pitha and Pitha, 1973). The conclusion of the latest of these trials is that "there is difficulty in assessing the antiviral activity[4] of an insoluble polynucleotide inducer whether the polynucleotide adheres to or is released from the support. We believe that the problem of whether polynucelotides must enter cells for an antiviral effect to occur requires further study with new approaches" (Hutchinson and Merigan, 1975).

The main problem with such studies has been "leaking" of polynucleotides from the supporting matrix or immobilization in an inactive configuration (Pitha and Hutchinson, 1977). Thus, in all of these experiments some polynucelotide was either available to cells in a soluble form or it was unable to induce antiviral activity.

While it is perhaps not clear whether polynucleotides *must* enter cells to induce interferon synthesis, it is apparent that polynucelotides *can* induce interferon from inside the cells (a statement that is obvious if one considers viral RNA as a polynucleotide).

In a series of elegant studies, Magee and his associates (Straub, Garry, and Magee, 1974; Magee et al., 1976) showed that poly rI·poly rC contained within liposome vesicles was a much more efficient inducer in mice than was naked poly rI·poly rC. This effect was also found *in vitro*: poly rI·poly rC entrapped within lipid vesicles was taken up by cells 5 to 10 times more than the free double-stranded RNA, and vesicle-entrapped polynucleotide complex enhanced interferon induction 5 to 10-fold in human cell cultures (Mayhew et al., 1977). Though coated RNA is more efficiently taken up, there is no reason to assume that naked polynucleotides cannot enter cells in intact forms. Many naked infectious viral RNA molecules have been shown to be taken up intact by a variety of cells, and naked interferon messenger RNA has been taken up by cells in a functional form (Section VI. A. 1.).

The initial interaction of polynucleotide complex with cells, binding nonspecifically and superficially, can be neutralized by antibodies to double-stranded polynucleotides (Johnston et al., 1976). Subsequent to short incubation at 37° C, polynucleotides bound to cells become resistant to ribonuclease and antibodies. Johnston et al. (1976) found that double-stranded RNA, rather than forming non-inducing triple-stranded complexes with added single-

---

[4] Antiviral activity induction by polynucleotides is often used as a more sensitive measure for determining interferon induction than measuring extracellular interferon. Several lines of evidence support the contention that antiviral activity of polynucleotides is due to interferon induction: Vero-like cells, which can respond to interferon but cannot produce interferon do not become virus resistant after poly rI·poly rC exposure (Stewart II, Scott and Sulkin, 1969; Schaefer and Lockart, 1970); cells incubated in medium containing antiserum to interferon did not develop virus resistance when induced with poly rI·poly rC (Vengris, Stollar, and Pitha, 1975), as the induced interferon was neutralized by the antiserum as it left cells and before it could interact with the cells to induce antiviral activity (see Section VIII. C. 1).

stranded RNA, as previously repeatedly proposed by Declercq and his associates (Declercq *et al.*, 1974a, b; Declercq, Janik, and Sommer, 1976; Declercq, Torrence, and Witkop, 1976), were merely displaced by single-stranded RNAs.

The plant lectin concanavalin A was able to inhibit induction of interferon by poly rI·poly rC in cultured cells, though it had no *quantitative* effect on poly rI·poly rC binding to these cells (Harper and Pitha, 1973). This suggests that cell surface membrane changes known to occur with concanavalin A contact altered the *specific* binding of polynucleotides. Similar results were reported with neuraminidase-treated cells (Pitha, Harper, and Pitha, 1974).

The interaction of polynucelotides with cells also appears to differ significantly with different cell species. Human and rabbit cell cultures respond to double-stranded polynucleotides by becoming virus resistant and producing interferon, but mouse cells (primary kidney cultures, L cells, 3 T 3 cells, mouse embryo cultures, etc.) and chick cells will not develop antiviral activity or produce interferon unless cells are first treated with DEAE-dextran or polynucleotide-DEAE dextran together (Dianzani *et al.*, 1968; Vilček *et al.*, 1968; Bausek and Merigan, 1969; Billiau *et al.*, 1969; Aksenov *et al.*, 1970; Billiau *et al.*, 1970; Borecky, Lackovic, and Fuchsberger, 1970; Dianzani *et al.*, 1970; Falcoff, Falcoff, and Catinot, 1970; Rice *et al.*, 1970; Rosztoczy and Mecs, 1970; Stewart II and Lockart, 1970; Tilles, 1970; Rosztoczy, 1971; Stewart II, Gosser, and Lockart, 1971b, 1972; Mecs and Rosztoczy, 1971; Wacker *et al.*, 1972). The requirement for DEAE-dextran is not understood, though it enhances binding and uptake of polynucleotides (Pitha and Carter, 1971a; Stewart II, Gosser and Lockart, 1971a) and increases ribonuclease resistance of the structure. Priming of cells with interferon removes this species barrier for polynucleotide interferon induction: interferon-treated L cells are able to produce interferon in response to poly rI·poly rC without DEAE-dextran (Rosztoczy and Mecs, 1970; Stewart II, Gosser, and Lockart, 1971a). The effect of priming on induction will be discussed later (Section X. C.).

Recently, Borden, Booth, and Leonardt (1978) reported that induction of mouse L929 cells by poly rI·poly rC was enhanced 10 to 100-fold by either pretreatment or simultaneous treatment of cells with polyene macrolides (amphotericin B, nystatin or filipin), but induction by Newcastle disease virus was not altered. The kinetics of interferon induction was not altered, and the macrolides did not enhance binding of the double-stranded RNA to cells. Further, Booth and Borden (1978) found that calcium chloride also enhanced induction of L929 cells by poly rI·poly rC.

3. Induction Lag Periods

Between the initial interaction of inducers with cells and the appearance of interferon there is, depending on the inducer-cell system, a period of from about 1 to 8 or more hours. This induction "lag period" has represented the black box into which interferonologists have been sticking their probes for answers for some twenty years, and to date no particularly enlightening information has surfaced.

a) The *in vitro* Lag

The length of the period between addition of an inducer and appearance of interferon has been suggested as depending on the steps that inducers such as single-stranded RNA viruses must perform to synthesize "the inducing structure" (supposedly a double-stranded RNA structure; Finkelstein, Bausek, and Merigan, 1968; Declercq and Merigan, 1970a, b; Tan et al., 1970). When certain cell cultures are induced with poly rI·poly rC, they produce interferon by about 2 hours while with Newcastle disease virus, interferon does not appear for several hours later (Finkelstein, Bausek, and Merigan, 1968; Mozes and Vilček, 1974, 1975; Stewart II, Gosser, and Lockart, 1971 b). However, this is a gross oversimplification, for in other cell cultures (L cells), interferons are induced by either poly rI·poly rC or Newcastle disease virus after the same, prolonged lag (Stewart II, Gosser, and Lockart, 1971 b; Youngner and Hallum, 1969; Kronenberg and Friedman, 1975; Borden, Booth, and Leonhardt, 1978).

Analogous arguments have been put forward to explain why poly rI·poly rC induces "early" interferon production *in vivo* while virus-induced interferon appears much later (Desomer and Billiau, 1966). Again, such generalizations can cause misinterpretations. Thus, I shall detail here a number of systems for which the lag period has been described, to indicate whether patterns of appearance of interferons are determined by inducers or by cells.

The data summarized in Fig. 7 illustrate the induction lag found with various inducers *in vitro*. It is apparent from these data that poly rI·poly rC can induce interferon earlier than can virus in certain cells such as primary mouse kidney cultures (Stewart II, Gosser, and Lockart, 1971 b), primary rabbit kidney cultures (Tan et al., 1970) or RK-13 rabbit kidney cell line (Mozes and Vilček, 1974), or human diploid cells (Mozes and Vilček, 1975). However, in mouse L cell cultures, both virus and poly rI·poly rC induce a later interferon response (Kronenberg and Friedman, 1975; Stewart II, Gosser, and Lockart, 1971 b; Borden, Booth, and Leonhardt, 1978). Thus, the induction lag period is dependent on both the inducer and the cell type induced. The interpretation that the longer induction lag with viruses in certain cells is due to need for virus to synthesize an inducer structure does not fit the data; it would rather appear that double-stranded RNA can induce different cells in some cultures and each of these cells have different lag periods.

An interesting aspect of the induction lags illustrated in Fig. 7 is that in each case, the interferon responses induced can be completely aborted if cells are treated with actinomycin D only a short time (1 to 2 hours) before appearance of interferon (Wagner and Huang, 1966; Ho and Breining, 1965; Stewart II, Gosser, and Lockart, 1971 b). This suggests that in the case of poly rI·poly rC-induced rabbit kidney, mouse kidney or human diploid cells, the messenger RNA for interferon is transcribed within the first hour after addition of the inducer, whereas with the same inducer in L cells, the transcription event has not occurred even 4 to 5 hours after addition of the double-stranded RNA. What is occurring in these cells during this several-hour lag between addition of a "preformed inducer structure" and the induction event (transcription of interferon messenger RNA)?

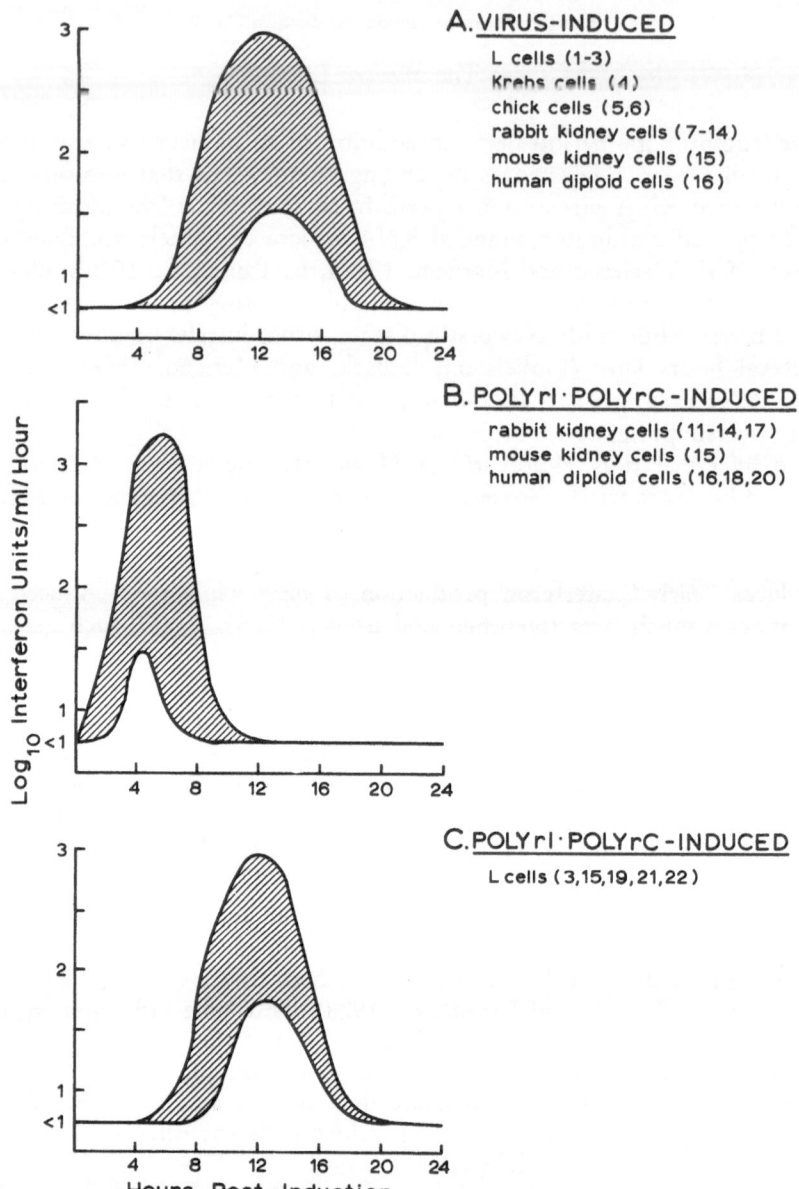

Fig. 7. Inducer-dependent and cell-dependent lag periods in cell cultures. Data illustrated are composites from low-to-high response ranges of the indicated references

1. Cantell and Paucker (1963 a)
2. Stewart II, Gosser, and Lockart (1971 a)
3. Kronenberg and Friedman (1975)
4. Wagner and Huang (1966)
5. Ho and Breinig (1965)
6. Burke, Skehel, and Low (1967)
7. Mozes and Vilček (1974)
8. Vilček et al. (1968)
9. Vilček, Rossman, and Varacalli (1969)
10. Field et al. (1972 a)
11. Vilček (1970 a, b)
12. Vilček, Barmak, and Havell (1972)
13. Tan et al. (1970)
14. Tan, Armstrong, and Ho (1971 b)
15. Stewart II, Gosser, and Lockart (1971 b)
16. Mozes and Vilček (1975)
17. Barmak and Vilček (1973)
18. Havell and Vilček (1972)
19. Margolis, Oie, and Levy (1972)
20. Myers and Friedman (1971)
21. Rosztoczy (1971)
22. Borden, Booth, and Leonhardt (1978)

One possibility is that different induction mechanisms are triggered by different inducers in different cells. The short lag with poly rI·poly rC in certain cultures which exhibit a long lag with viruses could represent different cell populations being induced by each inducer (Stewart II, Gosser, and Lockart, 1971 b). Thus, short-lag could represent a cell population whose induction mechanism requires fewer steps than those cells with longer lag periods, which would have multi-step induction mechanisms. There is some support for this interpretation. First, it has been observed that ability of cells to form interferon in response to viruses is more sensitive to actinomycin D-inhibition than is the ability of the same cells to form interferon in response to poly rI·poly rC (Finkelstein, Bausek, and Merigan, 1968; Bausek and Merigan, 1970 a, b; Vilček, 1970 a, b). This differential sensitivity could be a reflection of the multi-step induction mechanism having more potential targets for actinomycin D inhibition than the shorter induction process. Secondly, as will be described later (Section X. C.), cells which normally produce "late" interferon in response to either virus or poly rI·poly rC (e. g., L cells; Stewart II, Gosser and Lockart, 1971 b; Rosztoczy, 1971; Kronenberg and Friedman, 1975) produce "early" interferon response if they are primed (interferon-treated) prior to induction (Stewart II, Gosser, and Lockart, 1971 b; Rosztoczy, 1971; Margolis, Oie, and Levy, 1972). Thus, priming has been interpreted has performing part of a sequential multi-step induction process (Stewart II, Gosser, and Lockart, 1971 b; Stewart II and Declercq, 1973). Such accelerated induction of interferon in primed cells also makes it less likely that the lag for virus to induce interferon is owing to the need for virus to accomplish synthesis of the double-stranded RNA inducer structure, for it is difficult to conceive that virus could do so more quickly in an interferon primed cell, in which virus induced interferon more rapidly (Stewart II, Gosser, and Lockart, 1971 b).

b) Induction Lag *in vivo*

When animals are inoculated with an inducer the time until peak production of interferon varies significantly with different types of inducers. These responses have generally been lumped together as "early" or "late" (Declercq, 1974), or "virus-type" or "endotoxin-type" (Ho, 1964 a, b). Many of the inducing agents that give "virus-type" (late) interferon responses in the animal are unable to induce interferon in cell cultures. Thus, the polycarboxylates induce late interferon in mice but do not induce in cell cultures (Regelson, 1967; Merigan, 1967 a; Desomer, Billiau, and Declercq, 1968; Claes *et al.*, 1970; Billiau, Desmyter, and Desomer, 1970). On the other hand, polyribonucleotide double-strands, which like viruses are able to induce interferon both *in vivo* and *in vitro*, induce early "endotoxin-type" responses in animals (Haahr, 1971; Field *et al.*, 1967 a; Magee and Griffith, 1972; Allen and Cochran, 1972; Suzuki *et al.*, 1971; Matsuda *et al.*, 1971; Youngner and Stinebring, 1965; Youngner, 1972; Keleti, Feingold, and Youngner, 1974; Youngner, Stinebring, and Taube, 1965; Youngner, Taube, and Stinebring, 1966).

Again, as illustrated in Fig. 8, there can be no correlation with time of ap-

pearance of interferons and the replication events of viruses, as many nonviral
inducers also induce late interferon (Siminoff et al., 1973; Declercq and Merigan, 1971a; Stringfellow and Glasgow, 1972b). Many inducers do not fall into
these convenient classifications of "early" or "late". Galabov and Galabov
(1972, 1973) have reported that *Salmonella typhi* O-antigen injected into mice
induces an interferon peak at about 4 hours, while sonicated O-antigen induces
interferon at 1 to 2 hours. Grossberg et al. (1972) report that *E. coli* protein
induces interferon in mice at 2 hours whereas this inducer injected with
Freund's adjuvant gives a second interferon peak at about 6 hours. It is also interesting that while intact *Brucella abortus* gives rise to "late" interferon in
mice (Youngner and Stinebring, 1965; Desomer et al., 1970), *Brucella*
lipopolysaccharide induces ,,early" interferon (Youngner, 1972; Keleti, Fein-
bold, and Youngner, 1974). These data all suggest that different cell populations can become involved with different physical states of inducers.

c) Time of Appearance of Lymphocyte Interferons – Types I and II

Human leukocyte suspensions and mouse spleen cell suspensions have been
shown to produce interferons in response to 3 different inducers at 3 different
times (Table 4).

Human "buffy coat" leukocyte suspensions mixed with Sendai virus or
Newcastle disease virus produce interferon after an induction lag of about 3 to
4 hours (Tovell and Cantell, 1971; Matsuo, Hayashi, and Kishida, 1974).
Leukocyte suspensions exposed to mitogens produce interferons at 2 different
times depending on the type of mitogen (the target-cell specificity of the inducer): T-cell mitogens (e. g., phytohemagglutinin) induce an interferon peak
at 3 days after addition to cultures, and B-cell mitogens (e. g., pokeweed
mitogens) induce interferon only after incubation with cultures for *5 to 7 days*
(Epstein, Kreth and Herzenberg, 1974a, b; Epstein, Cline, and Merigan, 1970,
1971; Epstein, 1975). It is truly difficult to imagine what induction events must
be required that can take several days! These interferons have also been shown
to differ physically, antigenically and biologically (Section VII. C. 1.).

Mouse splenic lymphocytes stimulated with T-cell mitogens produced interferons within 24 hours of incubation (Stobo et al., 1974; Wietzerbin et al.
1977a, b), whereas B-cell mitogens did not yield interferon until 72 hours
(Wietzerbin et al., 1977a, b). Here again, T-cell and B-cell mitogen-induced
interferons were distinguishable antigenically and physically (Wietzerbin et al.,
1977; Johnson, Stanton, and Baron, 1977), the former being acid-labile and
not neutralized by antibodies prepared against virus-induced (Type I) mouse
interferon, the latter being related to Type I mouse interferon antigenically and
physically (Virelizier et al., 1977; Wietzerbin et al., 1977a, b; Section X.).

These data suggest that different cells can produce different interferons at
different times, suggesting that separate interferon genes may be derepressed.
Also, different inducers can induce similar (or identical) interferons at different
times, suggesting different induction mechanisms leading to derepression of the
same gene.

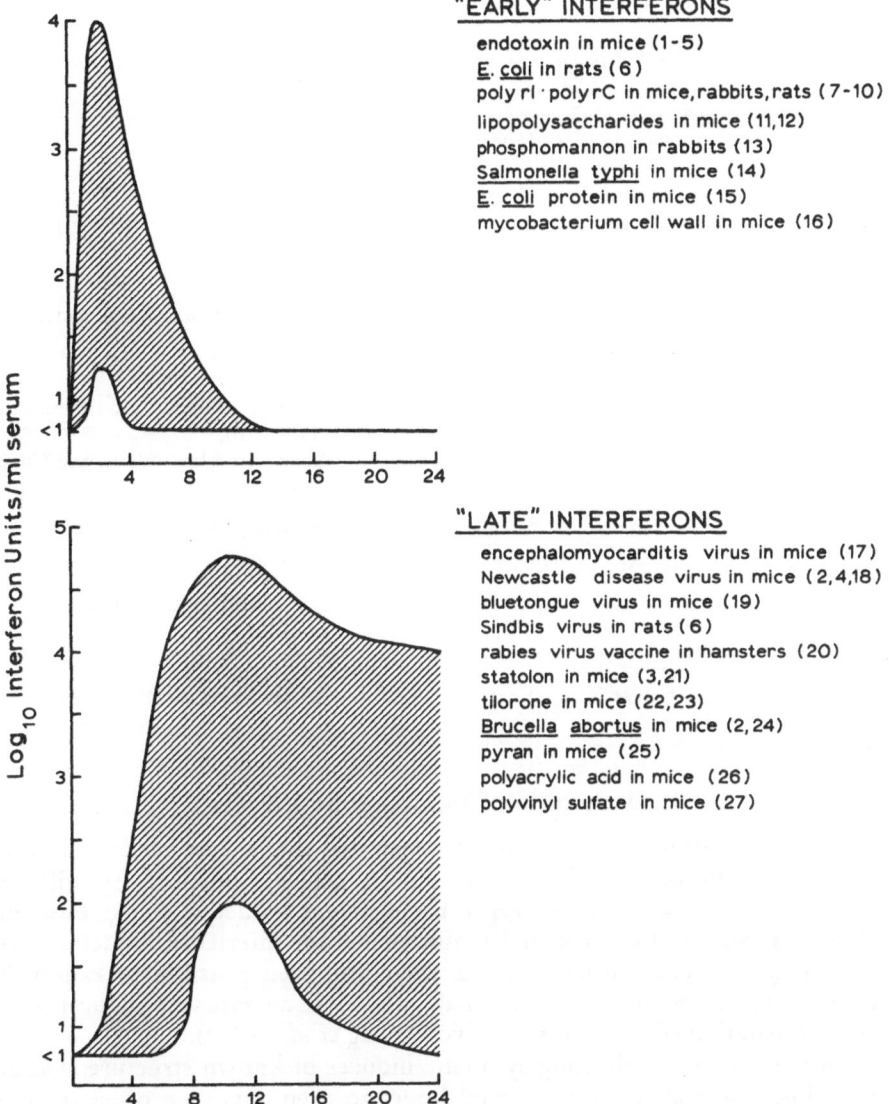

"EARLY" INTERFERONS

endotoxin in mice (1-5)
E. coli in rats (6)
poly rI · poly rC in mice, rabbits, rats (7-10)
lipopolysaccharides in mice (11,12)
phosphomannon in rabbits (13)
Salmonella typhi in mice (14)
E. coli protein in mice (15)
mycobacterium cell wall in mice (16)

"LATE" INTERFERONS

encephalomyocarditis virus in mice (17)
Newcastle disease virus in mice (2,4,18)
bluetongue virus in mice (19)
Sindbis virus in rats (6)
rabies virus vaccine in hamsters (20)
statolon in mice (3,21)
tilorone in mice (22,23)
Brucella abortus in mice (2,24)
pyran in mice (25)
polyacrylic acid in mice (26)
polyvinyl sulfate in mice (27)

Fig. 8. „Early" and „late" interferon inductions in animals. Data illustrated are composites from low-to-high response ranges of the indicated references

1. Youngner and Stinebring (1965)
2. Youngner, Taube, and Stinebring (1966)
3. Youngner and Stinebring (1966)
4. Havell, Holtermann, and Starr (1970)
5. Ito et al. (1971)
6. Desomer and Billiau (1966)
7. Haahr (1971)
8. Field et al. (1967 a)
9. Magee and Griffith (1972)
10. Suzuki, Suzuki, and Imaya (1971)
11. Youngner (1972)
12. Keleti, Feingold, and Youngner (1974)
13. Matsuda et al. (1971)
14. Galabov and Galabov (1972)
15. Grossberg et al. (1972)
16. Nagano et al. (1971)
17. Baron et al. (1966 a)
18. Baron and Buckler (1963)
19. Jameson, Schoenherr, and Grossberg (1977)
20. Wiktor et al. (1972)
21. Allen and Cochran (1972)
22. Declercq and Merigan (1971 a)
23. Stringfellow and Glasgow (1972 b)
24. Desomer et al. (1970)
25. Merigan (1967)
26. Desomer, Billiau, and Declercq (1968)
27. Came et al. (1969)

Table 4. *Inducer-cell dependent lag periods of interferons in leukocyte suspensions*

Type of cells	Inducer	Induction lag	References
	virus	< 1 day	Tovell and Cantell (1971); Matsuo, Hayashi, and Kishida (1974)
Human leukocyte suspensions	T-Cell mitogens	3 days	Epstein (1975); Buimovici-Klein, Weiss, and Cooper (1977)
	B-cell mitogens	5–7 days	Epstein, Kreth, and Herzenberg (1974 a, b); Buimovici-Klein, Weiss, and Cooper (1977)
Mouse spleen cell suspensions	virus	< 1 day	Wietzerbin *et al.* (1977 a, b)
	T-cell mitogens	< 1 day	E. Falcoff (personal communication, 1977)
	B-cell mitogens	3 days	Wietzerbin *et al.* (1977 a, b)

B. Mechanism of Induction by Viruses

The studies outlined above have demonstrated that a vast variety of structures can lead to derepression of interferon gene(s), possibly by different mechanisms and in separate cell-types for different inducers. It has been impossible to recognize the structural requirements for interferon induction even with synthetic polynucleotides. It has even not been possible to rationalize why one preparation of single-stranded poly rI is an efficient inducer while another preparation of poly rI is inactive (Thang *et al.*, 1977).

Even when a non-replicating synthetic inducer of known structure is added to cells, long intervals of time (several hours to even days) are often required before the interferon induction event occurs.

However, many years of work have gone into numerous studies searching for the common denominator in the viral inducers. Viruses of every size, RNA or DNA, double- or single-stranded, mutants with various replication defects, live or inactivated, have been used to probe the interferon induction mechanism.

As soon as it was realized that synthetic double-stranded RNA was able to induce interferon, the popular opinion was that all viruses able to induce interferons did so because they were able to form double-stranded RNA molecules during their replication cycle (Field *et al.*, 1967a; Declercq and Merigan, 1970a; Colby, 1971). However, as there is much unexplanable data on interferon-inducing potentials of single- and double-stranded synthetic polynucleotides, one would expect at least as much difficulty in generalizing with these more complex natural RNAs and DNAs.

1. Search for Double-Stranded RNA

Work on induction mechanisms by viruses have focused on the viral replication functions that must be accomplished for derepression of the interferon gene to occur; this has been done by trying to eliminate those events that are not required. So far, such work has suggested that with some viruses early replicative events are necessary and with other viruses, the input virus components can trigger production. Often, input virus double-stranded RNA is apparently insufficient for induction (Gauntt, 1973), while certain single-stranded RNA viruses are able to induce interferon without undergoing any detectable replicative processes (Dianzani, Pugliese, and Baron, 1975). The ability of single-stranded RNA viruses to induce interferon without forming the hypothetical inducing structure, double-stranded RNA, has been a center of controversy for several years, analogous to the story of whether single-stranded synthetic RNAs can induce interferons. Since it has now been confirmed that certain single-stranded synthetic RNA preparations can indeed induce interferons (Baron et al., 1969; Thang et al., 1977), it appears appropriate to review the literature on induction by viruses. Some which are apparently not able to produce „the common stimulus", double-stranded RNA are able to induce interferon (Dianzani et al., 1970; Goorha and Gifford, 1970a; Gandhi, Burke, and Scholtissek, 1970; Dianzani, Pugliese, and Baron, 1974, 1975; Levy and Wheeler, 1973; Azuma, 1976); in others, no correlation between formation of double-stranded RNA by virus and interferon induction could be found (Lockart et al., 1968; Thacore and Youngner, 1970; Lomniczi and Burke, 1970; Lai and Joklik, 1973; Atkins et al., 1974; Atkins and Lancashire, 1976; McKimm and Rapp, 1977a, b).

Dianzani et al. (1970) reported that Newcastle disease virus which was unable to replicate in mouse L cells was able to induce interferon even when protein synthesis inhibitor, cycloheximide, was present in the cultures during the induction period (and removed for production time). They interpreted these results to indicate that the stimulus for interferon induction was provided by the input virus. This was, of course, before it was known that virion RNA transcriptase accompanying such virions could have accomplished double-stranded RNA formation. Therefore, these authors subsequently repeated these experiments using an interferon-inducing virus which does not contain a virion-associated RNA transcriptase, Chikungunya virus, and again found that apparently an input component of the single-stranded RNA virus was able to induce interferon production (Dianzani, Pugliese and Baron, 1974, 1975). These authors suggest that the reason that double-stranded RNA is usually a more effective inducer than single-stranded RNA is because the latter inducing molecules are more sensitive to intra- and extracellular ribonucleases.

Several other reports using inactivated viruses unable to perform any detectable viral RNA synthesis in cells but able to induce interferon led authors to conclude that the input RNA of the virus was the inducer (Gandhi and Burke, 1970; Gandhi, Burke, and Scholtissek, 1970; Goorha and Gifford, 1970a), or at least some component present in the virion up to the regular uncoating process (Azuma, 1976).

Another approach has been to completely inhibit viral RNA synthesis by interferon treatment and to determine ability of virus to induce interferon. Stewart II, Gosser, and Lockart (1971a) found that MM strain of encephalomyocarditis virus was unable to replicate in interferon-treated L cells, yet induced much more interferon than did replicating virus. Field *et al.* (1972c) suggested that the ability of non-replicating single-stranded RNA viruses to induce interferon in cells can be explained by the presence of contaminating double-stranded RNA in crude concentrates of RNA viruses. However, Stewart II and his associates (1971a) found induction of interferon in interferon-treated (virus resistant) cells with highly purified preparations of MM virus and with infectious RNA extracted from these virions. Levy and Wheeler (1973) also reported interferon induction attributable to input virions of Chikungunya virus in interferon-treated chick cells.

Numerous publications have reported lack of correlation between ability of viruses to replicate viral RNA and to induce interferon, and concluded that viral RNA or its accumulation in cells as double-stranded RNA is probably not the actual inducer of interferon production (Lockart *et al.*, 1968; Thacore and Youngner, 1970). In many cases, inverse correlations were reported (Lomniczi and Burke, 1970; Lai and Joklik, 1973; Atkins and Lancashire, 1976). Such findings have led some to conclude that double-stranded RNA is an unlikely candidate for the interferon-inducing molecule (Meager and Burke, 1972).

In many cases, however, early viral replicative events were apparently necessary for induction (Huppert, Hillova, and Gresland, 1969; Clavell and Bratt, 1971; Fleischmann and Simon, 1974), and in many cases the ability of viruses to form double-stranded RNA and to induce interferon was correlated (Burke, Skehel, and Low, 1967; Skehel and Burke, 1968a, b), not surprisingly as viral replicative intermediate structures are formed during infections and interferon is induced during viral infection. It was surprising, however, that even DNA (vaccinia) virus-infected chick cells contained double-stranded RNA (Colby and Duesberg, 1969; Bakay and Burke, 1972). This double-stranded RNA could induce antiviral activity in cells. Interestingly, vaccinia virus-infected chick cells do not themselves produce interferon (Bakay and Burke, 1972). Interferon-inducing double-stranded RNAs have also been isolated from normal cells (DeMaeyer, DeMaeyer-Guignard, and Motagnier, 1971; Kimball and Duesberg, 1971) which were apparently not producing interferons. Thus it is not clear what relation these double-stranded RNA structures have to the interferon trigger, as they are residing in the cells without interferon induction occuring.

2. Viral Events Effecting Induction

Many factors besides the ability of virus to form double-stranded RNA, or whatever other inducing structure is relevant, seem to determine whether a virus will induce interferon in cells or not. Some viruses (herpesviruses, myxoviruses, picornaviruses, rhabdoviruses) are poor inducers apparently because they have the ability to rapidly inhibit cellular RNA and protein syntheses that would otherwise lead to transcription and translation of interferon messenger RNA (Wagner and Huang, 1966; Gandhi and Burke, 1970; Aurelian and Roizman, 1965; Johnson and McLaren, 1965; Wagner *et al.*, 1963; Wertz and Youngner, 1970).

Some workers have shown that synthesis of virus RNA is not always in itself sufficient stimulus to induce interferon. Most of these studies were based on replication events of temperature-sensitive (ts) mutants studied at nonpermissive temperatures. Lockart *et al.* (1968) found that Sindbis virus wildtype was able to induce interferon and to replicate in chick cells at 42° C, but a ts-mutant was unable to induce interferon at high temperature, though it could synthesize RNA. They concluded that viral events other than synthesis of new RNA are required for interferon induction. These results were supported by similar studies using ts-mutants of Semliki Forest virus, wherein synthesis of virus RNA was not accompanied by interferon induction (Lomniczi and Burke, 1970). In the latter study, however, the input virus RNA itself was apparently able to induce interferon when high multiplicites of infection were used. To date, no satisfactory explanation has appeared to define what replicative events are involved for induction in these situations.

Many investigators have attempted to use myxoviruses to study interferon induction mechanisms. These viruses are often better inducers after they have been partially inactivated by ultraviolet irradiation or heat (at least in chick cells), while complete inactivation inhibits their interferon inducing activity (Youngner *et al.*, 1966; Vilček, 1963; Ho and Breinig, 1965; Isaacs and Lindenmann, 1957; Burke and Isaacs, 1958b). This effect of mild inactivation has occasionally been attributed to the elimination of the ability of the viruses to inhibit cellular macromolecular syntheses (Gandhi and Burke, 1970). However, this attribute of myxoviruses (and others) may have little to do with interferon yields, for in some cells (mouse L cells), Newcastle disease virus can strongly inhibit cellular RNA and protein syntheses yet induce high yields of interferon (Youngner *et al.*, 1966). Also, some strains of Newcastle disease virus which do not inhibit cellular synthesis do not induce interferon (Lomniczi and Burke, 1970). Some experiments suggest that the replicating Newcastle disease virus produces an inhibitor of interferon induction or production (Sheaff, Meager, and Burke, 1972). It seems likely that the rapidity as well as degree of cellular syntheses inhibition would determine whether the virus would induce or not.

Ultraviolet-inactivation of Newcastle disease virus first causes loss of infectivity, followed in sensitivity by loss of polymerase activity, which was destroyed in parallel with interferon-inducing capacity (Youngner *et al.*, 1966; Meager and Burke, 1972). Similar parallel inactivation of polymerase and interferon-inducing activities have been reported with heat and β-propiolactone-inactivations (Sheaff, Meager, and Burke, 1972). These data suggest that some RNA synthesis is needed for induction.

In human and chick cell systems, reoviruses induced interferon, and it has been concluded that the input viral RNA was the inducer (Oie and Loh, 1968; Long and Burke, 1971), especially as double-stranded RNA extracted from reovirus was itself able to induce interferon (Tytell *et al.*, 1967). However, Lai and Joklik (1973) reported that several ts-mutants of the double-stranded

RNA-containing reoviruses were unable to induce interferon in L cells even though input virus double-stranded RNA, single-stranded and double-stranded replicative products were present. Again, UV-inactivation kinetics showed that loss of polymerase activity in reoviruses paralleled loss of interferon-inducing activity (Burke, 1973).

Adenoviruses have been shown to lose their ability to induce interferon in chick cells when treated with trypsin, though such treatment did not effect infectivity of the virions (Ho and Kohler, 1967; Beladi and Pusztai, 1967). Some authors reported that viral penton hemmagglutinin was able to induce, and neutralization or inactivation studies suggested parallel stabilities of this antigen and interferon-inducing activity (Pusztai *et al.*, 1969; Pusztai *et al.*, 1974). However, some studies did not reveal inducing activity in the protein fractions of adenoviruses (Ho and Kohler, 1967) and different adenoviruses showed inconsistent correlations with penton antigen and interferon-induction (Beladi *et al.*, 1970, 1974; Mucsi *et al.*, 1970; Ustacelebi, 1976). Clearly this intriguing involvement of a viral structure protein in interferon induction warrants further investigation.

C. Alternative Induction Mechanism Hypotheses

At least three distinct trigger mechanisms for interferon derepression can be proposed, with some data arguing for and against each being "the" induction mechanism. This probably suggests that cells can be induced by more than a single mechanism (not a particularly surprising realization in view of the many functions attributed to interferons).

1. The Double-Stranded RNA Hypothesis

As has been demonstrated throughout the previous discussions, interferon induction can result from interaction of various natural or synthetic double-stranded RNA complexes with cells. Clearly, also, many viruses form double-stranded RNA during replication. Thus, it was previously very tempting to speculate that double-stranded RNA was *the* way to interferon stimulation.

Such a unifying hypothesis was comfortable, particularly as it could be rationalized that those substances not stimulating interferon appearance via double-stranded RNA content or formation (endotoxins, etc.) were really not "true" inducers as they did not induce *de novo* synthesis but rather only caused cells to leak "preformed" interferons.

However, the downfall of the "preformed" interferon concept (as outlined in Section IV. A. 1.) clearly eroded support for the latter argument. The solid basis for the double-stranded RNA hypothesis deteriorated further in light of clear demonstrations of interferon induction by single-stranded RNAs (either viruses clearly unable to perform any replicative steps, or synthetic single-stranded polyribonucleotides). Also, the demonstrations of double-stranded RNA molecules in both viral-infected and normal uninfected cells which are not producing interferons, makes one wonder about the importance of this structure as the interferon initiator.

Studies for more than a decade have failed to show why some single – or double-stranded synthetic RNAs are able to instigate interferon reactions in cells while others are not. It seems a low probability that continued testings of further analogues will clarify this situation. In view of the many magnitudes of complexity increase with replicating RNAs (viruses) it seems even less likely that we will soon decipher the trigger mechanisms by looking for double-stranded RNA forms in virus-infected cells.

2. The Repressor-Depletion Hypothesis

Several of the inducer classes have been shown to correlate with functional properties of the interferons.

a) Viruses induce interferons, and interferons inhibit virus replication.

b) Mitogens induce interferons, and interferons inhibit cell multiplication.

c) Immune recognitions induce interferons, and interferons inhibit immune reactions.

d) Some toxins (diphtheria toxin, endotoxins) induce interferons (Marchenko et al., 1976a; Green, Cooperband and Kibrick, 1969; Smorodintsev et al., 1969) and interferons inhibit the effect of certain toxic substances (Yabrov, 1966, 1967, 1975, 1976; Smorodintsev et al., 1969; Moehring, Moehring and Stinebring, 1971).

Yabrov (1975, 1976) suggested that many of the inducers of interferons disturbed protein synthesis and that interferons' raison d'être was to protect against this perturbation. This inducer-action relationship has recently been formulated into an induction mechanism hypothesis by Tan and Berthold (1977), who suggested that all reversible inhibitors of cellular protein or RNA synthesis induce interferon, and all interferon inducers (viruses, double-stranded RNAs, cycloheximide and other macromolecular synthesis inhibitors) owe their ability to induce interferon to their abilities to inhibit a rapidly turning-over repressor which normally represses interferon gene(s).

Such an induction common-denominator would be more all inclusive than the double-stranded RNA hypothesis to explain induction by lectins, endotoxins and low molecular weight inducers. Clearly more work will better define this hypothesis that depletion of repressor content in cells leads to interferon synthesis.

3. The Basal-Level-Interferon Hypothesis

The repressor-depletion hypothesis can be related to the Basal-Level-Interferon hypothesis if it is assumed that the repressor that is depleted is interferon per se.

Styk et al. (1973) suggested that a part of an inducing virus was incorporated into the interferon it induced. Subsequently, Taborsky, and Stancek (1974) found that ^{3}H-uridine-labeled double-stranded RNA of E. coli f2 phage comigrated in polyacrylamide gel electrophoresis with the highly purified activity peak of the interferon it induced. These authors asked the intriguing question: "Can a part of an inducer become incorporated into interferon?"

The association of inducer with interferon (as repressor) leading to derepression of the interferon was previously proposed by Kleinschmidt (1972). If various inducers do indeed bind selectively to interferons, as suggested from earlier works of Styk *et al.* (1973) and Taborsky and Stancek (1974), it would be tempting to speculate that this relationship of inducer binding to the induced protein might be significant in the interferon induction mechanism.

Such an induction derepression mechanism would be contingent upon cells containing endogenous Basal-Level Interferons. This likelihood can be suspected from the many reports of ,,spontaneous" interferon production (Section III. D.), which suggest that cells constitutively produce endogenous interferons at normally subdetectable levels, which are elevated upon exposure to inducers.

Indeed, interferons have been demonstrated to bind with a high degree of selectivity to a number of inducer classes. Concanavalin A and other mitogens induce interferons (Section III. B. 5.) and have high affinities for the induced interferons (Besancon and Bourgeade, 1974). In fact these affinities have been widely exploited for affinity chromatographic purification of the interferons (Section VII).

Interestingly, it was incidental experiments on purification of interferons that provided strongest support for the Basal-Level-Interferon induction mechanism hypothesis. DeMaeyer-Guignard, Thang and DeMaeyer (1977) found that the displacement of interferon from blue-dextran-Sepharose columns was affected by the single-stranded polyribonucleotide poly rI but not by oligomers of nucleotides. Interferons were bound selectively to columns of immobilized poly rI or poly rU. Thus interferons also contain specific binding sites for this class of inducers. It clearly seems more than a coincidence that an inducible protein is very selectively bound to components of various classes of inducer molecules.

Accordingly, interaction of mitogens, virus input single-stranded RNA or their replicative intermediates, or polynucleotides, could trigger interferon production by binding basal levels of endogenous interferons which are perhaps necessary for normal cellular functioning.

Therefore, the relative efficiencies of different inducers might relate to their relative affinities to interferons. It will be interesting to determine the affinities of interferons to the various other classes of inducers, such as the low molecular weight compounds.

The events occurring between addition of an inducer to a cell and the derepression of the genes for interferon messenger RNA, the induction phase, terminate in the nucleus of the cell, where the genetic information for interferon synthesis begins to be expressed.

V. The Genetics of Interferon Production

As it is evident both from indirect evidence using inhibitors and direct evidence using enucleated cells that synthesis of interferon is dependent upon nuclear components, it should be possibly by using cytogenetic techniques to assign interferon structural genes to specific chromosomes.

Such analyses have been approached by two methods: (1) analyses of interferon production by series of hybrid cells which have sorted-out different chromosomes or combinations of chromosomes; (2) studies using aneuploid cells with multiple copies of a selected chromosome or which are deficient in certain chromosomes. It must be cautioned, however, that chromosomal assignments based on levels of production of interferon must be interpreted carefully, as there are numerous epigenetic factors modulating induction and/or production by cells, any of which can give misleading data on relative "abilities" of cells to make interferons.

A. Hybrid-Cell Analyses of Interferon Production

1. Production Regulation in Hybrid-Cells

Several investigators have used somatic cell hybrids for assigning the interferon synthesizing potentials to selected chromosomes. Some such hybrids preferentially lose chromosomes of one of the fusion partners, so that hybrid populations can be selected containing identifiable chromosomes; such populations can be induced for their abilities to make interferon of the type specified by the cell species being analyzed. (Thus the property of partial "species specificity", which was mentioned in Section I. B. 6 and which will be discussed in detail elsewhere [Section VII. A. 2] can be a valuable tool.) From such analyses of large series of cells containing various combinations of chromosomes, or lack of such, it is possible to compute which chromosome responds to induction by transcribing interferon-information.

The first use of such heterokaryons for analysis of interferon production mechanism was made by Guggenheim, Friedman, and Rabson (1968), who fused nucleated chick erythrocytes (which cannot produce chick interferon) with two different human cell lines, one able to produce human interferon, the other unable to produce interferon. Hybrids were tested for ability to produce either species of interferon when induced with Sendai virus. Heterokaryons of chick cells with the interferon-competent human cells were able to produce both human and chick interferon; those formed by fusion of chick erythrocytes and interferon-defective human HeLa cells produced neither interferon.

This study suggested that the human genetic components could activate latent interferon-producing components in the analogous gene of another species. A similar ability of human chromosomes in human-hamster somatic cell hybrids to activate normally dormant genetic information was recently reported by Morgan and Faik (1977), who found that hybrids formed with Chinese hamster cells, which could not normally be induced to produce hamster interferons with human cells were able to produce hamster interferon and human interferon if both human chromosomes 5 and 18 were present, and hamster interferon alone if human chromosome 18 were present. These studies suggest that certain cells which apparently lack genetic information for interferon production, such as the "Vero-like" cells previously described (Section IV. A. 1), may rather have such information in a repressed state and lack ability to derepress this gene. Similarly, hybrid clones of mouse-hamster cells were also found able to produce significantly more hamster interferon than could be produced by the parent hamster cells (Carver, Seto, and Midgean, 1968; Grossberg, Smith, and Sedmak, 1975). These data suggest that this enhanced expressibility of interferon genes in hybrids is a phenomenon which could be exploited for obtaining high interferon producing cells from low producing cells, by selection of fusion products of high producers of another species (Creagan et al., 1975).

2. Chromosomal Assignments for Interferon Production in Hybrid-Cell Lines

Hybrids that randomly lose chromosomes from one of the parent species have been studied to identify particular chromosomes involved in interferon production. Cassingena and his associates (1971) fused African green monkey cells with mouse cells and obtained a small number of hybrids which gradually lost monkey chromosomes while retaining mouse chromosomes. This study suggested a correlation of monkey interferon production with presence of a particular monkey chromosome. This chromosome was identified as monkey chromosome 22 (Chany, Ankel and Bourgeade, 1975).

Tan, Creagan, and Ruddle (1974 a, b) examined a large number of independently derived clones of mouse-human hybrids for ability to produce human interferon when induced with either poly rI·poly rC or Newcastle disease virus. Each hybrid was also tested for presence of other specific human markers (human chromosomes and human enzymes). Subcloning of interferon-producing clones revealed that no single human chromosome or linkage group could be correlated with human interferon production (Tan, 1977). Human chromosomes 2, 5, 15 and 18 were apparently present in all hybrid populations that were able to make human interferon. However, chromosomes 15 and 18 were ruled out, as some clones lacked known marker enzymes for these chromosomes. Thus, all hybrid clones containing human chromosomes 2 and 5 could make human interferon, but those which contained only chromosome 2 or 5 were unable to make human interferon.

The apparent requirement for two human chromosomes for production of human interferon has been rationalized (Creagan et al., 1975; Tan, 1977) as:

    1. One of the chromosomes codes for specific receptors for interferon inducers (or components of the "trigger" mechanism),

2. One of the chromosomes codes for a factor which converts interferon precursor into active interferon while one codes for interferon structural components,

   or

3. One chromosome counteracts the regulating mechanisms of heterologous genes in hybrid cells.

Recently, studies using hamster-human hybrids have shown that chromosome 2 is not necessary for human interferon production in those hybrids, suggesting that mouse genetic information regulating human interferon formation in mouse-human hybrids was suppressed by human chromosome 2. Alternatively, hamster elements might be able to provide information normally furnished by human chromosome 2, but mouse elements cannot.

B. Chromosomal Assignments for Interferon Production in Aneuploid Cells

Hybrid analyses suggested that chromosomes from different species may influence the ability of genes to be expressed in mixed genetic-element conditions. This was suggested further by reports that in reverse-segregating mouse-human hybrids (preferential loss of mouse rather than human chromosomes) human interferon production was greatly decreased by the presence of a single mouse chromosome but was restored after all mouse elements were eliminated (Tan, 1977).

In this regard, more recent studies have claimed that only human chromosome 5 is necessary for human interferon production in *human* cells (Tan, 1977; Tan and Berthold, 1977). Such data have all been obtained using aneuploid cell lines which contain imbalance in numbers of copies of specific chromosomes or pieces of chromosomes. One type of such aneuploid cells derived from persons with Cri-du-Chat syndrome contains partial deletions of chromosomes 5, in their short arms. Such cells could produce normal amounts of human fibroblast interferon, suggesting that interferon gene information resides in the long arm of human chromosome 5 (Tan, 1977).

In another approach to genetic assignments for human fibroblast interferon, Tan (1977) reported extensive examinations of a variety of aneuploid human fibroblast cell lines which contained different numbers of copies of chromosome 5, with some having more short arms than long arms of this chromosome, and some having more long than short arms. These data show that the amount of human interferon inducible in these cells correlated with the amount of chromosome 5 long arm, but no correlation with chromosome 2 was observed, again suggesting that in human cells as well as certain hybrids, only chromosome 5 is required for human fibroblast interferon production.

Further, Tan (1977) reported that the amount of human interferon produced varied inversely with the number of chromosome 5 shortarms and directly with the number of chromosome 5 long arms, suggesting that regulatory information for human interferon production is transcribed from the short arm while structural information is read from long arm products. This regulation component was further restricted to a specific chromosome 5 short arm segment, as Cri-du-Chat derived cells with partial short arm deletions seemed to have normal interferon regulation. It was further claimed that particular cell clones with multiple copies of chromosome 5 short arms were able to produce significantly increased levels of human fibroblast interferon (Tan and Berthold, 1977), with some clones reportedly producing extremely high levels of human interferon. Such cells could be useful as sources of human fibroblast interferons for purification studies; however, apparently owing to the unusual instabilities of such interferons, it has not yet been possible to confirm their quoted high levels of activity (W. E. Stewart II, unpublished data).

It should be emphasized at this time that all the assignments for chromosomes responsible for production of human interferons have been done with human fibroblasts, thus assignments are for production of human *fibroblast* interferons. As will be elaborated later (Section VI and VII), human leukocyte and fibroblast interferons are physically, chemically and biologically distinguishable and may be products of *different interferon genes*. This further studies must clarify whether chromosome 5 is also carrying structural information for human *leukocyte* interferon production.

C. Epigenetic Complications of Assessing Genetic Contributions to Interferon Production

It has been proposed that human fibroblastoid cells with more chromosome 5 long arms than short arms are more inducible for interferon production than those with the reverse ratio, and that this is because the former would be less strongly repressed than the latter by regulatory components synthesized from information coded from the short arm (Tan, 1977; Tan and Berthold, 1977). This hypothesis must await confirmation which will likely require isolation of the gene products involved in this regulation. Until then, it should be emphasized that evaluating the contribution of specific chromosomes to interferon production can be complicated by a number of epigenetic factors.

Expression of genetic potential for production of interferon can clearly reflect more than merely relative numbers of certain chromosomes coding for structural components. Fluctuations in production can also result from:

1. Defects in the induction processes. These could result from higher or lower concentrations of surface receptors for inducers, differences in levels of intracellular mechanisms (enzymes, membranes, etc.) involved in inducer processing and/or derepression "trigger"-events.

2. Regulation mechanisms involved in transcription of interferon messenger RNA.

3. Regulatory mechanisms modulating translation of interferon and/or its processing.

1. Age Effects on Interferon Production

It is often not possible to distinguish which of the above is involved in effecting levels of interferons produced, but it is clear that factors other than presence or absence of specific chromosomes are pertinent.

A significant example of factors affecting interferon formation which are not *genetically* attributable is the age effect, both *in vivo* and *in vitro*. The data on effects of age either *in vivo* or *in vitro* on abilities of cells to *produce* interferons are very similar to those reported for affect of age on *sensitivities* of cells to interferon action (Section II. D. 6), and generally suggest that it may not be to the advantage of rapidly growing cells to either produce or respond to a substance which can inhibit its growth.

a) *In vivo* Age and Interferon Potential

It has often been reported that tissues from young embryos are not able to produce as much interferon as those from older embryos or mature animals (Isaacs and Baron, 1960; Barbosa *et al.*, 1974; Soloviev *et al.*, 1972a; Mendelson, Kapusta, and Dick, 1970; Sawicki, 1961; Siegel, Brown, and Morton, 1973). Others, however, have reported the opposite, that more interferon was produced by younger animals than by older (Vilček, 1964b; Overall and Glasgow, 1970; DeMaeyer and DeMaeyer-Guignard, 1968; Carter *et al.*, 1971; Rinaldo, Overall, and Glasgow, 1975), and other have found no significant effect of age on interferon production (Banatvala, Potter, and Best, 1971; Gandhi and Stewart, 1968; Ray, 1970; Cantell *et al.*, 1968b).

It is difficult to interpret what accounts for these fluctuations in interferon potentials. On the one hand the increased replication of certain viruses in younger animals could enhance interferon production by providing more inducer to more cells. This seems a feasible explanation for enhanced interferon yields in younger animals in some of the *in vivo* studies but seems less likely in the studies of leukocytes or cell cultures derived from animals of different ages.

One study reported that during early pregnancy rats and their embryos were both equally unable to product interferon, but later in gestation both became equally able to product interferon. Explants of both maternal and embryo tissues of pregnant rats were able to produce interferon at all times (Mendelson, Kapusta, and Dick, 1970). These data suggest that hormonal influences, rather than age, determined interferon production potential *in vivo*. Obviously, the fluctuations in abilities of the cells to produce interferons could not be determined solely by numbers of chromosomes. On the other hand, Carter *et al.* (1971) claimed that tissue cultures derived from fetal human tissues were able to produce significantly more interferon than cultures of human cells derived from adult tissues. These tissues were taken from paired donors to diminish genetic variability. Supposedly the fetal-origin cells produced 300-fold more interferon than did adult-derived cells, this enhanced capacity for interferon production was consistent in fetal skins obtained between the 10th and 20th gestational weeks, and the responses were stable in the cell cultures for 18 generations.

b) Interferon Production and *in vitro* Aging

"Aging" in cell cultures, that is, prolonged cultivation without passage, has been consistently reported to increase the ability of cells to produce interferons. Human amnion cells maintained for 2 weeks or more produced more interferon than did fresh cultures (Ho and Enders, 1959b); HeLa cell cultures aged about a week produced more interferon than 1 to 3 day old cultures (Cantell and Paucker, 1963 b); chick embryo cell cultures incubated for 6 days produced markedly more (about 10-fold) interferon yields than at 3 days (Henslova and Libikova, 1966). Carver and Marcus (1967) reported that chick cells aged 1 week produced about 32-fold more interferon than cells at 1 to 2 days in culture, and suggested that such "aged" cultures exhibited a generalized state of "enhanced derepressibility".

Chick cells "aged" in culture were also found superior producers of interferons in comparison to young cultures, by Libikova (1973), who also reported that such cells grown *in vitro* for up to a week without medium change elaborated a "factor" (suggested to be a "chalone") which enhanced viral-induced interferon production when it was applied to young cultures (Libikova, 1975). A similar report was previously published by Kato and Eggers (1969 b) who found that the "factor" released from aged chick cell cultures enhanced interferon production and made the cells make interferon sooner. To my knowledge the only other substance reported to bring about both of these effects on interferon production is interferon itself, which primes cells both quantitatively and temporally (Section X. C). It seems possible that low levels of "spontaneous" interferon in "aged" chick cell cultures (as first described by Lockart, 1968) may accumulate to enhance their interferon production potential.

All these "aging" variations in interferon production of cells again demonstrate the difficulty in evaluating chromosomal contributions to interferon response-levels, as all these studies likely employ cells whose chromosomal components were not quantitatively altered by "aging" in cultures for 3 to 14 days but whose interferon-producing potentials varied significantly, as much as several hundred-fold.

2. Variations in Interferon Production by Human Diploid Cell Cultures

As indicated in the previous discussion on "aging" of diploid human fibroblasts, it was reported that diploid fetal human cells consistently produced significantly more (about 5-fold) interferon than the genetically-paired maternal diploid cells (Carter *et al.*, 1971). Other differences in abilities of a number of human diploid cell lines to produce interferons have been reported which did not relate to age discrepancies of the cells (Moehring, Stinebring, and Merchant, 1971). Also, human diploid cells from different tissues were studied by Spina *et al.* (1972), who found that fibroblasts produced more interferon than leukocytes, and Sreevalsan (1973) found that human diploid cells derived from various organs of a single embryo responded variably to poly rI·poly rC for interferon production.

Many laboratories that have developed large-scale human diploid fibroblast interferon production units have routinely tested many different human diploid cells, many from individual embryos, or neonatal skin, and it has been a concensus finding that considerable and significant quantitative differences in interferon production occur (Havell and Vilček, 1972; W. E. Stewart II, unpublished data). Of these, the FS-4 cell strain originating in Vilček and Havell's laboratories have proved to be the most consistent producers (Mozes *et al.*, 1974; Vilček and Havell, 1973).

These data again emphasize the difficulty encountered in assigning interferon-production levels to chromosomes, as variations in interferon yields can be so dramatic in genetically (in terms of chromosome numbers and their apparently physical completeness) identical cells.

D. Genetics of Interferon Production *in vivo*

In attempting to evaluate the role of interferon in animal virus disease and tumors, it has been difficult to sort out the contributions of interferon, specific immunity and the various other non-specific host factors contributing to recovery (Stewart II, 1973; Section XII. A).

1. Mendelian Analyses of Interferon Production

One approach has been to study genetic strains or different age of animals which exhibit high or low susceptibilities to such diseases and to determine relative abilities to manifest each of the specific and non-specific defense mechanisms. This approach has been used extensively and, as will be described in detail in Section XII, has shown that each of the factors may or may not be involved.

Another approach that has been employed recently is studies of mutants that have markedly different abilities to produce interferons. DeMaeyer and DeMaeyer-Guignard and their associates have described the existence of several such mutants (DeMaeyer and DeMaeyer-Guignard, 1969). By Mendalian analyses of recombinant inbred mice strains, these workers found that circulating interferon production in mice after inoculation with Newcastle disease virus was under control of a single autosomal locus, which they designated If-1. Two alleles were described, If-1^h and If-1^l, which determined high or low interferon responsiveness, respectively (DeMaeyer, DeMaeyer-Guignard, and Jullien, 1970). Characterization of comparative sizes of interferons made in the high and low producers indicates that the If-1 locus determines quantitative rather than qualitative effects on circulating interferon in response to Newcastle disease virus (Martelley, Bailey and DeMaeyer-Guignard, 1972; Bailey and DeMaeyer-Guignard, 1972).

Inoculation of mouse mammary tumor virus in different lines of mice revealed that mice with different mammary tumor virus sensitivities also produced different levels of circulating interferon, with the tumorvirus-resistant C57BL mice lines producing about 3 times more interferon than the tumor-virus-susceptible BALB/c lines. Importantly, the murine mammary tumor-virus-induced interferon locus segregated independently from the locus determining Newcastle disease virus-induced interferon levels (If-1), and so was designated If-2. If-2^l and If-2^h producers showed normal distributions of serum interferon responses of 1.29 to 2.77 log$_{10}$ units and 2.00 to 3.12 log$_{10}$ units, respectively (DeMaeyer *et al.*, 1974).

The levels of difference of interferon production in mice with If-1^l and If-1^h alleles when inoculated with Newcastle disease virus were about 10-fold; thus mouse strains genetically very similar can differ significantly in ability to produce interferons in response to a given inducer (DeMaeyer *et al.*, 1974). Of

6*

23 inbred lines reported in one study, 22 were either clearly If-1h or If-1l; only one was unclassifiable because of intermediate interferon response (DeMaeyer, DeMaeyer-Guignard, and Bailey, 1975; DeMaeyer et al., 1975). It was found that If-1 genotypes could be transferred to irradiated mice by grafting bone marrow from unirradiated mice. Thus, irradiated If-1l or If-1h mice grafted with marrow from If-1h or If-1l mice, respectively, acquired the If-1 character of the donor mice (DeMaeyer et al., 1975). These data show that interferon production in mice induced with Newcastle disease virus is expressed through hemopoietic stem cells, and, as will be described in detail in Section VI. B. 1, it has been shown that Newcastle disease virus-induced serum interferon is derived from radiosensitive and antilymphocyte-sensitive cells (DeMaeyer-Guignard and DeMaeyer, 1971).

Other If-loci have been reported, which segregate independently from If-1, that determine interferon production to Sendai virus (DeMaeyer et al., 1974), so that generalization of interferon control cannot even be made with closely related inducers.

The If-1l and If-1h congenic mice have been used as tools to determine the contribution of interferon to immunosuppression (Section X). Newcastle disease virus induced interferon and inhibited delayed-type hypersensitivity in If-1h mice, but did neither in If-1l mice, whereas Sendai virus, whose interferon induction is not determined by If-1 locus, was able to induce interferon and suppress delayed-type hypersensitivity responses equally in *both* If-1h and If-1l mice (DeMaeyer et al., 1975; DeMaeyer, 1976).

These *in vivo* analyses show that the ability to produce interferon may reflect the relative abilities of mice to proliferate specific cell populations responding to certain inducers. *In vitro* experiments with suspensions of different hemopoietic cells from high- and low-producer mice congenic at If-1 should clarify this possibility.

2. Non-Specific Factors Influencing in vivo Genetic Evaluations of Interferon Production

In addition to the age effect and normal variations in interferon production by chromosomally similar systems, there have also been a great number of factors described which influence interferon production *in vitro* and *in vivo*. Many of these might influence interferon responses by eliminating or effecting functioning of cell populations involved in production. Some genetic mutants might be more sensitive to such non-specific factors than others, and altered interferon responses in such animals could reflect increased sensitivity to the factor rather than true differences in interferon producing potentials. Clearly control of all these variables must be evaluated along with interferon titer fluctuations.

a) Temperature

Some studies on the effect of elevated temperature have suggested that interferon production in cell cultures is best at temperatures higher than those for virus replication (Ruiz–Gomez, and Isaacs, 1963b; Lab, Tinland, and Kirn, 1968). Others have found that optimal yields of human leukocyte interferons were obtained at 37° C (Strander and Cantell, 1966; Falcoff, Fournier, and Chany, 1966). Lackovic *et al.* (1967) and Waschke, Lackovic, and Borecky (1969) found that the ability of mouse peritoneal leukocytes to produce interferon in response to virus increased up to 40° C, while *E. coli* endotoxin or mannan in these cultures produced optimal interferon levels at 22–26° C. These authors later reported that precultivation of these cells at 36° C for 5 hours before infection raised the ability of the cells to respond to virus at 26° C (Waschke, Lackovic, and Borecky, 1969b).

Some authors also reported that temperature influenced interferon production in animals. Ruiz-Gomez and Sosa-Martinez (1965) claimed that adult mice infected with Coxsackie B 1 virus and kept at 4° C died from virus replicating to high titers because they were unable to produce interferon at 4° C, whereas mice kept at 25° C produced high levels of interferon, but little virus and survived. Others reported that rabbits maintained at an elevated body temperature of 41.1° C produced more interferon than those at room temperature when induced by virus, but similar levels when induced by endotoxin (Postic *et al.*, 1966), while endotoxin induced more interferon at lower temperature. Quite opposite results from those claimed by Ruiz-Gomez and Sosa-Martinez (1965) were reported by Haahr and Teisner (1973) who found that mice kept at 4° C had both higher virus and higher interferon levels than those kept at 25° C, an effect explained as due to more inducer forming to induce more interferon at the lower temperature.

b) Hormones

Numerous hormones, particularly corticosteroids, have been examined for their effects on interferon production *in vivo* and *in vitro* (Table 5) and in both animal and cell cultures these usually reduced the amount of virus-induced interferon produced, though in some studies no effect or even increased interferon production was found, perhaps as a consequence of increased virus growth providing more inducer (Rytel, 1969; Oh, 1970; Giron, Schmidt, and Pindak, 1971; Giron *et al.*, 1973 a). Talas and Stoger (1972) reported similarly that hydrocortisone depressed interferon production of viral-, endotoxin- and poly rI·poly rC-induced interferons. On the other hand, they (Talas and Stoger, 1972) reported that adrenocorticotropin and 3 estrogens produced different effects on interferon production in mice, depending on the type of inducer. Thus, hydrocortisone inhibited interferon synthesis induced by virus, endotoxin and poly rI·poly rC; adrenocorticotropin inhibited virus- and endotoxin-induced interferon but not poly rI·poly rC-induced interferon; and the estrogens had no influence.

In certain lines of EB virus-containing human lymphoblastoid cells, hydrocortisone treatment enhanced expression of the EB virus genome and "induced" the appearance of detectable interferon (Joncas *et al.*, 1973).

In some cases, hydrocortisone was much more inhibitory to endotoxin-induced interferon responses than to viral responses (Postic *et al.*, 1967; Corragio *et al.*, 1968) and in some cases the relative effect may depend on the particular animal used (Postic *et al.*, 1967; Solomon, Merigan, and Levine, 1967;

Table 5. *Influences of hormones on interferon production*

Hormone	Type of inducer	in vivo	in vitro	Interferon production	References
Hydrocortisone	Virus	+		decreased	Kilbourne, Smart, and Pokorny (1961); Smart and Kilborune (1966); Reinicke (1964); Postic et al. (1967); Corragio et al. (1968)
	Virus		+	decreased	DeMaeyer and DeMaeyer (1963); Reinicke (1965 a); Mendelson and Glasgow (1966)
	Virus	+		no effect	Desomer, Billiau, and Declercq (1968)
	EB Virus		+	increased	Joncas et al. (1973)
	Endotoxin	+		decreased	Postic et al. (1967); Desomer, Billiau, and Declercq (1968); Talas and Stoger (1972)
	Poly rI·poly rC	+		decreased	Talas and Stoger (1972)
Adrenocorticotropin	Virus	+		decreased	Talas and Stoger (1972)
	Virus	+		no effect	Desomer, Billiau, and Declercq (1968); Solomon, Merigan, and Levine (1967)
	Endotoxin	+		no effect	Desomer, Billiau, and Declercq (1968)
	Endotoxin	+		decreased	Talas and Stoger (1972)
	Poly rI·poly rC	+		no effect	Talas and Stoger (1972)
Cortisone	Virus	+		decreased	Rytel and Kilbourne (1966)
	Virus	+		increased	Rytel (1969); Oh (1970)
Corticosterone	Virus	+		no effect	Desomer, Billiau, and Declercq (1968); Solomon, Merigan, and Levine (1967)
	Endotoxin	+		decreased	Desomer, Billiau, and Declercq (1968)
Testosterone	Virus	+		no effect	Giron, Schmidt, and Pindak (1971)
	Virus		+	decreased	DeMaeyer and DeMaeyer (1963); Reinicke (1965 b); Zeitlenok et al. (1968)

Hormone	Type of inducer	*in vivo*	*in vitro*	Interferon production	References
Estrogen	Virus		+	decreased	Reinicke (1965 b)
	Virus	+		no effect	Talas and Stoger (1972)
	Endotoxin	+		no effect	Talas and Stoger (1972)
	Poly rI·poly rC	+		no effect	Talas and Stoger (1972)
Pituitary growth hormone	Virus	+		no effect	Reinicke (1965 b)

Desomer, Billiau, and Declercq, 1968). It is particularly pertinent in this regard that adrenalectomy has been shown to significantly increase the interferon production induced by endotoxin in rabbits (Postic *et al.*, 1967) and by virus in mice (Solomon, Merigan, and Levine, 1967).

Such influences could significantly effect interferon levels produced by mutant mouse strains, depending, for example, on the type of inducer or resulting from physical defects, for example, micro- or macro-adrenal mutations.

c) Other Factors Modulating Interferon Production

i) Stress. A few studies have been reported claiming that "stress" induces a transitory impairment in the ability of animals to produce interferons. Chang and Rasmussen (1965) reported that mice subjected to high intensity sound were more sensitive to virus infection and produced less interferon. Presumably this stress caused elevated levels of endogenously produced corticosteroids which, as previously discussed, can inhibit production of interferon. Jensen (1968a) claimed that mice subjected to electric punishment conditioning also exhibited depressed interferon when induced with virus, but this transitory impairment was not altered by adrenalectomy. This author (Jensen, 1968b) also reported a depression of interferon response in mice injected with serotonin, or various vasoactive amines (Jensen, 1969; 1973). However, others found a slight increase in interferon in mice similarly stressed (Solomon, Merigan, and Levine, 1967). In fact, neither the increases nor decreases reported seem significant ($\leq$ 2-fold).

Mice have been reported to produce more interferon when breathing air containing disproportionately high nitrogen-oxygen mixtures, and to produce less interferon at high or low atmospheric pressures (Huang and Gordon, 1968), and tracheal epithelium from mice living several days in an ozone enriched environment was not able to produce interferon (Ibrahim, Zee and Osebold, 1976). It is not clear what mechanisms are involved in any of these alterations of interferon production.

ii) Microbials. Viruses, bacteria, and mycoplasmas have all been reported to influence interferon production. Hermodsson (1963) reported that parainfluenza virus infection inhibited ability of calf kidney cultures to produce interferon when infected with Newcastle disease or foot-and-mouth disease virus. Cytomegalovirus infection (Osborn and Medearis, 1966) and lymphocytic choriomeningitis virus (Holtermann and Havell, 1970) depressed interferon responses in mice. Other viruses have been reported to enhance interferon pro duction induced by a second virus (Ho and Breinig, 1962; Mahdy and Ho, 1964), likely owing to ability of the first virus to induce low levels of interferon which primed for induction by the superinfecting virus (Section X. C.).

Considine and Starr (1967) and Havell, Holtermann, and Starr (1970) found that germ-free mice were better producers of interferon than conventional mice when stimulated with virus, but no difference was found in responsiveness of the groups of mice induced with endotoxins (Havell, Holtermann, and Starr, 1970).

Chronic infection of mice with *Mycobacterium lepraemurium* suppressed their interferon response to virus (Glasgow and Bullock, 1972). Mice injected with viable or non-viable *Corynebacterium acnes* produced lower interferon levels in response to viruses or poly rI·poly rC, but produced enhanced interferon levels when injected with endotoxin (Farber and Glasgow, 1972; Fischbach and Glasgow, 1975). Similarly *Eperythrozoon coccoides*-infected mice produced depressed interferon yields to viruses during the first 3 weeks of infection, but normal levels by 6 weeks (Glasgow et al., 1971; Glasgow, Murrer, and Lombardi, 1974).

Early studies on the effect of mycoplasmas on interferon production conflicted, some reporting that mycoplasma infection enhanced interferon production induced by virus in chick cells (Yershov and Zhdanov, 1965), others reporting that they had no effect on interferon responsiveness of mouse or human cells to virus (Armstrong and Paucker, 1966) and still others reporting that they decreased interferon yields in hamster cells induced by virus (Singer, Barile, and Kirschstein, 1969). More recently, mycoplasma have been shown to reduce "spontaneous" interferon production by human lymphoblastoid cells (Archer and Young, 1974) and to induce a marked hyporesponsiveness in mice to interferon induction by virus or poly rI·poly rC, but not tilorone (Cole et al., 1975).

iii) Leukemias, Lymphomas and Other Disease States. Interferon production has been reported to be depressed in mice with lymphoblastic and erythroblastic leukemias when induced with viruses or poly rI·poly rC, each known to induce different cells (DeMaeyer-Guignard, 1972). Leukocytes of patients with chronic *lymphocytic* leukemia produced lowered or normal interferon levels (Lee, Ozere, and Van Rooyen, 1966; Hadhazy et al., 1967; Strander et al., 1970) or delayed responses (Dennis et al., 1972), while leukocytes from patients with chronic *myelogenous* leukemia were reported to produce increased interferon levels (Lee, Van Rooyen, and Ozere, 1969; Hadhazy et al, 1967; Hadhazy et al., 1976). Zedginidze et al. (1975) reported that interferon production induced in patients by oral poliovirus type II vaccine was significantly depressed in acute leukemia.

Interferon responses have also been reported to be depressed in Stage IV Hodgkin's disease patients (Rassiga-Pidot and McIntyre, 1974; Veskova and Nemirowskaya, 1971), in infectious mononucleosis (Pidot, Maurer, and McIntyre, 1973), in patients with uremia (Sanders et al., 1971), in children with chronic hepatitis (Tolentino et al., 1975) or in cytomegalovirus infection (Emodi and Just, 1974 b).

iv) Miscellaneous Factors. Carcinogens from several different chemical classes have been reported to have depressing effects on interferon production in cell cultures (DeMaeyer and DeMaeyer–Guignard, 1963; 1964a, b, 1967; De-Maeyer–Guignard, and DeMaeyer, 1965 a), while structurally related non-carcinogenic compounds had no effect. Similarly, one carcinogen, urethane, reduced serum interferon levels in mice, but the structurally-related noncarcinogen, methylcarbamate, had no such effect (DeMaeyer–Guignard, and De-Maeyer, 1967)

A variety of chemicals effecting cell surfaces or metabolism, not surprisingly, effect interferon production. A few of these substances have been reported to increase interferon production. Vitamin A (Siegel, 1974), given orally, gave a slight (approximately 2-fold) increase in mice, though it suppressed induction of interferon *in vitro* (Blalock and Gifford, 1975; 1976 a, b; 1977). Emetine, an ipecac alkaloid, increased interferon production in mice inoculated with poly rI·poly rC (Schellekens, Hoffmeyer, and Van Griensven, 1975). Cyclophosphamide, an immunosuppressant drug, can increase or decrease interferon production in mice or cell cultures, depending on dosage administered (Robinson, Cureton and Heath, 1969; Robinson and Heath, 1968; Szalaty and Golubska, 1973), and Amphotericin B, a polyene antibiotic, increases ability of poly rI·poly rC to induce interferon in L cell (Borden and Leonhardt, 1976). Not all membrane function-altering chemicals, however, effect interferon production, for ouabain, which specifically inhibits membrane-bound ATPase activity, has no effect on interferon production (Link *et al.*, 1966; Lebon *et al.*, 1975). Heparin (Kato and Eggers, 1969 a; Mentkevich and Zhdanova, 1971), colchicine (Soloviev and Mentkevich, 1965; Ito *et al.*, 1976b) and cytochalasin (Ito *et al.*, 1976b), deuterium oxide (Mayer and Dobrocka, 1968), chloroquine (Kohno, Kohase, and Suganuma, 1968), adenine and guanidine (Mecs, 1964; Johnson and McLaran, 1965), Methotrexate and vitamin A (Tokumaru, 1967) have all been reported to depress interferon production through mechanisms unknown. Similarly, psychomimetic drugs (marijuana, peyote, hashish, mescaline, morphine) have been reported to inhibit interferon production *in vivo* but not *in vitro* (Hung, Lefkowitz, and Geber, 1973; Lefkowitz, Hung, and Geber, 1973; Lefkowitz, 1976; Geber, Lefkowitz, and Hung, 1975, 1976a, b; 1977). Lead poisoning in chickens suppressed interferon production, but subclinical intake for prolonged periods was without effect (Vengris and Mare, 1973). Arsenicals at high concentrations inhibited interferon production in mice (Gainer, 1972), and coal dust inhibited its production in human cell cultures (Hahon, 1974).

Treatment of mouse or rat cells with cyclic AMP or adrenaline plus theophylline (enhancers of cyclic AMP) strongly inhibited interferon production induced by poly rI·poly rC or viruses (Dianzani, Neri, and Zucca, 1972; Johnson, Blalock, and Baron, 1977), and cholera toxin inhibition of mitogen-stimulated interferon production was presumably mediated by this cyclic nucleotide (Epstein and Bourne, 1976).

v) Interferon. Interferon itself can also influence interferon production, both positively and negatively, but the effects will be discussed later in connection with non-antiviral functions and regulatory mechanisms of interferon production (Sections VI. X. C and X. D).

VI. Interferon Production

To recapitulate our progress through the interferon system to this point, it has been described that inducers of a wide variety can interact with most animal cells to directly or indirectly activate genetic information on specific chromosomes. The product of this sequence of events is interferon messenger RNA.

In this section, I shall describe interferon production from 3 different approaches: *1:* production mechanisms at the cellular and molecular level; *2.* production in the organism; *3.* large-scale production procedures for obtaining interferons on the scale necessary for the purifications and characterizations to be described in Section VII.

A. Interferon Production at the Cellular and Molecular Level

1. Interferon Messenger RNA

a) Indirect Evidence for Interferon Messenger RNA

The first suggestions that a messenger RNA for interferon was formed as a consequence of addition of inducer to cells was obtained by the findings that the inhibitor of DNA-dependent RNA synthesis, Actinomycin D, prevented production of interferon, if added up to shortly before first appearance of interferon (Heller, 1963; Wagner, 1963 b, 1964; Gifford and Heller, 1963) but if added after this lag period (Section IV. A. 1), interferon continues to form even though RNA synthesis is inhibited (Wagner and Huang, 1965, 1966; Levy, Axelrod, and Baron, 1965; Burke and Walters, 1966). Recent studies on interferon production by enucleated cytoplasts also suggest that the interferon message leaves the cell nucleus very soon after it is transcribed (Burke and Veomett, 1977).

Early attempts to detect radio-labelled interferon-specific messenger were unsuccessful (Burke and Walters, 1966) for, as the investigators concluded, the amount of interferon messenger RNA formed is below the limits of such direct detection methods.

b) Extraction of Interferon Messenger RNA and Its Translation in Heterologous Cells

The first direct evidence for existence of interferon messenger RNA was obtained by DeMaeyer–Guignard, DeMaeyer, and Montagnier (1972), who found that RNA extracted from mouse embryo cells which had begun produc-

Table 6. *Interferon Messenger RNAs*

Message source	Inducer	Translation System	References
Mouse embryo cells	Poly rI·poly rC or Newcastle disease virus	chick cells vero cells	DeMaeyer-Guignard DeMaeyer and Montagnier (1972)
Mouse bone marrow cells	Poly rI·poly rC or Newcastle disease virus	chick cells human cells	Orvola *et al.* (1974 a, b); Orvola *et al.* (1976); Georgadze *et al.* (1974)
Mouse C243 cells L cells	Poly rI·poly rC or Newcastle disease virus	chick cells	Montagnier *et al.* (1974)
Mouse L cells	Poly rI·poly rC	Hela cells vero cells hamster BHK 21 cells chick cells	Kronenberg and Friedmann (1975)
Mouse C243 cells	Poly rI·poly rC	wheat germ cell-free system (+spermine)	Thang *et al.* (1975)
Human fibroblasts	Poly rI·poly rC	chick cells	Reynolds and Pitha (1974)
Human fibroblasts	Poly rI·poly rC	syrian hamster cells	Greene, Diffenbach, and Tso (1978)
Human fibroblasts	Poly rI·poly rC	Xenopus oöcytes	Reynolds, Premkumar, and Pitha (1975); Sehgal, Dobberstein, and Tamm (1977); Cavalieri *et al.* (1977 a, b); Raj and Pitha (1977)
Human fibroblasts	Poly rI·poly rC	Krebs II cell-free system rabbit reticulocyte cell-free system	Reynolds, Premkumar, and Pitha (1975); Reynolds and Pitha (1974)
Human fibroblasts	Poly rI·poly rC	mouse Ehrlich ascites cell-free system	Pestka *et al.* (1975, 1977)
Human fibroblasts	Poly rI·poly rC	wheat germ cell-free system (+spermine)	Raj and Pitha (1977)
Human lymphoblasts	Newcastle disease virus	Xenopus oöcytes	Cavalieri *et al.* (1977 a)
Chicken embryo cells	Newcastle disease virus	mouse L cells	Georgadze *et al.* (1974)

Table 6 (continued)

Message source	Inducer	Translation System	References
Monkey ES1 cells	Newcastle disease virus	chick cells vero cells	DeMaeyer-Guignard DeMaeyer and Montagnier (1972)
Monkey BSC-1 cells	Poly rI·poly rC	mouse L cells	Kronenberg and Friedmann (1975)

ing maximal levels of interferon (12 hour after induction with either Newcastle disease virus or poly rI·poly rC) was able to enter chicken or Vero monkey cells and cause these to produce low levels (about 3 to 30 units) of interferon with the "species specificity" and antigenic-identity of mouse interferon, i. e. active on mouse cells but not active on the type of cells producing it. They also found that RNA extracted from interferon-producing monkey cells could be translated into monkey interferon by chicken cells. The production of interferon in the message-recipient cells was inhibited by protein-synthesis inhibitors but not by actinomycin D (the latter in fact increased interferon production), showing that it was translated from input RNA. Thus, a naked eukaryotic cell messenger RNA could be taken up, intact and in functional condition, by another cell and translated into a biologically active protein foreign to the translating cell.

The message activity was reported to be in a component sensitive to RNase, but not Pronase or DNase. RNA extracts from cells which had not been induced to make interferon or had been induced for only a short period were without activity, again confirming that interferon is a truly inducible protein (and that detectable message is not even transcribed until late in the lag period, as suggested in Section IV. A. 3).

This work was soon confirmed by Reynolds and Pitha (1974) using human diploid fibroblasts induced with poly rI·poly rC, with extracted RNA translated in actinomycin D-treated chick cells. These workers found that the interferon-message would bind to oligo (dT)-cellulose (poly A-containing) and sedimented at 7 to 10 S in sucrose. The level of interferon obtained in these studies (about 30 to 1500 units) was higher than those obtained with mouse interferon messenger RNA by DeMaeyer–Guignard et al. (1972), but did not correlate with the interferon levels obtained in the "natural" cell system. This will be discussed in detail in Section VI. A. 2. Interferon message activity was extracted at intervals after induction of the human fibroblasts and was found to peak at about 6 hours and to disappear by about 12 hours, the time used for message extractions by DeMaeyer–Guignard et al. (1972); however, examination of the differences in interferon induction-lags obtained with poly rI·poly rC in certain human and mouse cells suggests the timing of extractions may be important (Fig. 7).

Extraction of interferon messenger RNA from virus- or poly rI·poly rC-induced bone marrow cells of mice and chickens and their translations in actinomycin D-treated heterologous mouse, chicken and human cells was also reported by Orlova *et al.* (1974a, b, 1976), but these authors extracted the RNA from cells 17 hours after induction, a time when message-activity decline would be expected. Georgadze *et al.* (1974) also reported translation of bone marrow cell interferon messenger RNA in heterologous cells, and claimed that cells hyporesponsive to repeated induction produced markedly less interferon message. However, the low quantities of interferon produced in such experiments, the variability in times of extraction and of appearance of interferon messages in normal and primed cells, and the poor quantitative relations found between amounts of extracted RNA and interferon productions (DeMaeyer–Guignard *et al.*, 1972; Reynolds and Pitha, 1974) prevent validation of this interpretation.

Montagnier *et al.* (1974) reported that interferon-translating RNAs extracted from virus-induced mouse C_{243} cells or poly rI·poly rC-induced mouse L cells could be separated into two forms, one with poly A tails, one without. The former was sensitive to pancreatic RNase but resistant to RNase III, while the latter was resistant to pancreatic RNase but sensitive to RNase III, suggesting it was a double-stranded RNA or a "hairpin" single-strand. Both RNA forms, extracted 8 hours after induction, were able to produce mouse interferon in actinomycin D-treated chick cells, about 100 units (approximately 10 reference units).

Kronenberg and Friedmann (1975) also extracted RNA from induced mouse or monkey cells (in this study RNA was extracted at 16 hours after induction) and translated them into their paternal interferons in HeLa, Vero, chick or hamster cells. They claim a relatively quantitative assay for interferon message, with yields of interferon being proportional to amounts of RNA applied to translating cells. Unlike the results of DeMaeyer–Guignard *et al.* (1972), they report that actinomycin D treatment of message-recipient cells either had no effect on production or decreased it, but no explanation was offered. The RNA isolated in this study was also not bound by polyuridylic acid.

Human fibroblast interferon message has also been translated in Syrian hamster embryo cells (Greene, Dieffenbach, and Tso, 1978), and its uptake was facilitated by the use of $CaCl_2$ instead of DEAE-dextran. In these cells actinomycin D-treatment increased interferon translation and message was bound to oligo(dT)-columns. Again, interferon production was independent of the applied total RNA concentration from 10 to 100 μg/ml. However, by varying interferon messenger RNA at constant total carrier RNA concentrations of 50 μg/ml, a linear interferon yield was reported.

c) Translation of Interferon Messenger RNA in *Xenopus* Oöcytes

The translation of interferon messenger RNA in heterologous cell systems has the disadvantages of cells being variable in responses to applied RNA concentrations and of containing large reserve pools of amino acids to preclude preparation of specifically labelled translation products in them. However, translation of messenger RNAs in oöcytes from the frog *Xenopus leavis*, which have low amino acid pool levels, seemed a possibility for synthesizing labelled

interferon protein, Reynolds, Prekumar, and Pitha (1975) translated messenger
RNA from poly rI·poly rC-induced human fibroblasts in microinjected
Xenopus oöcytes and found this system to be much more efficient than the
chick cell recipient system, yielding about 50-times more interferon. When the
product of this translation was formed in ^{3}H-animo acid, a radioactive product
was obtained which, when electrophoresed in SDS-polyacrylamide gels, by the
procedure described by Stewart II (1974; Section VII. C), migrated at about
25,000 daltons, in the same position as human fibroblast interferon (Section VII. C). No labelled materials were seen at this position in translation
products of oöcytes injected with RNA from uninduced human fibroblasts.

RNA preparations for these studies (Reynolds *et al.*, 1975) were prepared
from human fibroblasts which were induced with poly rI·poly rC followed by
cycloheximide, for 1 hour and 5 hours, respectively. Titers of interferons obtained from 50 homogenized oöcytes in 1 ml of buffer were reported to be
64,000–128,000 units/ml. The amount of interferon mRNA again did not correlate well with interferon yields (Raj and Pitha, 1977).

Sehgal, Dobberstein, and Tamm (1977) found that *Xenopus* oöcytes injected with poly A-containing human fibroblast-derived interferon messenger
RNA doses of from 1 to 20 ng yielded linear interferon production. These authors extracted interferon message from fibroblasts $2\frac{1}{2}$ hours after normal induction and found more message activity than when extractions were made at
6 hours after induction. Cells induced ("superinduced") with poly rI·poly rC
and cycloheximide still contained high message activity levels at 6 hours. The
implication of these data will be discussed in Section VI. A. 2. Sehgal and his
associates (1977) also found that the oöcyte-produced interferon translated
from human fibroblast message was neutralized by an antiserum prepared
against human fibroblast interferon but not by antiserum against human leukocyte interferon.

Other workers (Cavalieri *et al.*, 1977a) reported that messenger RNA preparations derived from induced human fibroblasts and from induced human
lymphoblastoid cells (whose interferons are distinguishable antigenically) translated with fidelity into interferon distinguishable antigenically as human fibroblast or human leukocyte interferon. Oöcytes are able to carry out a number of
posttranslational processes such as glycosylation, polypeptide cleavage, acetyla-
tion, and phosphorylation (Cavalieri *et al.*, 1977a). These data suggest that
there are two interferon structural genes. In these studies, 10 oöcyte produced
about 12 units of lymphoblastoid interferon or 350 units of fibroblast interferon when injected with the respective messenger RNAs. Neutralization of
the lymphoblastoid interferon message product required a mixture of both antiserum to human fibroblast interferon and antiserum to human leukocyte interferon, suggesting that this preparation contained both types of interferon.
When these oöcyte-derived interferons were analyzed by SDS-polyacrylamide
gel electrophoresis they migrated the same as normal fibroblast and lymphoblastoid cell-derived interferons (Section VII. C. 1). These two oöcyte-produced
interferons were also distinguishable from each other in activity levels when assayed in heterologous cells, similar to their native forms, with the fibroblast
message-derived interferon and fibroblast interferon being about 500-times

more active on human than on bovine cells, while lymphoblastoid message-derived interferon and lymphoblastoid interferon were active on both human and bovine cells at about the same levels.

These authors later reported that, similar to the data of Sehgal, Dobberstein, and Tamm (1977) described above, amounts of interferon messenger RNA levels in poly rI·poly rC-induced human fibroblasts (as measured by translation in oöcytes) was highest at 1 to 1½ hours after induction and disappeared rapidly (half-life about 68 minutes), whereas with cycloheximide present, message was present in high levels for several hours longer (Cavalieri *et al.*, 1977).

No one has yet reported extraction of interferon messenger RNA from human fibroblasts induced with Newcastle disease virus, but owing to the markedly prolonged lag period as compared to poly rI·poly rC induction in these cells (Section IV. A. 3 and Fig. 7), it should be emphasized that searches for such messages should not necessarily be based on the times of extractions presented here that have been used for human fibroblasts induced with poly rI·poly rC.

d) Translation of Interferon Messenger RNA in Cell-Free Protein-Synthesizing Systems

Several laboratories have recently reported successful translation of interferon messenger RNAs in several cell-free protein synthesizing systems, thus making interferon the first biologically active eukaryotic cell protein to be so translated. Such systems may prove useful for studying the mechanisms of regulation of interferon production.

Reynolds and Pitha (1975) and Reynolds, Premkumar, and Pitha (1975) isolated human fibroblast interferon messenger RNA and translated it in both a preincubated cell-free ribosomal system prepared from Krebs II cells enriched with rabbit reticulocyte initiation factors, and in a rabbit reticulocyte cell-free system. After 1 hour incubation at 37° C or 45 minutes at 30° C, respectively, the antiviral activity titers were about 100 units/ml/cell-free system), or about 500-times lower than those achieved by translation of the same message in oöcyte.

Pestka *et al.* (1975) translated human fibroblast interferon message in cell-free mouse Ehrlich ascites cell extracts. Again, both in this study and that of Reynolds, Premkumar, and Pitha (1975), the cell-free-translated human fibroblast interferon was antigenically and biologically (low activity on bovine cells) identical to fibroblast-made human interferon. It is not clear whether such cell-free-produced interferons are glycosylated. The activity translated in this system after 1 hour at 30° C was again disappointingly low (about 68 units/ml).

Thang *et al.* (1975) were apparently more fortunate in choice of interferon species or translating systems, as they reported that poly A-containing mouse C243 cell-interferon messenger RNA could be translated in a wheat germ cell-free system with high efficiency. In this system the presence of spermine was absolutely required for synthesis of active interferon. In these studies and that of Montagnier *et al.* (1974), interferon message was extracted from the induced cells at about 9 hours after induction, rather than at 12 hours as previously reported (DeMaeyer–Guignard et al., 1972). However, as these data are reported in interferon units derived from assays on "aged" mouse embryo fibroblasts, which units are generally significantly higher than reference units, the translating efficiency cannot be determined. However, the system compared favorably with the in vivo translation of mouse interferon message in Vero cells.

Raj and Pitha (1977) also reported that spermine was essential for translation of human fibroblast interferon messenger RNA into biologically active interferon in the wheat germ system, although it did not increase label-incorporation. The spermine concentration between 80 to 100 μM was critical. Again, however, the wheat germ system was much less efficient than the oöcyte system, yielding only low levels of interferon. Interestingly, wheat germ extracts were unable to translate interferon from message obtained from poly rI·poly rC "normally" induced fibroblasts but translated interferon from message extracted from "superinduced" fibroblasts; however, Xenopus oöcytes translated about the same amount of interferon from both message preparations. This suggests that the Xenopus oöcyte system might be able to modify inactive interferon messenger RNAs whereas wheat germ cannot.

Pestka et al. (1977) translated human fibroblast interferon message in Ehrlich ascites system and added sparsomycin (an inhibitor of protein synthesis) at 30 minutes (a time prior to appearance of interferon activity but after amino acid incorporation was complete) and found that interferon activity was generated by further incubation to 2 hours. Therefore, it appeared that interferon activity was generated after synthesis of the primary polypeptide chain, suggesting that posttranslational modifications were required for activity.

In this regard it may be that the cell-free systems have yielded such low levels of interferon, as compared to the oöcytes, because the latter are able to perform several posttranslational modifications whereas the former are not. Another possibility appears trivial but is worth considering; most interferons, especially human fibroblast interferon, are inactivated by reducing agents; all the cell-free protein synthesis systems that have been reported, showing low interferon activity, have the reducing agents dithiothreitol or 2-mercaptoethanol in the translating cocktail.

e) Translation of Interferon Messenger in Bacteria?

One report has appeared claiming that chicken interferon messenger RNA could be applied to actinomycin D-treated bacterial (Escherichia coli) cells which would then produce low levels of chick interferon (Orlova et al., 1976, 1977). This report has, of course, not been confirmed, though the much more complex task of using recombinant-DNA technology to retrocopy interferon messenger RNA into bacteria is presently being pursued as a potential for large-scale interferon production.

Clearly more systematic and rational approaches to the kinetics of production of messenger RNAs for interferons are needed. These should be based on consideration of production curves with the particular inducer-cell system used (Fig. 7).

2. Superinduction or Superproductions?

Regulation of interferon production was early deduced from the observed production curves, as illustrated in Figures 6 and 7: interferon appears a few hours after inducer-cell interaction, is produced for only a short time and then production terminates completely. The mechanism of this shutoff of production could represent a destruction of newly formed interferons or an inactivation of messenger RNA. Either would imply a termination of transcription of interferon messenger RNA shortly after its initiation, suggesting an activation of a mechanism for interferon repression along with or shortly after its derepression, as defined in the excellent analyses of these data by Havell (1977) and by Sehgal (1977).

a) Interferon Enhancement by Metabolic Inhibitors

The early studies on the effects of metabolic inhibitors on interferon induction by endotoxins *in vivo,* as described in Section IV. A. 2, were first interpreted that viruses induced *de novo* synthesized interferons while endotoxins only caused release of "preformed" interferons. In fact, while interferon responses in mice inoculated with Newcastle disease virus were inhibited by cycloheximide, endotoxin-induced interferon was actually enhanced by this antimetabolite, being produced at higher levels and for a longer time than without the inhibitor (Youngner, Stinebring, and Taube, 1965). When similar experiments were repeated with poly rI·poly rC in mice similar results and similar interpretations were obtained (Youngner and Hallum, 1968).

Obviously, the possibilities for alternative interpretations derived from such *in vivo* studies based on using various inducers and various inhibitors, some of which were themselves interferon inducers, are limitless, but the possibility for deriving meaningful interpretations from such studies are extremely limited.

However, studies on induction of interferons in tissue cultures eliminated a number of the variables possible in intact organisms, and such studies soon began to provide a few clues to interferon production regulation. Poly rI·poly rC, which was found to induce "early" interferon *in vivo* which was apparently preformed on the basis of its resistance to inhibitors of protein synthesis, also induced "early" interferon in cultures of human fibroblasts, whereas virus induced a "later" interferon in these same cultures; the former interferon was resistant to actinomycin D and to puromycin at concentrations which inhibited the latter interferon (Finkelstein, Bausek, and Merigan, 1968). Similar observations were made with primary mouse kidney cell cultures induced with poly rI·poly rC or Newcastle disease virus: however, while lower levels of inhibitors prevented only virus-induced interferon, and occasionally even enhanced poly rI·poly rC induced interferon, both responses were inhibited at higher inhibitor concentrations (Stewart II, Gosser, and Lockart, 1970, unpublished data). Vilček and his associates (1969) first reported that poly rI·poly rC-induced interferon production in rabbit kidney cell cultures could be significantly enhanced by actinomycin D if the inhibitor were added at the appropriate interval after inducer, but inhibitor added prior to inducer prevented interferon synthesis. It was only with careful kinetics experiments that these paradoxically enhanced interferon yields obtained with inhibitors began to make sense. Vilček (1970a, b) reported that interferon yields in poly rI·poly rC-stimulated rabbit kidney cell cultures could also be enhanced by cycloheximide or puromycin. Enhancement of interferon was obtained when cycloheximide was present before interferon levels in the normal production curve had reached their peak, but if added later the inhibitor decreased yields. In such cultures interferon was produced over a prolonged period rather than the normal production curve peaking at about 5 hours (Fig. 7). These data suggested that partial inhibition of protein synthesis inhibited the interferon regulatory (shutoff) function of the cells, and that regulatory event had occurred before production had reached its peak.

It was also reported that when rabbit kidney cell cultures were treated for only an early period and then protein synthesis inhibition reversed, interferon yields were greater than if inhibitor were present throughout (Tan et al., 1970). Also addition of actinomycin D to cultures before protein synthesis inhibition was reversed further enhanced interferon production. These data suggested that induced interferon messenger RNA, unable to translate in the presence of protein synthesis inhibitor, had accumulated during this period, and enhancement was due to a prevention of the synthesis of the messenger RNA for the purported repressor protein responsible for terminating translation of interferon message (Vilček, 1970a, b; Tan et al., 1970; Vilček, Rossman, and Varacalli, 1969; Vilček and Ng, 1971; Vilček and Varacalli, 1971; Ho, Tan, and Armstrong, 1972).

Such protein synthesis inhibitors as emetine, Streptoviracin A and pactamycin similarly enhanced interferon yields (Youngner, 1970; Vilček and Ng, 1971; Ke and Ho, 1971; Tan et al., 1971a), as did cordycepin (Vilček and Havell, 1973) and 5,6–dichloro-1-β-D-ribofuranosylbenzimidazole and neutral red (Sehgal, Tamm, and Vilček, 1975a, b; 1976a, b, c; Sehgal and Tamm, 1976; Tamm and Sehgal, 1977; Sehgal, Dobberstein, and Tamm, 1977; Wiranowska–Stewart, Chudzio, and Stewart II, 1977). "Superinduction" has also been observed in mouse cells (Tovey, Begon-Lours, and Gresser, 1974; Edy, Billiau, and Desomer, 1973).

Havell and Vilček (1972) showed that human fibroblast interferon could be produced in large quantities by employing "superinduction" techniques, and such procedures have come into wide use (Billiau, Joniau, and Desomer, 1973; Billiau et al., 1977 a; Vilček and Havell, 1973; Wiranowska–Stewart, Chudzio, and Stewart II, 1977; Section VI. C). In each system, the superinduction scheme established for poly rI·poly rC-induced rabbit kidney cells has proven generally applicable. The sequence of a treatment illustrated in Fig. 9 is typical of a superinduction scheme of human diploid skin fibroblast cultures induced with poly rI·poly rI·poly rC according to the methods designed by Havell and Vilček (1972). Cultures are induced with poly rI·poly rC containing cycloheximide at a concentration sufficient to inhibit protein synthesis greater than 95%. Cycloheximide remains in the culture medium for 6 hours after initiation of the induction, fresh medium is added to washed cultures and interferon rapidly begins to accumulate in the medium and synthesis continues for several hours. Interferon production phase in the FS-4 strain of human diploid cells has been found to be enhanced and continues for longer periods if they are incubated during this production phase at lowered temperatures (32° C instead of 37° C), presumably because the interferon messenger RNA was stabilized (Vilček and Havell, 1973). Relevant to this, Kojima and Yoshida (1974) suggested that enhanced interferon production in rabbit cell cultures at 25° C was due to inhibition of synthesis of the putative repressor protein at the lower temperature.

Ultraviolet-irradiation could be substituted for the metabolic inhibitor actinomycin D in the superinduction scheme in both rabbit and human cells (Mozes and Vilček, 1975; Mozes et al., 1974; Lindner-Frimmel, 1974), but control of dosage apparently prevents reliable results with this method (Stewart II, unpublished data).

Mozes and Vilček (1975) found that human diploid fibroblasts induced with Newcastle disease virus produced only little "early" interferon before 5 hours but produced a large "late" peak: irradiation "superinduced" the "early" interferon but inhibited the latter. However, it is important to note that irradiation of these cultures as late as 10 hours after viral induction produced an enhanced yield of interferon. These data suggest that superinduction schemes must be adjusted to take account of the kinetics of the different interferon lag periods with different inducers in various cell cultures (Section IV. A. 3). In this regard, it seems pertinent that certain cells not superinducible by the scheme in Fig. 9 (Edy et al., 1973) may have protracted induction lags (Fig. 7). It is tempting to speculate that the optimal kinetics of the superinduction scheme in primed cells will be different from that for unprimed cells, for as will be discussed in detail (Section X. C.) priming shortens this lag period in many cell cultures.

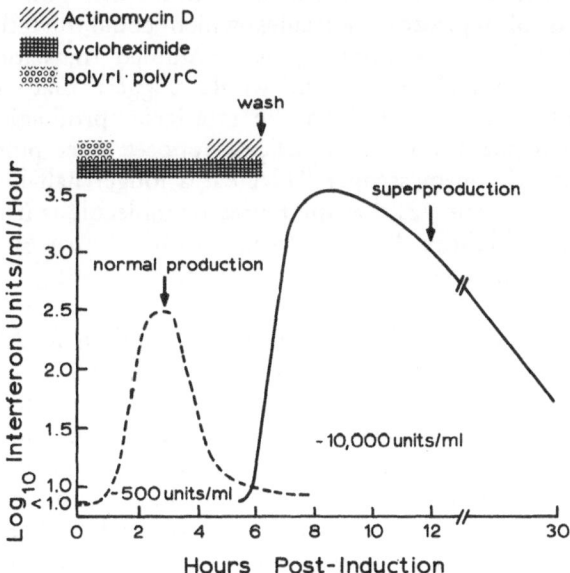

Fig. 9. Superproduction of interferon. The system illustrated is the human fibroblast method described by Havell and Vilček (1972)

On the basis of studies described, it can be hypothesized that, in those systems exhibiting an "early" (short-lag) interferon response to poly rI·poly rC (Fig. 7), the synthesis of interferon messenger RNA is largely complete within about 3 to 4 hours after inducer-cell contact, and superinduction suppresses a mechanism of post-transcriptional regulation. The evidence for this, outlined in the following Section, is becoming more convincing. If this regulation is truly post-transcriptional rather than acting on transcription (induction), then "superinduction" should actually be referred to as acting on the production phase, producing "superproduction".

b) Mechanisms of Superproduction

The model presented here for the so-called superinduction system for accentuation of interferon yields is based on the supposition that there are two distinct repression mechanisms controlling interferon production. One repression set controls *transcription* of interferon messenger RNA, and one terminates *translation* of this message once it is transcribed. To date most data suggest that the enhanced yields of interferon obtained by selective applications of anti-metabolites do not alter the derepression-repression constraint on transcription of interferon messenger RNA molecules but rather prolong interferon message functioning life-time. These data support the interpretation that so-called superinduction is actually superproduction. However, in some cases, as described below, *transcription* may also be increased, yielding a composite super[induction/production].

Previously, accentuations of production of tyrosine amino-transferase (TAT) by Actinomycin D had been described by Tomkins and his associates (1966) and was attributed to inhibition of synthesis of a new messenger RNA for the synthesis of repressor molecules which could directly interact with TAT-messenger RNA, thus inhibiting its continued translation. Analogy of this system to the interferon system would suggest that enhancement by metabolic inhibitors also worked on the interferon production phase rather than the induction phase. Such a model presupposes three points: (1) that the newly induced interferon-messenger RNA has a longer half-life than the messenger RNA for repressor, (2) that the repressor molecule is itself rapidly turning-over, (3) that inhibitors do not prevent normal return of the temporarily derepressed interferon gene to its repressed state.

i) Indirect Evidence: Metabolic Inhibitor Dose-Relations. Alternative explanations of "superinduction" phenomena could rationalize that enhancement is due to a decreased rate of degradation of intracellular interferon itself, or elimination of cellular messenger RNAs that would compete with interferon messenger RNA for available ribosomes (as reviewed by Havell, 1977). Recent studies have been directed at distinguishing which of these explanations is likely to apply in the interferon system. These studies have been pursued using alternative metabolic inhibitors (other than Actinomycin D) and by measuring, and attempting quantitation of, interferon messenger RNA.

In a thorough series of experiments Sehgal and his associates (1975a, b) used neutral red or chloroquine to inhibit intracellular protein degradation by lysosomal proteases, and found that both these agents enhanced interferon yields in poly rI·poly rC-induced human diploid fibroblasts. However, they also observed inhibition of cellular RNA and protein synthesis by these drugs, and by calculations from drug-dose plotted against percent of each effect observed, it appeared that enhanced interferon production was correlated with capacity of the drug to inhibit RNA and protein synthesis rather than with inhibition of protein degradation. Further, these investigators (Sehgal et al., 1976a) found similar correlations of effects of different dosages of actinomycin D and cycloheximide on superinduction with effects on cellular RNA and protein synthesis. Again, data suggest inhibition of protein synthesis (presumably repressor protein) was correlated with enhanced interferon production.

Sehgal and his colleagues (1975a) used the halogenated benzimidazole riboside 5,6-dichloro-1-β-ribofuranosylbenzimidazole (DRB) to study correlations of RNA synthesis inhibition and interferon accentuations, as this drug was found to specifically and reversibly inhibit the polymerase transcribing heterogeneous nuclear RNA molecules (hnRNA) presumed to become messenger RNA (Sehgal, Tamm, and Vilček, 1976a, b, c). DRB was able to enhance interferon yields if added at time of induction and maintained in the culture medium throughout the production. If added at later times (such as times optimal for addition of actinomycin D) DRB did not increase interferon production. These data suggest that the event responsible for early interferon shutoff in normal induced cells is triggered very soon after, or along with, the interferon message. These data also imply that the interferon messenger RNA is itself relatively resistant to inhibition by DRB while the repressor messenger RNA is relatively sensitive to DRB inhibition (Sehgal, Tamm, and Vilček, 1976c).

However, it was later suggested that DRB may on the one hand inhibit interferon messenger RNA synthesis by inhibiting transcriptase activity while on the other hand enhancing the transcription by increasing derepression (Sehgal et al., 1976c). Thus enhanced production of interferon in this case could be a true "superinduction" resulting from increased derepression. Or, alternatively, a marked superproduction could mask a marked inhibition of interferon message synthesis, with much more translation masking reduced amounts of message. Such alternatives can only be resolved by experiments on direct isolations and quantitations of interferon messenger RNA, as will be described below.

Cultures induced with poly rI·poly rC in the presence of DRB produce interferon for extended periods of time (Sehgal, Tamm, and Vilček, 1975a; 1976a, c; Tamm and Sehgal, 1977; Wiranowska–Stewart, Chudzio, and Stewart II, 1977), and removal of DRB from the medium at any time during this production rapidly terminates interferon production. Thus, both the process required for repression of interferon message *transcription* and the process for termination of interferon message *translation* seem to require new messenger RNA synthesis. These data further support the theory that interferon production is posttranscriptionally controlled.

The possibility that interferon synthesis termination was caused by production of competing cellular messenger RNAs was tested by adding actinomycin

D or DRB to cultures at the time when interferon production was beginning to terminate (Sehgal and Tamm, 1976). Presumably, if competing messages were thus inhibited, interferon message translation would begin to increase again. In fact, interferon synthesis under such conditions continued to decline, suggesting again that the most likely explanation of enhanced interferon production by superinduction/production is that interferon production is normally terminated by an early-induced regulation mechanism which operates by inactivation of interferon messenger RNA and induction of this inactivation process is prevented by the metabolic inhibitors.

ii) Direct Evidence: Quantitation of Extractable Interferon Messenger RNA. As the shutoff of interferon induction appears to be attributable to irreversible inactivation of interferon messenger RNA (Sehgal and Tamm, 1976; Kohase and Vilček, 1977), accentuation of production of interferon by inhibition of such a repression mechanism would imply an increased functional stability of the interferon messenger RNA, as hypothesized by Vilček and Havell (1973). Indirect studies employing inhibitors suggested that the shutoff mechanism is initiated within an hour of addition of interferon inducer (in human fibroblasts; Sehgal, Tamm, and Vilček, 1975; 1976a). These data indicate that the half-life of interferon messenger RNA would normally be about 12 hours but that of the repressor message would be only 3 to 4 hrs.

A more direct approach to proof of the translation repressor hypothesis for superproduction has been attempted by several investigators employing techniques for quantitation of extractable interferon messenger RNA. These experiments have so far only quantitated message for interferon in terms of ability to translate biological activity. Truly direct proof of a translational repressor must await isolation and assay of the repressor molecule itself.

Raj and Pitha (1977) reported that while the amount of interferon synthesized in human fibroblasts induced by poly rI·poly rC in „superinduced" cells was markedly increased over that produced in normally induced cells, the measurable amount of interferon messenger RNA as assayed by translation in the *Xenopus* oöcyte system was only slightly higher in extracts from the former system. These data suggested that no quantitative difference in translatable message was present in the presence of inhibitors. However, when compared in the wheat germ cell-free system, the message prepared from cells induced with poly rI·poly rC alone was inactive while that from superproducing cells was active.

Sehgal and his colleagues (1977), on the other hand, reported that the amount of interferon messenger RNA extractable in active form (translatable in oöcytes) from poly rI·poly rC-induced human fibroblasts was significantly higher at about 6 hours after induction in superproducing cells than in cells induced with poly rI·poly rC alone. These data support the interpretation that the shutoff of interferon production involves post-transcriptional inactivation or degradation of interferon messenger RNA. The linear relationship between the amount of messenger RNA injected into oöcytes and the interferon yields obtained suggest that the oöcyte translation correctly reflects the amount of message.

Similar data to those of Sehgal, Dobberstein, and Tamm (1977) were presented by Cavalieri *et al.* (1977a) who also found that the amount of translatable interferon message extractable at about 3 to 4 hours post-induction in superproducing cultures (the shutoff period in normal production curve) was significantly higher than in cells induced with poly rI·poly rC alone. As found by Sehgal, Dobberstein, and Tamm (1977) with message preparations obtained in "shutoff phase" extracts, mixing experiments with "early" messenger RNA and "late" message did not reveal any inhibitory molecules. These authors also reported that cycloheximide alone both prolonged *transcription* of interferon messenger RNA to about 3 hours and decreased rate of message inactivation, increasing its half-life from about 18 minutes to 49 minutes. Actinomycin additionally prolonged message half-life to about 68 minutes. These data suggest that the accentuation of interferon yields by metabolic inhibitors, depending on type of inhibitor and time of its addition, can result from both *superinduction* (i. e., increased *transcription* of interferon messenger RNA) *and superproduction* (i. e., increased *translation* of interferon messenger RNA).

3. Regulatory Mechanisms on Interferon Production: The Refractory State in vitro (Hyporesponsiveness and Blocking)

Several early publications reported that chick chorioallantoic membranes could be repeatedly stimulated to produce second yields of interferon (Lindenmann, Burke, and Isaacs, 1957; Burke and Isaacs, 1958b; Isaacs, 1959c), often second inductions yielding even more interferon than the first (Isaacs, 1959c; Isaacs and Burke, 1958). Isaacs and Westwood (1959b) reported that rabbit kidney cells could be stimulated to produce interferon by inactivated influenza virus, and a week later the same cultures could be re-induced to produce a new "crop" of interferon. These reports gave the impression that once cultures quit producing interferon after the first induction they could be repeatedly stimulated to produce more interferon, suggesting that interferon shutoff was merely a depletion of inducer. This was not found to be a generally applicable situation, however, for in most cases, first induction of interferon is followed by a period of refractoriness to repeated interferon induction during which time repeated exposure to inducer yields little or no interferon (Cantell and Paucker, 1963a; Burke and Buchan, 1965; Paucker and Golgher, 1969; Paucker *et al.*, 1970; Vilček and Rada, 1962; Vilček, 1962; Paucker and Boxaca, 1967; Stancek and Vilček, 1965; Lockart, 1963; Friedman, 1966a; Bausek and Merigan, 1970b; Youngner and Hallum, 1969; Stewart II, Gosser, and Lockart, 1971b; Lobodzinska, Biernacka, and Skurska, 1975; Oie *et al.*, 1975; Paucker, 1963). This period of hyporesponsiveness has been observed both in cell cultures and in animals, and apparently can be mediated by several mechanisms. The *in vivo* tolerance to repeated inductions will be discussed below (Section VI. B. 2). The *in vitro* refractory state seems to be mediated by a complex of mechanisms, associated with the normal posttranscriptional shutoff mechanism induced along with the interferon messenger RNA itself, and at least partially mediated by interferon itself, or perhaps a product produced along with interferon or induced by interferon itself. For the present discussion I shall refer to these regulations as "*in vitro* hyporesponsiveness" and those clearly involving interferon as "blocking".

Vilček (1962) and Vilček and Rada (1962) found that contact of chick cells with interferon blocked the ability of tick-borne encephalitis virus to induce interferon, presumably because the virus was unable to perform events required for induction. Paucker (1963) reported that when L cells were exposed to a second stimulation with inactivated Newcastle disease virus 25 hours after the first such exposure, they made no interferon. Interferon pretreatment had similar effects. The interpretation that this "blocking" of interferon production resulted from prevention of virus from performing viral functions responsible for initiation of interferon production (Declercq and Merigan, 1970a; Bausek and Merigan, 1970b), became seriously doubtful after it was found that interferon responses induced by poly rI·poly rC were also inhibited in interferon-treated cells (Youngner and Hallum, 1969; Stewart II, Gosser, and Lockart, 1971b; Golgher and Paucker, 1973; Rousset, 1974; Barmak and Vilček, 1973).

Several hours exposure of cells to interferon were required for cells to become "blocked" (Paucker and Boxaca, 1967; Stewart II, Gosser, and Lockart, 1971b; Barmak and Vilček, 1973; Rousset, 1974; Lobodzinska, Biernacka, and Skurska, 1975) and during this exposure, protein synthesis was required for "blocking" to develop, suggesting that "blocking" was an interferon-induced control mechanism on interferon production (Stewart II, Gosser, and Lockart, 1971b; Barmak and Vilček, 1973). Alternative interpretations for the mechanisms of interferon "blocking" have been suggested (Paucker and Boxaca, 1967; Golgher and Paucker, 1973; Kleinschmidt, 1972; Soloviev *et al.*, 1974; Rousset, Fournier, and Chany, 1970) but so far none of these can account for the diversity of effects observed in the complex systems.

Paucker and Boxaca (1967) suggested that "blocking" was due to a " repressor" molecule induced by interferon, presumably similar to the "blocker" reported earlier by Isaacs and his colleagues (1966), or the "enhancer" described by Kato and Eggers (1969b). It has been suggested repeatedly that the antiviral and "blocking" components in the interferon preparations can be separated physically (Paucker and Boxaca, 1967; Borden and Murphy, 1971; Borden *et al.*, 1975) or that interferon preparations could be enriched for "blocking" factor by collection at different intervals after induction (Borden and Murphy, 1971; Chadha *et al.*, 1974). However, the reported chromatographic separability now seems unlikely (Paucker and Golgher, 1970; Golgher and Paucker, 1973; Stewart II, Gosser, and Lockart, 1971b; Stewart II and Declercq, 1973; Rousset, 1974), and the claimed enrichments for "blocking" activity unit/antiviral activity unit of interferon preparations should be interpreted with caution as the differences reported are trivial (Borden and Murphy, 1971; Chadha *et al.*, 1974; Borden *et al.*, 1975). This blocking factor has been referred to as "refractoriness-inducing principle (RIP)" which was called one of the "extracellular acid-soluble cell products (EASCP)" induced by Newcastle disease virus in L cells (Chadha *et al.*, 1974; Borden *et al.*, 1975); it seems preliminary to assume these activity-measurements are separable principles from interferon.

It is conceivable that interferon induces a regulatory factor (protein?) which is responsible for degrading interferon messenger RNA, and viral RNAs, and that more of this factor is itself present in interferon preparations harvested later after interferon-induction. This interpretation would place interferon refractoriness at the posttranscriptional level of regulation. However, other data suggest that refractoriness may involve transcriptional regulation as well. Vilček, Barmak and Havell (1972) found that hyporesponsiveness to secondary induction with poly rI·poly rC in rabbit cell cultures could be overcome by addition of DEAE-dextran, suggesting hyporeactivity was related to poor uptake of the inducer. Here again, it could be argued that the interferon-induced refractory factor was merely degrading the inducer and that this was prevented by the DEAE-dextran.

Paucker (1963) reported that the hyporesponsive period following primary induction by Newcastle disease virus or treatment with interferon was relatively short, production potential being fully regained within one to two cell divisions, whereas loss of virus resistance was significantly slower. However, Chany and Vignal (1968) reported that hyporesponsiveness persisted as long as the antiviral state. Billiau (1970) reported that after a dose of poly rI·poly rC or single-stranded RNA inducer, rabbit kidney cells were hyporesponsive for about 3 days.

A few systems have been reported wherein hyporesponsiveness to repeated inductions did not occur. Chany and Vignal (1968) reported a line of mouse embryo fibroblasts transformed with Moloney sarcoma virus which could be repeatedly stimulated by Newcastle disease virus to produce interferon quantities at the same level as produced by the first induction. These cells were completely resistant to mouse interferon (confirmed by Stewart II, unpublished data), suggesting again that "blocking" is related to an interferon-induced factor, perhaps that involved in viral and interferon message inactivations. Others have reported that virus resistance and interferon hyporesponsiveness did not correlate, and that both primary rabbit kidney cell cultures and L cell cultures could be repeatedly stimulated to produce interferon in response to poly rI·poly rC (Margolis, Oie, and Levy, 1971). Stewart II, Gosser, and Lockart (1971b) reported that L cells became hyporesponsive after induction by Newcastle disease virus or poly rI·poly rC; primary cultures of mouse kidney cells could not be restimulated by Newcastle disease virus after a primary induction by either this virus or poly rI·poly rC, but these cultures could be repeatedly stimulated by poly rI·poly rC. These data suggested that different cell populations might produce interferon in response to the different inducers, and passage of these cultures produced cultures able to produce interferon when induced by virus but not by poly rI·poly rC. Hyporesponsiveness might be overcome in some systems by use of inducers of different natures. Yershov, Tazulakhova, and Novokhatsky (1976) have claimed that chick cell cultures became hyporesponsive to induction by a second dose of poly rI·poly rC but could be stimulated by Venezuelan equine encephalomyelitis virus after poly rI·poly rC.

Breinig, Armstrong, and Ho (1975) reported that while repeated exposure to poly rI·poly rC led to hyporesponsiveness in primary rabbit kidney cell cultures, interferon itself, even at very high doses (about 100,000 units), did not produce hyporesponsiveness. The reasons for this discrepancy with the results of Billiau (1970) and Barmak and Vilček (1973), which both reported that even modest doses of interferon induced hyporesponsiveness to induction by poly rI·poly rC in primary rabbit kidney cultures is not clear.

Kohase and Vilček (1977) recently reported that exposure of human fibroblast cultures to low doses (2 μg) of poly rI·poly rC induced a peak interferon response by about 3 to 4 hours which was shutoff by 6 hours. Reinduction with high doses (50 μg) of poly rI·poly rC before this shutoff did not prevent the first shutoff, but produced a second interferon peak at about 8 to 10 hours. In fact, a single exposure of cultures to the high poly rI·poly rC dose produced an early and a late peak of interferon. Other authors have also reported that human skin fibroblasts could be repeatedly induced by exposure to double-stranded RNA (Billiau, Van den Berghe, and Desomer, 1972).

Thus it seems that hyporesponsiveness to repeated induction at the cellular level may be mediated: (1) by interferon, or (2) by a regulator induced along with interferon, or (3) by a regulator induced by interferon; this regulatory mechanism may also be involved in the antiviral mechanism. Hyporesponsiveness may or may not develop in cells, depending on type of inducers used for primary or secondary stimulus, the dose of the inducer, time of addition of inducer, amount of interferon induced by the initial inducer, the sensitivity of the cells to the interferon induced, the types of cells in the cultures, and other less well-defined factors. Some authors have even imagined that making structural modifications of poly rI·poly rC could somehow circumvent the hyporesponsiveness to repeated stimulation (O'Malley et al., 1975 b). Such is the general state of understanding of why cells decide to quit making interferon and to not make it again for awhile.

It is interesting that interferon may itself be the communication between cells to tell them to quit making interferon, for, as will be described later (Section X) interferon can also spread the message for cells to make more interferon and to make it sooner (priming).

The selective use of metabolic inhibitors used for "superproduction" likely interfere with the development of antiviral resistance mechanism in the cells producing interferon, as these inhibitors act to accentuate interferon yields, apparently by aborting the interferon regulatory shutoff mechanism. It will likely be necessary to isolate this regulatory factor and develop in vitro assays for it before we can resolve whether the factors involved are separate or identical.

4. Posttranslational Processing of Interferons

The interaction of inducer with cell thus proceeds to derepression of genes coding for interferon messenger RNA which is translated and then degraded. Meanwhile, the translation product itself must be processed to become interferon. This posttranslational processing may require proteolytic cleavage of a pre-, or pro-, interferon and it apparently acquires extensive carbohydrate additions before it is secreted from the cells as the glycoprotein interferon.

a) Interferon Precursor?

The idea cannot yet be dismissed that interferon precursor is normally present in cells and that the protein synthesis required for interferon production is not de novo interferon structural protein but is rather the enzyme responsible for this proteolytic conversion of an inactive precursor to an active form, interferon. Little data is available to support this contention, but German, Quero, and Poindron (1971) reported that non-interfering extracts partially purified from uninfected fertile egg allantoic fluid ellicited the production of antibodies to chick interferon and suggested there may be an inactive precursor to interferon present in all cells capable of synthesizing the inhibitor.

Even if the structural polypeptide for interferon were synthesized *de novo* following induction, it could be translated into a larger precursor such as occurs with secretory polypeptide hormones, which must be proteolytically degraded for transport. Experiments with highly purified anti-interferon globulins used to precipitate interferon-producing polyribosomes should provide information about these possibilities. It should also be recalled that Pestka *et al.* (1977) suggested that interferon became activated *after* it was translated in a cell-free system.

b) Glycosylation of Interferon Proteins

Intracellular interferon was first reported by Isaacs and Lindenmann (1957) and later by others (Vilček, 1960; Cantell and Paucker, 1963a). It was not possible to determine whether this was merely contaminating extracellular interferon. In L cell cultures, in which extracellular interferon was not observed until 7 to 8 hours after induction by Newcastle disease virus, intracellular interferon was also not detectable until after 7 hours postinduction (Lancz and Johnson, 1969), suggesting that interferon was not activated until shortly before release or was not synthesized until late in the induction-production phase.

Tan and his associates (1971b) studied the kinetics of production and release of intracellular interferon in primary rabbit kidney cell cultures induced by poly rI·poly rC and claimed that both intracellular and extracellular interferon had the same molecular weight and heat stability. They showed that intracellular interferon was detectable about 20 minutes before its extracellular appearance; therefore, interferon was not activated only on release, but "release" was a time-dependent separate process. A large proportion of the cell-associated interferon was in the soluble cytoplasmic sap, but some interferon was sedimented in association with ribosomes, polysomes and membrane and nuclear fractions. This association was not due to non-specific binding, as addition of soluble interferon to normal cell extracts did not sediment.

Field *et al.* (1972a) also reported that intracellular interferon and extracellular interferon from poly rI·poly rC induced rabbit kidney cells were similar in trypsin sensitivity and "species-specificity", and again suggested release was a separate, active process from synthesis.

Ng, Berman, and Vilcek (1972) found that intracellular interferon in poly rI·poly rC-induced rabbit kidney cells was detectable about 30 minutes before extracellular interferon. The intracellular interferon was "species specific", however, most of the intracellular interferon was associated with cellular membranes, and interestingly, was completely resistant to digestion by trypsin. These authors suggested that the addition of carbohydrate moieties to interferon protein takes place within membranous structures prior to excretion.

The intracellular interferon induced in human fibroblasts by poly rI·poly rC was also reported by Falcoff et al. (1976) to be associated with membrane fractions and to be trypsin resistant.

Havell and his colleagues (1975 b) added the glycosylation inhibitors 2-deoxy-D-glucose or D-glucosamine to poly rI·poly rC-induced human diploid fibroblast cultures and found a dose-dependent inhibition of interferon production, both intra- and extracellular interferon, suggesting that synthesis of active interferon, not its secretion, was inhibited. These authors reported that the interferon produced in presence of partially inhibitory concentrations of glycosylation inhibitors was more heat-labile than control interferon and was less efficiently neutralized by anti-interferon antibody. However, as will be described later (Section VII) others have found that carbohydrate components apparently have little, if any, involvement in the antigenic recognition of this or other interferons.

Recently Havell, Yamazaki, and Vilček (1977) subjected the residual levels of interferon produced in the human diploid fibroblasts in the presence of glycosylation inhibitors to electrophoresis in SDS-polyacrylamide gels and found that a portion of this interferon was significantly smaller (about 16,000 daltons) than the native interferon (about 21,000 daltons). Stewart II and his associates (1978) found that mouse L cells produce nearly normal amounts of antiviral protein in the presence of D-glucosamine; however, the antiviral factor produced was significantly smaller (about 16,000 daltons) than interferons produced under normal glycosylating condition (about 38,000 and 22,000 daltons) and thus referred to this protein as an "interferoid" (discussed in detail in Section VII).

Thus, after translation, interferon proteins are apparently processed in membrane structures where they are embellished with carbohydrates.

c) Secretion of Interferons

The first suggestion that interferonogenesis was associated with secretory structures was by Khesin, Voronina, and Amchenkova (1970), who suggested that the lysosome apparatus of the cell participated in this process, as they observed that during interferon formation by mouse macrophages, Gomori-positive vacuoles formed and broke-off into the culture medium concurrent with extracellular interferon appearance.

The active process involved in release has been evidenced by the finding that release of interferon from induced cells was completely inhibited at 4° C, despite presence of high concentrations of intracellular interferon (Tan, Armstrong, and Ho, 1971 b; Field et al., 1972 a). Tan, Jeng, and Ho (1972) found that while exposure of induced rabbit cells to emetine stopped interferon synthesis it did not affect release of interferon; though such release could be blocked by cyanide or p-hydroxymercuribenzoate; the inhibition of release by cyanide suggests its dependence on an energy generating system, while the latter suggests involvement of SH-group-containing enzymatic processes in interferon transport.

Kohno *et al.* (1971) reported that phospholipase C efficiently inhibited the release of interferon, indicating involvement of cellular membrane in the processing of interferon, and Havell and Vilček (1975) found that the plant alkaloid vinblastine, which causes disaggregation of micro-tubule structures, caused a preferential inhibition of interferon secretion. Colchicine, however, even in high concentration was ineffective in inhibiting the release process.

In summary, it appears that once interferon-polypeptides are translated, or even while they are being translated on membrane-bound polysomes, they are discharged into the protective lumina of the rough endoplasmic reticulum where they are glycosylated during passage through the intracellular membrane-delineated structures, to be released into the extracellular environment as "mature" interferon glycoproteins, ready to turn-on the nearest receptive individual cell.

B. Interferon Production at the Organism Level

As we turn from the cellular system to the multicellular organism involved in production of interferon during a viral disease, I shall attempt to sort out this complexity by describing a number of *in vivo* interferon production systems that have been reported, indicating distribution of the interferons. This will be followed by evidence defining the possible cellular sources of the interferons produced.

1. Interferon Production in vivo

a) Production of Interferon in Viral Infections

Baron and Buckler (1963) were the first to report systemic induction of high titered circulating interferon. Chick embryos had been used previously (Wagner, 1960) but the site of interferon synthesis in this system would be difficult to ascertain, particularly as the chorion and amnion produce interferon themselves (Lindenmann, Burke, and Isaacs, 1957; Burke and Isaacs, 1958 b).

In many virus infections interferon production is highest in the target tissues. Thus interferon has been demonstrated in lungs of mice infected with influenza (Isaacs and Hitchcock, 1960; Sawicki, 1961; Link, Blaskovic, and Raus, 1963, 1965; Pollikoff, Lieberman, and Lem, 1965) and parainfluenza viruses (Craighead, 1966). Interferon is produced in the brain of mice infected with numerous encephalitogenic arboviruses (Hitchcock and Porterfield, 1961; Vainio, Gwatkin, and Koprowski, 1961; Vilček and Stanček, 1963 a; Finter, 1964 b, 1965; Tongaonkar and Ghosh, 1973; Bardos and Sefcovicova, 1966), in human cases of St. Louis and Western equine encephalitis (Luby *et al.*, 1969; Luby, Sanders, and Sulkin, 1971), and in hamsters with rabies (Stewart II and Sulkin, 1966). Gresser and Naficy (1964) reported that specimens of cerebrospinal fluid from many patients with infectious and non-infectious disease of the central nervous system contained interferons. Degre and his collaborators (1976) reported interferon in cerebrospinal fluids of patients with multiple sclerosis and acute encephalitis.

Interferon can also often be found at local inoculation sites, such as: in brains of mice inoculated intracerebrally with vaccinia virus (Verlinde and Dret, 1963), Newcastle disease virus (Blach–Olszewska, and Skurska, 1974) or herpes simplex virus (Bostandzhyan and Bikbulatov, 1967); in lungs of mice inoculated intranasally with vaccinia virus (Link *et al.*, 1965), respiratory syncytial virus (Grodnitskaya and Dreizen, 1975) or influenza virus (Singer *et al.*, 1973); in the skin of rabbits or mice infected with herpes simplex virus (Force, Stewart, and Haff, 1965; Sydiskis and Schultz, 1966); guinea pigs (Friedman and Baron, 1961) and humans (Wheelock, 1964) inoculated intradermally with vaccinia virus; in liver of mice injected intra-peritoneally with mouse hepatitis virus (Malucci, 1964); in wings of chickens injected with Rous sarcoma virus (Force and Stewart, 1966), or in fetal tissues of pregnant monkeys receiving intrauterine injection of Chikungunya virus (Barbosa *et al.*, 1974).

Several studies have followed the distribution of interferon and virus in various tissues at different times during pathogenesis. Most of these showed correlation of tissue levels of interferon with virus levels. Vilček and Stancek (1963 a) found high levels of interferon and virus in brain tissue of mice inoculated intraperitoneally with tick-borne encephalitis virus, but not appreciable amounts in blood, spleen, liver, pancreas, kidneys or lymph nodes. Stewart II and Sulkin (1966) found that hamsters inoculated intramuscularly with rabies virus developed high levels of interferon in the brain as virus reached its peak in that tissue, and lower levels of interferon in peripheral tissues later in the disease, paralleling the spread of virus to these tissues. Interferon and virus levels in brain and other tissue also corresponded in mice infected with West Nile virus (Subrahmanyan and Mims, 1966), whereas in adult mice infected with Coxsackie B 1 virus, virus and interferon levels were higher in kidneys, liver and spleen than in brain (Heineberg, Gold, and Robbins, 1964).

Highest levels of interferon usually coincide with highest levels of virus in that location. However, many viruses may produce circulating interferon as a consequence of either virus – or interferon – spillover from replication sites in primary or secondary foci of infections or may induce interferon in the blood stream directly during viremia (Reyes and Lerner, 1976; Rollag and Degre, 1976; Berensci, Beladi, and Juhasz, 1974). Baron and Buckler (1963) found that direct intravenous injection of high doses of Newcastle disease virus, Sindbis, Sendai or vaccinia virus induced circulating interferon within an hour in mice and peak production was reached within a few hours. A great number of other virus-animal systems produced similar results (Baron *et al.*, 1966 a, b; Kono and Ho, 1965; Van Rossum and Desomer, 1966; Campbell and Colter, 1967; Youngner and Stinebring, 1965; Hellmann and Kohlhage, 1973 a, b; DeMaeyer, DeMaeyer–Guignard, and Bailey, 1975; Jameson, 1977). The highest titer of circulating interferon yet found (or any other *in vivo* interferon level for that matter) was recently reported to be induced by intravenous injection of Bluetongue virus in mouse, yielding titers of over 10^5 units/ml of serum (Jameson and Grossberg, 1977).

Interferon can also be found in peritoneal washes of animals inoculated with viruses intraperitoneally (Lackovic and Borecky, 1965; Borecky and Lakkovic, 1967), with interferon also being produced in blood circulation following similar inoculation route (Rathova et al., 1975). Even following intravenous inoculation with virus, interferon in circulation may originate elsewhere, as spleen interferon levels are often significantly higher than serum levels (Desomer and Billiau, 1966; Van Rossum and Desomer, 1966; Borecky and Lackovic, 1966).

Local production of interferon can be assigned to specific cell types in the case of certain locally limited infections. Interferon has been found in ocular tissue from eye infections with herpes simplex virus (Oh, 1970). Gresser and Dull (1964) found interferon in pharyngeal washing from patients with acute influenza. Nasal interferon has been collected from nose-washings following intranasal infections of volunteers with influenza viruses (Jao, Wheelock, and Jackson, 1965; Smorodintsev et al., 1971a, b; Murphy et al., 1973, 1975; Danielescu et al., 1975; Stanley et al., 1976; Richman et al., 1976). Others reported nasal interferon production in volunteers infected intranasally with rhinovirus 21 (Gatmaitan et al., 1973; Panusarn et al., 1974) or rhinovirus 13 (Douglas and Betts, 1974).

Interferon is also produced in nasal secretions of calves after intranasal administration of infectious bovine rhinotracheitis virus (Todd, Volenec, and Paton, 1972; Fulton and Rosenquist, 1976b).

It should be mentioned also that interferon is not always formed, at least in detectable levels, during viral infections. As noted previously, however (Section II. A. 6) many agents previously presumed to not induce interferons have now been found to do so. Interferon was reported as not detectable in serum samples of acute phase of transfusion-associated hepatitis (Hill, Walsh, and Purcell, 1971), and the slow virus infection, scrapies, failed to induce interferon (Katz and Koprowski, 1968). In view of the recent demonstrations that anti-interferon globulins can accelerate pathogenesis of certain virus diseases (Section XI), it would be very interesting to see what effect anti-interferon serum might have on the course of such diseases. In systemic infections it is more difficult to determine which cells are responsible for interferon production, as will be discussed below.

b) Non-Viral Interferon Inducers in vivo

In contrast to many of the viral inducers which may replicate in selected tissues and induce interferon in these active target-tissue areas, the non-replicating non-viral inducers afford somewhat more definable systems for studies on interferon origins in vivo.

When animals are injected intravenously with several bacteria or bacterial endotoxins, interferon rapidly appears, peaks in about two hours and rapidly disappears (Fig. 7; Section IV. A. 3; Youngner and Stinebring, 1964, 1965; Ho, 1964; Desomer and Billiau, 1966; Ho et al., 1970; Kato, Nakashima, and Ohta, 1975; Talash et al., 1974; Talas et al., 1973; Giron et al., 1973b; Rathova, Kociskova, and Borecky, 1974). Large amounts of interferon are produced by the spleen (Desomer and Billiau, 1966; Declercq, Nuwer and Merigan, 1970a; Borecky and Lackovic, 1966).

Oh (1966) found interferon in serum, ocular aqueous humor, urine and cerebrospinal fluid of rabbits injected intravenously with typhoid endotoxin, though much higher levels were in serum than in other fluid, suggesting its production in the former and passage into the latter. *Bordetella pertusis* was able to induce interferon in mice serum and spleen when inoculated intravenously but not intraperitoneally (Borecky and Lackovic, 1967). However, Degre, and Dahl (1971) found serum interferon in mice inoculated intraperitoneally with a mixed bacterial vaccine, and Feingold, Keleti, and Youngner (1976) found circulating interferon after intraperitoneal inoculations of mice with *Brucella abortus*, or "BRU-PEL". Circulating interferon was also found in children with *Hemophilus influenzae* meningitis and bacteremia (Michaels, Weinberger, and Ho, 1965; Ho, 1967).

The reports on differential kinetics of production and effects of protein synthesis inhibitors on endotoxin-induced and virus-induced interferons (Section IV A) led to the designations of "endotoxin-type" and "virus-type" interferons (Youngner, Stinebring, and Taube, 1965; Ke *et al.*, 1966). In the former induction, inhibitors sometimes enhanced and prolonged interferon production (Youngner, 1970), while inhibiting the interferon production by the latter inducers. While the response of most animals to inoculations with most bacteria or bacterial products is characteristically only a few hundred units of interferon, peaking at about 1 to 3 hours (Merigan, 1973), the ether-extracted preparation from *Brucella abortus* (Youngner, Keleti, and Feingold, 1974), "Bru-Pel", given intravenously or intraperitoneally induced interferon levels comparable to those induced by viruses (several thousand units/ml serum), and the interferon was produced with "virus-like" interferon kinetics, peaking at about 6 to 9 hours (Feingold, Keleti, and Youngner, 1976; Kern *et al.*, 1976); thus the designations of "endotoxin-type" and "virus-type" responses become increasingly less meaningful.

Polyribonucleotide double-stranded inducers were found to induce an early "endotoxin-type" interferon response in animals (Section IV A 3). However, Field *et al.* (1970) found peaks of interferon at 12 to 48 hours after intravenous injection of poly rI·poly rC in man, but interferon levels were very low (10 to 30 units/ml). After intravenous injection in rabbits or mice, poly rI·poly rC rapidly induced high levels of serum interferon, but only low levels of brain and cerebrospinal fluid interferon (Cathala and Baron, 1970; Stringfellow, Overall, and Glasgow, 1974a, b), while local (intracerebral) injection of poly rI·poly rC gave higher brain interferon levels. Similar early productions of circulating interferons were observed in rabbits and mice inoculated with poly rI·poly rC or polyriboguanylic acid·polyribocytidylic acid (Vilner *et al.*, 1976; Matsuda *et al.*, 1971; Sharpe, Birch, and Planterose, 1971; Yokota *et al.*, 1975a, b) or bacteriophage- or mycophage-derived double-stranded RNAs (Borecky *et al.*, 1975; Declercq, 1974), either intravenously or intraperitoneally (Buckler *et al.*, 1971; Tazulakhova, Novokhatsky, and Yershov, 1973), or in cattle injected with poly rI·poly rC (McVicar *et al.*, 1973).

Interestingly, polyribonucleotide double-strands, though inducing early interferon, induced levels in some animals comparable to those induced by viruses; thus at least certain "early"-responding cells producing interferon are, unlike those producing early responses to bacterial products, able to produce high levels of interferons.

Levy, Duenwald, and Buckler (1973) showed that intraperitoneal injection of chlorite-oxidized amylose (COAM) into mice or cats increased the titers of serum interferon induced by intraperitoneally injected poly rI·poly rC (or Newcastle disease virus). The mechanism for this effect is obscure. However, complexing poly rI·poly rC to poly-L-lysine enabled the double-stranded RNA to induce circulating interferons in chimpanzees, in which poly rI·poly rC alone could not induce (Purcell et al., 1976), presumably by protecting it from hydrolytic activity of the primate serum (Levy et al., 1975). Mecs, Ganti, and Kotai (1976) found that intraperitoneal inoculation of mice with poly rI·poly rC and a polycationic modified polypeptide, poly-DMAE-glutamine, produced enhanced serum interferon levels. Magee and Griffith (1972) found interferon in livers of rats after intravenous injection with poly rI·poly rC, the livers releasing interferon after being placed in a perfusion apparatus. Tilles and Braun (1973) also found that poly rI·poly rC induced interferon in perfused rat-lung cultures whereas endotoxin or pyran copolymer did not.

In an imaginative approach to delivery of intact inducer, Straub, Garry, and Magee (1974) showed that enclosure of poly rI·poly rC in phospholipid particles greatly potentiated and extended its interferon inducing activity in mice.

Mayer et al. (1976) followed the distribution of radioactive double-stranded RNA in mice after intraperitoneal administration and found large portions of the undegraded inoculum in the blood stream and correspondingly decreasing levels of interferon and inducer in liver, brain and spleen, respectively. Olsen et al. (1976) reported that peak interferon induction by poly-L-lysine-complexed poly rI·poly rC in mice was both increased in titer and significantly prolonged. Similar results were observed in monkeys injected intravenously with poly rI·poly rC · poly-L-lysine in carboxymethylcellulose (Levy et al., 1976; Sammons et al., 1977).

Guggenheim and Baron (1977) reported treatment of virus-infected children with intravenous injections of 0.1 to 1.0 mg/kg poly rI·poly rC. Peak titers of interferon in serum were discouragingly low, ranging from 8 to 500 units/ml during the first 24 hour-period; the half-life of the inducer was less than half an hour. They found a poor correlation between dose of poly rI·poly rC (mg/kg) and interferon induction, possible related to drug breakdown.

Local induction of interferon by poly rI·poly rC was observed in nasal secretions following intranasal application (Hill et al., 1971). Similarly, Statolon was able to induce lung interferon when given intranasally (Kleinschmidt and Streightoff, 1971). Though neither interferon nor poly rI·poly rC efficiently cross the blood-brain barrier (Habif et al., 1975; Declercq et al., 1975; Cathala and Baron, 1970), direct injection of poly rI·poly rC in the central nervous system has been reported to induce high levels of local interferon (Cathala and Baron, 1970).

In a recent report by Cornell et al. (1977), all patients injected with more than 1 mg/kg of particular lot of poly rI·poly rC, intravenously, had detectable serum interferon within the first 12 hours, with a mean peak titer of 85 units/ml. However, *none* of the patients receiving similar doses of a different poly rI·poly rC lot produced detectable interferon. The latter lot of poly rI·poly rC was also less effective in inducing antiviral activity in human fibroblast cultures and had a melting point 10 degrees lower than the other lot. In another study, the unreliability of different lots of poly rI·poly rC to induce interferon in 24 patients was reported. Serum interferon levels were formed between 4 and 24 hours. Again, differences were apparent in ability of the poly rI·poly rC lots to induce interferon (Freeman *et al.*, 1977). McIntyre *et al.* (1977) administered 300 mg of poly rI·poly rC/m^2 intravenously to patients and found "significant" serum interferon levels in 28/33 patients (mean level of 41 units/ml). Borecky (1977) recently reviewed his and his associates' preliminary studies in man with double-stranded RNA interferon-inducers and concluded that due mainly to toxicological considerations, attempts to exploit interferon-stimulating potentials of such inducers in man should be limited to studies in localized diseases of skin and eyes (Buchwald, Borecky, and Doskocil, 1975).

Tilorone hydrochloride in a single intragastric dose in mice lead to production of interferon (Mayer and Krueger, 1970), which was demonstrable in brain and serum (Fornosi, Talas, and Weiszfeller, 1971; Barker, Rheins, and Wilson, 1971) but induced no interferon in chickens (Portnoy and Merigan, 1971) or man (Kaufman *et al.*, 1971). In mice, serum interferon was produced between about 8 and 40 hours after ingestion of Tilorone or after its intraperitoneal inoculation in dosages of 250 mg/kg and 75 mg/kg, respectively (Declercq and Merigan, 1971a; Stringfellow and Glasgow, 1972a, b), with interferon reaching levels of about 10^4 units/ml of serum; similar results were obtained following subcutaneous injection. Glaz and Talas (1973) reported that low serum interferon levels could be maintained for several weeks in mice during continual tilorone ingestion in drinking water. In view of its high activity as an interferon inducer by various routes *in vivo* it is somewhat surprising that tilorone is inactive in cell cultures.

U-25, 166 induces high levels of serum interferon in mice (Nichols, Weed and Underwood, 1976; Stringfellow, 1977a) and in cats (Stringfellow and Weed, 1977), levels of interferon remaining high from about 4 to 14 hours after a single oral dose of 200 to 1000 mg/kg. Little, if any, interferon was produced in lung or liver, and high levels were produced in spleen and thymus. Only low levels of interferon were induced by subcutaneous administration of U-25, 166 (Stringfellow and Weed, 1977).

BL-20803, i. e., 4 (3-dimethylamino-propylamino)- 1,3-dimethyl-1 H-pyrazolo [3, 4-b] quinoline dihydrochloride, induces serum interferon in mice when given orally or parenterally with high levels (about 10^4 units/ml) between about 7 to 32 hours (Siminoff *et al.*, 1973), with substantial amounts of interferon present in lungs, liver and lymph nodes (Siminoff, 1975, 1976). The related compound BL-3849A is active orally or intraperitoneally, inducing interferon peaks between 15 to 30 hours and 9 to 18 hours by the respective routes (Kern *et al.*, 1976).

Another oral-inducer, MA-56 (Bis-w-piperidinylacetyldibenzofuran-HCl) induces maximum serum interferon in mice between 8 and 24 hours of dosage (400 mg/kg), with lower levels in spleen, kidney, thymus and lymph nodes, but not in lungs (Soehner, Gambardella, and Hou, 1974).

In the following section I shall describe the literature indicating which tissues or cell types are responsible for production of interferon in each of these *in vivo* induction systems. .

c) Cell-Sources of Interferon

A great deal of work has been directed toward elucidating the cellular origins of the interferons produced in response to the different inducers. These attempts have been through direct separations of cell-types or by studying effects of direct or indirect eliminations of certain cell populations or sources on interferon production.

i) Macrophage-Derived Interferons. Peritoneal leukocytes from mice (Lakkovic and Borecky, 1965; Glasgow, 1965; Ash and Bubel, 1966) produce interferons *in vitro* in response to various viruses. Interferons are produced by virus-induced human (Wheelock 1965, 1966a; Lee and Ozere, 1965; Falcoff, Fournier, and Chany, 1966; Strander and Cantell, 1966; Szalaty, Lobodzinska, and Albin, 1977) and bovine (Kono, 1967) leukocyte or alveolar macrophage suspensions (Fulton and Rosenquist, 1976a, b) and in alveolar (Acton and Myrvik, 1966) and peritoneal (Smith and Wagner, 1967a, b) macrophages from rabbits and mice (Glasgow, 1970; Szolgay and Talas, 1976–1977). In some studies attempts were made to separate populations of mononuclear and polymorphonuclear cells. Lee and Ozere (1965) reported that magnetically-removed, iron-phagocytosing human cells and non-phagocytic cells both produced interferon in response to Sendai virus. Wheelock (1966a) separated lymphocytes from peripheral polymorphonuclear cells by glass beads and reported that the lymphocytes alone produced interferon in response to Newcastle disease virus. Similarly, mononuclear elements were reported to be better interferon producers than polymorphonuclear cells by Gresser and Lang (1966). In each of these cases the interferons produced were mostly acid-stable; however, Yamada *et al.* (1970) and Azuma, Yamada, and Nishioka (1970 a, b) and Azuma (1973) reported production by Newcastle disease virus-induced mouse peritoneal macrophage cultures of interferon that was acid-labile. Smith and Wagner (1967a, b) had reported that rabbit macrophage interferon induced by Newcastle disease virus was partially labile at pH2. Macrophages from mouse peritoneal washes have also been reported to produce interferon spontaneously (DeMaeyer, Fauve, and DeMaeyer-Guignard, 1971; Lackovic and Borecky, 1974).

Borecky and his associates (1970) reported that mouse peritoneal macrophages produced interferon in response to a wide variety of viruses, double-stranded RNA, polysaccharides, endotoxin and bacteria. Talas *et al.* (1973) claimed that radio-resistant macrophages in mouse spleens were the source of interferon in irradiated animals inoculated with Newcastle disease virus. In agreement with this interpretation Ito *et al.* (1973 a) found that the ability of splenectomized mice to produce interferon in response to injection of endotoxin could be restored by glass-adherent spleen cells (macrophages), but not by lymphocytes, from either mice or rats. However, the endotoxin-induced interferon in such mouse-rat chimeras was *mouse* interferon (as measured by "species-specificity" properties), suggesting that the macrophages were not the true source of the interferon but only facilitated its induction and/or production by other mouse cells. (This augmentation of interferon production by macrophages will be discussed further below.) Ito *et al.* (1973 b) reported that omentumectomy also eliminated the ability of endotoxin to induce interferon in mice. Rabbit peritoneal macrophages were reported to produce interferon in response to both virus and endotoxin (Smith *et al.*, 1973), and rabbit peritoneal macrophages "activated" by fibroma virus infection *in vivo* produced higher levels of interferon when stimulated with Newcastle disease virus than did normal macrophages (Pathak and Tompkins, 1974). Peritoneal cells were also able to produce interferon in response to endotoxin injected *in vivo* when endotoxin was given intraperitoneally or intravenously (Lackovic and Borecky, 1974). Fischbach and Glasgow (1975) reported interferon production by mouse peritoneal macrophages induced by viruses *in vitro;* this production was reduced by exposure of the cells to *Corynebacterium acnes* or its components. Mouse peritoneal macrophage interferon was also stimulated by lactic dehydrogenase virus (Lagwinska *et al.*, 1975) and influenza virus (Tsukui, 1977). Kolot *et al.* (1976) reported that glass-adherent rabbit alveolar macrophages produced higher levels of interferon when induced with viruses than did non-adherent cells; induced human alveolar macrophages were also able to produce low levels of interferon. Macrophages also produce interferon and become ,,activated" when exposed to bacterial lipopolysaccharide (Rabinovitch *et al.*, 1977; Maehara and Ho, 1977), virus or poly rI·poly rC (Maehara, Ho, and Armstrong, 1977), or polyanions (Acton, 1973; Ibrahim *et al.*, 1976; Schultz, Papamatheakis, and Chirigos, 1977).

ii) Contributions of the Spleen to Interferon Responses. In addition to the demonstrations of high levels of interferon in the spleen of animals treated with interferon inducers, several investigators have attempted to show the role of the spleen in interferon responsiveness by removing it (Table 7).

Subrahmanyan and Mims (1966) and Guttman and Sorokin (1973) found less interferon in influenza-injected mice and, Fruitstone *et al.* (1966) found that serum from splenectomized mice contained markedly less interferon after intravenously injected Newcastle disease virus than did serum from normal mice. Similar results were reported by Guttman and Sorokin (1973), while Borecky and Lackovic (1967) found no effect. Billiau (1969) reported that splenectomy also reduced interferon induction in rats by Newcastle disease virus, but interferon induction in either mice or rats by Sindbis virus was not effected (Billiau, 1969; Desomer and Billiau, 1966). On the contrary, Nagata, Kunii, and Ono (1967) reported that splenectomy reduced interferon production in rats induced with Sindbis virus. Interestingly, the converse disagreement between these authors was reported for the effect of splenectomy on the

Table 7. *Effects of organ-removals on serum interferons*

Organ removed	Animal	Inducer	Effect on interferon response	References
spleen	mice	Newcastle Disease virus	reduced	Fruitstone *et al.* (1966); Youngner (1968); Maehara and Nagano (1972); Gutman and Sorokin (1973)
spleen	mice	Newcastle Disease virus	none	Borecky and Lackovic (1967)
spleen	mice	Sindbis virus	none	Billiau (1969)
spleen	mice	Influenza virus	reduced	Subrahmanyan and Mims (1966); Gutman and Sorokin (1973)
spleen	rat	Newcastle Disease virus	reduced	Billiau (1969)
spleen	rat	Sindbis virus	none	Desomer and Billiau (1966)
spleen	rat	Sindbis virus	reduced	Nagata *et al.* (1967)
spleen	hamster	Venezuelan Encephalitis virus	delayed	Jahrling, Navarro, and Scherer (1976)
spleen	mice	Endotoxin	none	Youngner (1968)
spleen	mice	Endotoxin	reduced (temporarily: < 6 weeks)	Ito *et al.* (1971)
spleen	mice	Endotoxin	none (after 6 weeks)	Ito *et al.* (1971)
spleen	mice	Bordetella	reduced	Borecky and Lackovic (1967)
spleen	rat	Endotoxin	reduced	Desomer and Billiau (1966)
spleen	rat	Endotoxin	none	Nagata *et al.* (1967)
spleen	rabbit	Endotoxin	none	Hellmann and Kohlhage (1973 a, b)
thymus	mice	Sindbis virus	none	Nagata *et al.* (1967)
thymus	mice	Endotoxin	none	Nagata *et al.* (1967)
thymus	mice	Newcastle Disease virus	none	Woodruff and Kilbourne (1967)
omentum	mice	Endotoxin (Intraperitoneal)	reduced	Ito *et al.* (1973 a, b)
omentum	mice	Endotoxin (Intravenously)	none	Ito *et al.* (1973 a, b)

ability of rats to make interferon in response to endotoxin, Desomer and Billiau (1966) claiming reduced levels and Nagata *et al.* (1967) claiming no effect; Youngner (1968) agreeing with the latter effect, in mice. However, Ito *et al.* (1971) found that splenectomy had a marked but only temporary suppressive effect on production of circulating interferon in response of mice to endotoxin, so that by 6 weeks, interferon responses of splenectomized mice were normal (the time used for inductions by Nagata et al., 1967), while Borecky and Lackovic (1967) and Desomer and Billiau (1966) had used 1 to 4 days respectively. Hellmann and Kohlhage (1972, 1973 a)[5] reported that splenectomy seemed not to effect virus-induced interferon production in rabbits, and virus was injected only 1 day after splenectomy.

These data, taken together rather than individually, suggest that cell populations depleted by splenectomy may be replenished, perhaps by recruitment of new cells from precursor stem-cell populations. This interpretation is further supported by the findings of Guttman and Sorokin (1973) that inhibition of interferon responses in splenectomized mice induced by Newcastle disease virus and influenza virus were compensated 48–72 hours after operation and greater than 7 days, respectively. Jahrling, Navarro, and Scherer (1976) reported that splenectomy in hamsters delayed their interferon response to Venezuelan equine encephalitis virus.

Removal of the thymus was also reported not to effect interferon production in mice injected with Sindbis or endotoxin (Nagata et al., 1967). One report showed that omentumectomy reduced interferon response of mice to endotoxin if inducer was injected intraperitoneally, but was without effect when inducer was inoculated intravenously (Ito et al., 1973 b).

iii) Nude Mice: Contributions of the Thymus to Interferon Response. Yokota et al. (1975 a) were the first to study the ability of congenitally athymic (nude) mice to produce interferon. These apparently B-cell animals maintained in pathogen-free environment were induced with poly rI·poly rC intraperitoneally and blood and organs were assayed for interferon levels. These animals, either nude (nu/nu), heterozygous (+/nu) or normal, all produced normal interferon levels. However, when induced with Newcastle disease virus the nude mice produced significantly lower interferon levels than normal mice at all times after induction (Yokota et al., 1975 b). Pantelouris and Pringle (1976) also reported that nude mice had relatively little interferon in the serum when compared to normal mice at 4.6 and 6.5 hours after intraperitoneal injection of Newcastle disease virus, but by 10 hours levels were similar in both groups and both terminated production together. These data suggest that nude mice are deficient in a cell population (T-cells) responsible for "early" interferon, while another cell population responsible for the later interferon is present. Declercq (1977) reported that nude mice produced interferon when injected with poly rI·poly rC intraperitoneally; unfortunately this study had no control group of normal mice for quantitative interferon titer comparisons. Declercq claims that these animals could be repeatedly stimulated to maintain serum interferon levels of about 1000 units/ml by either 21 repeated doses of poly rI·poly rC or by a total interferon dose of only 1000 units/mouse, 3 injections/week. This is difficult to reconcile with either „tolerance" uniformly found

---

[5] This paper was, interestingly, published in identical form in two journals: Arch. Ges. Virusforsch. **39**, 396 (1972) and Nature New Biology **241**, 239 (1973 a).

with such repeated inductions *in vivo* (Section IV. B. 2) or rapid initial drop of titer (by distribution and clearance) after exogenous interferon injections (Section XII).

Merigan, Oldstone, and Walsh (1977), in contrast to the findings of Yokota *et al.* (1975b) and Pantelouris and Pringle (1976) found that nude mice inoculated intravenously with Newcastle disease virus produced significantly *more* interferon than normal mice. More interferon was produced also in nude mice injected intracerebrally with lymphocytic choriomeningitis virus, with higher levels of interferon in spleen, liver, kidney and serum but low (normal mouse levels) in the brain.

The increased interferon production in nude mice seemed to correlate with increased virus replication (therefore more inducer). Interestingly the nude mice with higher virus titers than normal mice survived the lymphocytic choriomeningitis virus infection whereas normal mice with much lower virus levels in tissues did not, possibly owing to the lower interferon levels in the latter group.

iv) Irradiation-Elimination of Interferon Producing Cells. The effect of irradiation on ability of animals to produce circulating interferon has been used to assess the contribution of cell populations with different radiosensitivities to interferon responses. Jullien and DeMaeyer (1966) reported that X-irradiation of mice (1000 R, whole-body) reduced their interferon responses to Newcastle disease virus and to Sindbis virus; however, inhibition was detectable with Sindbis virus by 24 hours, but did not develop to Newcastle disease virus induction until more than 48 hours after irradiation, suggesting that different cell populations are involved in production of interferon in response to each of these viruses. The interferon-producing capacity of mice to each of these inducers could be restored by transfers of bone marrow from normal mice immediately after irradiation (DeMaeyer, Jullien, and DeMaeyer–Guignard, 1967), again with different efficiencies for each inducer. DeMaeyer, Fauve, and DeMaeyer–Guignard (1971) and DeMaeyer, Jullien, and DeMaeyer–Guignard (1967) concluded, from X-irradiation studies of mice followed by transplanation with rat cells, that macrophages play a minor role – if any – in circulating interferon synthesis induced by myxoviruses, paramyxoviruses or encephalomyocarditis virus, but contribute to poly rI·poly rC induced interferon. In this transplantation of rat cells to irradiated mice, rat interferon was produced by the rat-mouse chimeras (These reports contrast with the situation of endotoxin-treated rat-mouse chimeras formed in splenectomized mice, where the interferon produced was mouse type). Solovyov *et al.* (1972b) and Mentkevich, Shcheglovatova, and Amchenkova (1974) also transplanted rat bone marrow into irradiated mice and found that Newcastle disease virus induced rat interferon in these chimeras. Mentkevich, Orlova, and Shcheglovatova (1973a) reported rat interferon produced in irradiation mouse-rat chimeras found in mice induced with influenza virus. Such xenogeneic chimeras produced both rat and mouse serum interferons when induced with vesicular stomatitis virus (Mentkevich *et al.*, 1973) and predominantly mouse type after injection with poly rI·poly rC.

DeMaeyer, DeMaeyer–Guignard, and Jullien (1970) found that interferon production by different viruses could be knocked-out at different doses of X-irradiation, myxovirus and paramyxovirus responses being significantly reduced by 125 R but encephalomyocarditis and vaccinia viruses still inducing in mice exposed to even 1000 R; Sindbis and Semliki forest viruses were intermediate. Similar data were reported by others (Murphy and Glasgow, 1967; Glasgow, 1971). Billiau (1969) reported that X-irradiation of rats did not effect interferon production induced by Sindbis virus. The interferon responses to vesicular stomatitis virus (Murphy and Glasgow, 1967) and herpesvirus (De-Maeyer–Guignard and DeMayer, 1971) were only partially depressed by irradiation.

Tilorone-induced interferon production potential was sensitive to irradiation, whereas poly rI·poly rC-interferon was resistant and endotoxin-interferon was significantly enhanced (Glasgow, 1971).

Thus there seems to be reasonably good agreement that myxovirus and paramyxovirus-induced circulating interferon are produced by radio-sensitive elements whereas vesicular stomatitis, encephalomyocarditis, vaccinia and herpesviruses induce interferon in radio-resistant cells.

It should perhaps be emphasized that all these measures are of circulating interferons, for while serum interferon levels in irradiated mice intravenously exposed to influenza virus were reduced, lung interferon was normal in irradiated mice inoculated intranasally with this virus (Hellman et al., 1968; Mentkevich et al., 1973). Talas et al. (1972) studied the effect of X-irradiation on poly rI·poly rC and endotoxin-induced interferon in mice and found slightly increased production with both, while response to Newcastle disease virus was decreased. Stringfellow and Glasgow (1972b) also found that poly rI·poly rC-induced interferon was slightly enhanced in X-rayed mice, while Newcastle disease virus-interferon was greatly inhibited, and tilorone-induced interferon was completely eliminated.

Jullien and the DeMaeyers (1974) grafted rat hemopoietic cells to irradiated mice and found that interferon response to poly rI·poly rC became of donor type whereas their response to encephalomyocarditis virus remained mouse-type. Reirradiation of chimeras depleted rat-type interferon induced by Newcastle disease virus but not rat interferon induction by poly rI·poly rC. These data point to a macrophage origin of poly rI·poly rC-induced interferon. DeMaeyer et al. (1975) reported that X-irradiated-mice with the If–1[l] genotype receiving marrow transplants from If–1[h] mice produced higher levels of interferon when induced with Newcastle disease virus, indiciating that the If–1 locus is expressed through hemopoietic stem cell-derived elements.

Recently, Sonnenfeld et al. (1977) have investigated the effect of whole-body X-irradiation on production of Type I and Type II interferons in BCG-immunized mice injected with old tuberculin or lipopolysaccharide. The Type II interferon response was inhibited by irradiation whereas Type I interferon induced by lipopolysaccharide was uneffected, even at much higher doses of X-rays.

v) Anti-Lymphocyte Serum. Hirsch and Murphy (1968) and Hirsch et al.

(1968) reported that anti-mouse lymphocyte serum (ALS) did not affect interferon production in mice injected with pyran, Rauscher virus or vaccinia virus. Borden et al. (1970) also reported no effect of ALS on Newcastle disease virus-induced interferon, and Blanden (1970) found increased interferon induction by ectromelia virus in ALS-treated animals, possibly due to increased virus replication. However, others reported that ALS depressed interferon production induced by poly rI·poly rC and Newcastle disease virus (Barth et al., 1969; Treagan, 1972) or West Nile virus (Haahr, 1969). Inglot and her associates (1970) found that a single intraperitoneal dose of ALS given 24 hours prior to Sindbis virus replicative RNA reduced serum interferon titers 4-to 10-fold. However, ALS had no effect on interferon production following injection of intact Sindbis virus, suggesting that different classes of cells participate in interferon responses to different types of inducers. DeMaeyer–Guignard and De-Maeyer (1971) confirmed this interpretation by finding that interferon induced by myxoviruses was quite sensitive to ALS, whereas Sindbis or encephalomyocarditis virus-induced interferon was not sensitive, and poly rI·poly rC interferon-response was enhanced.

Interestingly, tilorone, whose interferon response was strikingly sensitive to X-irradiation (Glasgow, 1971) was able to induce comparable interferon levels in normal and ALS-treated mice (Stringfellow and Glasgow, 1972a, b). These data suggest that radiosensitive cell populations other than lymphocytes may be important in production of interferon in response to this inducer.

These data demonstrate that lymphoid cells are involved in interferon responses to certain inducers, but that generalized assumptions that ALS-treated animals make less interferon in response to virus infection (Stevens et al., 1972) are not justified. Another caution in interpretation of data obtained with ALS is pointed out by the reports that ALS itself can induce interferons (Falcoff, E., et al., 1970; Falcoff, R., 1972; Falcoff, Oriol, and Iscaki, 1972).

vi) T- and B-Cell Interferons: Types I and II. Lymphocyte populations from peripheral blood and milk can produce ,,classical" Type I (acid-stable) interferons in response to many viral and non-viral inducers (Epstein, 1976a, b, 1977).

Wheelock (1966a) reported that human peripheral blood lymphocytes purified to 99% by siliconized glass bead column produced interferon in response to Newcastle disease virus. Emodi and Just (1974a) separated lymphocytes from human milk by Ficoll gradient and induced interferon in them with Newcastle disease virus. Human cord lymphocytes produced interferon with Sendai virus (Cantell et al., 1968b). The interferon produced in these systems is all produced within about 1 day (Table 4; Tovell and Cantell, 1971; Matsuo, Hayashi, and Kishida, 1974; Rassiga-Pidot et al., 1972) and is acid-stable. A lymphocyte-macrophage augmentation of production has been suggested, as mixed cultures of these cells produced more interferon than either separately (Rassiga-Pidot and McIntyre, 1974). Similar enhanced production of bovine interferon was found in mixed bovine leukocyte cultures (Kono, 1967). The involvement of lymphocytes in production of interferons in mouse systems *in vivo* in response to certain inducers is implicit from the data with antilymphocyte serum described previously. The T- or B-lymphocyte origins of these Type I interferons has not yet been determined. Yamaguchi et al. (1977) showed that high levels of interferon were produced by Sendai virus-induced mononuclear human leukocytes but not by polymorphonuclears. Removal of monocytes from the mononuclear suspensions did not inhibit virus-induced interferon levels but strongly suppressed poly rI·poly rC-induced response. Pure monocytes and T-lymphocytes were reported to produce no interferon in response to Sendai virus, and it was concluded that non-T lymphocytes produce interferon in response to the virus. On the other hand, Tsukui (1977) reports that treatment of mouse spleen cultures with antithymocyte serum and complement reduced their ability to make interferon when stimulated with influenza virus. T-cell-enrichment enhanced yields, which were also augmented by macrophages; the acid-stability/lability property of the interferon produced was not reported.

Wheelock (1965) reported that suspensions of human leukocytes produced an acid-labile interferon when stimulated with phytohemagglutinin. Acid-labile interferons have been reported in numerous systems (Section VII. A. 3) but are probably even more prevalent than is indicated by these reports, as most investigators working with interferons have, since the time that interferons were first reported to be acid stable, routinely pretreated all samples to be tested for interferons at pH 2, as a convenient method of eliminating inducer-virus activity. Inducers of Type II interferon include various mitogens and antigens triggering immune-recognition reactions (Section III. B. 5).

Epstein and her associates (as reviewed by Epstein, 1976 a, b, 1977) have contributed heavily to development of in vitro systems for production of Type II human interferons and to elucidation of the essential components of the induction-production system. Significant segments of these studies have involved development of techniques for isolation of pure populations of lymphocytes and macrophages (Epstein and Cline, 1974; Epstein, Kreth, and Herzenberg, 1974a, b; Epstein, Cline, and Merigan, 1970, 1971a, b) and separation of T and B lymphocytes.

These workers found no interferon in cultures of 96 to 100% pure macrophages stimulated with phytohemagglutinin, low levels of interferon in pure lymphocyte cultures, and a 5-fold increase in mixed lymphocyte-macrophage cultures (Epstein, Cline, and Merigan, 1970, 1971a, b). Interferon production peak occurred 3 days after addition of inducer. Medium from stimulated or unstimulated macrophages did not augment lymphocyte-interferon response; mouse macrophages could be substituted for human macrophages and interferon made in such cultures was human, not mouse; and there was no correlation between degree of lymphocyte transformation and interferon levels. Freeze-thaw of lymphocytes eliminated interferon production, whereas such treatment of macrophages did not effect their ability to augment interferon production.

Human T lymphocytes and B lymphocytes can both produce interferon in response to mitogens and both are enhanced by macrophages, T-cell-containing cultures producing interferon by 3 days and B-cell-containing cultures not producing interferon until 5 to 7 days (Epstein, Kreth, and Herzenberg, 1974a, b; Epstein, 1975; Epstein and Salmon, 1974).

Lymphocytes from human tonsil tissues have also been reported to produce interferon in response to mitogens (Sugiyama et al., 1972, 1974; Klimpel, Day, and Lucas, 1975). Plasma cell-enriched cultures from patients with multiple myeloma also produce interferon spontaneously, whereas normal plasma cells induced with phytohemagglutinin or pokeweed mitogen produce interferon after several days (Epstein and Salmon, 1974).

Wallen, Dean, and Lucas (1973) demonstrated that mouse lymphocytes produced interferon after incubation with phytohemagglutinin, concanavalin A or *Mycobacterium* PDD; this response could be eliminated by antiserum directed against the theta-antigen of mouse lymphocytes (anti θ serum), but the response to pokeweed mitogen could not. Similarly, Stobo et al. (1974) eliminated the ability of mouse splenic lymphocyte cultures to respond to phytohemagglutin by treating cultures with anti θ antibody, whereas antiserum against B-cells had no effect.

The types of mouse interferons induced by mitogens in T-cells and in B-cells are also different physically; T-cell-stimulating mitogens induce interferon antigenically distinct from type I mouse interferon and are acid-labile (i. e., Type II) whereas B-cell stimulants (lipopolysaccharide, tilorone, pokeweed mitogen) induce interferons exhibiting antigenic and stability properties of mouse type I interferons (Wietzerbin et al., 1976b). On the contrary, Maehara, and Ho (1977) reported that bacterial lipopolysaccharide induced interferons with different properties in mouse macrophages and B-lymphocytes, the macrophage interferon being neutralized by Type I antiserum and the B-cell interferon less efficiently neutralized; they were unable to detect interferon in T-cells induced with lipopolysaccharide. In another report, these authors claim that T and B lymphocytes induced with Newcastle disease virus or poly rI·poly rC, produce interferon antigenically distinct from macrophage or other Type I interferons; however all of these interferons induced in B-, or T-cell macrophages or fibroblast differed from those induced in sensitized mice by BCG by being acid stable whereas the latter was acid labile (Maehara, Ho, and Armstrong, 1977).

Leukocyte suspensions obtained from individuals sensitized to PPD or to tetanus or diphtheria toxoids were reported by Green et al. (1969, 1970) to produce interferon in response to specific antigens. Such immune-specific induction of interferon was also reported by Milstone and Waksman (1970) in leukocytes from tuberculin-sensitized mice exposed to PPD *in vitro*. Borecky and his colleagues (1971) found that mouse L cells induced interferon in cultures of mouse lymphocytes from mice immunized to L cells. In these mouse systems the interferon was produced within 1 day. The interferon in this case was acid stable.

The Falcoffs (Falcoff, E., et al., 1970; Falcoff, E., et al., 1972a; Falcoff, Oriol, and Iscaki, 1972; Falcoff, R., 1972) demonstrated that small human lymphocytes could be induced to make interferon by exposure to antilymphocyte globulins, producing acid-labile interferon by 48 hours.

Sensitized human lymphocytes stimulated with specific antigens also pro-

duced interferon (Epstein, Cline, and Merigan, 1971h; 1972) and these responses were increased by macrophages, interferon appearing only after 7 to
8 days with PPD-stimulation, or vaccinia virus antigen (Epstein, Stevens, and
Merigan, 1972; Merigan et al., 1973b). Similar results were obtained with
lymphocyte-macrophage cultures from patients with recurrent herpes simplex
induced with heat-inactivated herpesvirus hominis (Rasmussen et al., 1974,
Valle et al., 1975a, b; Fujibayashi, Hooks, and Notkins, 1975; Haahr, Rasmussen, and Merigan, 1976). Elimination of T-cells with antiserum and complement inhibited interferon responses. Also, memory for immune-specific interferon production was derived from the lymphocyte donor, not the macrophage donor (Valle et al., 1975b).

Immune-induced interferon produced by bovine macrophage-lymphocyte
cultures exposed to herpesvirus antigen was formed by T-lymphocytes (Rouse
and Babiuk, 1977). Antigen-antibody complex of this virus was at least as
good an inducer in this system as free antigen, suggesting that such complexes
could play a role in the in vivo induction of immune-interferon at local infection foci, thereby contributing to the recovery mechanism, in contrast to previous interpretations that virus mixed with specific antibodies are unable to induce interferon (Petralli, Merigan, and Wilbur, 1965b).

2. Hyporesponsiveness in vivo: Tolerance to Repeated Inductions

As was described in Section VI. A. 3, cells in culture become refractory to
repeated stimulations with interferon inducers, normally making much less interferon when reinduced. A similar situation is observed in vivo. This inability
of animals to respond to repeated inductions by producing high levels of interferons has been regarded one of the two major obstacles to overcome with regard to hopes of utilization of inducers in prevention and therapy of virus diseases (Anonymous, 1974; Galasso, 1974), the other obstacle being toxicity of
inducers. In this Section I shall describe studies on the in vivo hyporesponsive
period to interferon induction, emphasizing those reports giving some information as to whether it is, in fact, necessary to maintain detectable circulating
levels of interferon during repeated inductions in order to maintain a long lasting antiviral effect; or does tolerance decay at the same rate as decline of virus
resistance induced by the first interferon response? Can tolerance be explained
like "blocking" in vitro, interferon restricting its own synthesis?

a) Cross-Tolerance to Different Inducers

Ho, Kono, and Breinig (1965) observed that rabbits injected intravenously
with either Sindbis virus or endotoxin failed to mount a second interferon response when restimulated a few hours after the first injection with the same
inducer. This refractory period lasted for about 6 days. When injected first
with endotoxin, rabbits were hyporesponsive to secondary inductions with
either virus or endotoxin, but when first induced with virus, animals could
produce interferon in response to endotoxin (Ho, Kono, and Breinig, 1965).
Youngner and Stinebring (1965) also observed that endotoxin induction completely prevented interferon production in mice in response to either endotoxin

or *Brucella abortus* injected 48 hours later. The virus did not make mice tolerant to endotoxin induction, nor could tolerance be transferred in plasma of refractory mice (Youngner and Stinebring, 1966). Ho, Kono, and Breinig (1965) were also unable to transfer tolerance in serum. However, Siegert *et al.* (1967) found that tolerance to induction of interferon by virus could be transmitted passively by plasma of tolerant mice. This "serum hyporeactive factor" may be related to that described below. Lackovic and Borecky (1965) found that one intraperitoneal injection of Newcastle disease virus made mice tolerant to a second induction at 24 hours.

Statolon injected into mice induced a marked hyporesponsiveness to a second injection, lasting from 2 to 10 days (Kleinschmidt and Murphy, 1967), but did not induce tolerance to induction by endotoxin, and endotoxin did not cause tolerance to statolon (Youngner and Stinebring, 1966). Youngner (1968) speculated that these agents induced different cell populations. Borecky and Lackovic (1966) reported that *Bordetella pertussis* produced tolerance to Newcastle disease virus, but only in circulating interferon levels, as normal interferon levels were found in spleens of virus-challenged mice. Van Rossum and Desomer (1966) and Desomer and Billiau (1966) reported tolerance was reciprocal in rats with Sindbis virus and *E. coli.*

Ho (1967) postulated that either a refractoriness factor was produced in association with interferon, as first evidenced by Siegert *et al.* (1967) and espoused later by Borden and Murphy (1971) and others (see discussion below on "Serum Hyporeactive Factor"), or producing cells had been "exhausted". However, even small doses of endotoxin, too low to induce significant interferon levels, induced tolerance, so exhaustion of producers seems unlikely (Ho, Kono, and Breinig, 1965). Cells (leukocytes) from animals tolerant to induction were still able to produce interferon *in vitro* (Ho, Postic, and Ke, 1967; Ho, 1967). Other possible interpretations of tolerance were offered (Kono and Ho, 1965), but did not hold up to scrutiny (Ho, Postic, and Ke, 1967; Borecky, Lackovic, and Russ, 1969).

Ho *et al.* (1970) and Ho and Ke (1970) reported that injections of viruses, endotoxin or poly rI·poly rC produced cross tolerance in rabbits, except that poly rI·poly rC increased amounts of interferon induced by endotoxin. However, Absher, and Stinebring (1969) found that endotoxin and poly rI·poly rC induced cross-tolerance in mice. Chester, Declercq, and Merigan (1971) found both effects, depending on timing of inducers.

The hypothesis that interferon is "blocking" its own synthesis, as can be demonstrated *in vitro* (Section VI. A. 3), seems unlikely, as endotoxin is most efficient at inducing tolerance, yet is weakest of interferon inducers. Merigan and Finkelstein (1968) reported that mice inoculated with pyran copolymer intraperitoneally produced a primary interferon response for only 2 to 3 days, yet were tolerant to a second induction for more than 3 weeks, and there was no residual antiviral activity detectable at 6 days (Declercq and Merigan, 1969b; Declercq, Nuwer, and Merigan, 1970a; Declercq, 1972). Gresser *et al.* (1969c) also found that mice repeatedly injected 1 day and 3 days after initial interferon-inducing Newcastle disease virus dose were tolerant to reinduction and were no better protected than mice given only the first inducing injection.

However, Giron et al. (1973b) reported that poly rI·poly rC-induced protection against virus infection lasted longer than tolerance. Desomer, Billiau, and Declercq (1968) also observed hyporeactivity in mice injected with a second dose of polyacrylic acid after a 1-week interval.

Tolerance to repeated inductions by poly rI·poly rC has been reported in rabbits, mice and man (Hill et al., 1971; Centifanto et al., 1970). This data and others (DuBuy et al., 1970; Sharpe, Birch, and Planterose, 1971; Field et al., 1971; Guggenheim and Baron, 1977) are contradicted, however, by the claim (Declercq, 1977) that 21 repeated injections, 3/week, of poly rI·poly rC in mice maintained high serum interferon levels. Similar claims of repeated full-induction of interferon in mice by poly rI·poly rC-reinduction was reported by Tazulakhova et al. (1973), and by Slamon (1975).

Degre and Dahl (1971) reported that bacterial vaccine, inoculated intraperitoneally into mice induced partial tolerance, but still significant protective levels of interferon could be produced by serial inoculations on alternate days.

Tilorone induced marked homologous hyporeactivity and some tolerance to poly rI·poly rC which was reciprocal (Declercq and Merigan, 1971a). However, Glaz, and Talas (1973) reported that permanent serum interferon levels can be maintained in mice by continued administration of tilorone in drinking water. However, it should be emphasized that the maintained serum levels were always less than 50 units/ml (Glaz and Talas, 1973), as compared to several thousand units/ml attained by a single oral dose (Declercq and Merigan, 1971a).

BL-20803 was compared to tilorone and poly rI·poly rC for development of hyporesponsiveness in mice, by Siminoff et al. (1973) who found that mice became hyporesponsive after a single encounter with tilorone or poly rI·poly rC, but mice did not become tolerant to induction by BL-20803 until after second treatment. In fact, serum interferon levels stimulated by the second dose of this compound were somewhat higher than the first induction. Similar delayed hyporesponsiveness was seen when tilorone or poly rI·poly rC were given after the first dose of BL-20803. It is also important to note that the serum levels of interferon induced by the first dose of BL-20803 was higher than that induced by either tilorone or poly rI·poly rC, again suggesting no relation between ability to induce interferon and hyporesponsiveness.

Kern et al. (1976) reported that hyporesponsive state to a second injection of the related compound BL-3849A had developed sufficient to reduce yields of interferon to 10 to 20%, and after a fourth dose responses were about 3% of the original level.

Cole et al. (1975) also found no relation between interferon and hyporesponsiveness to Newcastle disease virus or poly rI·poly rC in mice infected with Mycoplasmas which made mice tolerant to induction by both these inducers.

MA-56 induced strong hyporesponsiveness to repeated stimulation for at least 3 days after the first induction with this compound in mice (Soehner et al., 1974).

The capsular polysaccharide of Klebsiella pneumoniae (CPS-K) shown to induce interferon in mice also induced homologous and heterologous tolerance to reinduction of interferon by lipopolysaccharide; again no simple correlation was found between interferonogenic and tolerogenic capabilities of the substances (Kato et al., 1975). Kern, Glasgow, and Overall (1976) also found that the *Brucella* extract BRU-PEL induced hyporesponsiveness after a first injection, inducing 600–900 units of interferon/ml serum instead of 4800, and only 50–225 units after a third and fourth injection.

Glaz and Talas (1975) reported that the hyporesponsiveness of mice to repeated inductions with the acridine-related drugs was similar to that seen with tilorone, but the dye was able to induce interferon after a previous tilorone dose, but not the reverse.

Hyporesponsiveness to poly rI·poly rC·poly-L-lysine in mice was pronounced after the first injection (Olsen et al., 1976) but residual titers were significant even after several dosages. The hyporesponse to poly rI·poly rC in children given daily doses of inducer was marked (Guggenheim and Baron, 1977) and persisted for 6 to 8 days. Sammons et al. (1977) reported that tolerance developed to poly rI·poly rC·poly-L-lysine after the third injection in rhesus monkey, and lasted until the sixth injection, at which time the interferon levels became somewhat more elevated, though still significantly depressed.

Yershov et al. (1976) reported that it might be possible to circumvent hyporesponsiveness by alternating types of inducers. They report that a first injection with poly rI·poly rC in mice followed by a second injection with inactivated Venezuelan equine encephalitis virus gave a second response greater than the first (about 3000 and 5000 units/ml serum, respectively).

Stanley et al. (1976) reported that the propanediamine inducer produced hyporesponsiveness in levels of nasal interferon after 3 days of daily intranasal treatment. Also the vehicle for this drug, a mixture of polysorbate 80 in glycerol and saline was reported to induce interferon and tolerance.

Tilorone also induced hyporesponsiveness in nude mice (Gibson et al., 1976), indicating that the hyporesponsive factor, as well as interferon, is a product of cells other than T-lymphocytes.

Stringfellow (1977a, b) recently found that U-25, 166, poly rI·poly rC and tilorone each produced hyporesponsiveness in mice. However, tolerance developed more slowly to U-25, 166 and poly rI·poly rC than to tilorone. Hyporesponsiveness in each case lasted 5 to 6 days. In cats, orally administered U-25, 166 maintained interferon levels over an 18-week period in which 9 doses of compound were given; if daily doses were given, however, hyporesponsiveness developed rapidly.

Rathova, Kociskova, and Borecky (1974, 1975) suggested that interferon production in mice occurs in different separated „compartments", depending on the route of inoculation of inducer. They found that Newcastle disease virus induced hyporesponsiveness when inoculated intravenously but did not do so when inoculated intraperitoneally. Singer et al. (1973) found high levels of interferon in the lungs of influenza virus infected mice shown to be hyporesponsive to induction of serum interferon by poly rI·poly rC. Blach–Olszewska and Skurska (1974) found that Newcastle disease virus induced hyporesponsiveness in mice following intravenous injection, which lasted about 1 week, but tolerance to production of local interferon was not observed after a second intracerebral inoculation of this virus. Repeated intranasal application of the virus stimulated interferon in some mice but others became tolerant. These authors make the candid assessment that these experiments failed to clarify anything. Unfortunately that seems to have been the general situation with most studies on hyporesponsive states. It has usually been the case that hyporesponsiveness has been measured only as circulating interferon, and local interferon levels have not been determined, and it has not been resolved whether these circulating levels of interferon represent spill-over of excess levels not necessary for virus resistance. It is also not clear whether the marked hyporesponsiveness, often more than 99% decrease in serum interferon levels, still allows sufficient circulating titers to maintain resistance to virus, as it is not even known what levels of serum interferon are needed for resistance. There seems to have been a general panic over the observation that lowered interferon levels are produced, on the assumption that lower levels are bad, when even such lowered levels may in fact be higher than those needed. As emphasized by Blach–Olszewska and Skurska (1974) this problem may not even be a problem, for tissue levels of interferons do not always reflect antiviral resistance and hyporesponsiveness does not necessarily mean lower resistance (Sharpe, Birch, and Planterose, 1971).

It is clear that induction of at least partial tolerance to repeated interferon induction is a general phenomenon. Its significance is not clear, but its very general occurences in many species suggests that the systems have evolved a way of saying "that's enough of that stuff for a while!". Clearly interferon is an induced product, and there are likely to be reasons which are advantageous to the host for its not being constitutive. Tolerance may be the mechanism whereby the animal makes sure it doesn't get an overdose. Several of the non-antiviral effects induced by interferons are likely related to the necessity for controlling interferon overproduction (Section X).

b) Serum Hyporeactive Factor

A number of observations have shown that virus-infected animals rapidly become unable to produce interferon in response to the various inducers (De-Maeyer–Guignard, 1972; Holtermann and Havell, 1970; Stringfellow et al., 1977a, b; Stringfellow, 1977b; Osborn and Medearis, 1966). Similar refractoriness to induction of interferon in man is suggested by the findings that leukocytes obtained from virus-infected patients produced lowered interferon levels (Emodi and Just, 1974b; Tolentino et al., 1975). Stringfellow and Glasgow (1972a) found that mice infected with encephalomyocarditis viruses could not produce normal interferon levels in response to poly rI·poly rC, Newcastle disease virus or tilorone. These workers (Stringfellow and Glasgow, 1974) found that such infected mice had a circulating factor in their serum at a time when all virus-induced interferon had been cleared from the blood, which could induce hyporesponsiveness in cell cultures. This factor, termed "Serum hyporeactive factor (SHF)" was similar to Type I mouse interferon in size, heat lability, pH 2 stability, sensitivity to proteases, and "species-specificity"

(Stringfellow, 1975), but lacked antiviral activity and was not neutralized by antiserum to mouse interferon. SHF has also been demonstrated in sera of mice with leukemias (Stringfellow, 1976) and various virus infections (Stringfellow *et al.*, 1977a, b). This factor may be the same as that described by Siegert *et al.* (1967) which transferred tolerance in mice, or to the factor in "late" interferon preparations obtained from mice inoculated with interferon inducers (Borden and Murphy, 1971; Borden *et al.*, 1975).

Mentkevich and Shcheglovitova (1974) have made the interesting observation that repeated administration of poly rI·poly rC in xenogenous rat-mouse chimeras induces hyporesponsiveness of mouse-type interferon whereas the level of rat-type interferon is unreduced. In view of the "species-specificity" of SHF (Stringfellow, 1975), it is tempting to speculate that host mouse SHF is unable to regulate synthesis of interferon in the donor cells.

Thus interferon inducers *in vivo* (as well as *in vitro*: Section VI. A. 3) may induce a regulatory protein which represses interferon production, or interferon may itself perform this task, or interferon may induce a substance which does this regulating. In either case, *in vivo* or *in vitro*, cells become induced to make interferon, do so for a short period, stop doing so and decline to do so again for a while.

C. Mass Production of Interferons

Interferons must be produced in large-volume production systems to obtain sufficient amounts for the purifications and characterizations described in Section VII. Large-scale production systems have so far been developed for only four interferons: mouse fibroblast interferon, human leukocyte interferon, human fibroblast interferon and human lymphoblastoid cell interferons. The systems described here are "pilot-plant" productions; other means for mass-production will be required to make available interferon for wide clinical applications rather than only purification studies and limited clinical trials.

1. Mouse Interferon

More than a decade ago Finter (1964b, 1965) stressed the practical importance of realizing what are good sources of interferon. At that time a "rich source" of mouse interferon was described as the brains of mice infected with West Nile virus, yielding a "wealth" of about 17,000 units/brain. This type of interferon production system has indeed been used to provide interferon for several mouse protection experiments, but the limitations of such a supply system are apparent.

Graff, Kassel, and Kastner (1971) devised an elaborate scheme for large-scale production of mouse interferon in a "cytogenerator" and reported that suspension L929 cells induced with Newcastle disease virus yielded about one unit of interferon per 200 to 3000 cells. Likely owing to the complexity of this system noone has adopted it.

Stewart II, Gosser, and Lockart (1971a) reported that a much less intricate system of roller-bottles of L cells primed with interferon and induced with MM strain of encephalomyocarditis virus yielded crude interferon titrating $10^{4.0}$

units/ml or about 1 unit of interferon per 100 cells. This system enables a pilot-plant scale production of about 10^9 units of mouse interferon/week. Introduction of the multisurface glass roller bottles recently described by Knight (1977a) could boost production potential of this system by about 10-fold. This production system has been used by Stewart II (1974) and Knight (1975) to obtain large batches of crude mouse interferon for purification and characterization studies (Section VII). Newcastle disease virus can be substituted in this system for MM virus. Oie *et al.* (1972b) found a line of Moloney sarcoma virus-transformed 3T3 cells designated C-243-3, which produced about 10^4 to 10^5 units of crude interferon/ml, or about four- to tenfold more than produced by L cells in their laboratory. These cells were used by Tovey and his colleagues (1974), who developed a method for large-scale interferon production in suspension cultures, consistently yielding more than 10^5 units of crude interferon/ml. This scheme includes priming with interferon, induction with Newcastle disease virus, and super-production with sequential cycloheximide and actinomycin D. Though the authors claim the system obviates the necessity for highly skilled operatives, it is my experience that only such personnel can make it work satisfactorily. This production system has provided potent interferon preparations for many purification and characterization studies (Stewart II *et al.*, 1976; Stewart II, LeGoff and Wiranowska–Stewart, 1977) and for production of potent antiserum to mouse interferon (Gresser *et al.*, 1976b, c). This production system has been used for the commercial production of mouse interferon. Sano, Matsui, and Kobayashi (1974) reported large-scale production of mouse interferon from Newcastle disease virus-induced L cells in suspension cultures.

Thus, several systems are presently available that can conveniently be adapted to laboratory-scale production of mouse interferons for *in vivo* experiments or purification and characterization studies.

2. Human Leukocyte Interferon

If the production of interferons on sufficient scale for animal experiments and for purification and characterization studies were referred to as large-scale, production in large enough quantities to allow these studies and to provide interferon sufficient for clinical trials must be considered a massive-scale production. Presently there are few such facilities. Human interferon intended for clinical use must be prepared from human diploid cells. Dr. Kari Cantell and his associates (Cantell, 1977; Cantell and Hirvonen, 1977) in Helsinki, Finland, have developed a mass production facility for human leukocyte interferon in sufficient quantities for small-scale clinical studies (Section XIV). Present techniques, which have evolved over more than 10 years of experience in Cantell's laboratories, provide about one or two million units from leukocytes derived from one blood donor, about 1 unit/50 cells (Cantell *et al.*, 1968a, 1974; Strander and Cantell, 1966; Mogensen and Cantell, 1977; Kauppinen, Myllyla, and Cantell, 1977; Tovell and Cantell, 1971); thus the supply has obvious limitations. However, multiple "units" of leukocytes can be extracted from a single donor by the leukophoresis process, thus expanding supplies somewhat.

"Buffy coat" leukocytes are primed with interferon and induced with Sendai virus at a high multiplicity (after erythrocytes are lyzed with ammonium chloride). Interferon is produced in medium supplemented with human plasma protein fraction, as contrary to other reports (Goore et al., 1973), the interferon yields are lower in serum-free medium. Crude leukocyte interferon harvested 16 to 20 hours later is purified (by procedures described in Section VII) to the stage designated "P-IF" with a specific activity of about 10^6 units/mg of protein. This is the material utilized clinically in trials described in Section XIV. Interferon batches of several liters are prepared from pools of buffy coat products, so that one hepatitis-positive donor can render hundreds of millions of units of interferon unacceptable for the clinic; such clinically-worthless batches are currently utilized for purification and characterization studies (Stewart II and Cantell, unpublished). The present production capacity of the Finnish Red Cross is about 10^{11} units annually being produced from about 65,000 buffy coats. A facility of similar size has recently been established by the Memorial Sloan-Kettering Cancer Center. Many more such production centers will likely be developed to meet the need merely of material for clinical trials; wide clinical use will clearly require alternative supply processes.

3. Human Fibroblast Interferon

One possibility for overcoming the limitations on numbers of available cells, as encountered in use of buffy coat leukocyte suspensions, is the use of cells that will replicate in culture. Human fibroblast cultures for this purpose can be prepared from available human diploid fibroblasts obtained in large numbers from child-birth procedures, either stillbirth materials of embryonic origin or from after-birth material, the amniotic membrane, or can be obtained from surgical procedures such as circumcision. Fournier, Falcoff, and Chany (1967) described "mass production" of interferon from human amnion cells. This material is biologically and antigenically identical to other human fibroblast interferon but is distinct in these respects from human leukocyte interferon (Fournier, Falcoff, and Chany, 1967; Stewart II, unpublished data). This source of cells has not been used for large-scale interferon production.

Havell and Vilček (1972) applied the technique of "superproduction" to cultures of neonatal human foreskin fibroblasts, designated FS-3, and obtained about 10^4 units of interferon/ml or about 1 unit/100 cells. This procedure includes priming of "aged monolayer" cells with interferon before induction with poly rI·poly rC in medium containing cycloheximide and actinomycin D for 2 hours, wash and incubate with growth medium about 24 hours. This system has been adapted to large-scale production in roller-bottles or stationary cultures in FS-3, or FS-4 cells (Havell and Vilček, personal communication; Knight, 1976a) and several other laboratories have used this process for large-scale production of human fibroblast interferons with similar results from various other diploid human fibroblast cell strains (Billiau, Joniau, and Desomer, 1972, 1973; Edy et al., 1975; Wiranowska–Stewart et al., 1977; Horoszewicz et al., 1977). Such materials have been used for purification and characterization studies (Knight, 1976; Section VII) and for a limited number of very pre-liminary clinical trials (Section XIV).

Variations on the superproduction scheme have included substitution of ul-traviolet irradiation for the metabolic inhibitors, which would provide inter-feron free of such agents (Lindner–Frimmel, 1974; Mozes et al., 1974); how-ever, technical difficulties such as uniform application of irradiation doses has prevented large-scale application of this method. Others have substituted the reversible DNA-dependent RNA synthesis inhibitor DRB for actinomycin D, which allows repeated superinduction–superproduction from the same cultures (Wiranowska–Stewart, Chudzio and Stewart II, 1977a). However, owing to the presently restricted supplies of such inhibitors, this method has not been used for large-scale production. Transformed human cell lines have been de-scribed which reportedly produce somewhat higher per cell yields of human fibroblast interferon (Billiau et al., 1977a). Such cells, while having the advan-tage of unrestricted culture-life span, have the disadvantage that interferon ob-tained from them cannot be used in the clinic.

Interferons produced from human diploid fibroblast cultures are presently being produced on a large-scale in a few research centers, but the present methods, with its main restrictions being housing facilities for large numbers of anchorage-dependent (monolayer or multilayer) cultures and the numbers of hands required for manipulations will foreseeably not be able to provide more interferon than for purification and characterization and small clinical trials. An alternative immediately exploitable is the method for growing the anchor-age-dependent fibroblasts on microcarriers (Levine, 1977); thus pseudosuspen-sion cultures could be superinduced on a large-scale by a scheme similar to that developed for mouse interferon by Tovey et al. (1974). The life-span of human diploid fibroblasts in culture is usually about 50 doublings and optimal yields of interferon are produced only during a limited period, usually between 20 to 30 passages, usually declining with increasing passage level (Havell, per-sonal communication; Horoszewicz et al., 1977). Thus to have available fully-characterized, interferon-competent cells for large-scale, long-term production requires large banks of frozen stocks of low-passage cells and large cell back-up cultures. For example, to progress from a frozen vial of about 10^6 (low-passage) fibroblasts to a weekly production of 100 roller bottles (yielding about 10^8 units), requires about 12 population doublings at which time cul-tures are at about 20-doublings. There are also the tasks of constant monitor-ing such cultures for growth properties, morphological stability, karyology, oncogenicity in mice, and contaminants (viral, bacterial, fungal and mycoplas-mal); only such controls can produce material acceptable for clinical investiga-tions.

4. Human Lymphoblastoid Cell Interferon

It has been recognized for some time that a continuous leukocytic line would overcome the problem of limited numbers of leukocytes available from buffy coat-suspensions (Strander and Cantell, 1974; Strander, Mogensen, and Cantell, 1975). The "Namalwa" cell line from Burkitt's lymphoma patient which release low levels of interferon spontaneously (Section III. D) were found to produce moderate levels of leukocyte-type interferon in response to Sendai virus (Gresser *et al.*, 1974; Strander, Mogensen, and Cantell, 1975) or Newcastle disease virus (Finter, personal communication; Bridgen *et al.*, 1977; Stewart II, unpublished data). These cells can be grown in large vat-cultures and the supply of interferon from such cultures would be sufficient for clinical utility. Bridgen *et al.* (1977) reported production of 800 liter batches (2.6×10^9 units). However, at least for the immediate future such material, derived from transformed cells would be acceptable only for laboratory studies and possibly for administration to patients with neoplasia.

5. Alternatives to Large-Scale Production

It is tempting to speculate or hope that the present production facilities will become obsolete in the near future, through the introduction of mass-production based on either direct chemical synthesis of interferon, or an interferon active core or "interferoid", or by use of the rapidly evolving recombinant-DNA techniques.

The isolation of pure interferons has apparently recently been achieved (Section VII) and studies on its essential composition are underway. Sequencing of different interferons may reveal a common active sequence of sufficiently small size to enable chemical synthesis.

Insertion of interferon information into bacteria by retro-copy of interferon messenger RNA is a presently pursued possibility in several research centers. It is envisioned that human interferons could be produced from huge vats of bacteria.

6. Which Human Interferon Should Be Produced?

Each laboratory producing a human fibroblast interferon or a human leukocyte interferon understandably expounds the virtues of their interferon, the leukocyte interferon being simple to make and stable, the fibroblast being unlimited by cell sources and more likely to be pathogen-free. However, I should like to emphasize the present importance of having large-scale production facilities for *both* types of human interferons. We do not presently know the physiological significance of the distinct molecular species of human interferons, but tissue specificities have been hypothesized (Stewart II and Desmyter, 1975; Stewart II, LeGoff, and Wiranowska–Stewart, 1977; Einhorn and Strander, 1977). If such were the case, one type of interferon might be much more efficient in a given clinical situation than another, and the reverse could apply for another disease. Only after extensive studies comparing both types of interferons can the argument for exclusive production of a given type of human interferon be rational.

VII. Interferons: Their Purification and Characterization

Cells which encounter a variety of substances called (by interferonologists) "interferon-inducers" begin to produce and release substances which are called (perhaps again only by interferonologists, but maybe other names by investigators of different orientation) "interferons", which among other activities, induce cells to become virus resistant. In this Section, I shall try to define interferons, describe how they have been purified and present evidence that they are responsible for the pleiotypic activities attributed to them in subsequent Sections.

A. Defining Interferons

The discovery of interferon resulted from searches for a virus-induced antiviral substance. Thus, by definition, interferons are substances that make cells resistant to viruses. Had Isaacs and Lindenmann been cell-biologists looking for a mitogen-induced factor that restricted cell growth, the same substance, interferon, might have been called "restricton", or had they been immunologists looking for a factor induced by immune-recognition reactions which modulated immune responses, interferons could have been referred to as "modulons". It is, in fact, possible that certain of the various factors that have been identified in various disciplines, and which are identified by their abilities to perform a specific function, are the same factor expressing pleiotypic effects. It will only be with proper purification and characterization that the relations of each of these lymphokines will be clear. Certainly interferons are more thoroughly characterized than most of these factors, owing largely to the recent progress that has been made in their purifications, which itself results from advances in interferon production methods.

The criteria for acceptance of a factor as an interferon were first carefully enumerated by Lockart (1966). The properties include biological and physicochemical measures, and have been continually modified by the accumulation of data. Many of the properties thought to be distinctly useful in classifying substances as interferons have been found to be variable. Previously assignments of properties to interferons were tenuous as the described property was often attributed to noninterferon substances in preparations containing interferons as trace components; thus, the definition of interferons has only been possible definitively as preparations of interferons have been obtained which approach purity.

1. *Induction of Antiviral Activities*

All interferon preparations, by definition, must be able to exert antiviral activity. The antiviral activity is not directly due to interferon but rather is induced by interferon in sensitive cells through processes requiring new cellular RNA and protein synthesis (Section IX will describe antiviral activities in detail). Interferon-induced antiviral activity is characteristically broad-spectrum, making cells refractory to a wide variety of RNA and DNA viruses (Stewart II, Scott, and Sulkin, 1969) and the relative sensitivities of viruses to the resistance induced is determined by the species of the interferon treated cell (Stewart II and Lockart, 1970; Ahl and Rump, 1976; Ito and Montagnier, 1977; Section IX, Table 14).

2. *"Species Specificity" of Interferons*

Interferons were early shown to usually exert less activities on heterologous cells, having predilections for cells of the animal producing them (Isaacs and Westwood, 1959b; Tyrrell, 1959; Sutton and Tyrrell, 1961; Andrews, 1961). However, even many early reports gave clear evidence that at least some interferons were active on phylogenetically related cells (Sutton and Tyrrell, 1961), or even quite distant cells, i. e., monkey and rabbit interferons on rabbit and monkey cells, reciprocally (Andrews, 1961). Then it was reported that virtual complete activity barriers existed between mouse and chicken interferons on, respectively, chicken and mouse cells (Friedman *et al.*, 1962; Levy *et al.*, 1963; Baron, Barban, and Buckler, 1964; Merigan, 1964), and previous reports of cross-species activities were attributed to non-interferon inhibitors in the preparations. It was even suggested that the property of strict species-specificity be a criterion for acceptance as an interferon (Baron, Barban, and Buckler, 1964). In fact, had this house-rule been inacted, we would today have no interferons! None of the virus inhibitors would qualify, as all interferons that have been tested in a variety of cell-species have been found to exert antiviral activity in some of these cells, often being more active than in homologous cells (Table 8).

The finding that mouse interferons could exert a small amount of activity on rat and hamster cells (Buckler and Baron, 1966) and monkey and human interferons would cross-react (Bucknall, 1967) brought the concept of "species-specificity" to doubt in some minds (Bucknall, 1967), while in others it suggested a phylogenetic relationship of heterospecific activities (Buckler and Baron, 1966). Clinging to the latter notion became increasingly difficult as crossings by interferons from less closely related cells caused stretches of the imagination to create terms like "genus specificity" (Zimmerman *et al.*, 1972; Hilfenhaus, Thierfelder and Barth, 1975) or even "family" (Anfinsen *et al.*, 1974; Johnson, Smith, and Baron, 1975) or "order specificity" (Moehring and Stinebring, 1970). The persistence of this misconception about interferons is evidenced by statements encountered in recent literature that " the biological effect of interferon is restricted to the homologous cell species" (Bourgeade, 1977) or that Interferons are "species-specific cellular glycoproteins" (Pitha, 1977). And even after it had been repeatedly reported that human interferons

Table 8. *Cross-species activities of interferons*

Interferon	Assayed on	Crossing*	References
Human fibroblast	monkey	–	Polikoff *et al.* (1962)
		+ to ++++	Chany (1961); Bucknall (1967); Stewart II and Lockart (1970); Duc-Goiran, Galliot, and Chany (1971); Gresser *et al.* (1974); Neumann-Haefelin *et al.*, (1975); Lerner and Bailey (1976); Desmyter and Stewart II (1976); Scott *et al.* (1977c)
	rabbit	+ to ++++	Andrews (1961); Pollikoff *et al.* (1962); Desmyter, Rawls, and Melnick (1968; 1970); Paucker *et al.*, (1975); Desmyter and Stewart II (1976)
	hamster	–	Pollikoff *et al.* (1962)
	chick	–	Pollikoff *et al.* (1962); Merigan, Winget, and Dixon (1965); Pestka *et al.* (1975; 1977)
	bovine	– to ±	Stewart II (unpublished); Babiuk and Rouse (1977); Cavalieri *et al.* (1977 a, b)
		+ to ++	Gresser *et al.* (1974); Pollikoff *et al.* (1962)
	mouse	–	Merigan, Winget, and Dixon (1965); Bucknall (1967); Levy-Koenig *et al.* (1970 a); Berman and Vilcek (1974); Pestka *et al.* (1975)
		+	Ito and Kobayashi (1974)
	rat	+++	Duc-Goiran, Galliot, and Chany (1971)
	cat	– to ±	Rodgers *et al.* (1972); Rodgers and Merigan (1974); Desmyter and Stewart II (1976); Billiau *et al.* (1977a)
		++	Edy *et al.* (1977)
	pig	+	Babiuk and Rouse (1977)
		–	Desmyter and Stewart II (1976)
Human leukocyte	monkey	+ to +++	Gresser *et al.* (1974); Hilfenhaus *et al.* (1975; 1977); Lerner and

* Degree of cross-reactivity: –, no detectable activity reported; ±, trace activity ≤ 1% of activity on homologous cells: +, less than 10% homologous activity; ++, about 25–50%; +++, 50–75%; ++++, titers as high as those obtained in homologous cells; +++++, titers significantly higher than those on homologous cells.

Table 8 (continued)

Interferon	Assayed on	Crossing*	References
			Bailey (1976); Desmyter and Stewart II (1976); Jameson, Dixon, and Grossberg (1977); Scott et al. (1977); Samuel and Farris (1977)
	rabbit	− to ±	Duc-Goiran et al. (1971); Jameson, Dixon, and Grossberg (1977)
		+ to ++++	Desmyter et al. (1968; 1970); Stewart II and Desmyter (1975); Paucker et al. (1975); McGill et al. (1976); Desmyter and Stewart II (1976); Pinto et al. (1970)
	chick	−	Duc-Goiran et al. (1971)
	rat	−	Duc-Goiran et al. (1971)
	mouse	−	Jameson, Dixon, and Grossberg (1977); Duc-Goiran et al. (1971); Imanishi et al. (1975)
		+	Borecky et al. (1974); Hilfenhaus, Thierfelder, and Barth (1975); Stewart II et al. (1976); Dahl (1977a); Greenberg and Mosny (1977); Paucker et al. (1977); Samuel and Farris (1977)
	hamster	+	Borecky et al. (1974); Jameson, Dixon and Grossberg (1977)
	bovine	+ to +++++	Gresser et al. (1974); Cavalieri et al. (1977 a); Babiuk and Rouse (1977); Jameson, Dixon, and Grossberg (1977); Paucker et al. (1977); Lin et al. (1978)
	pig	+ to +++	Gresser et al (1974); Jameson, Dixon, and Grossberg (1977); Paucker et al. (1977)
	cat	+ to +++++	Desmyter and Stewart II (1976); Edy et al. (1977); Jameson, Dixon, and Grossberg (1977); Billiau et al. (1977a)
	dog	+ to ±	Desmyter and Stewart II (1976); Jameson, Dixon, and Grossberg (1977)
Human lymphoblastoid	bovine	++ to ++++	Gresser et al. (1974); Cavalieri et al. (1977 a); Stewart II (unpublished)
Human (Type II)	bovine	−	Stewart II (unpublished)

Table 8 (continued)

Interferon	Assayed on	Crossing*	References
	cat	−	Epstein, Stevens, and Merigan (1972)
	pig	+++	Babiuk and Rouse (1977)
	rabbit	−	Lai, Alpers, and Mackay-Scollay (1977)
Monkey	human	+ to +++++	Sutton and Tyrrell (1961); Pollikoff et al. (1962); Jones, Galbraith, and Al-Hussaini (1962); Bucknall (1967); Desmyter et al. (1970); Stewart II and Lockart (1970); Wright, Falk, and Deinhardt (1974); Thacore (1976); Desmyter and Stewart II (1976); Stephen et al. (1977 a); Samuel and Farris (1977)
	bovine	+	Pollikoff et al. (1962)
	rabbit	−	Wright, Falk, and Deinhardt (1974)
		+ to +++	Pollikoff et al. (1962); Desmyter et al. (1970)
	rat	++	Uhlendorf et al. (1973); Zimmerman et al. (1972)
	chick	−	Pollikoff et al. (1962); Desmyter et al. (1970); Wright, Falk, and Deinhardt (1974); DeMaeyer-Guignard, DeMaeyer, and Montagnier (1972)
	cat	+++	Desmyter and Stewart II (1976)
	hamster	−	Pollikoff et al. (1962); Wright, Falk, and Deinhardt (1974)
	mouse	−	Kronenberg and Friedmann (1975); Samuel Farris (1977)
Rabbit	human	−	Pyhala and Cantell (1974); Desmyter and Stewart II (1976); Babiuk and Rouse (1977); Pollikoff et al. (1962)
	monkey	−	Pollikoff et al. (1962); Desmyter and Stewart II (1976)
	bovine	−	Pollikoff et al. (1962); Gresser et al. (1974)
	pig	−	Gresser et al. (1974); Babiuk and Rouse (1977)
	chick	−	Isaacs and Westwood (1959 a); Pollikoff et al. (1962)

Interferon	Assayed on	Crossing*	References
	cat	−	Desmyter and Stewart II (1976)
	mouse	−	Ngan, Lee, and Kind (1976)
		±	Ito and Kobayashi (1974)
Bovine	human	−	Pollikoff et al. (1962)
		±	Gresser et al. (1974)
		+ to ++	Ahl and Rump (1976); Babiuk and Rouse (1977); Tovey et al. (1977 a)
	monkey	−	Pollikoff et al. (1962)
		+ to +++	Babiuk and Rouse (1977); Tovey et al. (1977 a)
	pig	+ to +++++	Rosenquist and Loan (1967); Ahl and Rump (1976); Babiuk and Rouse (1977)
	sheep	+++++	Rinaldo et al. (1976)
	horse	−	Babiuk and Rouse (1977)
	dog	−	Babiuk and Rouse (1977)
	rabbit	−	Babiuk and Rouse (1977)
	hamster	−	Pollikoff et al. (1962)
	chick	−	Pollikoff et al. (1962)
Bovine (Type II)	human	++	Babiuk and Rouse (1977)
	monkey	++	Babiuk and Rouse (1977)
	pig	++++	Babiuk and Rouse (1977)
	rabbit	++	Babiuk and Rouse (1977)
	horse	+	Babiuk and Rouse (1977)
	dog	±	Babiuk and Rouse (1977)
Chicken	partridge, quail, turkey	+ to ++++	Moehring and Stinebring (1970)
	duck, goose	−	Wagner (1961); Moehring and Stinebring (1970)
	mouse	−	Baron et al. (1964); Merigan (1964); Weber and Stewart (1973); Orlova et al. (1976)
		± to +	Gifford (1963 c)

Interferon	Assayed on	Crossing*	References
	rabbit	− to ±	Isaacs and Westwood (1959 b); Desmyter *et al.* (1970); Pollikoff *et al.* (1962)
		+	Andrews (1961)
	monkey	− to ±	Tyrrell (1959); Pollikoff *et al.* (1962)
		+	Andrews (1961)
	human	−	Pollikoff *et al.* (1962); Merigan (1964)
	bovine	− to ±	Tyrrell (1959); Pollikoff *et al.* (1962)
Duck	chick	− to ±	Wagner (1961); Moehring and Stinebring (1970)
	goose	+++	Moehring and Stinebring (1970)
Pig	bovine	++	Hermodsson (1964); Pollikoff *et al.* (1962); Torlone, Titoli, and Gialletti (1965)
	monkey	−	Pollikoff *et al.* (1962)
	human	−	Pollikoff *et al.* (1962); Gresser *et al.* (1974)
	hamster	−	Pollikoff *et al.* (1962)
	rabbit	−	Pollikoff *et al.* (1962)
	chick	−	Pollikoff *et al.* (1962); Torlone, Titoli, and Gialletti (1965)
Hamster	mouse	+	Henle and Henle (1963); Stewart II, Scott, and Sulkin (1969); Umino and Kohno (1976)
	bovine	+	Pollikoff *et al.* (1962)
	monkey	−	Pollikoff *et al.* (1962); Jahrling (1975)
	human	−	Pollikoff *et al.* (1962)
	rabbit	−	Desmyter *et al.* (1970)
		+	Pollikoff *et al.* (1972)
	chick	−	Pollikoff *et al.* (1962); Jahrling (1975)
Sheep	mouse	−	Rinaldo *et al.* (1975)
Rainbow trout	goldfish	+ to ++	DeSena and Rio (1975)

Interferon	Assayed on	Crossing*	References
	fat head minnow	−	Kinkelin and LeBerre (1974)
Dog	bovine	+	Pollikoff et al. (1962)
	rabbit	+	Pollikoff et al. (1962)
	cat	−	Desmyter and Stewart II (1976)
	monkey	−	Pollikoff et al. (1962)
	human	−	Pollikoff et al. (1962)
	chick	−	Pollikoff et al. (1962)
Cat	dog	+	Desmyter and Stewart II (1976)
	monkey	−	McCullough (1972); Rodgers and Merigan (1974); Desmyter and Stewart II (1976)
	human	−	McCullough (1972); Rodgers et al. (1972); Desmyter and Stewart II (1976)
	mouse	−	Rodgers et al. (1972)
	rabbit	−	Desmyter and Stewart II (1976)
	hamster	−	McCullough (1972)
Rat	mouse	± to +	Soloviev et al. (1972 b); Mentkevich et al. (1973; 1974); Vassef et al.
	monkey	−	Lobodzinska et al. (1973 a, b)
	chick	−	Lobodzinska et al. (1973 a, b)
	human	−	Lobodzinska et al. (1973 a, b)
	bovine	−	Lobodzinska et al. (1973 a, b)
Rat (type II)	mouse	+++ to ++++	Lobodzinska et al. (1973 a, b); Lobodzinska et al. (1975)
	human	++	Lobodzinska et al. (1973 a, b)
	bovine	+	Lobodzinska et al. (1973 a, b)
	monkey	−	Lobodzinska et al. (1973 a, b)
	chick	−	Lobodzinska et al. (1973 a, b)
Mouse	hamster	−	Blalock and Baron (1977); Pantelouris and Pringle (1976); Grossberg et al. (1975)

Table 8 (continued)

Interferon	Assayed on	Crossing*	References
		± to +	Umino and Kohne (1976); Buckler and Baron (1966); Stewart II, Scott, and Sulkin (1969)
	rat	± to ++	Buckler and Baron (1966); Soloviev et al. (1972 b); Mentkevich et al. (1973); Beck et al. (1974); Oie et al. (1975)
		−	Pantelouris and Pringle (1976)
	chick	−	Baron et al. (1964); Merigan (1964); Merigan et al. (1965); Buckler and Baron (1966); DeMaeyer-Guignard et al. (1972); Weber and Stewart (1973); Youngner and Salvin (1973); Oie et al. (1975)
		+	Gifford (1963 c)
	human	−	Merigan et al. (1965); Oie et al. (1975); Blalock and Baron (1977)
		+	Bodo, Palese and Lindner (1971); Samuel and Farris (1977); Wiranowska-Stewart and Stewart II (1977)
	monkey	−	Buckler and Baron (1966); DeMaeyer-Guignard et al. (1972); Samuel and Farris (1977); Kronenberg and Friedmann (1975)
	rabbit	−	Desmyter et al. (1970); Youngner and Salvin (1973); Stewart II et al. (1972 b); Oie et al. (1975); Ngan et al. (1976)
	guinea pig	+ to ++++	Youngner and Salvin (1973); Umino and Kohno (1976); Stewart II, LeGoff, and Wiranowska-Stewart (1977)
	bovine	−	Gresser et al. (1974); Stewart II (unpublished)
	pig	−	Gresser et al. (1974)
Mouse (type II)	guinea pig	−	Youngner and Salvin (1973)
	chick	−	Youngner and Salvin (1973); Saito et al. (1976); Virelizier et al. (1977)
	monkey	−	Virelizier et al. (1977)
	rabbit	−	Youngner and Salvin (1973); Saito et al. (1976)

were highly active on rabbit cells (Polikoff *et al.*, 1962; Desmyter, Rawls, and Melnick, 1968, 1970), investigators were proposing to use interferon sensitivities of cells as adjuncts for determining the genus of origin of cell cultures (Zimmerman *et al.*, 1972; Uhlendorf *et al.*, 1973). As illustrated in Table 8, it appears rather that interferons have "defined host-ranges" of cells which are receptive to them, some interferons being much more omni-active than others. The host-range can differ significantly even for different interferons from the same animal. For example, human leukocyte interferons are highly active on a large number of unrelated animals whereas human fibroblast interferon is significantly active on only a relatively limited number of these cells.

The apparent degree of cross-reactivity of interferon that have been repeatedly reported to cross react can vary tremendously, depending on both the cells used to obtain homologous titers and the cells used to determine heterologous titers. Desmyter and Stewart II (1976) found that different types of cat cells were all sensitive to human leukocyte interferon, yet the titers obtained on a number of cat cells differed several hundred-fold. The apparent degree of cross-species activity can also be tremendously influenced by the challenge virus used. Ahl and Rump (1976) found that bovine interferon titers determined on bovine cells challenged with vesicular stomatitis virus were higher than those obtained for bovine interferon in porcine cells challenged with this virus; however, when other viruses were used for challenge in porcine cells, bovine interferon titers were much higher in the pig cells than in the homologous cells. This host cell dependence of relative sensitivities of different viruses to interferon has been observed repeatedly (Stewart II, Scott, and Sulkin, 1969; Ito and Montagnier, 1977) and will be discussed in detail later (Section IX).

The accumulated data on cross-species activities demonstrate a number of important points:

First, the phyllogenetic relationship has little relation to cross-species activity, as many interferons are more active on cells of distantly related animals than on those of close kins (human leukocyte interferon being uniformly more active on bovine cells and on cat cells than on monkey cells; Gresser *et al.*, 1974; Desmyter and Stewart II, 1976). Also, it cannot be argued that because only one-way crosses are observed between some species that humans are more closely related to cows than cows are to humans.

The differences in host-ranges can also apply to different molecular forms of interferons produced by cells of a single species, human leukocyte interferons being highly active on cat and bovine cells, while human fibroblast interferons are much less active on these (Gresser *et al.*, 1974; Desmyter and Stewart II, 1976). However, this is not to imply that human leukocytes are generally able to cross-react better than human fibroblast interferons, as the latter are the more active on rat cells (Duc-Goiran, Galliot, and Chany, 1971). The defined host ranges of various human interferons can be used to distinguish them, as human leukocyte and lymphoblastoid cell interferon exhibit identical cross-species properties which are different from the host-range of fibroblast interferon. The difference between leukocyte and fibroblast interferons seen in human species has not been found with bovine leukocyte and fibroblast interferons (Tovey *et al.*, 1977a).

Even the different molecular species of given types of interferon can differ in host-range. Human leukocyte interferon preparations resolve into 21,000 dalton and 15,000 dalton components in SDS-polyacrylamide gel electrophoresis and exert about 100% and 5%, respectively, of homologous titers on rabbit cells (Stewart II and Desmyter, 1975); similarly mouse interferon gel-isolates at 38,000 daltons and 22,000 daltons are slightly (about 5%) and significantly (more than 100% of mouse cell activity levels) active on guinea-pig cells (Stewart II, LeGoff, and Wiranowska–Stewart, 1977). Bodo and his associates (1971) also found that a smaller component of mouse interferon was more cross-reactive on human cells.

The acid-labile interferons (designated Type II) have different host-ranges than the Type I (acid-stable) interferons of the same species. In the cases of bovine Type II interferon (Babiuk and Rouse, 1977) and rat Type II interferon (Lobodzinska et al., 1973 a, b; 1975) these were significantly more cross reactive than the Type I interferons, but in the case of human Type II interferon (Epstein et al., 1972; Stewart II unpublished data; Lai et al., 1977) and mouse Type II interferon (Youngner and Salvin, 1973; Virelizier, Allison, and De-Maeyer, 1977), they were less cross-active than the Type I interferons.

The cross-species activities found in cell culture systems have also been found to apply in the animals, as human interferons active in rabbit and monkey cell cultures are also active in rabbits (Pinto et al., 1970; McGill et al., 1976; Desomer et al., 1977) and in monkeys (Hilfenhaus et al., 1975; 1977; Scott et al., 1977 c; Neumann–Haefelin et al., 1975) and monkey interferon, active in human cell cultures, was active in human eyes (Jones, Galbraith, and Al-Hussaini, 1962).

It is also worthwhile mentioning that the terms "monkey" interferon, "fish" interferon, etc., are greatly oversimplified. In fact, some monkey interferons are only fractionally active on human cells and cells from other types of monkeys (Wright, Falk, and Deinhardt, 1974), and fish interferons distinguish between different species of fish cells (DeSena and Rio, 1975; Kinkelin and LeBarre, 1974). Similarly, Mexican free-tailed bats and big brown bats both produce interferons, neither of which will exert activity in the other bat's cells (Stewart II, 1969).

The cross-reactivity of interferon activities is not limited to induction of antiviral activities, as similar host-ranges are observed for the non-antiviral activities, "priming" and "blocking" actions (Levy–Koenig et al., 1970a; Stewart II et al., 1971a; Weber and Stewart, 1973; Lobodzinska et al., 1975; Ito and Kobayashi, 1974; Beck et al., 1974), cell multiplication inhibition (Gresser et al., 1973; Borecky et al., 1974; Stewart II et al., 1976; Babiuk and Rouse, 1977), and immunomodulations (Ngan et al., 1976; Greenberg and Mosny, 1977; Imanishi et al., 1975) and double-stranded RNA toxicity-enhancement (Stewart II et al., 1972).

The "defined host-ranges" of interferons are useful for characterization of interferons, even more than true "species-specificity" would be. Thus interferons made from messenger RNAs from various cells can be identified not only by species of origin (DeMayer–Guignard, DeMaeyer, and Montagnier, 1972; Kronenberg et al., 1975; Reynolds and Pitha, 1974; Orlova et al., 1977), but also as to type of cell of origin, even within the given species. Human fibroblast interferon message translated in various heterologous cells, oöcytes or cell-free systems gives interferon with host-range characteristic for human fibroblast interferon (Pestka *et al.*, 1975; 1977; Cavalieri *et al.*, 1977a), while human lymphoblastoid interferon message RNA translated in each of these systems produces an interferon exhibiting the host-range characteristic of human leukocyte interferon (Cavalieri *et al.*, 1977a).

The total of data definitely show that the concept of "species-specificity" should be superceded by *"defined host-ranges"* of interferons.

3. Acid-Stability of Interferons

For many years stability of a virus inhibitor to pH 2 treatment was considered a requirement for classification as an interferon. This property was not only useful for characterization but was a convenient method to rid suspected interferon preparations of the infectivity of inducing viruses and to facilitate selective precipitations of extraneous proteins (Stewart II, Gosser, and Lockart, 1971a). However, a number of publications began to appear reporting "interferon-like" inhibitors which induced virus resistance through interferon-like mechanisms, showed interferon-like defined host-ranges, but which were distinct from classical interferons in being destroyed by treatment at pH 2. A number of these acid-labile interferons are listed in Table 9 to demonstrate the types of systems reported to produce them. These have often been referred to as "endotoxin-type" interferons, to distinguish them from interferons induced by viruses, which were presumed to be uniformly acid-stable (Ke and Ho, 1967; Ke, Ho, and Merigan, 1966). However, again the term "endotoxin-type" is misleading as some viruses also induce acid-labile interferons (Maehara and Nagano, 1970; Yamada *et al.*, 1970; Higashihara, 1971; Biernacka and Lobodzinska, 1973; Lobodzinska *et al.*, 1973a, 1975; Fujibayashi, Hooks, and Notkins, 1975; Trubina *et al.*, 1975) and some endotoxin-induced interferons were acid-stable (Matisova *et al.*, 1970; Saito *et al.*, 1976).

As indicated previously (Sections III. B. 5 and VI. B. 1) interferons can be produced by specifically sensitized immunocompetent cells after such cells are exposed to the specific sensitizing antigen (Falcoff, 1972; Salvin *et al.*, 1973, 1974, 1975a, b; Youngner and Salvin, 1973; Fujibayashi *et al.*, 1975; Trubina *et al.*, 1975; Azuma *et al.*, 1970; Falcoff, Oriol, and Iscaki, 1972; Epstein, Stevens, and Merigan, 1972; Valle *et al.*, 1975a, b). These interferons are distinct from "classical" interferons in being acid-labile, and were designated "immune" interferon (Falcoff *et al.*, 1970). However, this nomenclature was, again, a misrepresentation as many other acid-labile interferons are not induced by immune-recognition sets (Maehara and Nagano, 1970; Higashihara, 1971; Biernacka and Lobodzinska, 1973; Lobodzinska *et al.*, 1973a, 1975; Wheelock, 1965; Suzuki *et al.*, 1971; Epstein *et al.*, 1971a, b; Klimpel, Day, and Lucas, 1975), and some immune-induced interferons are not acid labile (Glasgow, 1966).

More recently all these acid-labile interferons have been grouped as "Type II" interferons to distinguish them from the acid-stable "classical" in-

Table 9. *Type II interferons*

Species	Production system	inactivated by*			References
		pH2	56° C	Type I-interferon antiserum	
Human	Cerebrospinal fluid in CNS diseases	+			Gresser and Naficy (1964)
	Cerebrospinal fluid in CNS diseases	+	+		Larke (1967)
	Leukocytes + PHA	+	+		Wheelock (1965)
	Lymphocytes + anti-lymphocytic serum	+	0		Falcoff, R. (1972); Falcoff, E. *et al.* (1972 a)
	Lymphocytes + macrophages + mitogens	+	+		Epstein *et al.* (1971 a, b; 1974 a, b); Epstein and Cline (1974); Epstein and Ammann (1974)
	Tonsil lymphocytes + mitogens	+	+		Klimpel *et al.* (1975)
	Herpesvirus-sensitized lymphocytes + macrophages + herpes virus antigen	+	+	0	Haahr, Rasmussen, and Merigan (1976); Valle *et al.* (1975 b)
	Rubella-virus-sensitized lymphocytes + rubella virus	+	+		Buimovici-Klein, Weiss, and Cooper (1977)
	Lymphoblastoid cells	+			Archer and Young (1974)
	Bone marrow of multiple myeloma patients	+	+		Epstein and Salmon (1974)
Mouse	*Toxoplasma gondii* (serum)	+	+		Freshman *et al.* (1966)
	Trypanosoma cruzi (serum)	+	+		Rytel and Marsden (1970)
	Rift valley fever virus (1.5-hour serum)	+	+		Higashihara (1971)
	Newcastle disease virus + macrophages (immune or normal)	+	+		Yamada *et al.* (1970); Azuma *et al.* (1970 a, b), Azuma (1973; 1976)
	Spleen cells + hemagglutinating virus of Japan	+	+		Ito *et al.* (1974)
	Sensitized spleen cells + cytomegalovirus	+			Rytel and Hooks (1977)
	Sensitized leukocytes + L cells	+	0		Borecky, Lackovic and Russ (1970)
	BCG-sensitized (serum) + BCG	+			Clinton *et al.* (1976)

Table 9 (continued)

Species	Production system	inactivated by*		Type I-interferon antiserum	References
		pH2	56° C		
	BCG-sensitized (serum) + BCG + BCG or old tuberculin	+	0	0	Salvin et al. (1973; 1974; 1975 a); Youngner and Salvin (1973)
	BCG-sensitized (serum) + BCG	+		0	Maehara, Ho, and Armstrong (1977)
	Endotoxin (serum)	+	+		Higashihara (1971)
	9-Methylstreptimidone (serum)	+	+		Saito et al. (1976)
	Spleen cells + mitogens (Con A, staphylococcal enterotoxin A)			0	Johnson, Stanton, and Baron (1977)
	Spleen cells + PHA	+		0	Wietzerbin et al. (1977 a, b)
	Candida albicans mannan (serum)	+			Borecky et al. (1967)
Rabbit	Endotoxin (serum)	+	+		Ke and Ho (1967)
	Phosphomannan (serum)	+	+		Suzuki et al. (1971)
	Newcastle disease virus (serum)	+	+		Maehara and Nagano (1970)
	Tuberculin-sensitized (skin) + PPD	+			Lodmell et al. (1976)
	Measles-virus-immune (serum) + measles virus	+	+		Trubina et al. (1975)
	Sensitized splenic leukocytes + herpes virus-antigen	+	+		Fujibayashi et al. (1975)
Rat	Sindbis virus or Newcastle disease virus (early serum) or Newcastle disease virus + rat embryo cultures	+	+		Lobodzinska et al. (1973 a); Biernacka and Lobodzinska (1973)
Bovine	Spleen cells + infectious bovine rhinotracheitis virus	+	+		Fulton and Rosenquist (1976 b)

* Inactivated, +; not inactivated, 0.

terferons which are designated "Type I" (Salvin et al., 1973, 1974, 1975; Youngner and Salvin, 1973). Of course, this designation is not uniformly applied by all investigators, as some chose to classify Type II interferons on the basis of heat (56° C)-stability or neutralization by anti-Type I interferon antisera rather than acid-lability (Sonnenfeld, Mandel, and Merigan, 1977; Johnson, Stanton, and Baron, 1977; Maehara, Ho, and Armstrong, 1977). However, as many acid-labile interferons are also heat labile while others are heat stable (Table 9), I prefer to emphasize the pH 2 lability property or antigenicity. In this tentative classification system a paraphrase of Milton seems appropriate: differences of opinions among informed individuals represent knowledge in the making.

Several other interferons likely to be Type II have been reported, but these are not included in Table 9 because neither acid-labilities nor antibody neutralizations were apparently determined: Wallen, Dean, and Lucas (1973) induced interferons in sensitized mice be injection of PPD antigen and various T-cell mitogens; similarly Rasmussen et al. (1974) reported that herpes virus antigen specifically stimulated interferon in lymphocytes-macrophage cultures from patients with recurrent Herpes virus hominis disease; and Babiuk and Rouse (1976) specifically induced interferon in virus- and tuberculin-immune bovine lymphocyte-macrophage cultures. Johnson, Stanton, and Baron (1977) induced interferon in mouse spleen cultures with either of two T-cell mitogens, concanavalin A or staphylococcal enterotoxin A; these interferons were, however, antigenically distinct from Type I poly rI·poly rC-induced mouse interferon though their stability properties were not reported. Kirchner et al. (1977) reported that Corynebacterium parvum induced interferon in mouse spleen cell cultures, but did not characterize the interferon as to pH 2-stability or antigenic properties. O'Reilly and his colleagues (1977) found interferon was specifically induced by Herpes simplex virus antigen in lymphocyte cultures from patients during convalescence from herpes virus-induced vesicular eruptions; the interferon was not characterized as to Type I or II. Of course, it is also likely that many acid-labile interferons have not been observed merely because many investigators routinely adjust samples to pH 2.0 to qualify, "sterilize" and purify them.

It should be mentioned that "acid-lability" may be a misleading term. Many interferons that are labile at pH 2 are completely inactivated (greater than 99.9% loss of activity: Youngner and Salvin, 1973), while others are only partially inactivated (about 50 to 90%: Fulton and Rosenquist, 1976). Also, pH 2-labile Type II mouse-interferon is stable at acid pH of 4.0 (Wietzerbin et al., 1977a; E. Falcoff, personal communication). This stability at moderately acidic pH values is important for purification of Type II interferon (Wietzerbin et al., 1977a).

These pH 2-labile and antigenically distinct interferons can be produced spontaneously, or in response to viruses or microorganisms in either sensitized or normal animals, in response to mitogens or specific viral or bacterial antigens, or in response to antibiotics, endotoxins or other microbial products. It is interesting that viruses which induce acid-stable, Type I, interferons at later times, can induce acid-labile, Type II interferons at earlier times (Maehara and

Nagano, 1970; Lobodzinska et al., 1973; Higashihara, 1971). Rabbits injected with Newcastle disease virus produced an acid-labile interferon at 2 hours postinjection, but by 6 hours the interferon produced was acid-stable (Maehara and Nagano, 1970). Mice also had circulating Type II interferon at $1\frac{1}{2}$ hour after inoculation with Rift valley fever virus, but Type I interferon by 8 hours (Higashihara, 1971). In rats, either Sindbis virus or Newcastle disease virus induced acid-labile early interferon that was active on mouse, human and bovine cells; later interferon was active only on homologous cells and was acid-stable (Lobodzinska et al., 1973; Biernacka and Lobodzinska, 1973). These authors also report that Newcastle disease virus-induced rat embryo cell culture interferon was acid-labile.

These data cumulatively show that both pH 2-stability and heat-stability are worthless for classification of a virus-inhibitor as interferon. However, it is only in the last 3 or 4 years that acid-labile interferons have become recognized as a general occurrence, and the vast majority of purifications and characterizations of interferon involve studies using Type I, acid-stable interferons.

4. Physiochemical Properties Generally Applicable to All Interferons: Protein Nature of Interferons

The fact that cellular RNA and protein synthesis are required for interferon production (Section VI. A), plus the uniform observation that activities of interferon preparations are destroyed by proteolytic enzymes (Lockart, 1973), and the generation of interferon activity from messenger RNA preparations extracted from induced cells and translated in cellular or cell-free protein synthesizing systems (Section VI. A), all point to the conclusion that interferons are proteins. Treatments of interferons with nucleases, either DNase or RNase, have no affects on their activities, and recent studies to be described below (Section VII. B) demonstrate that the carbohydrate moieties present on at least some of the interferons are merely embellishments, not needed for any of the activities of the protein core (Stewart II et al., 1977; Stewart II et al., 1978; Wiranowska–Stewart et al., 1978; Lin et al., 1978). More recent evidence has directly confirmed the assumption that interferons are proteins, for as will be demonstrated in detail below (Section VII. B. C), interferons have now been purified in sufficient quantities to visualize the interferon proteins by the high--resolution two-dimensional gel electrophoresis technique (Lin and Stewart II, 1978; Lin et al., 1978).

The interferon proteins are small enough to remain in solutions even during prolonged ultracentrifugation and are large enough to remain within dialysis tubings. Size estimates have ranged from about 10^4 to 10^5 for practically each interferon species (Fantes, 1973). Rather than present an exhaustive list of these mostly meaningless numbers, suffice it for me to assure the reader that nearly any number one chooses in this range has been reported as the molecular weight of some interferon. However, as most of these estimates are based on data obtained under nondissociating conditions, the "large" interferons likely represent aggregates of interferons with other proteins in the preparations. The imaginative claim by Carter (1970, 1971)[6] that the interferons with larger molecular weights could be dissociated into basic "subunits" and that these units could then be reassociated into "dimers", has been repeatedly discredited (Stewart II, 1974; Knight, 1975; Reynolds and Pitha, 1975; Tarodi et al., 1975; Yamamoto and Kawade, 1976; Vilček, Havell, and Yamazaki, 1977). It is, however still, being expounded (Carter et al., 1975 a, b) and is often assumed correct (Rodgers and Merigan, 1974; Declercq, 1974; Zuckerman, 1976), thus causing considerable confusion about this research field. The molecular heterogeneities of interferons will be dealt with in detail below; it should be emphasized that the different molecular forms of interferons are not composites of common subunits.

5. Antigenicities of Interferons

The early reported attempts to induce animals to make antibodies to interferons were unsuccessful (Isaacs, 1959a; Burke and Isaacs, 1960; Lindenmann, 1960); this lead to the premature assumption that interferons were weakly- or non-antigenic, and tempted speculation that this would enhance its therapeutic value (Isaacs, 1959a, b). Ironically, the observations were wrong, but conclusion was right: interferons are antigenic, but not in homologous systems. Levy–Koenig et al. (1970a, b) inoculated rabbits and guinea-pigs with about 10^4 units of rabbit interferon each week subcutaneously for several months; guinea-pigs developed high-titered neutralizing antibody to rabbit interferon; rabbits developed no anti-rabbit interferon. Strander et al. (1973) reported injecting 1 to 3×10^6 units of human leukocyte interferon intramuscularly into volunteers each week for several months without eliciting a detectable antibody response. These studies have since been extended in a number of clinical trials with human subjects often being injected with several million units of human interferons each day for months (Section XIV); no one has yet found human interferon-neutralizing activity in sera of any of these patients.

With the usual improved vision of hindsight, it is now possible to realize that the early reported negative antibody stimulation attempts are attributable to the extremely low antigenic mass of interferon protein being inoculated (with a specific activity of about 10^9 units of interferon/mg of protein, the few thousand units injected would represent nanograms of interferon protein). As larger doses of interferons became available the apparent antigenicity of each of the interferons has increased, with potent antisera now being produced in a number of laboratories (Table 10). Recently the United States National Institutes of Health has offered a contract for production of antisera to human leukocyte interferon, human fibroblast interferon and mouse interferon, each to titrate at least 10^5 interferon neutralizing units/ml of antiserum[7].

It is also interesting that, though not antigenic in homologous hosts, interferons are antigenic in heterologous species in which they are also active. For

---

[6] Another interesting phenomenon of interferonology is that, as pointed out in footnote 5, certain identical papers, such as these, seem to appear in two journals!

[7] RFP #NIH-NIAID-DAB-78-5: Production of antisera to interferons, issued November 29, 1977.

instance, rabbit cells *in vitro* and rabbits *in vivo* are sensitive to the human interferons (Table 8) yet human interferons are antigenic in rabbits (Table 10; Levy–Koenig *et al.*, 1970a; Duc–Goiran, Galliot, and Chany, 1971; Mogensen, Phyala, and Cantell, 1975; Berg *et al.*, 1975; Havell *et al.*, 1975a).

The first successful demonstration of neutralizing antiserum to an interferon was reported by Paucker and Cantell (1962). As the amounts of interferons available have increased and their purification have improved, the titers of antisera to the interferons have increased. Mogensen *et al.* (1975) reported that by injecting a sheep with a total of about 300 million units of human leukocyte interferon, a neutralizing antibody titer of about 10^6 was obtained (i. e., at a 1/1,000,000 dilution the antiserum was able to neutralize the antiviral activity of about 10 units of human leukocyte interferon). Using a similar injection scheme, M. Tovey was able to obtain antibodies of similar potency to mouse interferon (Gresser *et al.*, 1976b). Generally, the antigenicity of interferon preparations has been found improved with more highly purified interferons, likely because the noninterferon antigenic-mass is not competing with interferon for cells to convert to antibody factories. Highest antibody titers have been achieved by primary immunizing sequences with injections of relatively crude interferon, without adjuvant, followed by a booster injection of highly purified interferon with adjuvant to elicit a specific anti-interferon anamnestic reaction (Mogensen *et al.*, 1975; Gresser *et al.*, 1976b).

The antiserum to a given interferon is able to neutralize its antiviral activity and its various non-antiviral activities, equally. Thus, priming activity (Levy–Koenig *et al.*, 1970b), cell multiplication inhibitory activity (Gresser, Bandu, and Brouty-Boye, 1974), phagocytosis-enhancing action (Donahoe and Huang, 1973) and immunosuppressive effects (Johnson, Smith, and Baron, 1974) of interferons are all neutralized by antisera able to neutralize their antiviral activities. These data suggest that all these activities share a common active site which was antigenic. Alternatively, the antigenic site could be adjacent to the active site so that steric hindrance would result with antibody binding. It is difficult to imagine that the active site is the actual immunogen as the human interferon which is antivirally active on rabbits is also antigenic in them. Indeed Paucker and his associates (1975) have reported that certain rabbit antisera to human leukocyte interferon were able to neutralize its activity for human cells but not its activity for rabbit cells. Generally, however, homologous-cell activity and heterologous-cell activity are both neutralized by antiserum to interferons (Gresser, Bandu, and Brouty-Boye, 1974; Levy–Koenig *et al.*, 1970b).

The antigenic properties are, as indicated in previous discussions, useful not only for identification of interferon as to species, but also within species they can differentiate between types of interferons. Levy–Koenig *et al.* (1970a) and Duc–Goiran *et al.* (1971) reported that antisera prepared against human leukocyte interferon were more active against human leukocyte interferon than against human amniotic membrane interferon. Anti-human leukocyte interferon antibodies were also less efficient against human fibroblast interferon, and antisera to human fibroblast interferon had no activity against human leukocyte interferon (Vilček *et al.*, 1977; Berg *et al.*, 1975; Havell *et al.*,

Table 10. *Antigenicities of interferons*

Inter-feron species	Animal inoculated	Route[a]	Dose and frequency	Total units inoculated	Neutral-izing antibody titer[b]	References
Chick	chick rabbit	im.	$<10^3$ units; $\times$ <4 weeks	?	none	Isaacs (1959 b)
	rabbit	im.	$<10^3$ units/week; $\times$ 2 weeks (+ adjuvant)	?	none	Burke and Isaacs (1960); Linden-mann (1960)
	rabbit	sc.	$\sim 10^3$ units/dose; $\times$ 10 to 20 weekly doses	$\sim 2 \times 10^4$	$\sim 10^2$	German, Quero, and Poindron (1970)
Mouse	guinea pig	ip. im.	$\sim 10^3$ units/dose $\times$ 13 doses over 5 months + 3 doses	$\sim 2 \times 10^4$	$\sim 10^2$	Paucker and Cantell (1962)
	guinea pig rabbit	im. ip.	$\sim 10^3$ units/dose/ week $\times$ 20–30 weeks	$\sim 2 \times 10^4$	$\sim 10^2$	Paucker (1965)
	rabbit	sc.	$\sim 10^3$ units/dose/ week $\times$ 20 weeks	$\sim 2 \times 10^4$	$\sim 10^3$	Fauconnier (1967 a, b)
	rabbit guinea pig	sc. sc.	3–10×10^3 units/ week $\times \sim 25$ weeks	$\sim 2 \times 10^5$	$\sim 4 \times 10^3$	Levy-Koenig *et al.* (1970 a)
	sheep	sc.	4×10^6 units/ week $\times$ 35 weeks	$\sim 10^8$	$\sim 10^3$	Sipe *et al.* (1973)
	rabbit	im. sc. footpad	10^7 units/dose/ month (+ adjuvant) $\times \sim 1$ year	$\sim 10^8$	$\sim 3 \times 10^4$	Ogburn *et al.* (1973)
	rabbit	sc.	1°) 10^3 units/ week $\times$ 10 months – 1.3 year 2°) 6–8×10^3 unit/dose $\times$ 20 doses	$\sim 2 \times 10^5$	$\sim 3 \times 10^2$	Skurkovich, Eremkina, and Klinova (1974)
	goat	sc.	1°) 40×10^3 units/week $\times$ ~ 1 year 2°) additional 20 weeks	$\sim 3 \times 10^6$	$\sim 10^2$	Skurkovich *et al.* (1974)
	sheep	sc.	1°) $\sim 10^6$ units/ dose $\times$ 24 dose/ 13 months (adju-vant) 2°) $\sim 10^7$ unit/	1°) 24×10^6	$\sim 6 \times 10^3$	Gresser *et al.* (1976 b)

Interferon species	Animal inoculated	Route[a]	Dose and frequency	Total units inoculated	Neutralizing antibody titer[b]	References
			week × 2 weeks (+adjuvant)	2°) 20 × 10⁶ ∼4 × 10⁷	∼2 × 10⁶	
	rabbit	im.	∼10⁴ units/week × 13–28 weeks + 2–4 doses insolubilized interferon	∼3 × 10⁵	∼10²	Inglot and Chudzio (1976)
	rabbit	im.	∼10⁴ units/week × ∼1 year	∼5 × 10⁵	∼10³	Inglot and Chudzio (1977)
	rabbit	im.	1.2–6 × 10⁶/ dose × 21 doses/ year	∼10⁸	∼5 × 10⁴	Hajnicka et al. (1976)
	rabbit	im. ip.	1°) 1.2–6 × 10⁶ units/dose × 13 doses (+adjuvant) 2°) 8 doses (−adjuvant)	∼10⁸	∼3 × 10⁴	Fuchsberger et al. (1976)
Rabbit	rabbit guinea pig	sc.	3–10 × 10³/week ∼25 weeks	∼10⁵	none 4 × 10³	Levy-Koenig et al. (1970 a)
Human leukocyte	rabbit	sc.	10³ units/week × ∼25 weeks	∼25 × 10³	∼10³	Levy Koenig et al. (1970 a)
	rabbit	sc.	10⁵ units/week (adsorbed on acrylic particles) × at least 11 weeks	≧10⁶	+	Duc-Goiran et al. (1971)
	human	im.	1–3 × 10⁶ units/ week × >20 weeks	>20 × 10⁶	none	Strander et al. 61973)
	rabbit	ip.	10⁵ units/week × 26 weeks	∼3 × 10⁶	∼2 × 10³	Mogensen and Cantell (1973/74)
	donkey	sc.	∼10³ units/10-day interval × 23 doses + 15 boosters after 6 month delay	∼10⁵	∼10²	Skurkovich et al. (1974)
	sheep	sc.	10⁶ units/biweekly × 8 doses „after initial immunization"	10⁷	10³	Anfinsen et al. (1974)
	guinea pig	sc.	6 × 10⁵ units/ week × 8–16 weeks (−adjuvant) or 2.4 × 10⁶	∼10⁷	∼3 × 10⁴	Mogensen, Pyhala, and Cantell (1975)

Table 10 (continued)

Inter-feron species	Animal inoculated	Route[a]	Dose and frequency	Total units inoculated	Neutral-izing antibody titer[b]	References
			units/month (+ adjuvant)			
	rabbit	sc.	3×10^6 units/week $\times$ 8–16 weeks (–adjuvant) or 12×10^6/week (+adjuvant)	$\sim 5 \times 10^7$	$\sim 10^5$	Mogensen, Pyhala, and Cantell (1975)
	sheep	sc.	1°) crude interferon: 16×10^6 unit/week $\times$ 13 weeks (–adjuvant) 2°) 6×10^6 units/week $\times$ 4 weeks (–adjuvant) 3°) purified interferon booster: 30×10^6 units (+adjuvant)	$\sim 3 \times 10^8$	$\sim 10^6$	Mogensen, Pyhala, and Cantell (1975)
	rabbit	sc.	1°) crude interferon: 10^6 units/month $\times$ 3 months (+adjuvant) 2°) 8×10^6 units/week $\times$ 13 weeks (–adjuvant) 3°) purified interferon: 3×10^6 units/week $\times$ 4 weeks (–adjuvant)	$\sim 10^8$	$\sim 10^4$	Berg et al. (1975)
Human fibroblast	guinea pig	im.	10^2 units/week $\times$ 20–30 weeks	$\sim 3 \times 10^3$	none	Paucker (1965)
	rabbit	sc.	250 unit/week $\times$ 25 weeks	$\sim 10^4$	$\leq 10^2$	Levy-Koenig et al. (1970 a)
	chicken	iv.	2.5×10^4 units/week $\times$ ~ 9 weeks	$\sim 2 \times 10^3$	$\sim 10^2$	Vengris, Stollar, and Pitha (1975)
	rabbit	sc.	1°) 32×10^3 units/week $\times$ 3 (+ freund's complete adjuvant) 2°) 32×10^3 units/dose $\times$ 7 (+ freund's incomplete adjuvant)			

Table 10 (continued)   Defining Interferons   155

Interferon species	Animal inoculated	Route[a]	Dose and frequency	Total units inoculated	Neutralizing antibody titer[b]	References
			3°) 32 × 10³ units/dose × 8 (−adjuvant)	∿6 × 10⁵	∿10³	Havell et al. (1975 a)
	rabbit	sc.	10⁶ units/week (multiple)	>10⁶	∿5 × 10³	Berg et al. (1975)
	rabbit	sc.	1.1 × 10⁶ units/ 3 doses at 2 week intervals (first and second + freund's complete adjuvant; third + freund's incomplete adjuvant)	∿10⁶	∿2 × 10³	Vilcek, Havell, and Yamazaki (1977)

[a] Route of inoculation: im, intramuscular; sc, subcutaneous; ip, intraperitoneal; iv, intravenous.
[b] Neutralizing titers of antisera expressed as dilutions neutralizing antiviral activity of approximately 10 units of same species of interferon used as immunogen.

1975 a). Human amnion and fibroblast cell interferon were antigenically indistinguishable (Stewart II, unpublished). Havell and his colleagues (1975) immobilized human fibroblast interferon on a Sepharose column and, by passing anti-human leukocyte interferon antiserum through this column, separated two antibody populations from it, one neutralizing only human fibroblast interferon and one neutralizing only human leukocyte interferon, the former component amounting to only about 1% of the total.

Antigenic identity of human leukocyte interferons and human lymphoblastoid interferons have been reported by a number of investigators (Strander, Mogensen and Cantell, 1975; Adams et al., 1975), with the latter containing perhaps slightly (about 10%) more of the fibroblast interferon component (Havell, Yip, and Vilcek, 1978a; Paucker, 1977). Antibodies to Type I interferons have, as demonstrated in Table 9, also been useful to distinguish Types I and II interferons, the latter not neutralized by antisera to the former (Valle et al., 1975a; Youngner and Salvin, 1973; Maehara et al., 1977; Johnson and Baron, 1976a, b; Wietzerbin et al. (1977a).

Antibodies to interferons have helped to reveal the essential role of interferon in the natural recovery from virus diseases. Antiserum to interferon has been shown to enhance virus replication both in vitro (Fauconnier, 1970; Vilcek, Yamazaki, and Havell, 1977) and in vivo (Fauconnier, 1971; Gresser et al., 1976b, c; Riviere et al., 1977). This involvement in pathogenesis will be described in detail elsewhere (Section XII).

Anti-interferon has also been useful in characterizing products of translation of interferon messenger RNAs (Section VI. A. 1). Such studies have revealed that interferons translated from human fibroblast-derived interferon messenger RNA is antigenically identical to homologous cell-derived human fibroblast interferon whether it is translated in heterologous cells, oöcytes, or cell-free systems. These studies also suggest that the contribution of carbohydrates to antigenicity of interferon glycoproteins are insignificant.

In this regard it is relevant to note that some investigators have reported that neither human leukocyte nor human fibroblast interferons showed any change in binding to anti-interferon antibody columns as a result of treatment with glycosidases (Bose *et al.*, 1976). Such columns of immobilized antisera to interferons have been increasingly useful for purification and characterization of various interferons (as will be described in subsequent Sections.

6. Induction of Non-Antiviral Activities

Each of the non-antiviral functions attributed to interferons (as are described in Section X) have for many years been the focus of controversy, as it was not possible to definitively resolve their association with interferons rather than with other factors in the interferon preparations (see for reviews of this topic: Stewart II and Declercq, 1973; Desomer and Stewart II, 1975; Stewart II, 1977; Gresser, 1977a). However, with the achievement of interferon preparations of apparent homogenous purity, it has recently been possible to assign at least certain of these activities (priming, blocking, double-stranded RNA toxicity-enhancement and cell-multiplication inhibition) as truly functions of interferons. As described in detail in Sections VII. C, IX and X, the list of other alterations induced by interferons will likely increase greatly as research continues. With each of the activities induced by interferons, the ratio of each activity to all the other activities will be invariable with increasing purity, and abilities of interferons to induce these actions will be lost in parallel during inactivations.

7. A Summary Definition of Interferons

The criteria for accepting a viral inhibitor as an interferon are, thus, as originally proposed by Lockart (1966), modified by Lockart (1973), and amended here:
  (i) The virus inhibitor must be a protein.
 (ii) Its antiviral effect must not result from non-specific toxic effects on cells.
(iii) It must be active against a wide range of unrelated viruses, their relative sensitivities being determined by the treated cells.
 (iv) It must inhibit virus replication through an intracellular effect which must involve synthesis by the cells of both RNA and protein.
  (v) It must exhibit activity on a defined host-range of cells.
 (vi) It must also induce the following non-antiviral alterations in cells: priming, blocking, double-stranded RNA-toxicity enhancement, and cell-multiplication-inhibition, always in constant ratios.

B. Purification of Interferons

The subject of interferon purification has been reviewed many times over the past 20 years (Fantes, 1966, 1973; Kleinschmidt, 1972; Ng and Vilček,

1972; Stewart II, 1977), yet it was only in the very recent period that there was any significant new progress to report. For some years the area of interferon purification was considered a scientific quagmire, with most analyses of progress being reiterations of rationalizations for the incredibly slow progress toward cleaning up the interferon preparations. Early workers were operating with no conception as to the specific activity of interferons, assuming it to be modest; in fact it turned out to be exceptionally high. Thus, while for years it was assumed that by starting with what seemed like reasonably large volumes of starting materials (for example, 50 liters of crude allantoic fluid; Lampson et al., 1963), one could achieve a reasonably well-purified interferon preparation in which interferon would be, if not the only component, at least a major one. In reality, such purification studies only repeatedly revealed that the specific activity of interferon was higher than had been expected. An extensive review of each of the methods and results obtained with each of the various interferons whose purification have been attempted would add next to nothing to knowledge of interferons and would contribute only to the bulk of this book; therefore, I shall in this Section primarily cover only the purification of the interferons which have been extensively studies in recent years, mouse and human interferons, referring only tangentially to relavent research on other interferons for analogies. For a thorough description of earlier studies, I refer the reader to the review by Fantes (1973).

The concerns for success of interferon purification seemed to grow with each new realization that interferons' specific activity was yet higher than predicted. Essentially, by starting with several liters of interferons of what at times were the highest titers attainable, one would purify until it was no longer possible to detect protein. This problem of high specific activity (which could imply either that interferons are exceptionally active, or, more likely that the assay for interferon is exceptionally sensitive) was complicated by the normal problem of purification of a trace protein: once the protein finds itself alone in solutions (high diluted and highly purified) it seems to suffer a stability problem (i. e., its activity disappears unexpectedly), though this may merely represent its seeking something to cling to (this "stickiness" of interferons will be discussed in detail below).

The main reasons for the recent rapid progress in purification and characterizations of interferons (and in being able to determine that purity has been achieved) have been:

i) Development of Methods for Increasing Amounts of Interferons Produced by Cells. The findings that "priming" (Stewart II et al., 1971a) and "superproduction" (Tan et al., 1971a; Vilček and Ng, 1971) could be applied to significantly increase large-scale productions, often in combination (Tovey et al., 1974; Billiau, Joniau, and Desomer, 1973), meant that rather than starting purification studies with a few hundred units of interferon/ml of solution, one could begin with a hundred-or thousand-times more interferon per volume, in both human and mouse interferon production facilities (Cantell, 1977; Havell and Vilček, 1972; Tovey et al., 1974).

ii) The Recognition of Needed Starting Bulks. When it was eventually realized that even high total amounts of interferon activity represented extremely small amounts of interferon protein, it was possible to predict that an initial large-scale production period for stock-piling of interferon would be required to realize pure interferon.

iii) Isolation of Interferons Under Dissociating Conditions. The demonstration that interferons could be denatured under dissociating conditions in hot (100° C) anionic or cationic detergent solutions and restored to active forms (Stewart II et al., 1974a, b, c; 1975a) has allowed isolation of various interferons by the techniques of SDS-polyacrylamide gel electrophoresis (Stewart II, 1974; Stewart II and Desmyter, 1975; Knight, 1975; 1976a; and others as described below) and application of the two-dimensional electrophoresis technique to obtain apparently homogeneously pure interferons (Lin and Stewart II, 1978).

1. Purification of Mouse Interferons

As with the other interferons described in this Section, mouse interferon for purification studies is produced in large batches which must be initially concentrated to workable volumes before purification can be initiated. The most convenient way to do this with large volumes of several liters is with an ultrafiltration apparatus, as originally described by Bradish and Allner (1970). This method has been used by Knight (1975), and in our laboratories is performed with centrifuge-clarified pH 2-treated interferon to eliminate infectious inducer Newcastle disease virus. Some investigators have used chemical precipitations, with zinc acetate (Bodo et al., 1971; Kawade, 1973; Yamamoto et al., 1974; Fuchsberger, Hajnicka, and Borecky, 1975) or ammonium sulfate for initial or secondary concentrations (Stewart II et al., 1971a; Knight, 1975). Others have reported use of glass beads for batch concentration of mouse interferon (Edy et al., 1976).

Once reduced to workable volumes, mouse interferon preparations have been processed through nearly every conceivable type of precipitation scheme or chromatographic separation available (for lists of such methods used in early studies see Fantes, 1973). The purification scheme used in my laboratory consists of a composite of the techniques selected from the vast literature and from several years of personal practice and prejudice. The methods used have been modified from the indicated sources to fit into a large-scale production scheme with high efficiency. It is presented here as a simple model purification scheme composed of individually 30 to 100-fold purification-steps each separately reliable, yielding about 30 to 80% total recovery over the entire sequence. It should be emphasized that all of these steps can be performed with reagents that are commercially available. Essentially, 20 liters of crude interferon harvested from primed, Newcastle disease virus-induced L-cell cultures is adjusted to pH 2.0, clarified by centrifugation and concentrated to about 2 liters by ultrafiltration in an Amicon unit using UM-10 membranes. Concentrates are fractionally precipitated with ammonium sulfate at pH 2.0 at 4° C (Stewart II *et al.*, 1971a). Precipitate at 40 to 60% saturation, containing more than 90% of total starting activity is dissolved in about 200 ml of phosphate buffer, pH 7, dialyzed against acetate buffer, pH 5.0, and loaded on a column of Af-figel-202 (Bio-Rad) which is eluted sequentially with the acetate buffer, phosphate and phosphate containing sodium chloride (Bekesi *et al.*, 1976). Interferon eluted with the salt is dialyzed against ammonium bicarbonate, lyophilized, dissolved in Tris buffer and loaded onto a column of poly U-Sepharose, from which it is eluted with salt, dialyzed against bicarbonate, lyophilyzed and stored at –70° C as highly purified mouse interferon. It is important to note, as illustrated in Fig. 10, that at each step of the purification, interferon components identical to those present in crude preparations are retained, as demonstrated by SDS-polyacrylamide gel electrophoresis. This 10,000-fold purification scheme will increase specific activities of crude mouse interferon preparations (about 10^4 units/mg of protein) to about 10^9 units/mg of protein (Fig. 10). This degree of purity of mouse interferon has recently

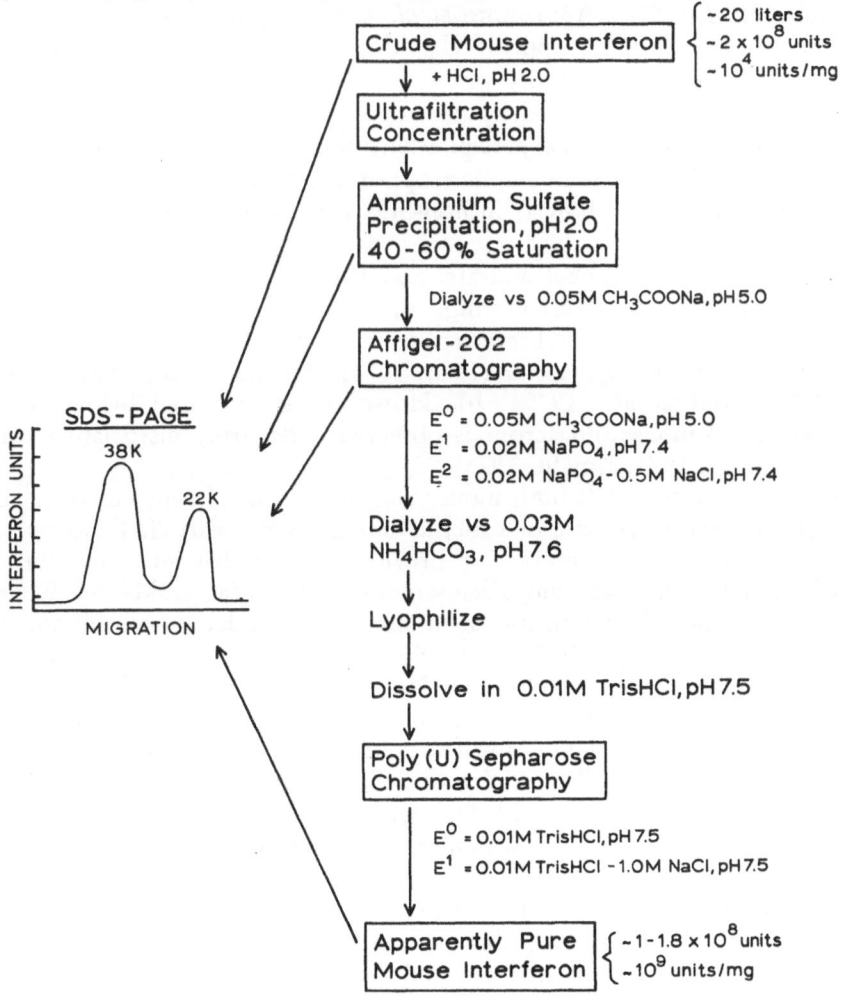

Fig. 10. Purification of mouse interferon

been reported by a number of investigators using the various approaches outlined below.

The purification of mouse interferon by SE-Sephadex chromatography and
polyacrylamide gel electrophoresis to more than 10^6 units/mg of protein was
reported by Paucker and his associates (Stancek, Gressnerova, and Paucker,
1970; Paucker and Stancek, 1972); this material was heterogeneous on the
non-SDS-polyacrylamide gels. Golgher and Paucker (1973) purified mouse interferon to about 3×10^6 units/mg protein by CM-Sephadex chromatography,
and Paucker and his associates (Gresser et al., 1973) combined CM-Sephadex
and non-SDS-polyacrylamide gel electrophoresis to achieve about 10^7 units/mg
protein. Bodo and his colleagues (Bodo, Palese, and Lindner, 1971)
chromatographed mouse interferon sequentially on SP-Sephadex, DEAE-cellulose and CM-Sephadex to achieve a similar purity. Others have achieved
similar specific activities on CM- and/or DEAE-Sephadex chromatographs, often achieving somewhat higher activity/protein ratios (Kawade, 1973;
Yamamoto et al., 1974). Yamamoto et al. (1974) reported that such preparations analyzed on non-SDS polyacrylamide gels "began" to have perceptible
protein at the interferon activity peaks. Fuchsberger, Hajnicka, and Borecky
(1975) obtained a specific activity of about 3×10^8 units of mouse inter-
feron/mg of protein by zinc precipitation, chromatography on SP-Sephadex
and non-SDS polyacrylamide gel electrophoresis. It is significant that in these
studies reporting electrophoresis in non-SDS gels, mouse interferons have uniformly resolved into slow- and fast-migrating components (Fuchsberger et al.,
1975; Kawade, 1973; Paucker and Stancek, 1972; Yamamoto et al., 1974). As
these systems were non-dissociating, the authors were unable to resolve
whether the heterogeneities observed were caused by aggregates of interferon
"subunits" as claimed by Carter (1970; 1971; Marshall et al., 1972; Pitha et
al., 1973; Carter et al., 1975a, b). However, as discussed below, similar
heterogeneity of mouse interferons is observed under truly dissociating conditions (Stewart II, 1974; Knight, 1975).

The demonstration that both mouse and human interferons could be renatured after boiling in anionic or cationic detergents (Stewart II, Desomer, and
Declercq, 1974a, b, c) – contrary to previous reports that interferons are destroyed in SDS (Merigan and Kleinschmidt, 1965; Yamazaki and Wagner,
1970a) – has enabled investigations on interferons under protein-dissociating
conditions. Thus Knight (1975) was able to purify mouse interferon by a
scheme involving sequential ultrafiltration, acid ammonium sulfate precipitation, gel filtration, ion-exchange chromatography and SDS-polyacrylamide gel
electrophoresis, obtained highly purified mouse interferon in physically detectable amounts with a specific activity of at least 3×10^8 units/mg of protein.
He concluded, in accordance with Stewart II (1974) that the mouse interferon
activity was present in distinct molecular species which were not attributable to
aggregated forms of a basic interferon subunit as claimed by Carter (1970;
1971). Yamamoto and Kawade (1976) also found that the purified mouse interferon preparations obtained by the method of Yamamoto et al. (1974) were
heterogeneous when electrophoresed under either non-dissociating conditions
or in SDS gel. Knight (1975) was able to stain the interferons isolated in

SDS-gels by the periodic acid-Schiff base procedure, suggesting that these interferons were glycoproteins. It remains to be determined whether pure mouse interferons were achieved by this process, but application of the two-dimensional gel electrophoresis technique will allow this question to be settled shortly.

Lengyel and his associates (Graziadei, Weideli, and Lengyel, 1973) reported that a preparation of mouse interferon induced in Ehrlich ascites tumor cell cultures by Newcastle disease virus could be purified by a specific activity of 1.5×10^9 NIH reference units/mg of protein and that this preparation contained an endonuclease of high specific activity (similarly Taylor–Papidimitrious et al., 1971, claimed that chick interferon preparations contained endonuclease activity). Unfortunately the purification scheme, reported to be published elsewhere ("Weideli et al., in preparation", 1973), has not appeared, and more recently, Lengyel and his associates (1978) have reported that a mouse interferon preparation, produced again in Ehrlich ascites tumor cell cultures induced with Newcastle disease virus, could be purified to a specific-activity of 1.6×10^9 NIH reference units/mg of protein, and this interferon was apparently free of nuclease activity. Unfortunately the purification scheme is at this writing unpublished and reported by be "Kawakita et al., in preparation". This material is reported to comigrate with a major broad protein band in SDS gel electrophoresis.

Likely owing at least in part to its carbohydrate content, mouse interferon was found to bind to concanavalin A covalently linked to Sepharose beads (Besancon and Bourgeade, 1974) and to be displaced from this lectin by α-methyl-D-mannoside (Carbohydrate components of interferons will be discussed below, Section VII. C. 1). The use of immobilized gangliosides for purification by elution with specific sugars has also been proposed (Besancon, Ankel, and Basu, 1976; Besancon, Basu and Ankel, 1976). It is possible that specific binding of interferons to lectins may be sugar-recognitions in some cases and hydrophobic bindings in other cases. Thus, by trying to use lectins for purification of human fibroblast interferons, Carter and his collaborators (Davey et al., 1974) have inadvertantly found that certain interferons bind to lectins by hydrophobic affiliations, rather than carbohydrate recognitions, as they could not be recovered, contrary to anticipations, by elution with specific sugars but rather required ethylene glycol for liberation. Mouse interferon is, however, eluted from concanavalin A by the lectin-preferred sugar (Besancon and Bourgeade, 1974), and mouse interferon also did not share the hydrophobic binding property of human fibroblast interferon seen on carboxypentyl-agarose (Davey et al., 1975) or albumin immobilized on agarose (Huang et al., 1974). However, these authors (Davey, Sulkowski, and Carter, 1976a, b) have envoked hydrophobicity of mouse interferons to explain their bindings to certain hydrocarbon-coated agaroses, i. e., affigel-202.

The mouse and human interferons, both fibroblast and leukocyte, all bind to the blue chromophore Cibracron Blue F3GA of the substituted dextran, blue-dextran (Cesario et al., 1976; DeMaeyer–Guignard and DeMaeyer, 1976; Jankowski et al., 1976). This observation, also inadvertantly made in other laboratories (Stewart II, unpublished observation), could be used to purify interferons either by elution with high salt solutions or polarity reversing solvent (Cesario et al., 1976; DeMaeyer–Guignard and DeMaeyer, 1976; Jankowski et al., 1976). DeMaeyer–Guignard, Thang, and DeMaeyer (1977) speculated that the binding of interferon to blue-dextran-Sepharose might result from the interferon having a supersecondary structure called the "dinucleotide fold" in which case it would bind to the chromophore because of the latters structural resemblance to nucleotide cofactors, and in which case the interferon should elute by desorption with nucleoside phosphates. In fact, none of the nucleoside phosphates were able to displace mouse interferon from the blue-dextran columns, suggesting that interferon lacks the dinucleotide fold. However, mouse interferon could be released from blue-dextran by desorption with certain polyribonucleotides, poly rI or poly rU, while double-stranded RNAs, poly A or poly rC were ineffective. The displacement was not due to a stronger affinity of the polyribonucleotide for the blue-dextran, but was a strong affinity of the interferon for the polyribonucleotide. Thus interferon could be chromatographed on ligand columns of agarose-immobilized poly rI or poly rU, giving elution in salt with a specific activity reported at about 2×10^9 units/mg of protein. Interestingly these authors also claim that the poly rI and poly rU confer a significant degree of stability to the interferon against thermal denaturation rendering it almost completely stable to heating at 60° C under conditions which inactivated normal mouse interferon by about 99% (this causes reflection back to the first suggested interaction of inducer and interferon, Section IV. C. 3, in which it was asked: "Can a part of an inducer become incorporated into interferon?"; Taborsky and Stancek, 1974).

These data also suggested that mouse interferon might also have an affinity for other types of RNA, and Thang, DeMaeyer–Guignard, and DeMaeyer (1977) subsequently reported that mouse interferon could also be desorbed from blue-dextran-agarose by certain tRNAs, and that mouse interferon could be purified through columns of immobilized tRNA with significant purification and more than 100% (apparent) recovery. Certain tRNAs, i. e., tRNA[Phe], tRNA   , tRNA[Val], and tRNA[Asp] were efficient, while, others (tRNA[Lys], and tRNA[Tyr]) were totally inactive. Further, those tRNAs efficient for elution from blue-dextran conferred heat stability to the interferon whereas the inactive tRNAs did not. As suggested by these authors, it is difficult to imagine that the highly selective interaction of interferon with polyribonucleotides or tRNAs is devoid of physiological significance (also Section IV. C. 3).

In addition to the many physicochemical schemes that have been applied and derived for purification of mouse interferons, the technique of antibody affinity chromatography has also been employed. The limitations to application of this technique were initially the low levels of antibodies specific for interferon that could be obtained. However, as antibodies titer against interferon are now significant (Table 10) it is possible to foresee large-scale purification of interferon by immobilized antibodies.

Mouse interferon was first chromatographed by antibody affinity by Sipe et al. (1973) who reported a purification of about 2000-fold in a single step; however, as the starting interferon was only about 200 units/mg of protein, even this purification factor was not very impressive. Ogburn and his associates

(1973), on the other hand, obtained an impressive 50-fold purification using this technique but starting with antibodies that had been purified by adsorbing against normal cellular and viral proteins before immobilized and chromatographing mouse interferon already at a purity of about 10^7 units/mg of protein, to a final purity of about 3×10^8 units/mg protein.

It is likely that a double-chromatography technique could now be applied to achieve large-scale antibody affinity chromatography. Highly purified interferon isolated by the previously described physicochemical techniques (specific activities about 10^9 units/mg of protein) could be covalently immobilized to agarose; antiserum prepared against semi-purified interferon passed through columns of this bound interferon could be eluted as highly purified antibodies by acid wash. Such highly interferon-specific antibodies could in turn be immobilized and used to batch-purify crude interferon preparations. Alternatively, the highly purified interferons could themselves be used as immunogens to prepare interferon-specific antiserum.

Mouse Type II interferon, of course, could not be purified by antibodies against Type I mouse interferon (Wietzerbin et al., 1977a) but was found to chromatograph in the same manner as Type I interferon on Affigel-202, fortunately being stable to the pH 5.0 acetate buffer (Falcoff, personal communica-

Table 11. *Recent progress in purification of mouse interferon*

Purification scheme	Approximate[a] specific activity achieved	References
Mouse interferon antibody affinity chromatography	3×10^8	Ogburn, Berg, and Paucker (1973)
?b	1.5×10^9	Graziadei, Weideli, and Lengyel (1973)
$(NH_4)_2SO_4$, pH2; biogel-P150, CM-sephadex; SDS-page	3×10^8	Knight (1975)
Zinc acetate; SP-sephadex; page	3×10^8	Fuchsberger, Hajnicka, and Borecky (1975)
BSA-agarose	3×10^8	Davey, Sulkowski, and Carter (1976 a)
Zinc acetate; DEAE- and CM-sephadex; SDS-page	2×10^8 to 1.3×10^9	Yamamoto and Kawade (1976)
$(NH_4)_2SO_4$, pH2; HClO4; poly rI-agarose	2×10^9	DeMaeyer-Guignard, Thang, and DeMaeyer (1977)
?b	1.6×10^9	Lengyel et al. (1977)
$(NH_4)_2SO_4$, pH2; affigel-202; poly rU-agarose	1×10^9	Stewart II et al. (1978)

[a] Units of interferon/mg of protein
[b] Purification procedure not published

tion). And, Type II mouse interferon apparently also binds to polyribonuc-leotides (DeMaeyer–Guignard, Thang, and DeMaeyer, 1977).

Thus as summarized in Table 11, mouse Type I interferon has very recently been purified to very high specific activities, attaining or approaching purity, in a number of laboratories employing a number of techniques. On the basis of theoretical (and somewhat vague) calculations, it is estimated that pure interferon should have a specific activity of about 2.5×10^9 units/mg of protein (Ng and Vilček, 1972). It will soon likely be resolved whether purity of mouse interferon has been achieved.

2. Purification of Human Leukocyte (and Lymphoblastoid) Interferons

It has already been pointed out that human leukocyte and lymphoblastoid interferons and human fibroblast interferons are antigenically distinguishable and that they are distinct in their defined host-ranges. In later discussions I shall describe that they also have different stability properties, and distinct physical and chemical properties. It is, therefore, not surprising that they must be purified by separate schemes.

The production of human leukocyte interferon has virtually entirely been developed by Dr. Kari Cantell and his coworkers in Helsinki, and during their decade of experience in large-scale production of this material they have developed methods suitable for its large-scale purification to a degree acceptable for injections into patients at dosages of several million units/day (Cantell, Pyhala, and Strander, 1974; Mogensen and Cantell, 1977). Practically all of the purification and characterization studies on human leukocyte interferon reported from other laboratories begin by using interferon preparations already purified to the stage of what is commonly called "Cantell P-IF", i. e., as supplied by his laboratories, at about 10^6 units/mg of protein. The scheme illustrated in Fig. 11 for purification of human leukocyte interferon was performed with interferon which left Dr. Cantell's laboratory as P-IF.

Crude human leukocyte interferon, after clarification by centrifugation was originally treated at pH 2 to inactivate the Sendai virus inducer, but as human leukocyte interferon is soluble in acid-ethanol (Fantes, 1970, 1974), but insoluble in neutral alcohol (Graff, Kassel, and Kastner, 1971), this virus inactivation is now performed by dissolution of acidic potassium thiocyanate-precipitated interferon and debris in acid-alcohol. A second acid-alcohol extraction from re-precipitated material yields interferon which is dissolved in phosphate buffered saline as P-IF, purified approximately 100-fold from the crude interferon. Crude human leukocyte interferon can also be purified by ammonium sulfate precipitation, CM- and DEAE-cellulose chromatography and gel filtration to achieve about the same purity as P-IF (Matsuo et al., 1974). Human leukocyte interferon preparations at this stage of purity have been shown to contain a contaminating ribonuclease activity not correlated with interferon activity levels (Winchirch et al., 1977) and to be free of migration inhibitory activity (Mogensen and Cantell, 1977; Block et al., 1977).

Human leukocyte interferon was found to be stabilized against heat denaturation by SDS (Mogensen and Cantell, 1974; Stewart II et al., 1975 a) and

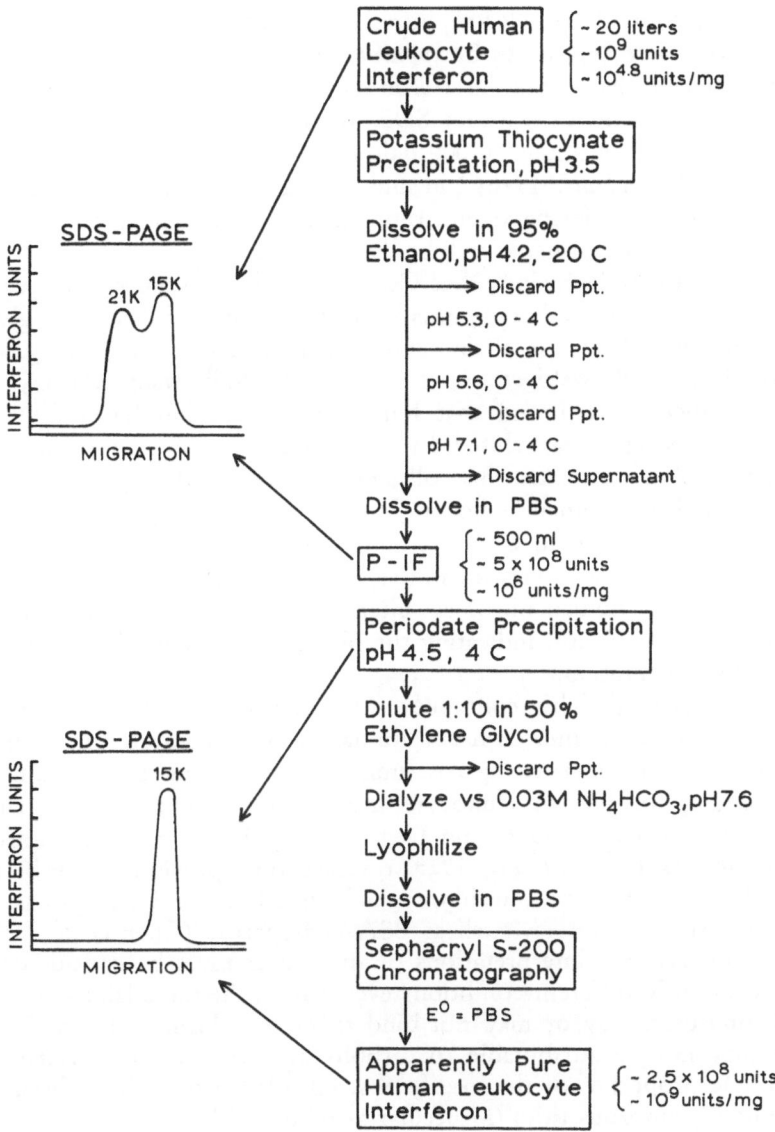

Fig. 11. Purification of human leukocyte interferon

such treatment allowed resolution of interferon preparations in SDS-polyacrylamide gels giving two components with *apparent* molecular weights of about 21,000 and 15,000 daltons (Stewart II and Desmyter, 1975; Desmyter and Stewart II, 1976). Similar size populations have been revealed in SDS-gel electrophoresis by Vilček, Havell, and Yamazaki (1977) and others (as discussed below). Torma and Paucker (1976) used chromatography on Sephadex G 100 columns in the presence of SDS to resolve interferon from contaminants, obtaining a 50-fold purification, to a specific activity of about 5×10^7 units/mg protein. These authors also resolved two components from these preparations in SDS-polyacrylamide gel electrophoresis at about 20,000 and 16,000 daltons. The key word here appears to be *apparent* molecular weights in SDS-gels, for when the human leukocyte interferon is chromatographed in Sephadex or Sephacryl S-200, with or without SDS, it invariably elutes as an apparently homogeneous peak at about 26,000 daltons (Torma and Paucker, 1976; Chen *et al.*, 1976; Bose *et al.*, 1976; Lin and Stewart II, 1978). This anomalous sizing relation in the sieving vs electrophoretic systems is suggestive of glycoprotein nature of interferons, as will be discussed below.

In this regard it is curious that Carter and his colleagues have repeatedly concluded that human leukocyte interferon is in all probability not a glycoprotein, because it did not, in their hands, bind to lectins recognizing terminal sugar residues (Jankowski *et al.*, 1975; Davey, Sulkowski, Carter, 1976c). However, others have found that human leukocyte interferon did bind to Concanavalin A and was eluted by α-methyl-D-mannoside (Besancon and Bourgeade, 1974). Carter and his colleagues (Davey, Sulkowski, Carter 1976c) also interpreted that human leukocyte interferon had no exposed carbohydrates because it failed to bind to Concanavalin A while human fibroblast interferon could bind, and the latter was thus interpreted to be a glycoprotein. However, the "stickiness" of human fibroblast interferon to the lectin could only be reversed by ethylene glycol, indicating the binding was hydrophobic rather than carbohydrate recognition.

Initially Carter and his colleagues (O'Malley *et al.*, 1975 c) also claimed that human leukocyte interferon and human fibroblast interferon bound in an indistinguishable manner to agarose-immobilized bovine serum albumin. A similar binding of human leukocyte interferon to bovine serum albumin-agarose was reported by Dahl and Degre (1975). Later, however, Carter and his associates (Jankowski *et al.*, 1975) reversed their previous claim be reporting that human leukocyte interferon would not bind to BSA-agarose, unless there was a spacer inserted, such as BSA-CH-agarose (Chen *et al.*, 1976). It seems, therefore, that interpretations of these data must be considered tentative. Under subtly different conditions even within the same laboratory a given type of interferon may or may not bind to a given ligand, and such binding may or may not be attributable to carbohydrate contents or electrostatic or hydrophobic properties of the interferons. Clearly such studies, though often touted under glamorous titles (Molecular Structure of Human Interferons) have not even resolved whether human leukocyte interferons are glycoproteins.

Mogensen, Pyhala, and Cantell (1975) have produced high-titered antibodies to human leukocyte interferon in sheep, capable of neutralizing about 10 units of human leukocyte interferon at 1/1,200,000 dilution. These investigators made the important observation that this antiserum, immobilized on agarose, had a much greater interferon binding capacity than its neutralizing capacity. Human leukocyte interferon has been purified on anti-human leukocyte interferon-sepharose columns to about 3×10^7 units/mg of protein, by Berg *et al.* (1975) and several thousand-fold by Torma and Paucker (1976). Others applied this technique, but did not report specific activities achieved (Anfinsen *et al.*, 1974). Recently Berg (1977) described purification of human leukocyte interferon by sequential antibody affinity chromatography to achieve a "direct" specific activity of about 5×10^7 units/mg of protein, which was about 75% due to albumin, bringing calculated "indirect specific activity" up to about 2×10^8 units/mg protein.

The major contaminating proteins in human leukocyte interferon, P-IF, preparations are albumin, 67,000 daltons, and unidentified protein chromatographing in the area of the interferon i. e., at about 26,000 daltons on Sephacryl or Sephadex with or without SDS (Kauppinen, Myllyla, and Cantell, 1977; Lin and Stewart II, 1978; Lin, Wiranowska–Stewart, and Stewart II, 1978). Stewart II and his coworkers (Stewart II et al., 1977) found that the size and charge heterogeneities of human leukocyte interferons could be eliminated by mild acid-periodate treatment, converting the interferon to an homogeneous size-band in SDS-gel electrophoresis with an apparent molecular weight of about 15,000 dalton. When batches of PIF are incubated with acid-periodate buffer the major contaminant in the size-range of interferon is selectively precipitated and the interferon stays in solution with most of the albumin, giving an increase of specific activity of PIF to about 10^7 units/mg protein (Fig. 11). The albumin can be separated from the interferon by a sizing gel of Sephacryl S-200 yielding a specific activity of about 3×10^8 units/mg protein. The eluted interferon preparations have recently been concentrated and analyzed by the two-dimensional gel electrophoresis technique of O'Farrell (1975) and the interferon activity separated from remaining contaminants, migrating as an isolated spot of protein at pI 5.7 and *apparent* molecular weight 15,000. Activity could also be completely eluted from SDS-polyacrylamide gels after they had been stained with coomassie blue in acetic acid (as also recently published by Bridgen et al., 1977 for human lymphoblastoid interferon). The specific activity of the apparently homogeneous human leukocyte interferon was approximately 10^9 units/mg of protein (Lin and Stewart II, 1978). Recent progress in purification of human leukocyte interferons is summarized in Table 12: again several laboratories using various techniques have apparently approached purity.

Table 12. *Recent progress in purification of human leukocyte interferons*

Purification scheme	Approximate specific activity achieved[a]	References
SDS-Sephadex G-100	5×10^7	Torma and Paucker (1976)
Sequential antibody affinity chromatography	5×10^7 ("direct") 2×10^8 ("indirect")	Berg (1977)
PIF; periodate-precipitation; sephacryl S-200	3×10^8	Lin, Wiranowska-Stewart, and Stewart II (1978)
PIF; periodate precipitation Sephacryl S-200; two dimensional gel electrophoresis	$\sim 10^9$	Lin and Stewart II (1978)

[a] Units/mg of protein

Human lymphoblastoid interferons have only recently become available in large quantities for purification studies. From all available information it is identical in all respects to human leukocyte interferon, though perhaps having a little more of the fibroblast-type component (Havell, Yip, and Vilček, 1978a). It can be purified on anti-leukocyte interferon antibody affinity columns (Bose and Hickman, 1977; Havell, Yip, and Vilček, 1978a). Lymphoblastoid cell interferon has recently been precipitated by trichloroacetic acid, chromatographed on antibody-affinity columns, SP-Sephadex and electrophoresed in SDS-polyacrylamide gels (Bridgen et al., 1977). These studies and those of Cavalieri et al. (1977b), Havell, Yip, and Vilček (1978a, b) and Wiranowska–Stewart et al. (1978) show that human leukocyte and lymphoblastoid cell interferons are composed of identical interferon components, though perhaps the latter are somewhat less heterogeneous. Wiranowska–Stewart and her colleagues (1978) have also reported that the elimination of size- and charge-heterogeneities seen with human leukocyte interferons treated with periodate was also found with lymphoblastoid cell interferon. Again, lymphoblastoid cell interferon with an apparent molecular weight of 15,000 daltons in SDS polyacrylamide gel electrophoresis had a molecular weight of about 26,000 in Sephacryl S-200 sizing-columns (Stewart II and Lin, unpublished data).

3. Purification of Human Fibroblast Interferon

The products of several years of work on the purification of human fibroblast interferon has clearly demonstrated its distinctness from human leukocyte interferon in being less stable to denaturation by physical and chemical means (see below), in antigenicity, in defined host range, and in the purification schemes that have been applicable.

Human fibroblast interferon was reported by Carter (1970, 1971) to be purified about 1500-fold by a process of differential precipitation, gel chromatography and isoelectric focusing; the human fibroblast interferon was also (as with mouse interferon) claimed to dissociate into its subunit form, being dimers of 24,000 daltons and monomers of 12,000 daltons. Again, as with mouse interferon "subunits" this phenomenon could not be reproduced in a number of laboratories (Stewart II, unpublished data; Knight, personal communication; Vilček and Ng, personal communication). Further, with the demonstration that human fibroblast interferon could be reactivated after boiling in SDS, mercaptoethanol and urea (Stewart II et al., 1975a), it was possible to electrophorese human fibroblast interferon in SDS-polyacrylamide gels. In such gels human fibroblast interferon migrates as a single peak at about 20,000 daltons (Knight, 1976a, b; Reynolds and Pitha, 1975; Havell, Yamazaka, and Vilček, 1977; Vilček, Havell, and Yamazaki, 1977; Cavalieri et al., 1977a; Wiranowska–Stewart et al., 1978). Thus the human fibroblast interferon, like mouse interferon does not dissociate into monomeric subunits even under conditions known to dissociate all non-covalently bound proteins; it is difficult to imagine that it would do so merely by dialysis against low-salt buffer. It is also interesting that human fibroblast interferon gives approximately the same molecular weight in gel filtration and electrophoresis systems (see below).

Knight (1976a) has used a combined process of acid-ammonium sulfate precipitation, gel filtration, ion-exchange chromatography and SDS-polyacrylamide gel electrophoresis, similar to that he used to purify mouse interferon (Knight 1975), to purify human fibroblast interferon about 5000-fold to apparent homogeneity at a specific activity of about 2×10^8 units/mg of protein, in physically detectable quantities (Fig. 12). Periodic açid-Schiff base stain indicated this interferon was also a glycoprotein. Further resolution of this material by the two-dimensional gel electrophoresis technique should allow certification of its purity.

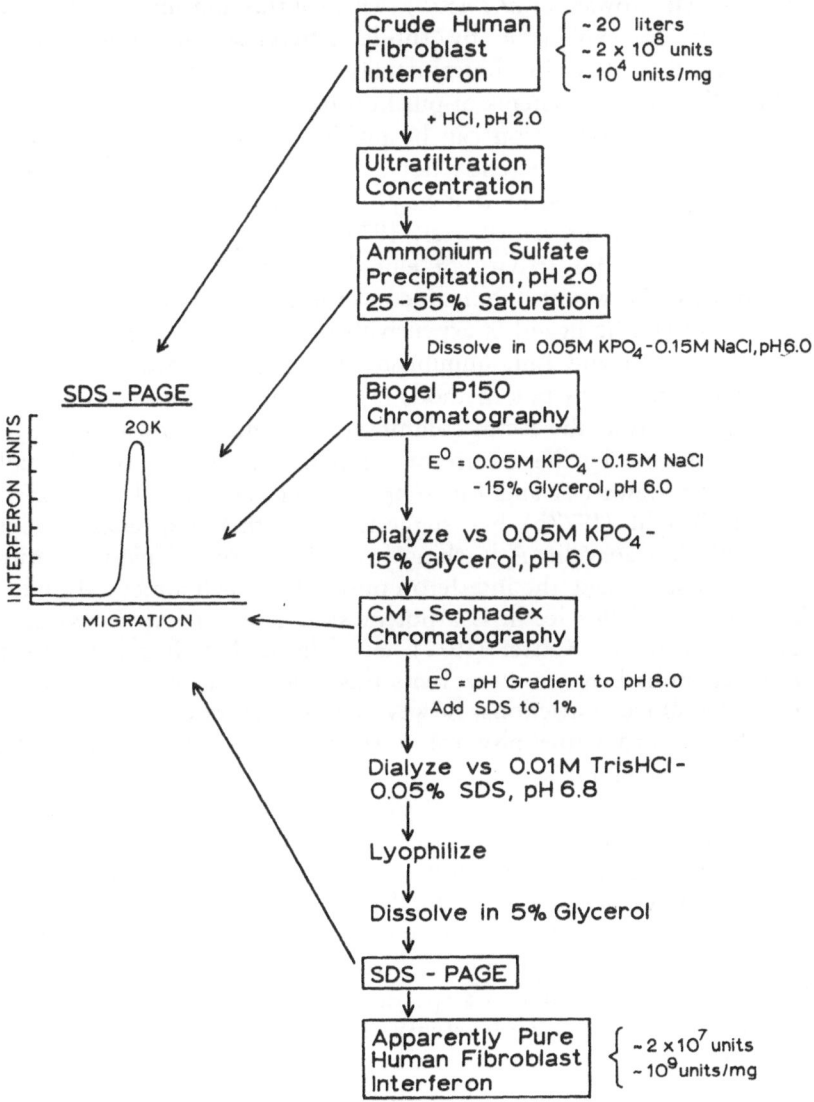

Fig. 12. Purification of human fibroblast interferon

Human fibroblast interferon and human leukocyte interferon were both found to bind to blue-dextran agarose (Cesario *et al.*, 1976; Jankowski *et al.*, 1976). Jankowski *et al.* (1976) reported that human leukocyte interferon would elute with salt-wash, whereas human fibroblast interferon would not; however, Cesario *et al.* (1976) reported elution of the fibroblast interferon by salt-wash. The basis for such discrepancies in binding properties is unclear, but they are not limited to interlaboratory observations, for as mentioned above, one laboratory first reported that human leukocyte and fibroblast interferons bind indistinguishably to BSA-agarose (O'Malley *et al.*, 1975c) and later reported that human fibroblast interferon would bind to BSA-agarose and to CH-Sepharose, whereas human leukocyte interferon would not bind to either of these supports (Jankowski *et al.*, 1975). These intra- and inter-laboratory contradictions may be explanable by subtle differences in commercial versus homemade ligands or trivial technical details; in any event they reduce the general applicability of such systems of purification.

Human fibroblast interferon can be purified by chromatography on Concanavalin A-agarose, but apparently not as a result of carbohydrate recognition as it is not efficiently eluted by α-methyl-D-mannoside but rather by ethylene glycol (Davey, Sulkowski, and Carter, 1976c). This purification procedure reportedly gives a specific activity of eluted interferon of about 5×10^7 units/mg of protein. However, the main concerns that have been expressed about this process are: (1) the ligand is expensive to purchase or prepare, and cannot be reused (Stewart II and Lin, unpublished); (2) it is difficult to purify large batches of interferon with this method; (3) some investigators have found that interferon eluting from the lectin-columns is contaminated with protein components not present in the interferon preparations loaded on the columns (Knight, 1977b; Stewart II and Lin, unpublished data; Vilček, personal communication). Knight (1977b) has suggested that this new contaminant is a component of Concanavalin A leaching from the agarose. This is a serious restriction as it would make the interferon purified by such a method undesirable for clinical use since this lectin is a potent stimulator of lymphocytes, among other effects. However, Carter (1977) has claimed that thorough and careful washing of columns before use prevents this contamination problem. For one or more of the above restrictions, however, most laboratories previously using Concanavalin A-chromatography for purification of human fibroblast interferons are no longer doing so.

Sulkowski, Davey, and Carter (1976) reported that a 2000-fold purification of human fibroblast interferon resulted from its selective binding to and elution from immobilized hydrophobic amino acids, to a specific activity of about 4×10^6 units/mg of protein. Also the "stickiness" property of human fibroblast interferon has been utilized by Edy *et al.* (1976) for purification by its adsorption to controlled pore glass beads, from which it can be eluted to yield a purification of about 100-fold to a specific activity of about 5×10^6 units/mg protein, with good recovery of activity. Human leukocyte interferon would not bind to the glass. This process can be performed on large-scale batch samples. Recently, Edy, Billian, and Desomer (1977) have shown that human fibroblast interferon binds to zinc which is chelated by imminodiacetic acid to an insoluble matrix at neutral pH and can be purified about 3000-fold by elution at lower pH, giving a specific activity of about 2×10^8 units/mg of protein, with about 60% recovery of activity.

Human fibroblast interferon has not been extensively purified by antibody-affinity chromatography, likely because the titers of antisera specific to it are so far much lower than those achieved with mouse or human leukocyte interferons (Table 10). Anfinsen et al. (1974) reported that both human leukocyte and human fibroblast interferon could be purified on columns of anti-human leukocyte interferon antibodies, but purification factors were not reported. This binding is likely due to the small proportion of anti-fibroblast interferon in the antileukocyte interferon antibodies (Havell et al., 1975a; Berg et al., 1975). Berg and his collaborators (1975) purified human fibroblast interferon to a specific activity of about 10^7 units/mg of protein on Sepharose-bound globulins from rabbits immunized with human fibroblast interferon.

It seems likely that certain of the various recently described methods for purification of human fibroblast interferon (Table 13) will be used in sequence to achieve even better results.

Table 13. *Recent progress in purification of human fibroblast interferon*

Purification scheme	Approximate specific activity achieved[a]	References
Controlled pore glass	10^6	Edy et al. (1976)
Hydrophobic amino-acid chromatography	4×10^6	Sulkowski, Davey, and Carter (1976)
(NH4)2SO4; pH2; bio gel P150; CM-Sephadex: SDS-page	2×10^8	Knight (1976 a)
Antibody-affinity chromatography	10^7	Berg et al. (1975)
Concanavalin-A-agarose chomatography	5×10^7	Davey, Sulkowski, and Carter (1976 c)
Zinc chelate chromatography	2×10^8	Edy, Billiau, and Desomer (1977)

[a] Units/mg of protein

C. Characterization of Interferons

1. Heterogeneities of Interferons

As indicated in the previous discussions it has repeatedly been apparent that not all interferons even from a given animal species behave in the same manner. These differences can be measured in terms of stabilities, sizes, stickinesses, antigenicities, host-ranges for activities, and other ways. In the following Section I shall emphasize each of the differences that have been observed between interferons from a given animal species, and attempt to rationalize their origins and speculate on implications of the multiple forms of interferons.

a) Molecular Weights of Interferons

Multiple forms of many enzymes have been recognized, and isomeric forms of certain structural proteins have also been reported (Whalen et al., 1976; Bray, 1976). However, early reports of significant molecular weight differences were easily attributable to non-interferon materials in preparations adhering to the interferons or aggregation of interferons themselves, as all these studies were performed under non-dissociating conditions (Merigan and Kleinschmidt, 1965; 1967; Youngner and Stinebring, 1966), since it was believed that interferon was destroyed by SDS (Merigan and Kleinschmidt, 1965; Yamazaki and Wagner, 1970). Certain reports that subtle size variables existed between interferons induced by endotoxins, mannans, statolons and antilymphocytic serum seemed to be more consistent with the interpretation that molecular size heterogeneities reflected distinct interferon populations (Ke, Ho, and Merigan, 1966; Smith and Wagner, 1967b; Ke and Ho, 1967; Matisova et al., 1970; Falcoff, R., 1972).

On the other hand, Carter (1970, 1971) and his associates (Marshall, Pitha, and Carter, 1972; Pitha, Marshall, and Carter, 1973; Carter et al., 1975a, b) claimed that the apparent molecular weight heterogeneities of interferons was attributable to associations of basic interferon "subunits" into dimers, or oligomers. Supposedly, both human fibroblast interferon and mouse interferon was able to dissociate into subunits of 12,000 and 19,000 daltons, respectively, merely by dialysis against low-salt buffer, and it was even claimed that reassociation of monomers into dimers was possible, though less efficient (Carter, 1970, 1971).

This imaginative model could not, however, be confirmed in other laboratories (Stewart II, unpublished data; Vilček and Ng, personal communication; Anfinsen et al., 1974; Knight, personal communication). And with the demonstration that both mouse and human interferons could be reactivated from boiling SDS solutions (Stewart II, Declercq, and Desomer, 1974; Stewart II, Desomer, and Declercq, 1974a, b, c) it was possible to directly determine the dissociability of these proposed dimeric interferon forms. Stewart II (1974) found that mouse interferon boiled in SDS, mercaptoethanol and urea resolved into two molecular-size populations by electrophoresis in SDS-polyacrylamide gels, one at 38,000 daltons and one at 22,000 daltons (Fig. 13). Knight (1975) also found that mouse interferon preparations contained distinct molecular forms of interferon when analyzed by SDS-polyacrylamide gel electrophoresis; similar results were reported by Yamamoto and Kawade (1976). In each case the larger molecular weight interferon also comprised most of the activity (Stewart II, LeGoff, and Wiranowska–Stewart, 1977). In some SDS-gel electrophoresis systems mouse interferon did not resolve into well-defined peaks but rather exhibited heterogeneity as a wide band from about 20,000 to 40,000 daltons, suggesting variable carbohydrate contents (Lengyel et al., 1977). It is important to point out that the distribution of activity of mouse interferon in SDS-gel is similar to the profile seen in Fig. 13 whether mouse interferon preparations were obtained from L cells, C$_{243}$ cells, mouse brain, or Ehrlich ascites cells, and irrespective of the stage of purity.

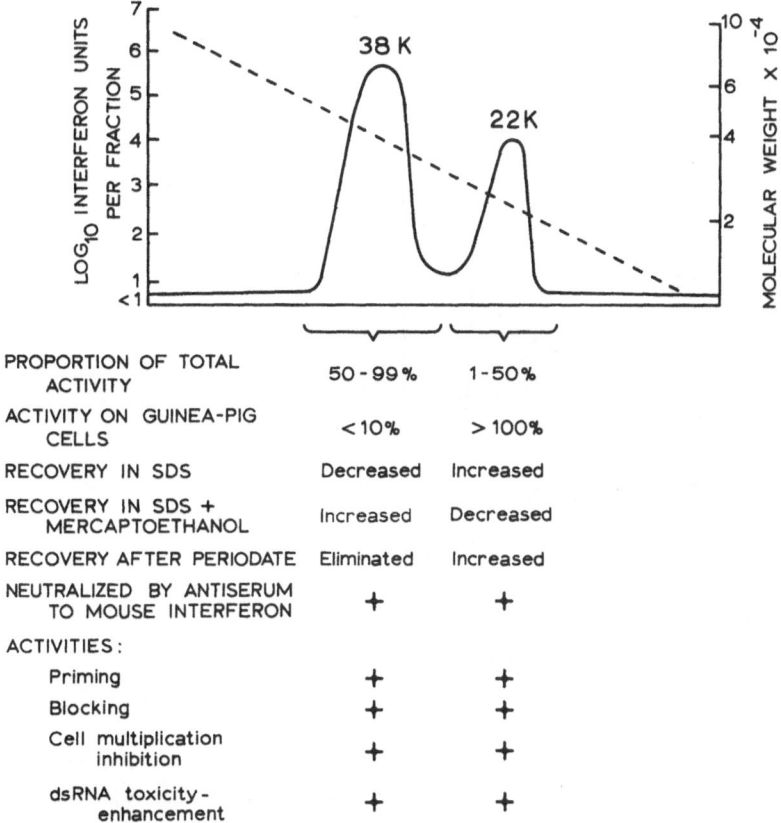

Fig. 13. Heterogeneity of mouse interferons in SDS-polyacrylamide gel electrophoresis

Thus the claim that mouse interferon at 38,000 daltons is a dimer of 19,000 dalton subunits (Carter 1970, 1971) is clearly untenable.

Similarly, the claim that human fibroblast interferon could be dissociated from dimers at 24,000 daltons to monomers at 12,000 daltons (Carter 1970, 1971) has been discredited by the numerous reports that this interferon migrates in SDS polyacrylamide gels, after boiling in SDS in the presence or absence of mercaptoethanol and urea, as a single band at about 20,000 daltons (Fig. 14; Reynolds and Pitha, 1975; Knight, 1976a, b; Reynolds et al., 1975; Vilček, Havell, and Yamazaki, 1977; Cavalieri et al., 1977a; Havell, Yamazaki, and Vilček, 1977; Wiranowska–Stewart et al., 1978).

Human leukocyte interferon has also been analyzed by SDS-polyacrylamide (Fig. 14) gels and resolved into two components at 21,000 and 15,000 daltons (Stewart II and Desmyter, 1975; Desmyter and Stewart II, 1976). Similar sizeheterogeneity of human leukocyte interferon has been reported by Torma and Paucker (1976), Vilček, Havell, and Yamazaki (1977), Berg (1977), Havell, Yip, and Vilček (1978a, b), Paucker et al. (1977), Stewart II et al. (1976) and Lin et al. (1977, 1978).

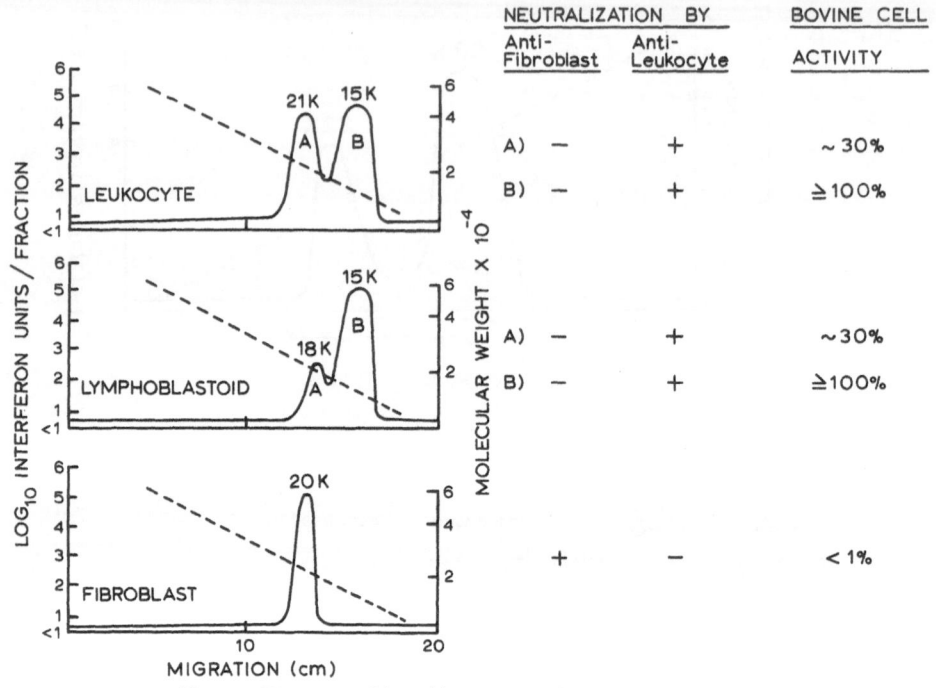

Fig. 14. Heterogeneities of human interferons in SDS-page

Human lymphoblastoid cell interferon also resolves into similar activity distributions on SDS-polyacrylamide gel electrophoresis (Bridgen *et al.*, 1977; Havell, Yip, and Vilček, 1978a; Wiranowska–Stewart *et al.*, 1978).

Thus the native mouse interferon preparations contain at least the two molecular forms of interferon illustrated in Fig. 13. The human fibroblast interferon contains only one form, which can be distinguished from the human leukocyte interferons or human lymphoblastoid cell interferons, which are composed of at least two interferon populations.

b) Stabilities of Interferons

The stabilities of interferons have already been described in regard to the distinctions between Types I and II interferons, demonstrating that in addition to the molecular heterogeneities on the basis of sizes seen in the acid-stable interferons there are yet other interferons that are acid-labile (Table 9).

The acid-stable human leukocyte and fibroblast interferons can be distinguished from one another on the basis of their stabilities to repeated freezing and thawing or shaking (Edy *et al.*, 1974; Cartwright, Senussi, and Grady, 1975). This difference was earlier suggested to be due to different impurities in the preparations (Mogensen and Cantell, 1973), but in view of the widespread observance that human fibroblast interferons are significantly less stable than leukocyte interferons at various degrees of purity, and that fibroblast interferons stick to so many surfaces, it seems possible that the lability of the fibroblast interferon may reflect its loss by attachment to purification and assay equipment (Anfinsen *et al.*, 1974). Clearly no better explanation has appeared, though it seems likely that scrambling of disulfide bonds could account for the relative ease of losses with the fibroblast interferon, if it is rationalized that the interferons both have essential disulfides whose placements differ in accessibility to disruptive agents (Mogensen and Cantell, 1973, 1974, 1973–1974; Cartwright, Senussi, and Grady, 1977 a, b). The hydrogen bond stabilities of mouse and human fibroblast interferon are also apparently important; interestingly, loosening of these at lower pH values significantly increases the stabilities of interferons to heat (Pitha, Marshall, and Carter, 1973; Jariwalla, Grossberg, and Sedmak, 1975, 1977).

The combination of detergent treatment and reducing agents can also be used to distinguish human leukocyte interferons and fibroblast interferons, often having different effects than either alone. Human leukocyte interferon is active after exposure to mercaptoethanol alone or after exposure to SDS alone (Mogensen and Cantell, 1974; Stewart II et al., 1975 a) but the combination of these agents caused partial loss of activity (Mogensen and Cantell, 1974; Stewart II and Desmyter, 1975; Vilček, Havell, and Yamazaki, 1977; Torma and Paucker, 1976; Allen and Stewart II, 1976; Desmyter and Stewart II, 1976; Stewart II et al., 1976). On the other hand, human fibroblast interferon is partially inactivated by exposure to either agent alone (Stewart II et al., 1974 c; 1975) yet it is stable in the combination of SDS and mercaptoethanol (Stewart II et al., 1974 b, c; 1975; Vilček, Havell, and Yamazaki, 1977; Reynolds and Pitha, 1975; Knight, 1976 a, b). The two molecular-size populations of human leukocyte interferons were found to both be sensitive to reduction in the presence of SDS, but the 15,000 dalton form was more labile than the 21,000 dalton interferon (Stewart II and Desmyter, 1975; Desmyter and Stewart II, 1976; Stewart II et al., 1976). Paucker et al. (1977) found they were both equally labile in this combination.

The two molecular-size species of mouse interferon isolated in SDS-gels exhibit markedly different sensitivities to reducing agents in combination with SDS, the 38,000 dalton interferon being significantly more active than in SDS alone, the 22,000 dalton interferon being less active than in SDS alone (Stewart II, 1974; Knight personal communication; Stewart II et al., 1976, 1978; Stewart II, LeGoff, and Wiranowska-Stewart, 1977).

Human fibroblast interferon was reported to be unstable when incubated in human serum, saliva, cerebrospinal fluid, stool extracts or bile (Cesario, Mandell, and Tilles, 1973; Cesario, 1977) and Harmon, Greenberg, and Couch (1976) found that nasal secretions from normal humans contain an inhibitor of human fibroblast interferon which had no effect on human leukocyte interferon.

It also appears that not all interferons from human fibroblast cells are equally labile, as Edy et al. (1977) have suggested that a stable component of fibroblast-type interferon accounts for the residual activity of human fibroblast interferons after shaking. In this regard it is interesting that Ng and Vilček (1973) found that rabbit kidney cell interferons made in the presence of the adenosine analogue toyocamycin was more labile at 56° C than normal rabbit kidney cell interferon, and suggested that the analogue was incorporated into the interferon messenger RNA, thus translating an altered, labile interferon.

c) Ligand Affinities of Interferons

The previous descriptions of purification schemes have given some suggestions that different interferons from the same animal do not always bind identically to the same ligand. While it apparently cannot generally be extrapolated that results from one laboratory will apply in another, direct comparisons of affinities of different interferons within each laboratory offer considerable evidence of heterogeneities. Certain consistencies exist, even in different laboratories.

Thus, human fibroblast interferon consistently will bind to albumin immobilized on agarose (Jankowski et al., 1975; Huang et al., 1974, 1975) whereas human leukocyte interferon will not (Jankowski et al., 1975) or at least only sometimes will (O'Malley et al., 1975c; Dahl and Degre, 1975). Human leukocyte and fibroblast interferons also bind differently to CH-sepharose 4 B (Jankowski et al., 1975) and to Concanavalin A (Davey, Sulkowski, and Carter, 1976b), the fibroblast sticking, the leukocyte not. Human fibroblast interferon also adheres to controlled-pore glass beads (Edy et al., 1976), blue dextran (Jankowski et al., 1976), agarose-immobilized L-tryptophan (Sulkowski, Davey, and Carter, 1976) and zinc-chelate affinity chromatographs (Edy, Billiau, and Desomer, 1977), under conditions where human leukocyte and lymphoblastoid cell interferon was eluted.

It was suggested that the two molecular-size populations of human leukocyte interferons that are resolved in SDS-gels could be eluted separately from DEAE-BioGel or BSA-CH-agarose, as two components eluted from human interferon preparations chromatographed on these columns (Chen et al., 1976). However, Lin et al. (1977) found that each of the two components of human leukocyte interferon that eluted from these ligands also contained each of the size-components when analyzed on SDS-gels. Similarly, the conclusion that the two populations of mouse interferons that eluted from ligands were the separated size forms (Davey, Sulkowski, and Carter, 1976b) seen in SDS-gels was also found to be incorrect, as each of the peaks that eluted from the ligand contained both the size-forms of mouse interferon (Chudzio and Stewart II, unpublished data).

On the basis of these observations it is possible to conclude that each of the different interferons can be distinguished on the basis of relative "stickiness", the human fibroblast interferons being "stickier" than the leukocyte or lymphoblastoid cell interferons. Within each of the size populations of human leukocyte interferons and mouse interferon it is also possible to have different adhesiveness, indicating that the size and charge heterogeneity is more extensive than merely two size-populations, each with respectively different charge properties. As will be discussed below, these data again suggest carbohydrate component complexities.

d) Biological Heterogeneities of Interferons

Some of the interferons produced by a given species of animal can be distinguished on the basis of biological properties.

i) Defined Host-Ranges. It has been described previously (Table 8) that human fibroblast interferons can exert antiviral activity on rat cells whereas human leukocyte interferon does not (Duc–Goiran, Galliot, and Chany, 1971), whereas human leukocyte and lymphoblastoid interferons are highly active on bovine, porcine, and feline cells while the fibroblast interferon is not (Gresser *et al.*, 1974; Cavalieri *et al.*, 1977a; Desmyter and Stewart II, 1977; Edy *et al.*, 1977; Billiau *et al.*, 1977a; Paucker *et al.*, 1977). Also human Type II interferon was reported to not be active on rabbit cells (Lai, Alpers, and Mackay–Scollay, 1977); whereas both fibroblast and leukocyte Type I human interferons are (Desmyter *et al.*, 1968, 1970; Paucker *et al.*, 1975).

Bovine Type I and II interferon also had distinct host-ranges (Babiuk and Rouse, 1977), and rat Type I interferons were reported to have different host-ranges than rat Type II interferons (Lobodzinska *et al.*, 1973a, b, 1975).

The heterogeneities of interferon is further extended by the findings that each of the size-populations in human leukocyte interferons showed different cross-species antiviral activity, the 15,000 dalton form only slightly active on rabbit cells, the 21,000 dalton fully active (Stewart II and Desmyter, 1975). The 15,000 dalton and the 21,000 dalton forms were both about equally active on bovine cells, but at the small side (more rapidly migrating portion of the faster peak (about 13,500 daltons), the interferon was about 100-times more active on cat cells (Desmyter and Stewart II, 1976) and on bovine cells (Lin *et al.*, 1978) than on human cells. Similarly, the two molecular size-forms of mouse interferon resolved in SDS-gels at 38,000 and 22,000 daltons were significantly different in their abilities to induce antiviral activity in guinea-pig cells, the smaller form being more than 100% cross-reactive, the larger interferon being less than 10% cross-active (Stewart II, LeGoff, and Wiranowska-Stewart, 1977). In this regard it is interesting that Bodo *et al.* (1971) found that mouse interferon eluting from a Sephadex column toward the lower molecular weight size was more active on human cells than the larger mouse interferon forms. Borecky and his associates (1974) have also found displacements of homologous and heterologous cell activities of interferons isolated in non-SDS polyacrylamide gels.

ii) Antigenic Heterogeneities. As described previously (Section VII. A. 5) human leukocyte interferons can be distinguished from human fibroblast interferons by cross-neutralizing capacities of antisera prepared against each. Thus antiserum to human leukocyte interferon was unable to efficiently neutralize human amnion cell interferon (Duc–Goiran *et al.*, 1971; Levy–Koenig *et al.*, 1970a). Human leukocyte interferon cannot be neutralized by antiserum prepared against human fibroblast interferon (Havell *et al.*, 1975a; Berg *et al.*, 1975; Vilček, Havell, and Yamazaki, 1977). However, both of the molecular size-forms of human leukocyte interferons isolated in SDS-polyacrylamide gels were equally neutralized by antiserum to human leukocyte interferons (Havell, Yip, and Vilček, 1978b).

iii) Action Heterogeneities. It has been reported (Havell, Berman and Vilček, 1975; Edy, Billiau, and Desomer, 1976a; Hilfenhaus, 1977) that human leukocyte interferons and human fibroblast interferon induce antiviral activities in human fibroblast cells with different mid-range dose-response curves (Section II. B). Thus, human leukocyte and fibroblast interferons may have different antiviral mechanisms. However, the relative sensitivities of different viruses to the activities induced by each of these interferons, as well as the rates of decays of the antiviral mechanisms were indistinguishable (Vilček, Havell, and Yamazaki, 1977; Havell, Berman, and Vilček, 1975). Thus it seems likely that these different forms of human interferons induce similar antiviral mechanisms, but differ in their efficiencies at the cell surface. Similar studies on the distinct molecular forms of human leukocyte interferons and mouse interferons should soon show whether their activities decay together and whether they induce similar relative orders of antiviral resistances against various viruses.

e) Origins of Heterogeneities of Interferons

The heterogeneities observed between different interferons of the same animal species could owe their individuality to their respective messenger RNAs, hence being products of different interferon genes, perhaps with separate chromosomal assignments. Alternatively, the differences could result from divergent posttranslational modifications of the products of identical messages, which could reflect proteolytic cleavages of preinterferon, prointerferon or even preprointerferon. Or the differences might represent additions of variable amounts or conformations of carbohydrates. Still it is also possible that the heterogeneities result from combinations of these modification- and origin-differences: human fibroblast interferons which are antigenically as well as physically distinguishable from human leukocyte interferon could represent gene→ message→product differences, whereas the physically different but antigenically similar human leukocyte interferons could represent variations in extraneous carbohydrate embellishments. In the former case, conversions from one to another would be unlikely; in the latter case convertibilities should be possible, enzymatically or by chemical cleavage.

i) Genetic Origins of Heterogeneities. It has been described previously that a number of laboratories have achieved translation of interferon messenger RNAs in heterologous cells, in *Xenopus* oöcytes and in cell-free protein translating systems (Section VI. A. 1). It has been repeatedly demonstrated that interferon messenger RNA isolated from human diploid fibroblast can be translated in chick cells (Reynolds and Pitha, 1974) or in Syrian hamster cells (Greene, Dieffenbach, and Tso, 1978), in *Xenopus* oöcytes (Reynolds, Premkumar, and Pitha, 1975; Sehgal, Dobberstein, and Tamm, 1977; Cavalieri *et al.*, 1977a, b; Raj and Pitha, 1977) and in various cell-free protein synthesizing systems (Reynolds, Premkumar, and Pitha, 1975), and in each case the interferon produced has been identifiable as human fibroblast interferon on the basis of at least one of the several traits that have been described above which distinguish it from human leukocyte interferon: neutralization by antiserum against human fibroblast interferon, one size-species at about 20,000 daltons on SDS gels, and low activity on bovine cells.

It was only recently speculated that, were human fibroblast interferon messenger RNA and human leukocyte interferon messenger RNA (which message had not been isolated at that time) translated in the same systems, the type of product obtained would indicate the origins of their heterogeneities as genetic or post-genetic (Stewart II, 1977). In fact, this experiment has since been described, using the messenger RNA derived from the Namalwa human lymphoblastoid cell line, which produces mostly interferon identifiable as human leukocyte interferon and a minor component identifiable as human fibroblast interferon. Cavalieri and his collaborators (1977 b) found that this lymphoblastoid cell-derived interferon message-mix translated in oöcytes into interferon preparations which were only partly neutralized by antisera against either fibroblast or leukocyte interferon, but was completely neutralized by a mixture of these antisera. Further the oöcyte-made human fibroblast and lymphoblastoid cell interferons were distinguishable as to their origins by SDS-gels and host-ranges (low and high activities, respectively, on bovine cells). These data strongly support the interpretation that human fibroblast interferons and human leukocyte-type interferons are products of different interferon genes. While the gene responsible for human fibroblast interferon has been reported to reside on C-5, the assignment for human leukocyte interferon is at present unknown.

Some evidence has been reported that there may also be different forms of messenger RNA for mouse interferons, one being RNase sensitive and one resistant (Montagnier et al., 1974); however, no characterization distinctions have been reported for the products of these messages.

ii) Contributions of Carbohydrates to Interferon Heterogeneities. Data on the chemical composition of interferons have been published along with ultraviolet spectra, amino acid contents, carbohydrate and lipid contents and subunit structures (Wagner, 1960; Burke, 1961; Davies, 1965; Fantes, 1966; Dima et al., 1967; Carter, 1970, 1971). Of course it is now clear that these interpretations are of historical curiosity value only.

In a great number of early publications it was also shown that various interferons were sensitive to periodate (Schonne, 1966; Nagano, 1967; Fantes and Furminger, 1967; Ke and Ho, 1968), implying that carbohydrate components were essential for interferons' active conformations. Several more recent reports using more highly purified interferons have also reported inactivations of interferons by periodate (Besancon and Bourgeade, 1974; Huet et al., 1974; Lindahl et al., 1974; Imanishi, 1975; Rossi et al., 1975; Booth et al., 1976; Cesario, Schryer, and Tilles, 1977; Brouty–Boye, and Little, 1977; Tovey et al., 1977 a). Again these findings have generally been interpreted that the interferons contain essential carbohydrates. However, even mild periodate oxidation can also inactivate proteins by attacking essential amino acids, and in fact, the bulk of data now indicate that carbohydrate moieties are apparently uninvolved in activity or antigenicities of interferons, though they may facilitate adhesion to cell surfaces preparatory to receptor binding (Section VIII. C. 1).

There is an accumulation of contradictory data on the presence or absence of carbohydrates on interferons. On the one hand Mogensen et al. (1974) reported that treatment of human leukocyte interferon with neuraminidase, acid hydrolysis and periodate did not alter its clearance rate when injected into rabbits (which are sensitive to this interferon (Table 8), nor did such treatment alter its charge heterogeneities as evidenced by isoelectric focusing. On the other hand, Bose and Hickman (1977) have reported that removal of terminal sialic acid from human lymphoblastoid interferon significantly reduced its survival time in circulation of rats (which are not sensitive to this interferon; Table 8). Curiously further removal of carbohydrate residues reversed this rapid serum clearance of the interferon. Bose and her colleagues (1976) have also found that enzymatic removal of carbohydrates reduced the charge heterogeneities of human leukocyte interferon in isoelectric focusing. These authors (Bose et al., 1976; Bose and Hickman, 1977) also claim that over 85% of carbohydrate is removed by such treatment. This interpretation assumes that the carbohydrate label removed from relatively crude interferon preparations was originally equally associated with interferon and other glycoproteins in the preparations.

Isoelectric heterogeneity of rabbit interferon was also reported to be reduced by neuraminidase treatment, and to be restored by enzymic incorporation of labelled acetylneuraminic acid into the asialointerferon (Dorner, Scriba, and Weil, 1973). Moreover, these authors reported that asialointerferon treated with galactose oxidase and sodium borohydrate was also equally active. Similar removal of sialic acids from rabbit interferon and associated reductions in their charge heterogeneities had been reported (Bocci et al., 1971; Schonne, Billiau, and Desomer, 1970), and such desialylated rabbit interferon was more rapidly cleared from circulation by rabbit liver tissue (Bocci et al., 1977a, b).

Carter and his colleagues (see discussion above; Jankowski et al., 1975) have presumed that human leukocyte interferon, in all probability, was not a glycoprotein, on the basis of its weaker binding to certain lectins under conditions in which human fibroblast interferon was bound firmly. This could suggest that fibroblast and leukocyte interferons differed because of the differences of glycosylating potentials of their respective cells of origin. This seems unlikely as the messages for each translates in its own image in numerous cells, in oöcytes and in cell-free systems. Also, the carbohydrate moieties of neither interferon seem important for antigenicities, as the ability of each to bind to anti-human leukocyte interferon antibody columns is unaltered under deglycosylation treatments reported to reduce both their molecular weights (Bose et al., 1976).

Direct demonstration of carbohydrate content of interferon proteins has been presented in the studies of mouse and human fibroblast interferons by Knight (1975; 1976a). The heterogeneous mouse interferon proteins separated in SDS gels were stainable by Coomassie blue and could also at least partially be stained by oxidation with periodic acid and Fuchsin base, as could the homogeneous peak of human fibroblast interferon isolated in SDS gels.

Recently, Stewart II et al. (1977) have found that the size and charge heterogeneities of human leukocyte interferons as revealed in SDS-polyacrylamide gel electrophoresis and isoelectric focusing, respectively, could be eliminated by periodate oxidation. The larger 21,000 dalton interferon was apparently converted to the smaller 15,000 dalton form. Similarly the size and charge heterogeneous forms of human lymphoblastoid cell interferons were also converted to the 15,000 dalton species, and both human leukocyte and lymphoblastoid cell interferons focused at pH 5.7 after periodate cleavage (Stewart II et al., 1977; Lin et al., 1978; Wiranowska–Stewart et al., 1978). Anfinsen and his associates (Bridgen et al., 1977) similarly reported that human lymphoblastoid interferon was converted to the smaller interferon species by treatment with mixtures of glycosidases, and such enzymes also reduced the charge heterogeneity of the lymphoid cell interferon, to focus at about pH 5.7. Thus, by either chemical or enzymatic modifications, human leukocyte-type interferons can be converted, without significant activity losses, from size and charge heterogeneous forms to apparently homogeneous interferons. However, further studies are needed to determine whether these molecules are in fact carbohydrate-free. Stewart II *et al.* (1978) have found discrepancies in the apparent sizes of these chemically cleaved interferons when measured in SDS-gels and in sieving columns, still suggesting glycoprotein character. Similarly, Lin *et al.* (1978) have found evidence of heterogeneity of these apparently homogeneous interferons by assays on heterologous cells.

Havell and his colleagues (1977) have used another approach to determine carbohydrate contributions to human fibroblast interferons. On the basis of their earlier finding that the glycosylation inhibitors 2-deoxy-D-glucose and D-glucosamine partially inhibited interferon production in human fibroblast cultures (Havell *et al.*, 1975b), they determined the size and charge properties of the residual interferon made under such conditions. The interferon made in the presence of either inhibitor was somewhat less charge-heterogeneous than the native interferon in isoelectric focusing gels, focusing at about pH 7.4, and instead of a single peak at about 20,000 daltons in SDS-gels as seen with native fibroblast interferon, small peaks were found at both 20,000 and 16,000 daltons. This suggests that glycosylation of human fibroblast was partially inhibited in glycosylation inhibitors. However, Wiranowska–Stewart and her associates (1978) were unable to reduce the size of human fibroblast interferon by periodate cleavage and such presumably heavily glycosylated fibroblast interferon gave similar molecular weights in SDS-gels and in sizing columns.

Recently, Stewart II *et al.* (1978) have found that treatment of mouse interferons with periodate will apparently convert the SDS-gel pattern of 38,000 dalton interferon to the 22,000 dalton interferon and a small amount of activity appears at 15,000 dalton (Fig. 15). However, when measured in Sephacryl S-200 sizing columns both preparations elute as broad peaks at about 30,000 daltons, suggesting again that the periodate-treated interferon was still behaving anomalously, as would be expected if it were still a glycoprotein. Taking a lead from the earlier finding of Havell *et al.* (1975b) that D-glucosamine or 2-deoxy-D-glucose inhibited most interferon production in fibroblasts, these investigators attempted to determine the size of any residual interferon possibly made in mouse cells in the presence of such inhibitors. In fact, we found that nearly normal quantities of interferons were produced, but virtually all of this interferon migrated at 15,000 daltons in SDS-gels, instead of the normal sizes of 38,000 and 22,000 daltons for mouse interferon, and these preparations of interferon made in glycosylation-inhibitors were also 15,000 daltons in Sephacryl S-200 sizing columns, suggesting they were carbohydrate-free. The aglycointerferon, or "interferoid" behaves identically to native 38,000 and 22,000 dalton apparent molecular weight forms in terms of hydrophobicity on Affigel 202 columns suggesting, in contrast to the finding of Jeng (1977), that carbohydrate content is not related to hydrophobicity of the interferons.

These data suggest that carbohydrate-free interferons are equally as active as native glycosylated interferons. These results are quite important in terms of pending plans for efforts to obtain a small active-core polypeptide of inter feroid which can be chemically synthesized. It is tempting to speculate that a common active-core exists even for those interferons which are apparently products of different genes; for, as will be described below (Section VII

C. 1), even heterologous interferons appear able to share a common receptor on some cells.

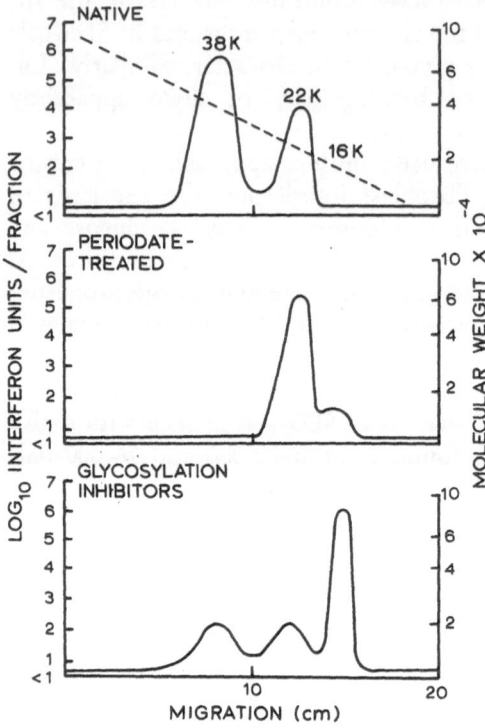

Fig. 15. Contributions of carbohydrates to heterogeneities of mouse interferons. Top panel: Native mouse interferon; Middle panel: mouse interferon treated with periodate according to Stewart II *et al.* (1977; 1978); Bottom panel: mouse interferon preparation obtained from mouse cells incubated with glycosylation inhibitors during production phase

f) Significance of Interferon Heterogeneities

As it has become apparent that our bodies deem it desirable to make different forms of interferons, it has become increasingly tempting to speculate that there are reasons for this. One possibility that has been posed is that the different interferons have different tissue affinities, which might explain the differences in dose response curves seen with human leukocyte and fibroblast interferons (Havell, Berman, and Vilček, 1975; Edy, Billiau, and Desomer, 1976a; Vilček, Havell, and Yamazaki, 1977). It has been suggested that interferons have specific tissue affinities on the basis of relative abilities of human leukocyte and fibroblast interferons to induce antiviral and cell-multiplication inhibitory activities (Einhorn and Strander, 1977); however, these data should be interpreted with caution, as the differences obtained are subtle, and difficult parameters must be employed in such studies. Skurkovich *et al.* (1976a) have reported that lymphoid cells may have increased sensitivity to immune-induced interferon. Others have reported that both leukocyte and fibroblast interferons are equally active in epithelial cells (Harmon *et al.*, 1977).

It is possible that interferons are produced in different forms to allow survivals (or timely eliminations) in particular environments. Local interferons produced by fibroblasts at site of viral entry might act locally and thus not be adapted for stability, whereas interferons produced in response to systemically circulating virus infections (leukocyte interferons) might be adapted for more stability to allow their transportation to distant target tissue. Studies on pharmacokinetics of interferons will be described later (Section XI).

Presently we do not know what different interferons mean to the animal producing them.

2. Non-Antiviral Activities of Interferons

The possibility that interferons can induce effects in cells other than inhibition of viruses has been a controversy for many years (Desomer and Stewart II, 1975; Gresser, 1977a; Rozee and Lee, 1977) and it has only recently been possible to satisfactorily resolve this dispute. Each of the non-antiviral functions of interferons are described in detail in Section X and will only be discussed here in regard to the possibility that interferons might be heterogeneous in functional aspects.

Each of the human leukocyte interferon preparations which segregate into two peaks of interferon activity on SDS-gels also separate into two peaks of cell-multiplication-inhibitory activity with the same size and the same effects of chemical reduction on both antiviral and this non-antiviral function, and each of these forms of interferon was about 1% cross-reactive on mouse cells, for both antiviral and cell-multiplication-inhibitory action (Stewart II et al., 1976). Knight (1976b) also reported that the human diploid fibroblast interferon purified to apparent homogeneity in SDS-gels was also able to inhibit cell-multiplication.

Recently, Gresser (1977a) and Stewart II et al. (1978) have reported that mouse interferon purified to more than 10^9 units/mg of protein was equally as active as crude or partially purified interferons for cell-multiplication-inhibition.

Each of the molecular forms of mouse interferon isolated in SDS-gels were equally able to induce priming, and double-stranded RNA toxicity enhancement (Stewart II, 1975b), and, recently, we have found that the 38,000 dalton, 22,000 dalton interferons and the 15,000 dalton interferoid were equally able to induce priming, toxicity-enhancement and blocking (Stewart II et al., 1978).

In studies in which human leukocyte and fibroblast interferons have been directly compared they are equally able to inhibit cell multiplication (Knight, personal communication; Hilfenhaus et al., 1976; Stewart II, unpublished data), and Type II human interferons are also able to induce equal unit ratios of cell-multiplication inhibition and antiviral action (Epstein and Epstein, 1976).

It, thus, appears that at least priming, double-stranded RNA toxicity-enhancement, blocking and cell-multiplication-inhibition, are measures of alterations induced by interferon *per se*, all interferons being equally able to induce each of these actions in cells able to be so altered. It remains to be determined if all interferons are equally able to induce other alterations (as discussed in Section X).

To recapitulate our progress through the interferon system to this point, an inducer interacts with a cell, induces transcription and translation of proteins which are processed and excreted from the cells as interferons, which can be purified and characterized to be heterogeneous proteins able to induce a number of effects in cells sensitive to them. In the remaining Sections I shall describe what interferons do and how they do it.

VIII. The Genetics of Interferon Action

As is the case for interferon production being under cellular genetic control, the actions of interferon are also under cellular genetic regulation, in this case the inducer of the actions being interferon itself. It will be described in detail in Sections IX and X that the interferon must induce new cellular messenger RNA and protein synthesis for cells to become refractory to viruses (Lockart, 1964; Taylor, 1964) and to develop some of the non-antiviral functions, and the cell nucleus must be present at the time of interferon treatment but not afterwards (Radke et al., 1974; Young, Pringle, and Follett, 1975). Thus it has been possible to employ the same basic approaches that were described in Section V to determine the cellular chromosomal compliments necessary for response to interferon. These, again, include studies in hybrid cells whose parents produce interferons with different host-ranges which have eliminated different chromosomes and involve making correlations with presence or absence of specific chromosomes and sensitivities to the interferons. After such studies show such correlations it is also possible to perform gene-dosage experiments in aneuploid cells with abnormal numbers of particular chromosomes. Again, it is necessary to interpret such data carefully, for as described for studies on genetic controls of interferon production (Section V), numerous epigenetic factors can modulate interferon sensitivities of cells or their abilities to express antiviral or non-antiviral actions. As will be pointed-out, it is often difficult to resolve interferon action mechanisms to its inductive phase and its expressive phase. In the following discussions I shall distinguish the binding of interferon to cells and events up to derepression of gene(s) producing messenger RNAs for interferon actions as the action-inductive phase and those events involved with translation and expression of the activities as the action phase. Such a conceptual breakdown of the action mechanism is helpful to distinguish data showing for example inhibition of interferon action by substances that merely prevent interferon's binding to cells from substances that can interfere with the mechanism of action induced within cells.

A. Hybrid-Cell Analyses of Interferon Action

Chany and his associates (Cassigena et al., 1971; Chany et al., 1973, 1975; Chany, 1976) were the first to demonstrate that the genes for the production of interferon and the action of interferon are asyntenic. This was also found to be the case in the human interferon system (Tan et al., 1973, 1974). Tan and his associates (1973) employed a large number of mouse-human hybrids, which gradually lost human chromosomes while retaining mouse chromosomes, and made correlations of residual human components with sensitivity to the antiviral action of interferon. The antiviral state could be induced in all the clones by mouse interferon but only a few were protected by human interferon. The sensitivity to human interferon showed a positive correlation with expression of the human isozyme of indophenoloxidase A, and the human chromosome 21. The assignment of antiviral action-induction by human interferon to human chromosome 21 was confirmed in a number of subclones showing syntenny between antiviral action of interferon and chromosome 21 (Tan et al., 1973; Tan, 1975; Creagan et al., 1975). Morgan and Faik (1977) have confirmed that human chromosome 21 is required for the antiviral effect of human interferon in human-hamster hybrids. Confirmation of the involvement of human chromosome 21 in sensitivity of human-mouse hybrids to antiviral action of human interferon has been provided by Revel, Bash, and Ruddle (1976). Chany and his colleagues (Chany et al., 1975; Chany 1976) found that if only human chromosome 21 were present in mouse-human hybrid, they were not responsive to human interferon; if any other human chromosome were also present, the hybrids were human-interferon responsive. However, Slate and her associates (1978) found that the presence of chromosome 21 alone was sufficient to render human-mouse hybrids sensitive to the antiviral action of human interferon, though the presence of additional human chromosomes further increased the human-interferon sensitivity of such hybrids.

B. Chromosomal Assignments for Interferon Actions in Aneuploid Cells

1. Antiviral Action of Human Interferon in Aneuploid Cells: Chromosome 21 Dosage Effect

The assignment of human interferon antiviral action sensitivity to chromosome 21 has been confirmed in a number of studies using cells containing abnormal numbers of specific chromosomes. Among the most common of such disorders in human cells is trisomy 21, as found in Down's syndrome. Tan and his coworkers (1974) demonstrated that monosomic 21 human aneuploid cells were appreciably less sensitive to human interferon than were normal diploid human cells, whereas cells trisomic for chromosome 21 were significantly more sensitive to the antiviral activity of human interferons. This observation has been confirmed repeatedly in a number of laboratories (Chany et al., 1975; Tan, Chou, and Lundh, 1975; Tan 1975, 1977; Revel, Bash, and Ruddle, 1976; Wiranowska–Stewart, and Stewart II, 1977; Slate et al., 1978), and trisomic 21 human cells are currently used in a number of laboratories for highly sensitive human interferon assays.

Importantly, this relationship also applies to antiviral action induced by type II human interferon (Epstein and Epstein, 1976), by human leukocyte as well as human fibroblast interferon (Tan, 1977; Slate et al., 1978; Wiranowska–Stewart, 1977), and by each of the molecular size-forms of human leukocyte interferons isolated in SDS-polyacrylamide gels (Stewart II, 1977). Furthermore, Wiranowska–Stewart, and Stewart II (1977) found that trisomic-21 human cells were also more sensitive to heterologous (mouse) interferon than were diploid human cells, which were more sensitive to mouse interferon than were monosomy-21 cells. It has apparently not been determined whether the presence of human chromosome-21 in the mouse-human hybrid cells correspondingly increased their sensitivities to mouse interferons as it did to human interferons. It would also be interesting to determine whether cells trisomic for human chromosome 21 were also more sensitive to other substances, for example, either toxins or other lymphokines.

It was shown that the increased sensitivity was not a non-specific effect associated with loss or gain of any chromosome because cells trisomic for any of several other human chromosomes were not more sensitive to human interferon (Tan, 1977; Epstein and Epstein, 1976). Further, Epstein, and Epstein (1976) and Tan and Greene (1976) showed that the interferon-sensitivity gene for both types I and II human interferons was localized to the distal portion of the long-arm of chromosome 21.

2. Relationship of Non-Antiviral Actions of Human Interferons to Chromosome 21

Declercq and his collaborators (1975) have claimed that there was no correlation between the interferon-induced antiviral sensitivity of human cells monosomic, disomic or trisomic for chromosome 21 and their sensitivities to the non-antiviral activities induced by interferon in such cells, namely double-stranded RNA toxicity-enhancement and priming, and thus pretended that the non-antiviral activities of human interferon are not controlled by chromosome 21. This interpretation itself can be refuted solely on a rational basis (Wiranowska–Stewart, and Stewart II, 1977; Chany, personal communication) but has also been discredited with data. Tan (1976, 1977) has shown that the sensitivity of cells to the cell-multiplication-inhibitory action of human interferons is controlled by chromosome 21. It was also demonstrated that chromosome 21 determines sensitivity to inhibition of mitogen-induced lymphoblastogenesis by human interferon (Cupples and Tan, 1977), and recently, Frankfort and his associates (Frankfort et al., 1978) have directly contradicted the claim of Declercq et al. (1975) by showing that priming activity is controlled by human chromosome 21.

3. Regulatory Chromosomes for Interferon Actions

It has been observed repeatedly that the increase in sensitivity to interferons in gene-dosage studies is not linearly related to the numbers of chromosomes but rather increases exponentially (Tan, 1977; Wiranowska–Stewart, and Stewart II, 1977). Thus it is likely that the regulatory genetic factor controlling interferon action(s) is located on separate chromosome(s) and the increase in chromosome 21 creates an imbalance between the product of the action gene and its regulator. Chany et al. (1975) have shown that human triploid cells (three copies of the entire human genetic set) were normal in interferon sensitivity, suggesting that the effect of an extra chromosome 21 is offset by other elements. These workers also found that human trisomic-16 cells were less sensitive than diploid cells to human interferon, suggesting regulatory control of interferon sensitivity is on this chromosome. Recently Blach–Olszewska and Cembrzynska–Nowak (1977) have hypothesized that the reason HeLa cells were not sensitive to interferon was related to disproportions between numbers of chromosomes connected with action of interferon and those controlling this process.

C. Role of Chromosome 21 in Interferon Actions: Interferon Binding

The previous data have shown that sensitivity to human interferon actions, both antiviral and non-antiviral are determined by human chromosome 21. Clearly this chromosome codes for some product that makes cells more sensitive to interferons (human or others: Wiranowska–Stewart, and Stewart II, 1977). In this Section data are presented indicating that this chromosome-21 product is not involved in the mechanism of these actions but rather codes for an interferon-receptor component.

1. Interaction of Interferons With Cells: Initiation of Interferon Actions

The nature of the initial interaction of interferons with cells remains obscure. It has been suggested that various membrane components bind to interferon but its specificity remains speculative. It should be recalled from previous discussions (Section VII) that interferons are quite selectively able to strongly adsorb to a large number of quite unrelated substances, including proteins, simple hydrocarbons, or polynucleotides, either electrostatically or hydrophobically. Thus it is not particularly attractive to surmise the nature of specific interferon receptor materials on cells on the basis of interferons being able to adhere to such isolated substances.

a) Indirect Studies on Interferon Binding

Early attempts to determine adsorption of interferon to cells by measuring its loss from medium were conflicting. Some investigators found that interferon activity disappeared from the medium after cell contact (Burke and Buchan, 1965; Gifford, 1963c; Lindenmann, Burke, and Isaacs, 1957; Merigan, 1964; Sellers and Fitzpatrick, 1962; Wagner, 1961). However, such losses could be attributed to inactivation of interferons (Merigan, Winget, and Dixon, 1965) or its sticking to various surfaces (Lampson et al., 1963). And others reported that interferons could repeatedly induce antiviral activity in cultures without appreciable loss of activity (Buckler, Baron, and Levy, 1966; Friedman, 1967).

Indirect evidence for interferon binding to cells was obtained in studies showing that resistance induced in cells by contact with interferon in cold was not removed by washing, but cells treated with trypsin after exposure to interferon in the cold failed to develop virus resistance (Freidman, 1967; Goldsby, 1967; Levine, 1966; Vilček and Lowy, 1967; Berman and Vilček, 1974; Stewart II, 1975a). These data suggest that interferons bind firmly to cells at a superficial site.

Interferon treatment has been reported to alter binding of cholera toxin and thyrotropin to plasma membranes (Kohn et al., 1976). Similarly, interferon-treated cells are less sensitive to the toxicity of diphtheria toxin (Yabrov, 1966, 1967; Moehring, Moehring, and Stinebring, 1971). These reports could suggest that interferons compete with these substances for common receptors (which seems unlikely) or that interferon binding altered the membrane such that their binding was obstructed. In fact, Knight and Korant (1977) have demonstrated that surfaces of interferon-treated cells are electrophorectically different from normal cells but only after several hours, suggesting it is not related directly to initial interferon interaction, but rather to interferon-induced alterations.

It has been repeatedly suggested that interferon receptors are gangliosides or ganglioside-like structures or are receptor-activators of ganglioside-glycoprotein complexes (Besancon and Ankel, 1974b; 1976; Vengris et al., 1976; Pitha, Vengris, and Reynolds, 1976a, b; Kohn et al., 1976; Pitha, 1977; Friedman, 1977). It has been reported that pretreatment of cells with plant lectins can block the action of interferon (Besancon and Ankel, 1974a, 1976). Similarly gangliosides were able to "coat" interferons bound to Sepharose and Sepharose-bound gangliosides were able to bind interferon (Besancon and Ankel, 1974b; Besancon, Ankel, and Basu, 1976). Further, addition of gangliosides to certain mouse cells deficient in these structures increased their interferon sensitivities. Interpretation of these data are difficult in view of the known host-range specificity of interferons and in view of the marked affinities of interferons to numerous structurally unrelated substances (Section VII).

It appears likely that interferon triggers all its actions from the exterior of cells, or at least pseudo-externally. Interferon immobilized on Sepharose has been shown to be able to induce antiviral (Ankel et al., 1973; Chany et al., 1974; Knight, 1974a) and non-antiviral (Knight, 1974b) activities. However, it is impossible to exclude the possibility of leakage of interferon or its direct removal from the beads by cell contact.

b) Direct Studies on Interferon Binding

If interferon sensitivities were determined by the amounts of interferon receptors on cells, positive correlations should be found between interferon binding to cells (as measured by recovery of interferon from such cells) and the sensitivities of cells to the interferons. Wagner (1961) treated chick cells with low levels (64 units) of interferon and was unable to recover interferon from cells of such cultures. Levine (1966) was also unable to detect interferon in cells exposed to 180 units of interferon, but found about 10 units in those treated with 900 units of interferon, and Friedman (1967) recovered trace levels of antiviral activity from chick cells exposed to 2000 units of interferon/ml. However, there were no attempts to correlate these bindings with sensitivities of the cells to the interferon they bound.

Stewart II, Declercq, and Desomer (1972b) found that mouse interferon could be recovered from homologous cells to which it was applied but could not be recovered from heterologous cells. The amounts of interferon recovered from three types of mouse cells correlated directly with their sensitivities to the antiviral activity of the interferon. Interferon was bound to cells rapidly at 4° C or 37° C though somewhat more slowly at the lower temperature, and was bound to actinomycin-D treated cells, but was not detectably bound to rabbit cells or to human cells. It was further found that interferon bound to cells at 4° C was still sensitive to destruction by trypsin whereas interferon bound at 37° C rapidly became trypsin resistant (Stewart II, 1975). Berman and Vilček (1974) also found human interferon could be recovered from interferon-sensitive human cells but it could not be recovered from mouse cells. Treatment of human cells with trypsin prior to interferon exposure inhibited binding of interferon. These authors also confirmed that cell-bound interferon was trypsin resistant. Cell-bound interferon eluted into medium at 37° C but did not do so at 4° C (Berman and Vilček, 1974; Stewart II, 1975). Stewart II (1975) also found that part of the applied interferon rapidly became internalized in cell-sap and nuclear-membrane fragments, but it was not possible to determine whether such uptake of interferon was necessary for the activities induced. Kohno et al. (1975a, b), also found that cell-bound interferon eluted from cells after removal of extracellular interferon, but these authors reported a lack of "species-specificity" in binding of mouse interferon to a human cell line. However, one of these investigators later found that the binding of interferon did determine the spectra of antiviral activity of rodent interferons in mouse, guinea-pig and hamster embryo cells and of hamster interferon in hamster and mouse cells (Umino and Kohno, 1976). Gresser, Bandu, and Brouty–Boye (1974) also found that mouse leukemia L1210 cells which were resistant to the antiviral and cell-multiplicationinhibitory actions of mouse interferon did not bind mouse interferon, whereas L1210 cells sensitive to these actions of mouse interferon did bind mouse interferon. These cells have also been found to be resistant and sensitive, respectively, to the double-stranded RNA toxicity-enhancing effect of interferon (Werenne and Rousseau, 1976a; Gresser and Stewart II, unpublished data).

In some cases, binding of interferon apparently is largely unrelated to induction of subsequent actions. Chany and Vignal (1968) have described a mouse embryo cell line transformed by murine sarcoma virus which became completely resistant to the antiviral action of interferon after more than 200 passages in the continued presence of interferon. These cells have been found to bind mouse interferon to the same extent as normal mouse L cells (Stewart II, unpublished data). Kuwata et al. (Kuwata, Fuse, and Morinaga 1976; Kuwata et al. 1976, Fuse and Kuwata, 1976) have described two lines of transformed human embryonic cells which were both sensitive to the antiviral effect of interferon, but were markedly different in sensitivities to the cell-multiplication-inhibitory action of interferon; the cells resistant to cell-multiplication-inhibition bound much less interferon. These reports suggest that there are some systems in which control of sensitivities to particular functions of interferons are determined subsequent to binding; certain cells may be receptor-competent yet action mechanism-defective.

2. Chromosome 21 and Interferon Binding

Alternative interpretations have been proposed for the possible role of human chromosome 21 in relation to the sensitivity of cells to interferon which it promotes. Tan (1975) suggested that chromosome 21 controls the synthesis of an intracellular antiviral protein. On the other hand, Chany *et al.* (1975) and Revel, Bash, and Ruddle (1976) suggested that this chromosome carries the structural gene for human interferon receptors, as antiserum prepared against chromosome-21-directed cell surface components made human cells resistant to the action of human interferons. Chany and his colleagues (Chany *et al.*, 1975; Chany, 1976) have suggested that the interferon host-specificity is due to receptor-interferon interactions, determined by chromosome 21 in human systems, whereas the antiviral machinery in mouse-human hybrids containing this chromosome is of mouse origin. Recently, Slate and her colleagues (1978) have shown that mouse-human hybrids containing human chromosome 21 as the only detectable human element were sensitive to human interferons (both leukocyte and fibroblast) but the presumed antiviral mechanism components activated by these interferons (specific phosphorylated proteins; see Section IX) were of mouse origin. All these data suggest that human chromosome 21 codes for an interferon receptor.

At variance with these data Declercq, Edy, and Cassiman (1976), as with their previous claim that human cells mono-, di- and trisomic for chromosome 21 were all identically sensitive to the non-antiviral actions of interferons, claimed that human cells trisomic, disomic and monosomic for this chromosome also all bound the same amounts of human interferons. However, this claim was also recently confuted by Wiranowska–Stewart and Stewart II (1977) who found that human cells with one, two or three copies of chromosome 21 bound increasing amounts of human interferons.

D. Epigenetic Complications to Assessing Genetic Contributions to Interferon Actions

The evaluation of genetics of the interferon system at the level of interferon production is complicated by a number of non-chromosomal contributions, as discussed previously (Section V. C); the genetic evaluations of interferon actions are similarly confused. Thus, as expression of genetic potential for production of human interferon can reflect more than merely the numbers of copies of chromosome 5, so the expression of interferon action can reflect more than numbers of chromosome 21. Action potentials can be modulated by varieties of influences that can act at various levels to give the same measurable effect: factors influencing interaction of interferons with receptors, those effecting subsequent transcription or translation events after interferon binding and those altering any of the interferon-induced products can all give results indicating action modulation without specifying which part of the process is involved.

1. Age Effects on Interferon Action

The relation of *in vivo* or *in vitro* ages of cells has been shown to effect the amount of interferon produced by the cultures (Section V. C. 1) and to effect the apparent titers obtained in interferon assays (Section II. D. 6). Thus to briefly recapitulate, it has been reported that tissues from very young chick embryos were much less sensitive than tissues from older eggs (Isaacs and Baron, 1960; Cantell et al., 1965; Grossberg and Morahan, 1971), similar differences being found with human embryonic tissues (Siewers, John, and Medearis, 1970). Several investigators have also reported that cultures of the same cell lines aged for increasing time in culture become increasingly sensitive to interferon (Cantell and Paucker, 1963a; Carver and Marcus, 1967; Lockart, 1963, 1968; Rossman and Vilček, 1969; Billiau and Buckler, 1970; McLaren, 1970; Korsantiya et al., 1967; Lvovsky and Levy, 1976). These differences in interferon sensitivities are significant, ranging from about 10-fold to 100-fold. And it is clearly not rational to relate these alterations to numbers of particular chromosomes as the same cells can again become less sensitive to interferon after passage before the new cultures have themselves "aged".

At least three mechanisms can be suggested for this aging effect:

(i) Cells may elaborate interferon receptors continually and, hence, their surfaces become increasingly more nearly saturated with these molecules. No direct experiments have yet been done to test this possibility, and efforts have been made to perform binding studies with fixed numbers of cells at similar culture age (Wiranowska–Stewart, and Stewart II, 1977). It has, however, been reported that interferon receptors are removed by trysinization (Berman and Vilček, 1974).

(ii) Younger cells may be more able to inactivate interferons, as proposed by Korsantiya et al. (1967).

(iii) Younger cells might elaborate a repressor of interferon action. Several reports of such substances have appeared, referred to as "stimulons" (Chany and Brailovsky, 1965, 1967; Brailovsky and Chany, 1965), virus "enhancers" (Kato et al., 1965a, b, 1966; Kato and Ota, 1966), or "interferon antagonists" (Truden, Sigel, and Dietrich, 1967; Fournier et al., 1968, 1969, 1972, 1974; Galliot et al., 1973; Rytel, 1975; Lidin and Adams, 1975; Cembrzynska–Nowak, 1977). Grossberg and Morahan (1971) have reported that younger chick embryo cells elaborated more of this factor which was antagonistic to interferon action when added to older cells. These action-modulating factors will be described below.

2. Cell Density Effect

It is also clear that interferon sensitivities are influenced by cell densities (Rossman and Vilček, 1969). Dianzani and his associates have performed several elaborate experiments to show that antiviral resistance developing in cells induced to make interferon develop more rapidly and to higher levels in the more concentrated cells. This could be a consequence of higher local levels of interferon transferred from one cell to another (Dianzani et al., 1975, 1976, 1977; Dianzani and Baron, 1975, 1977). On the other hand, Blalock and Baron (1977) have also recently reported that interferon-treated cells can apparently elaborate part of the antiviral machinery which can be transferred to adjacent cells (Section IX). It is feasible that dense cell cultures, perhaps "aged" cultures, could better share the amount of interferon-induced activities.

3. Variations in Interferon Sensitivities of Diploid Cells

As further evidence that factors other than chromosome numbers can effect interferon actions, some investigators have found that even different human diploid cell lines can vary considerably among themselves with respect to interferon sensitivities (Moehring, Stinebring, and Merchant, 1971). Gifford (1974) reported that spleen cells were markedly resistant to the antiviral effects of interferon, being at least 500 times less sensitive than L929 cells, which are normally somewhat less sensitive than primary mouse embryo fibroblast or mouse kidney cultures (DeMaeyer–Guignard et al., 1977; Stewart II, Declercq, and Desomer, 1972).

4. Other Factors Modulating Interferon Actions

The following discussion presents a number of assorted factors which have been reported to influence the apparent sensitivities of cells to interferons. These are presented here to emphasize the difficulties in assigning interferon action mechanism contributions to specific genetic components of cells. Each of these variables must also be controlled in studies on the mechanisms of the action of interferons.

a) Antagonists

A number of factors inhibitory to the action of interferons have been described. However, certain of these substances, which were presumed to be interferon action-antagonists because they enhanced virus growth, have been shown to enhance virus growth by decreasing interferon production (Kato and Eggers, 1969a; Kato et al., 1969). Other factors may effect apparent activity of interferon by stimulating growth of viruses through mechanism unrelated to interferon action (Sheaff and Stewart, 1969).

Chany and his associates (Brailovsky and Chany, 1965; Chany and Brailovsky, 1965, 1967; Chany, Lemaitre, and Gregoire, 1969; Galliot et al., 1973; Fournier et al., 1968, 1969, 1972, 1974; Chany–Fournier, Pauloin, and Chany, 1977) have described a protein isolated from virus-infected or non-infected tissues which when added to cells before or after interferon treatment lowers the virus-resistance of such cells. Other such factors have been isolated in several laboratories (Ghendon, 1965; Ghendon et al., 1966; Truden et al., 1967; Brodeur, Legar, and Brailovsky, 1973; Rytel, 1975; Cembryznska–Nowak, 1977). These have been found in normal serum and tissue extracts and from various sources, and it is difficult to imagine that it has any specific relation to eradication of interferon action. Recently, Chany and his colleagues (Chany–Fournier et al., 1977; Pauloin et al., 1977) have reported that plant lectins eradicate the interferon-induced antiviral state, and suggest that tissue antagonist of interferon is a mammalian lectin-like substance.

b) Factors Influencing Early Interferon-Cell Interactions

A number of agents which alter structural integrity of cell membranes have been shown to alter interferon responsiveness of cells, presumably by influencing binding and/or activation events (Chany, 1976; Bourgeade and Chany,

1976). Thus, various substances with affinities for gangliosides have been shown to affect interferon activity (sensitivity) in cells (Besancon and Ankel, 1974b; Besancon, Basu, and Ankel, 1976), as have gangliosides themselves (Vengris *et al.*, 1976). As there is no host-range specificity for these effects it is implied that these events are associated with adhesions other than to receptor sites.

Cholera toxin has been shown to partially inhibit the development of antiviral activity if added to cells together with interferon (Friedman and Kohn, 1976), but had no effect if added after interferon. Similar effects were found with gonadotropin (Besancon and Ankel, 1976) and thyrotropin (Kohn *et al.*, 1976). These data also suggested a two-step binding-initiation event for interferon action.

Isoprinosine, a p-acetanidobenzoic acid salt of N,N-dimethylamino-2-propanolinosine, which apparently affects membranes of cells, was reported to increase the antiviral potency of interferon in mice, but was ineffective *in vitro* (Chany and Cerutti, 1977a, b).

Cytochalasin B, colchicine and vinblastine were shown to decrease the action of interferon when added to cells with interferon, presumably by disrupting microtubes and microfilaments (Soloviev and Mentkevich, 1965; Bourgeade and Chany, 1976). Ouabain, which is known to inhibit function of membrane adenosine triphosphatase, also inhibits establishment of interferon induced antiviral state (Lebon *et al.*, 1975). Mercaptopyridethylbenzimidazole, which apparently inhibits membrane transport of nucleosides, blocked the development of antiviral action induced by interferon (Friedman and Pastan, 1969). On the other hand dibazole, a benzimidazole derivative, was reported to enhance interferon action (Yabrov *et al.*, 1971). Vitamin A has been reported to inhibit action of interferon if added to cells together with the interferon (Blalock and Gifford, 1974). However, this apparently results from direct inactivating interaction of the retinoic acid with interferon (Blalock and Gifford, 1975, 1976a, b, 1977).

Poly-L-ornithine, which enhances adsorption of various macromolecules to cells and their uptake, has been shown to increase interferon action (Kleinschmidt and Ellis, 1967; Tilles, 1967). Histones also enhanced interferon activity (Stancek and Matisova, 1968). Extracts from *E. coli* were also reported to enhance interferon action (Vilček and Ng, 1967).

Steroid hormones have been variously reported to enhance, not effect, or inhibit interferon action, though mechanisms are unknown (Kilbourne, Smart, and Pokorny, 1961; Reinicke, 1964, 1965a, b; Mendelson and Glasgow, 1966; DeMaeyer and DeMaeyer, 1963).

c) Miscellaneous Factors

i) Temperature. The temperature at which interferon assays are performed seems to have little influence on the titers obtained. Gifford (1963a) and Ruiz–Gomez, and Isaacs (1963a) found constancy within the ranges of 35–39° C, and Stewart II and Desmyter (unpublished data) found similar activity levels with 31° C and 37° C.

ii) Oxygen. Isaacs, Porterfield, and Baron (1961) reported that interferon action was influenced by oxygen tension, but others have found no such effect (Gifford, 1963a; Burke and Buchan, 1965; Zemla and Schramek, 1962).

iii) pH. Gifford (1963a) found that pH changes had no effect on interferon titers. Similar data were reported by Burke and Buchan (1965) within the range of pH 6.6 to 8.1. However, DeMaeyer, and Desomer (1962) reported that lower bicarbonate concentrations gave higher interferon titers. Hallum *et al.* (1968) found that below pH 6, interferon was unable to induce virus resistance, possibly because polyribosomes disaggregated at this pH. Similarly, Brown, and Besancon (1972) and Brown, Besancon, and Chany (1973) found an inhibitory effect of pH 6 on induction of antiviral action by interferon, but related this effect to membrane-transport arrest rather than solely inhibition of intracellular metabolism.

iv) Heavy Ions. Gainer (1972) reported that high concentrations of arsenicals inhibited the action of interferon in cell cultures if added before interferon or shortly after interferon, whereas low concentrations increased the activity of interferon. It was also reported (Gainer, 1977) that near toxic concentrations of cadmium, mercuric or nickel salts reduced interferon action in cell cultures.

v) Cyclic AMP. Cyclic 3'5' adenosine monophosphate was reported to slightly increase the sensitivity of chick cells to interferon (Friedman and Pastan, 1969), but no effect was seen with several analogues of cyclic AMP. Allen *et al.* (1974) found that, whereas cyclic AMP produced only a 2-fold increase in interferon action in mouse L_{929} cells, various related cyclic nucleotides had a more pronounced effect; one compound, 6-MT-PRcP (6-methylthio-9-β-D-ribofuranosylpurine 3', 5' cyclic phosphate), enhanced interferon action 16- to 32-fold at concentrations of 10^{-2} M. It was suggested that the cyclic nucleotides alter cells such that they behave as "aged" cultures, under limited growth conditions. Weber and Stewart (1975) also reported that cyclic AMP potentiated interferon action on L-cells; L-epinephrine and theophylline treatment of these cells elevated cellular cyclic AMP levels and potentiated interferon-induced antiviral activity. Dahl and Degre (1976a) also reported that vitamin C (ascorbic acid) slightly enhanced the antiviral activity of human leukocyte interferon in human fibroblast cells, and suggested this effect resulted from increased production of cyclic AMP. Recently, Meldolesi, Friedman, and Kohn (1977) demonstrated that interferon induced an increase in cyclic AMP levels in interferon-sensitive cells but not in interferon-resistant cells; and the elevation of cyclic AMP preceded induction of antiviral activity. Mecs *et al.* (1974), on the other hand, reported that interferon preparations raised levels of cyclic AMP in L cells, but this activity did not parallel the antiviral activity, and DEAE-Dextran was also effective.

vi) Viruses. A number of reports have demonstrated the abilities of viruses to abort the action of interferons, and it has been suggested that this is a mechanism whereby one virus can enhance the growth of another (Paucker and Henle, 1958; Cantell, 1968). Hermodsson (1963, 1964) demonstrated that calf kidney cultures infected with parainfluenza virus became resistant to interferon. Diderholm and Dinter (1966) reported a similar effect of bovine diarrhea virus. Mumps virus infection reduced the sensitivity of chick cells to interferon (Frothingham, 1965). Libikova (1965) found that chick cell infected with tick-borne encephalitis virus were refractory to interferon during the early phase of infection. Also, L cells persistently infected with tick-borne encephalitis virus (Vilček and Stancek, 1963 b), and HeLa cells infected with Sendai virus (Maeno *et al.*, 1966) were not sensitive to interferon action.

In a series of elaborate and elegant experiments Thacore and his colleagues (Thacore and Youngner, 1970, 1972, 1973 a, b; 1975; Thacore, 1976) have demonstrated that one virus can rescue another from interferon-induced inhibition. It has been reported that several viruses induce antagonists of interferon action (see discussion above), and it appears that established interferon-induced antiviral resistance can be eradicated by such antagonists. It would be interesting to determine this relationship to rescue of viruses.

Thus it is clearly not possible to attribute all fluctuations in interferon responsiveness to genetic determinants of the interferon-treated cells, as modifications can be affected at a number of stages in the alterations induced in cells by interferons.

13*

IX. Mechanisms of Antiviral Actions of Interferons

In this Section, I shall describe the antiviral actions of interferons at the cellular and molecular level. I have chosen to separate *in vivo* antiviral activities to be described in the Section after discussion of each of the non-antiviral mechanisms, as it seems likely that the involvement of interferon in natural recovery processes from viral infections represents a composite of each of the antiviral and non-antiviral actions (Stewart II, 1973).

A. General Considerations of Antiviral Actions of Interferons

Interferons have been defined largely in terms of the antiviral activities they induce in cells (Section VII. A. 7). This antiviral activity does not result from a non-specific toxic effect on the cells, but it inhibits the replication of a wide range of viruses and the development of this inhibition requires *de novo* cellular protein synthesis. Though the initial interaction of cells with interferon is sufficient for determining the subsequent development of virus resistance and though the magnitude of this antiviral state is achieved rapidly, binding being complete within minutes (Stewart II, Declercq, and Desomer, 1972b; Stewart II, 1975a; Berman and Vilček, 1974), the full expression of antiviral resistance usually requires several hours of incubation. The antiviral state once developed is maintained for a period of hours to days, depending on such variables as growth rate, after which cells return to their previous virus-sensitive condition. This Section will detail the events occurring subsequent to binding of interferon to cells, their conversion to the virus resistant state, the mechanisms by which they exert these inhibitory effects on viruses and their return to normal.

1. Conversion to the Antiviral State

a) Kinetics of Development of Antiviral Activity

Lindenmann, Burke, and Isaacs (1957) observed that no resistance to virus infection was detectable in chicken cells that were simultaneously exposed to interferon and virus, that some resistance had developed in cells exposed first to interferon for 6 hours prior to infection with the virus, and that maximal virus resistance had been established in cells exposed to interferon for 24 hours prior to virus. Some investigators have found that interferon can often induce some inhibition of virus replication when added for only short periods before virus (Vilček, 1969) and others have found inhibition by interferon treatment even when it was added after some viruses (Wagner, 1961; Desomer *et al.*, 1962; Grossberg and Holland, 1962; Lerner and Bailey, 1974), but usually several hours of incubation after initial contact with interferon is found necessary for full antiviral activity to develop (Fig. 16).

The length of period that is required for attainment for the antiviral potential has often been reported to be independent of interferon concentration (Lockart, 1966; Baron *et al.*, 1967). In one study the response rate for induction of resistance was found to be the same for several viruses in interferon-treated chick cells, but development of resistance to these viruses was slower in interferon-treated mouse cells (Jordan, 1972a). Dianzani *et al.* (1976) reported that in most strains of human foreskin cells, maximum resistance was reached at 6 hours after exposure to 3 to 10 units/ml of interferon, whereas some human fibroblasts did not develop maximum resistance until 17 to 20 hours.

In a series of recent studies, Dianzani and his associates (Dianzani *et al.*, 1976, 1977; Dianzani and Baron, 1977, 1975) have studied the effect of high concentrations of "local" interferon on development of virus resistance. They found that when cells were treated with interferon at "physiological conditions" (which amounts to using pre-warmed interferon preparations rather than room temperature interferon), antiviral resistance developed fully within only a few minutes, whereas with lower temperature preparations several hours were required. When cells were treated with warm interferon for 15 minutes, washed and exposed to antiserum to interferon, cells develop full antiviral ac-

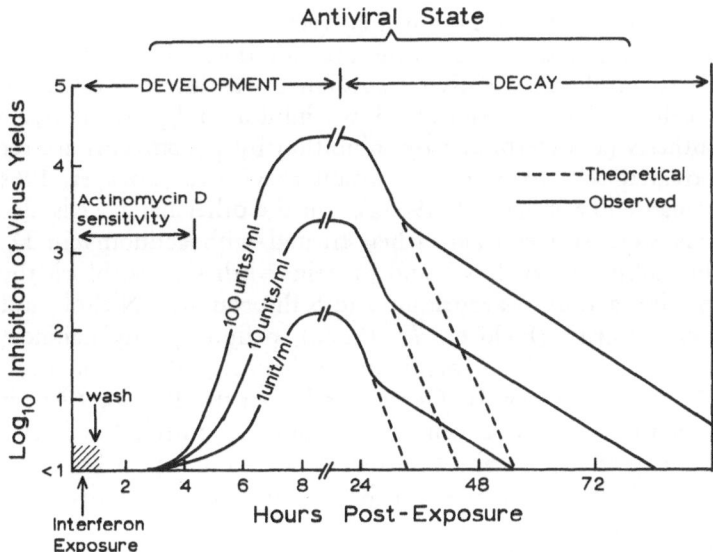

Fig. 16. The rise and fall of interferon-induced antiviral activity. The experiment designed is for mouse L cells challenged with vesicular stomatitis virus infection. After interferon treatment, at the indicated concentrations, cells were washed and challenged with virus at intervals thereafter. The decay tailing effect observed is apparently related to the elution of previously cell-bound interferon to reestablish antiviral state at a lower level. Addition of actinomycin D during the early period aborts development of virus resistance

tivity. These investigators (Dianzani et al., 1977) also reported that cells exposed to high concentrations of interferon (about 300 units/ml) developed antiviral activity much more rapidly than those exposed to low (2 to 4 units/ml) interferon levels. These studies, while confusing in terms of previous reports (Lockart and Horn, 1963; Baron et al., 1967; Dianzani et al., 1968), offer important implications for *in vivo* involvement of interferon in pathogenesis. For example, Declercq (1977) has pretended that interferon induction by poly rI·poly rC can be eliminated as the mechanism of its antitumor effect in mice because administration of amounts of exogenous interferon "mimicking" interferon blood levels induced by poly rI·poly rC failed to duplicate the poly rI·polyrC effect. Such unfortunate interpretations tend to unnecessarily confuse and delay true evaluations of the role of interferon as an antitumor agent and are naive in the assumption that circulating interferon levels reflect actual total production, and ignore the fact, as pointed out by Dianzani et al. (1977), that local levels of induced interferon, liberated from producing cells, effect significantly higher antiviral states than those induced by circulating interferon levels.

b) Metabolic Requirements for Development of Virus Resistance

It should be emphasized that it is necessary to cautiously evaluate data on kinetics of development of interferon induced antiviral effect in view of the fact that if metabolic processes are required for resistance to develop, such events could occur during the lag period, usually of several hours, of the virus replication. Thus only those events which can be selectively inhibited after interferon treatment-intervals can be timed correctly.

The interpretation that interferons are not themselves antiviral but rather induce cells to produce an antiviral substance was inferred from the observations that cellular RNA (determined by inhibition by actinomycin D), and protein synthesis (as determined by inhibition by puromycin) are required for interferon-treated cells to become resistant to viruses (Lockart, 1964; Taylor, 1964; Friedman and Sonnabend, 1965a). On the other hand, cells already resistant to virus were still resistant when treated with actinomycin D (Lockart, 1964). Other inhibitors of RNA and protein synthesis also block the development of antiviral action: 6-azauridine and 5 fluorouracil (Nichols and Tershak, 1967), mercaptopurine (Field et al., 1967a), p-fluorophenylalanine (Friedman and Sonnabend, 1964; Sonnabend and Friedman, 1973), or cycloheximide (Field et al., 1967a; Stewart II, Gosser, and Lockart, 1971a). Also, it has been demonstrated that enucleated cells cannot develop antiviral activity (Radke et al., 1974; Young et al., 1975). With the use of actinomycin D, Dianzani et al. (1976) suggested that the messenger RNA presumably required for the "antiviral protein" was produced before 1 hour after first contact of cells with interferon. These results clearly show that cellular RNA and protein synthesis are required after exposure to interferon for cells to develop virus resistance.

The interpretation of these data are not so easy as appears at first. Most investigators have assumed that these data demonstrate that interferon induces transcription of a cellular messenger RNA which translates "the antiviral protein". This model is comfortable but simplistic, but to date it has not been testable, for apparently no antiviral protein-messenger RNA has been isolated (though one has recently been suggested; Ershov *et al.*, 1976, 1977), nor has the "antiviral protein" yet been identified (though suggestions are at hand; see below). Alternatively, it has been proposed that interferon may itself be involved in the antiviral machinery and that the processes requiring cellular RNA and protein synthesis are merely involved in production of a permease to relocate interferon from its superficial binding site (Sheaff and Stewart, 1969, 1970a, b, c; Stewart and Sheaff, 1972). However, if this were the case, such "permease" must only be activatable from external of cells, as interferon-producing cells themselves apparently only become resistant when exposed to interferon from without (Vengris *et al.*, 1975).

c) Duration of the Antiviral State

Cells can remain in a virus resistant state for extended periods so long as interferon levels are maintained in the extracellular environment. However, once interferon is removed from culture media, cells return to the virus-sensitive state. The rate of decay of interferon-induced resistance is influenced by a number of factors, such as initial interferon concentration in the medium and the metabolic activity of the cells.

Isaacs and Westwood (1959a) reported that chick cells maintained their virus resistance for several days if incubated in serum-free maintenance medium after interferon removal, whereas they rapidly lost resistance if incubated in growth medium. Paucker and Cantell (1963) found that L cells regained full virus susceptibility only after several generations after interferon removal. Friedman and Sonnabend (1964) observed partial loss of antiviral activity after chick embryo cells were incubated in interferon-free medium for about 14 hours. In these reports it may be pertinent to recall that cell-bound interferon elutes from cells (Section VIII. C. 2); thus, after washing of interferon from cells, lower levels of interferon elute into culture medium, so that maintenance of interferon in "interferon-free" medium may prolong apparent decay of virus resistance by inducing new resistance. It should be possible to test true decay rates by incorporation of anti-interferon antiserum in medium after interferon removal. The decay of virus resistance in some cultures appears to vary considerably, perhaps owing to the original magnitude of resistance, which reflects original concentration of interferon treatment, which in turn would determine levels of residual (released) interferon in refed cultures.

Baron, Buckler, and Dianzani (1968) reported that interferon treated mouse embryo cells lost their virus resistance gradually over a 48 hour period. Recently, however, Dianzani *et al.* (1978) reported that resistance stayed at maximal levels for about 12 hours after removal of interferon, then rapidly plummeted to undetectable levels over a 2-hour period.

If actinomycin D, cycloheximide, or fluorophenylalanine were added to the medium after interferon removal, Baron, Buckler, and Dianzani 1968) claimed that resistance decay was much more rapid, suggesting that cellular RNA and protein are required for maintenance of antiviral resistance. However, several investigators have reported the contrary. Potentiation of the antiviral state has been reported by actinomycin D treatment of interferon treated L cells (Chany, Fournier, and Rousset, 1971) and chick cells (Lab and Koehren, 1972). Further, Radke *et al.* (1974) found that enucleated chick cells maintained virus resistance significantly longer than chick cells with nuclei. Recently, Lab, and Koehren (1976) reported that the antiviral state decays rapidly after removal of interferon from chick cell cultures, and had completely disappeared within about 72 hours. When cycloheximide was added at 18, 32, 48 or 72 hours after removal of interferon, cells fully or partially recovered their antiviral resistance depending on time of addition of inhibitor (as much as 3.5 $\log_{10}$ recovery of inhibition of Sindbis virus replication). These authors suggest that cycloheximide acts by blocking synthesis of a postulated regulatory protein which reversibly inactivates the antiviral protein or its expression. Thus it is possible to imagine that the induction of virus resistance by interferon, like the induction of interferon itself, is under posttranscriptional control and can similarly be "superinduced".

It should be emphasized at this point that the apparent decay of antiviral state may also depend on the type of virus being inhibited. On the one hand, viruses whose replications are dependent on rapidly turning-over (labile) mechanism components may be eliminated as production centers during the antiviral state and would thus not be able to restore production of virus after interferon-induced virus-resistance had decayed (Marcus and Sekellick, 1976; Friedman and Costa, 1976); on the other hand, viruses with persistent essential components could rapidly restore virus production as soon as interferon-induction restrictions faded. As will be described below, production of certain tumorviruses is arrested by interferon, but within a few hours after removal of interferon full virus production is resumed (Friedman *et al.*, 1976; Oxman *et al.*, 1967; Oxman, Rowe, and Black, 1867).

2. Character of Interferon-Induced Virus Resistance

The interferon-induced antiviral resistance is distinguishable by its ability to inhibit viruses of virtually every type known (see Table 15, Section X). This character was initially important to rule out the nonspecificity of inhibition of viruses by interferon as opposed to the absolute specificity of antibodies for the viruses used to stimulate their production. However, this property of virus non-specificity has now evolved to the point that it is possible to characterize interferon-induced virus resistance not only by the inhibition of the replication of many unrelated viruses, but also by their rankings in sensitivities in the particular animal cells involved.

Cells treated with a given concentration of interferon will become extremely resistant to some viruses, less resistant to other viruses and little, if at all, resistant to some viruses. Generalizing from particular selected data has sometimes led to the interpretation that certain types of viruses are interferon-sensitive, whereas some types of viruses are interferon-resistant (Grossberg, 1972). In fact, this is not the case. Rather each species of animal develops its particular characteristic spectrum of relative virus resistance (Stewart II, Scott, and Sulkin, 1969). Thus, a given virus can be quite sensitive to the resistance induced by interferon in one species but quite resistant to the interferon activity in cells of another animal species.

The results listed in Table 14 illustrate the relative sensitivities of a number of viruses to the antiviral activities induced in cells of various animal species by interferons. Such comparisons are only illustrated for those reports using the same assay method for each virus. Some authors have made comparisons of interferon sensitivities of viruses by using different assay methods for each virus (Rodgers et al., 1972; Hilfenhaus, Thierfelder, and Barth, 1975; Adams, Strander, and Cantell, 1975; DuBuy et al., 1973; Harris, Coleman, and Morahan, 1974); such data cannot be meaningfully compared (Stewart II and Sulkin, 1968). Some authors have also determined relative sensitivities of viruses to poly rI·poly rC (Hill, Baron, and Chanock, 1969; Oh, 1971; Thacore and Youngner, 1973c; Kern et al., 1975; Smetana, Eylan, and Weinberg, 1977), as these data have been shown to correlate with interferon sensitivities (Stewart II, Scott, and Sulkin, 1969) and to be due to interferon (Schafer and Lockart, 1970). These data emphasize a number of important points[7a]. First, the type of resistance induced is characterized by the cells, not the interferon. This was first illustrated by Stewart II and Lockart (1970) who found that monkey interferon induced human-type relative virus resistance on human cells and human interferon induced monkey cell-specified resistance in monkey cells. Others have since found similar cell species-related relative virus resistances (Ahl and Rump, 1976; Ito and Montagnier, 1977). An extreme example of this effect is that vesicular stomatitis virus is about 1,000 times more sensitive than bovine enterovirus to the interferon-induced antiviral state in bovine cells, yet is about 20-fold less sensitive than this virus to interferon-induced resistance in porcine cells (Ahl and Rump, 1976). Further evidence that the interferon-action mechanism is determined by the treated cell rather than the interferon was provided by the finding that human interferons induced mouse-type phosphorylated protein on mouse-human hybrids in which the proposed human interferon receptor-coding chromosome is the only human component. This protein may be a marker for the antiviral mechanism (see below).

Allen and his collaboratories (1976) have demonstrated that the host-dependent sensitivity of type C oncornavirus in two BALB/c mouse cell lines varies significantly as a feature of the cell line rather than the virus or the cell species.

Though it has been suggested that differential decay rates of established interferon-induced resistance against different viruses might produce artifactual differences in virus resistance obtained using plaque reduction techniques (Hallum, Thacore, and Youngner, 1970), many investigators have obtained identical results with simultaneous assays using plaque reduction, single-cycle yield reduction and cytopathic effect inhibition (Stewart II, Scott, and Sulkin, 1969; Stewart II and Lockart, 1970; Gallagher and Khoobyarian, 1971, 1972; Ito and Montagnier, 1977).

The relative sensitivities of viruses to the resistance induced by interferons

---

[7a] Perhaps the most amazing point of these data is the amount of agreement among different laboratories.

Table 14. *Relative sensitivities of viruses to interferon-induced antiviral activity*

Species of treated cell[a]	Interferon species	Assay method[b]	Relative sensitivities[c]	References
Human	human	CPE	Sindbis > echo-9 > vaccinia > herpes simplex	Ho and Enders (1959b)
	human	PR/SCYR	Sindbis > VSV > SFV > vaccinia	Stewart II and Lockart (1970)
	human	CPE	Sindbis > VSV > vaccinia > CMV	Glasgow et al. (1967)
	human	PR	Sindbis > VSV > SFV > vaccinia	Stewart II, Scott and Sulkin (1969)
	human	SCYR	Sindbis > VSV	Oie et al. (1972a)
	human	CPE	Sindbis = VSV > herpes simplex > adeno-2 = CMV	Glasgow et al. (1967)
	human	PR	Sindbis = VSV > SFV	Field et al. (1971)
	human	PR	VSV > vaccinia = adeno 2, 7, 12	Gallagher and Khoobyarian (1969)
	human	PR	VSV > adeno 1, 3, 4, 11, 18 > adeno 8, 5	Gallagher and Khoobyarian (1969)
	human	SCYR	VSV > adeno 2, 7, 12	Gallagher and Khoobyarian (1972)
	human	TAgR	SV40 > adeno 2, 7, 12	Oxman, Rowe, and Black (1967)
	human	PR	VSV > CMV	Rabson, Tyrrell, and Levy (1969)
	human	PR	VSV > vaccinia	Armstrong and Merigan (1971)
	human	SCYR	VSV > rhino-2	Fiala (1972)
	human	PR	Middleburg > VSV	Bodo, Palese, and Lindner (1971)
	human	CPE	VSV = rhino-HGP-corona 229E	Stewart II and Desmyter (Unpublished data)
	human	PR	VSV-clone 12 > VSV-clone 3	Ito and Montagnier (1977)
	human	PR/CPE	V-Z (infected cells) > V-Z (cell-free)	Rasmussen et al. (1977)
	human	CPE	VSV > clinical isolate-CMV > davis-CMV	Postic and Dowling (1977)
	human	PR	VSV = rubella	Desmyter et al. (1967)
	human	CPE	,,cold-loving" Adeno-1, 2, 3, 4, 7 > initial adeno-1, 2, 3, 4, 7	Selivanov et. al (1970)
	human	CPE	rhino-HGP > vaccinia	Smorodintsev et al. (1971a)
	human	SCYR	,,cold-strain" adeno-1, 2 > original adeno-1, 2	Lysov et al. (1971)
	human	SCYR	rhino-20 > VSV = rhino-14 > rhino-13	Stoker, Kiernat, and Gauntt (1973)

Table 14 (continued)

Species of treated cell[a]	Interferon species	Assay method[b]	Relative sensitivities[c]	References
	human	CPE	VSV = rhino-2 = rhino-4 > influenza A2 = influenza B	Merigan et al. (1973a)
	human	SCYR	VSV > herpesvirus-1	Rasmussen and Farley (1975)
	human	CPE	V-Z > macaque herpesvirus	Neumann-Haefelin et al. (1975)
	human	SCYR	Sindbis = parainfluenza-1	Murphy et al. (1975)
	human	SCYR	influenza A 1968 > influenza A 1974 > influenza A 1972 = Sindbis	Richman et al. (1976)
	human	CPE	herpesvirus-1 = herpesvirus-2	Menezes et al. (1976)
	human	SCYR	VSV > vaccinia = parainfluenza-3 = coxsackie B-1 > SV40 > adeno-1	Marchenko, Povolotsky, and Krivokhatskaya (1976)
	human	PR	VSV = rhino-3, 9, 16, 20, 36 > rhino-2, 17, 19, 24, 28, 45 > rhino-1A, 1B, 12, 13, 14, 22, 26, 38, 41, 60	Came, Schafer, and Silver (1976)
Human	monkey	PR/SCYR	Sindbis > VSV > SFV > vaccinia	Stewart II and Lockart (1970)
Human	mouse	PR	Middleburg > VSV	Bodo, Palese, and Lindner (1971)
Monkey	monkey	PR/SCYR	Sindbis > SFV > VSV > vaccinia	Stewart II and Lockart (1970)
	monkey	CPE	VSV > herpes saimiri	Barahona and Melendez (1971)
	monkey	SCYR	Sindbis = SFV = VSV > polio I	Buckler, Wong, and Baron (1968)
	monkey	TAgR	SV40 > adeno-2, 7, 12	Oxman, Rowe, and Black (1967)
	human	CPE/PR	herpesvirus-1 > herpesvirus-2	Lerner and Bailey (1976)
	human	CPE/SCYR	rhino-2 > influenza A2 = rhino-4 = influenza B	Merigan et al. (1973a)
	human	TAgR	SV40 > adeno-2 = adeno-2-SV40 hybrid	Oxman, Levin, and Lewis (1974)
	human	CPE	herpesvirus ateles > herpesvirus saimiri	Laufs et al. (1974)
	human	CPE	SFV > herpesvirus-1 > vaccinia	Hilfenhaus, Thierfelder, and Barth (1975)
	human	YR	SFV > Rabiesvirus	Hilfenhaus et al. (1975)
Chicken	chicken	PR	O'nyong-nyong > Chikungunya > vaccinia: SFV > VSV: fowl plague > NDV	Ruiz-Gomez and Isaacs (1963a)

Species of treated cell[a]	Interferon species	Assay method[b]	Relative sensitivities[c]	References
	chicken	PR	Chikungunya > vaccinia > SFV > NDV	Friedman (1964)
	chicken	PR	Chikungunya > vaccinia	Gifford, Mussett, and Heller (1964)
	chicken	PR	Bunyamwera > vaccinia > fowl plague > NDV	Isaacs, Porterfield, and Baron (1961)
	chicken	CPE	WEE = EEE > vaccinia > NDV > pseudorabies	Vilcek and Rada (1962)
	chicken	CPE	WEE = EEE > vaccinia = fowl plague > NDV > pseudorabies = herpes simplex	Vilcek (1962)
	chicken	PR	WEE > vaccinia > NDV	Vilcek and Rada (1962)
	chicken	PR	WEE > vaccinia = Japanese encephalitis > NDV	Grossberg and Scherer (1964)
	chicken	SCYR/PR	WEE > herpes simplex	Brown (1966)
	chicken	PR	Japanese encephalitis 423 > Japanese encephalitis hotta	Yamazaki (1968)
	chicken	CPE	WEE > Sendai	Balducci, Verani, and Balducci (1963)
	chicken	HAYR	Sendai > Mel-influenza > NDV	Isaacs, Lindenmann, and Valentine (1957)
	chicken	YR	Sendai > PR8-influenza > Mel-influenza > fowl plague	Burke and Isaacs (1960)
	chicken	YR	Sendai > NDV	Portnoy and Merigan (1971)
	chicken	PR	vaccinia > VSV > pseudorabies	Youngner, Thacore, and Kelly (1972)
	chicken	PR	vaccinia > SFV > VSV	Riley, Toy, and Gifford (1966)
	chicken	PR	vaccinia > VSV	Bader (1962)
	chicken	PR	vaccinia > fowl pox	Asch and Gifford (1970)
	chicken	POXR	vaccinia > herpes simplex	Isaacs, Burke, and Fadeeva (1958)
	chicken	PR	vaccinia > herpes simplex	Fruitstone, Waddell, and Sigel (1964)
	chicken	PR	VSV = fowl plague > NDV	Portnoy and Merigan (1971)
	chicken	PR	VSV > NDV pi	Hallum, Thacore, and Youngner (1970)
	chicken	SCYR	VSV = NDV pi	Hallum, Thacore, and Youngner (1970)
	chicken	PR	$VSV_{sp} = VSV_{1p}$	Wagner et al. (1963)
	chicken	YR	Rous sarcoma = lymphoid leukemia	Kuznetsov et al. (1972)
	chicken	PR	VEE (TC-83) > VEE (Trinidad)	Jordan (1973)

Table 14 (continued)

Species of treated cell[a]	Interferon species	Assay method[b]	Relative sensitivities[c]	References
	chicken	YR	pseudorabies (avirulent) > pseudorabies (virulent)	Lomniczi (1974b)
	chicken	PR	VSV > vaccinia	Radke et al. (1974)
Mouse	mouse	PR	vaccinia > Sindbis > EMC = EEE = herpes simplex = VSV	Glasgow and Habel (1962b)
	mouse	PR	vaccinia > Sindbis = VSV >SFV	Stewart II, Scott, and Sulkin (1969)
	mouse	HAYR	GD-7 > Sindbis	Oie et al. (1972a)
	mouse	PR/SCYR	NDV_{pi} > VSV	Hallum, Thacore, and Youngner (1970)
	mouse	PR/SCYR	VSV > pseudorabies	Youngner, Thacore, and Kelly (1972)
	mouse	PR	VSV_{sp} > VSV_{1p}	Wagner et al. (1063)
	mouse	PR	EMC > murine-CMV	Osborn and Mediaris (1966)
	mouse	YR	high oncogenic polyoma > low oncogenic polyoma	Gottlieb-Stematsky, Rotem, and Karby (1966)
	mouse	PR	VEE (TC-83) > VEE (trinidad)	Jordan (1973)
	mouse	SCYR	VSV > pseudorabies > vaccinia	Thacore and Youngner (1973c)
	mouse	YR	Sindbis > murine-CMV	Oie et al. (1975)
	mouse	PR	VSV > Sindbis > EMC > herpesvirus-2 > vaccinia > herpesvirus-1	Kern, Overall, and Glasgow (1975)
	mouse	PR/SCYR	mengo (sensitive mutant) > mengo (wild type)	Simon et al. (1976)
	mouse	PR	VSV clone-3 > VSV clone-12	Ito and Montagnier (1977)
Rabbit	rabbit	CPE	NDV PR8-influenza = VSV > WEE > vaccinia = herpes simplex	Oh and Gill (1966)
	rabbit	PR	SFV = Sindbis = VSV > vaccinia	Stewart II, Scott, and Sulkin (1969)
	rabbit	SCYR/PR	VSV > pseudorabies > vaccinia	Youngner, Thacore, and Kelly (1972)
	rabbit	CPE	NDV > Sindbis > VSV > vaccinia = herpes simplex	Schachter et al. (1970)
	rabbit	SCYR	VSV > mengo > herpes virus 1 and 2	Billiau and Schonne (1970)
	rabbit	PR	VSV > pseudorabies	Youngner, Thacore, and Kelly (1972)
	rabbit	SCYR	VSV > pseudorabies = vaccinia	Thacore and Youngner (1973c)
	rabbit	PR	VSV > foamy virus	Hooks et al. (1976)

Table 14 (continued)

Species of treated cell[a]	Interferon species	Assay method[b]	Relative sensitivities[c]	References
Bovine	bovine	PR	SFV > vaccinia > bovine enterovirus-M6	Finter (1968)
	bovine	PR	VSV > parainfluenza-3	Rosenquist and Loan (1967)
	bovine	YR	SFVMB > SFVCK	Finter (1964 a)
	bovine (type II)	PR	VSV > infectious bovine rhinotracheitis	Babiuk and Rouse (1976)
	bovine	CPE	NDV > VSV > SFV > FMDV > pseudorabies > bovine enterovirus	Ahl and Rump (1976)
Porcine	bovine	CPE	NDV > bovine enterovirus > FMDV > SFV > VSV > pseudorabies	Ahl and Rump (1976)
Hamster	hamster	PR	vaccinia > VSV > Sindbis = SLE = japanese encephalitis > SFV	Stewart II, Scott, and Sulkin (1969)
	hamster	YR	VEE (avirulent-BeAr) > VEE (virulent-Trinidad) = VEE (virulent-TC-83)	Jahrling, Navarro, and Scherer (1976)
Rat	rat	CPE	vaccinia > Sindbis = herpes ·	DeMaeyer and Desomer (1962)
	rat	SCYR	VSV > REO-3	Vassef et al. (1974)
Cat	cat	CPE	VSV > vaccinia	McCullough (1972)
Bat	bat	PR	Japanese encephalitis > VSV = SFV > Sindbis > vaccinia	Stewart II, Scott, and Sulkin (1969)

[a] Specific cells treated with indicated interferon.
[b] All viruses in each report were compared by indicated assay method: CPE = inhibition of cyto-pathic effect; PR = plaque reduction; SCYR = single-cycle yield reduction; TAgR = tumor-antigen reduction; YR = yield reduction; HAYR = hemagglutinin yield reduction.
[c] Viruses are listed from left to right in decreasing order of interferon-sensitivity in indicated assay system.
Abbreviations: VSV = vesicular stomatitis virus; SFV = Semliki Forest virus; CMV = cytomegalovirus; V-Z = varicella-zoster; NDV = Newcastle disease virus (NDVpi = NDV persistent infection); VSVsp and VSV 1p = VSV small and large plaque isolates; VEE = Venezualan equine encephalitis; EMC = encephalomyocarditis; FMDV = foot-and-mouth disease; SLE = St. Louis encephalitis; EEE = Eastern equine encephalitis; WEE = Western equine encephalitis.

has also been used to characterize different molecular species of interferons. Vilček, Havell, and Yamazaki (1977) found that both human leukocyte and human fibroblast interferons induced similar types of antiviral activities in human cells as measured by relative sensitivities of viruses to these activities. Similarly, each of the molecular size species of human leukocyte interferons isolated in SDS-polyacrylamide gels induce the same orders of resistance, as did the size-species of mouse interferons isolated in SDS-gels (Stewart II, unpublished data).

Any antiviral mechanism proposed must take these relative sensitivities to interferons into consideration and must be able to account for the fact that virus A may be more sensitive than virus B to the resistance induced in the cells of one animal species, yet virus B may be more sensitive than virus A to interferon-induced antiviral mechanisms in cells of another animal species. Such complexities nicely match the myriad mechanisms that have been proposed to explain "the" mechanism of interferon action.

B. Antiviral Mechanisms: Sites of Interferon Actions Against Viruses

The most interesting aspect of interferonology from the view of molecular mechanisms of action over the past decade or so has been the periodic rise and fall of attractive models of interferon action. Reviews dedicated to the materials published on the interferon action mechanisms have appeared frequently, but this frequency in no way reflects progress in understanding of the mechanisms (Colby and Morgan, 1971; Kleinschmidt, 1972; Sonnabend and Friedman, 1973; Metz, 1975a, b; Friedman, 1977; Joklik, 1977; Friedman and Chang, 1977; Lewis, Falcoff, and Falcoff, 1977). Rather, with each new hypothesis of antiviral mechanism, there has been a rush of research to prove or disprove it, with the ensuing glut of publications often doing both. Likely some of the contradictions have been caused by the fact that interferon preparations were often crude; this problem has been overcome with advances in purification and recent studies have usually been performed using interferons with high specific activities. Considerable information has accumulated on the ability of interferons to inhibit virus specific protein synthesis (Joklik and Merigan, 1966; Marcus and Salb, 1966, 1968; Carter and Levy, 1967a, b, 1968; Levy and Carter, 1968; Kerr, Sonnabend, and Martin, 1970; Kerr, 1971; Esteban and Metz, 1973; Metz and Esteban, 1972; Friedman, 1968; Friedman et al., 1972), indicating clearly that interferon can exert its action at the level of translation of viral messages. Other studies have reported that interferon can inhibit transcription of viral messenger RNA in polymerase-containing viruses (Marcus et al., 1971; Oxman and Levin, 1971; Bialy and Colby, 1972; Manders, Tilles, and Huang, 1972), perhaps through an inhibition of viral polymerase function. Most reports have indicated that interferon exerts its action at one of these earliest possible steps in virus replication, and even some suggestions have indicated this may involve uncoating of viruses (see below). Recently it has also been suggested that, at least in the case of C-type tumor viruses, inhibition of virus may occur at the latest possible step in virus replication, their maturation and/or release from cells (Billiau, 1977).

One school of thought would have it that all these effects are merely multiple manifestations of a single unifying mechanism: translation inhibition; others interpret that there may be multiple mechanisms of interferon action (Stewart II, Scott, and Sulkin, 1969; Stewart II and Lockart, 1970; Hallum, Thacore, and Youngner, 1970; Stewart II, Declercq, and Desomer, 1973; Marcus et al., 1971; Friedman, 1977; Friedman and Chang, 1977). In the following

Section, I shall review the evidence for and against interferons exerting inhibition on each of the events involved in virus replication processes.

1. Inhibition of Virus Attachment, Penetration and Uncoating

Early evidence was obtained with a few viruses that interferon-treated cells were able to normally adsorb these viruses (Ho and Enders, 1959a; Wagner, 1960; Cantell and Paucker, 1963a; Stewart II and Sulkin, 1966; Morgan, Colby, and Hulse, 1973) and it has been generalized that adsorption is unaffected. However, in view of the diversity of effects of interferons on various viruses (as will be described), and the apparent alterations of cell membranes after interferon treatment (Section X), this generalization merits questioning.

It has also been extrapolated widely that interferon-action does not inhibit virus uncoating. Again this represents a generalization from limited indirect data and very limited direct data. Indirect evidence leading to this assumption was obtained by observations that interferon not only inhibited virus replication in cells infected with intact virions but also inhibited infections with infectious RNA extracted from certain viruses (Ho, 1961; Ho, 1962; Desomer *et al.*, 1962; Mayer, Sokol, and Vilček, 1961, 1962; Grossberg and Holland, 1962). These data have been supposed to prove that interferon must act at a site beyond the uncoating step (Sonnabend and Friedman, 1973; Friedman, 1977). In fact, these data show that interferon *can* act after uncoating; additionally the interferon effect may act at more than one site. Direct studies showing lack of effect of interferon on uncoating have been reported for reovirus (Wiebe and Joklik, 1975; Galster and Lengyel, 1976). Additional studies seem worthwhile.

Indeed, some recent data have suggested that in certain virus infections uncoating may be effected by interferon treatment. Yamamoto, Yamaguchi, and Oda (1975) found that SV40 virus replication was only slightly sensitive to interferon inhibition if infection were initiated with infectious SV40 viral DNA, whereas intact SV40 virion-initiated infection was quite interferon-sensitive, as demonstrated repeatedly by Oxman and his colleagues (Oxman and Black, 1966; Oxman and Levin, 1971; Oxman, Levin, and Lewis, 1974; Oxman, Rowe, and Black, 1967; Oxman *et al.*, 1967; Metz, Levin, and Oxman, 1976; Metz, Oxman, and Levin, 1977), and others (Yakobson *et al.*, 1977; Yakobson, Revel, and Winocour, 1977). This suggests that interferon treatment had blocked uncoating or another early event. While this report has not been confirmed, and other interpretations are possible, it clearly points to the prematurity of decisions that "the" antiviral action uniformly does not block uncoating.

2. Inhibition of Virus Transcription

I previously pointed out that interferon-action hypotheses, once proposed, rapidly give rise to a plethora of publications both confirming and confuting the mechanism. The interpretation that interferon can inhibit primary transcription is such a case. The complexity of such systems virtually eliminates the possibility to choose sides on this issue at this time. The pitfalls of basing conclusions on partial data have recently been detailed with clarity by Friedman (1977).

The first observed inhibition of primary transcription by interferon was reported by Marcus et al. (1971) with vesicular stomatitis virus in chick cells. This effect was soon seemingly confirmed in human cells (Manders, Tilles, and Huang, 1972) and was later reported in monkey cells (Marcus and Sekellick, 1976). However, others have found significant discrepancies between interferon sensitivities of early vesicular stomatitis virus transcription products and those resulting from secondary transcriptions (Baxt, Sonnabend, and Bablanian, 1977) and it has been interpreted that the apparent primary transcription effect of interferon was due to trivial effects. Similarly, Wiebe, and Joklik (1975) found that whereas reovirus yields were inhibited significantly by interferon, primary reovirus transcription was only slightly depressed.

Repik, Flamand, and Bishop (1974) also attributed apparent primary inhibition in transcription of RNA in influenza virus infection of interferon-treated cell to insignificant differences and concluded that inhibition of transcription was not a primary one.

Transcription inhibition was also reported by Bialy and Colby (1972) in chick cells treated with interferon. However, this effect seems likely to result from the effect of cycloheximide (Jungwirth, Kroath, and Bodo, 1977). In fact analysis of the synthesis of poxvirus-specific RNA in interferon-treated cells showed that all "early" RNAs of vaccinia virus are synthesized, and in fact, transcription is rather enhanced than inhibited by interferon (Joklik and Merigan, 1966; Jungwirth et al., 1972a, b; Osterhoff et al., 1976; Esteban and Metz, 1973b Horak, Jungwirth, and Bodo, 1971; Metz, Esteban, and Danielescu, 1975; Metz and Esteban, 1972; Metz, 1975b). Reasons for this discrepancy are not clear.

Transcription inhibition by interferon of frog polyhedral cytoplasmic DNA virus in fish cells was also interpreted from data obtained by Gravell and Cromeans (1972), but these results seem to be, again, unavoidably complicated by the use of the antimetabolite and the relatively minor effect on primary transcription as compared to total effect on virus synthesis.

Clearly the most convincing evidence for primary transcription inhibition by interferon has come from extensive studies on SV40 virus replication by Oxman and his associates. Early viral RNA synthesis in monkey cells was markedly inhibited (Oxman and Levin, 1971), whereas virus adsorption, penetration, and uncoating were apparently not (Metz, Levin, and Oxman, 1976). However, as pointed out above, Yamamoto, Yamaguchi, and Oda (1975) presented data which indicated that inhibition of SV40 virus uncoating in interferon-treated cells might be responsible for the apparent transcription-inhibitory activity. Metz, Levin, and Oxman (1976) have suggested that inhibition of SV40 virus in interferon-treated cells is due to either reduced transcription of viral genome, or to enhanced degradation of newly synthesized viral RNA within the nucleus. They also reported that the accumulation of viral RNA is blocked in nuclei isolated from cells pretreated with interferon, an effect which could be reversed in 300 mM KCl but not by 100 mM KCl, suggesting the latter conditions were the more physiological.

Marcus, Terry, and Levine (1975) attempted an all-encompassing mechanism of interferon inhibition of viruses by reporting that a membrane-bound ribonuclease activity could be recovered from interferon-treated chick cells, and suggested that degradation of viral RNA was a unifying concept of interferon antiviral action. However, such an enzyme could not be found in hamster or monkey cells, and was found in untreated chick cells (Maenner and Brandner, 1976).

Thus to date the interpretation of whether interferon is able to inhibit virus transcription is confused, primarily by the complexities of the measurement techniques. Generally, it appears that the modest amounts of inhibitions of primary transcriptions are not sufficient to account for the marked inhibitions of virus replications.

3. Inhibition of Virus Translation

Whereas relatively few studies have reported effects of interferon on the adsorption, penetration, uncoating and transcription events of virus replications, an overwhelming amount of material has been published on interferon-induced translational regulation of viruses. The studies on virus translation inhibition have the advantage that it is possible to prove that interferon-action is exerted at the translational level in two ways: 1) studies of message function of input viral RNA in interferon – treated cells; 2) studies of viral RNA translation in cell-free protein – synthesizing systems prepared from interferon-treated cells. While with both these systems it has been possible to prove that interferon can act by translation-inhibition, it has not been possible to prove that it acts exclusively at this stage.

a) Inhibition of Virus Translation in Cells

The data revealing that interferon-treatment inhibits early viral synthesis in cells is extensive. These data overwhelmingly agree that translation inhibition is the major mechanism of arrest. However, the mechanisms by which viral proteins can be inhibited at the level of translation are themselves multiple. These possible mechanisms of translation inhibition will be described in relation to unifying mechanism of interferon action in Section IX. C.

Several early studies showed that formation of viral RNA was inhibited in interferon-treated cells (Lockart, Sreevalsan, and Horn, 1962; DeSomer et al., 1962; Taylor, 1965; Friedman and Sonnabend, 1965b; Gordon et al., 1966; Mecs et al., 1967) and with a given virus it was shown that certain classes of viral RNAs were more sensitive than others (Friedman, 1967; Mecs et al., 1967). These viral RNA replications were dependent on the specific synthesis of a viral RNA polymerase coded by the virus itself, thus inhibition of viral RNA synthesis could result from a primary effect of interferon on translation of viral polymerase from the parental viral RNA (Friedman et al., 1967; Friedman and Sreevalsan, 1970). Subsequently, it was reported that the amount of viral RNA polymerase activity in chick cells infected with Semliki Forest virus (Martin and Sonnabend, 1967; Sonnabend et al., 1967) and in L cells infected with Mengo virus (Miner, Ray, and Simon, 1966) was depressed, likely due to less of it being translated. Friedman (1968) showed that RNA of temperature-sensitive mutant Semliki Forest virus was unable to translate in interferon-treated cells.

Levy and Carter (1968) speculated that the mechanism of translation inhibition in Mengovirus-infected interferon-treated cells resulted from the inability of viral RNA to associate with viral ribosomal subunits to form functional polyribosomes. On the other hand, Friedman and Sreevalsan (1970) found that association of viral RNA with replication complexes was not inhibited by interferon treatment. Interferon treatment has also been shown to inhibit all vesicular stomatitis virus proteins in rabbit kidney cells (Yamamoto, Yamaguchi, and Oda, 1975), in which case it is clear that the slight transcription inhibition would not account for such effect.

Inhibition of viral proteins by interferon was also observed in reovirus infected cell (Wiebe and Joklik, 1975); again where protein inhibition was strongly inhibited, transcription inhibition was minimal.

Several studies have been reported showing that interferon inhibits the early thymidine kinase induction by vaccinia virus in chicken cells (Bodo and Jungwirth, 1967; Ghosh and Gifford, 1965; Levine et al., 1967; Ohno and Nozima, 1964) but it did not do so in mouse cells (Barban and Baron, 1968). It was suggested that interferon inhibited the secondary (virus-directed) uncoating of vaccinia virus (Magee et al., 1968), as virus remained in core particles; however, primary uncoating (which is controlled by cellular functions) proceeded normally. While vaccinia viral messenger RNA formed in interferon-treated cells is normally polyadenylated (Klesel et al., 1974) it apparently does not form stable polysomes (Bodo et al., 1972; Joklik and Merigan, 1966; Metz and Esteban, 1972; Metz, Esteban, and Danielescu, 1975). However, studies with vaccinia virus in some interferon-treated cells are complicated by the phenomenon that even when virus is inhibited the cytotoxicity is enhanced by interferon treatment and interferon-treated cells are destroyed even more rapidly than untreated vaccinia virus-infected cells (Joklik and Merigan, 1966; Horak, Jungwirth, and Bodo, 1971; Stewart II, Declercq, and Desomer, 1973). As double-stranded RNA is synthesized in vaccinia virus-infected cells (Colby and Duesberg, 1969), this phenomenon is likely related to the non-antiviral effect, double-stranded RNA-toxicity-enhancement (Stewart II et al., 1972) and will be discussed later (Section X). The rapid inhibition of cellular and viral proteins seen in interferon-treated cultures (Joklik and Merigan, 1966; Metz and Esteban, 1972; Suh et al., 1974) are difficult to distinguish due to polyribosomal breakdown or total cell breakdown.

In interferon pretreated cells SV 40 virus T antigen synthesis is inhibited (Oxman and Black, 1966). While this has been suggested to perhaps relate to inhibition of uncoating of the SV 40 virions (Yamamoto, Yamaguchi, and Oda, 1975) or to inhibition of transcription (Oxman and Levin, 1971), it was also found that translation of SV 40 viral cRNA was inhibited in interferon-treated cells when it was introduced by microinjection (Graessmann et al., 1974). Further, it has recently been shown that interferon is able to fully induce the antiviral state in monkey cells even when added when cells are already infected and producing SV 40 T antigen (Yakobson, Revel, and Winocour, 1977). By

18 to 24 hours after addition of interferon to such cultures both early and late SV 40 protein synthesis was arrested, though synthesis of viral messenger RNAs continued unabated (Yakobson *et al.*, 1977). In this system viral messages did not associate with polysomes, though host polysomes were not degraded and the bulk of cellular protein synthesis continued. Thus the suicide approach to virus limitation seen in interferon -treated vaccinia-virus-infected cells is not attempted by SV 40-infected cells.

An original approach to explaining the ability of interferon to inhibit viruses has been the suggestion that interferon-treated cells distinguish between cellular RNA and viral RNA by making modified messenger RNAs which apparently are somewhat larger than normal (Levy and Riley, 1973). It was proposed that the requirement for protein synthesis in interferon-treated cells is to make enzymes required to make these modifications (Riley and Levy, 1977). It is tempting to dismiss these data as artifactual, but this puzzling observation could perhaps prove pertinent.

Thus, even if attachment is, or is not, effected by interferon-induced virus resistance, and whether or not penetration and uncoating can proceed normally, and should viruses be, or not be, inhibited at transcription, they can then be restricted at the level of translation.

b) Inhibition of Virus Translation in Cell-Free Systems

Cell-free studies on mechanisms by which interferon can prevent production of viral products were undertaken more than a decade ago, but the early studies preceded the evolution of systems able to reliably perform translations of viral messages. The following discussion will briefly review these simplistic early studies and will then present the maze of mechanisms revealed by modern methods. In view of the complexity existing in the cell, with respect to interrelations of effects, it should not be particularly surprising that, even with the miracles of modern molecular biology, it has been difficult to reproduce many of the subtleties in a test tube by addition of certain isolated components (see Section IX. C. and Figure 17). Translation of proteins being a huge composite of processes, it should also be expected that many mechanisms for antiviral action of interferon would be revealed by such studies, even among those who have consensus that translation inhibition is "the" mechanism.

Marcus and Salb (1966) proposed that interferon induced a "translational inhibitory protein [TIP]" that combined with ribosomes and inhibited their ability to both bind and translate viral messenger RNA, but not cellular messenger RNA. It was claimed that treating inhibited ribosomes with trypsin restored their ability to translate viral RNA (Marcus and Salb, 1968). Carter and Levy (1967a, b, 1968) soon provided support to the interpretation that the site of interferon action was on the ribosome as they claimed that Mengo virus RNA would not bind to ribosomes from interferon-treated L cells. However, Kerr, Sonnabend, and Martin (1970) and Lockart (personal communication) reported there was no difference in binding of viral RNA to ribosomes from control and interferon-treated cells, and others (Content *et al.*, 1975) have found opposite results from Carter and Levy (1967). Thus, the ribosome-binding restrictions proposed by Marcus and Salb (1966) and Carter and Levy (1967a, b) have not yet been confirmed. Carter and Levy (1968) further reported that, whereas translation of Mengo RNA was inhibited in cell-free systems prepared from interferon-treated cells, translation of polyuridylic acid and tobacco mosaic virus RNA were not inhibited. These data have apparently also not been reproducible in other laboratories (Friedman, 1977).

It has only been with the development of partially-defined reliable cell-free protein synthesizing systems (Kerr, 1971) that investigators have begun to sort out the various influences of interferons on virus RNA translation (or to realize the many variables influencing interpretations of results obtained in such systems).

i) Infection-Activation of Antiviral Action. Friedman *et al.* (1972) found that extracts from normal and interferon-treated cells were both equally able to translate viral messenger RNA; however, vaccinia and EMC virus-infected interferon-treated cells provided extracts which would not translate viral messages in the cell-free system, though translation of polyuridylic acid was not inhibited. These investigators then interpreted that the interferon-induced antiviral action requires virus infection to activate translation inhibition (Kerr *et al.*, 1973, 1974).

Other workers have, however, reported systems in which infection of interferon-treated cells was not essential for their extracts to inhibit translation of viral messenger RNA (Falcoff *et al.*, 1972b; 1973; Gupta, Sopori, and Lengyel, 1973; Gupta *et al.*, 1964; Samuel and Joklik, 1974; Samuel, 1976; Mayr *et al.*, 1977; Hiller *et al.*, 1976; Zilberstein *et al.*, 1976a). These investigators reported that the interferon-treated cell extracts were normally able to translate polyuridylic acid but were unable to translate viral messenger RNAs. A factor inhibiting translation was apparently resident on ribosomes which could be removed by salt-wash.

Falcoff and his associates (1973), Gupta and his colleagues (1973, 1974) and Hiller *et al.*, (1976) found that translation of both viral RNAs and cellular (hemoglobin) messages were inhibited in such extracts. However, Samuel and Joklik (1974) reported that their translation system was able to discriminate between viral and cellular RNAs, allowing the latter to translate normally. They reported that a 48,000-dalton protein isolated from ribosomal washes of interferon-treated cells was able to inhibit translation of viral messenger RNAs when added to normal cell extracts. This translation-inhibiting protein has recently been reported to lack the "species-specificity" demonstrated by the defined host-range of interferons, as it was active in cell-free systems derived from heterologous cells (Samuel and Farris, 1977). This is reminiscent of the lack of host-range-specificity of the transfer of virus resistance from interferon-treated cells by close contact (Blalock and Baron, 1977). To my knowledge the selectivity of viral protein translation inhibition observed by Samuel and Joklik (1974) exhibiting similar specificity to that seen in intact cells treated with interferon has not been observed in any other laboratories. Recently, Eppstein, and Samuel (1977) reported that the inhibitor of translation isolated from ribosomal salt-wash fraction prepared from interferon-treated cell possessed nucleolytic activity.

ii) Double-Stranded RNA Activation of Antiviral Action: Protein Phosphorylation, Endonuclease Activation, and a Low Molecular Weight Inhibitor of Translation. Kerr and his colleagues (Kerr, Brown, and Ball, 1974; Kerr *et al.*, 1976) found that the interferon-treated cell extracts, which were not active in inhibition of translation unless activated by virus infection, could also be activated for translation-inhibition by adding double-stranded RNAs. This inhibitory effect required also addition of adenosine-5'-triphosphate (ATP), but after incubation of interferon-treated cell-extracts with double-stranded RNA and ATP, the two latter agents could be removed and translation-inhibitory activity was maintained; thus a translation inhibitory factor had been generated in the reaction mix (Roberts, Clemens, and Kerr, 1976), apparently by a phosphorylation process. As double-stranded RNA replicative-intermediates are formed during RNA virus infection and as double-stranded RNA has been observed to form even during DNA virus infection (Colby and Duesberg, 1969), it seems likely that the activation of translation inhibition previously performed by virus infection is attributable to double-stranded RNA.

Lengyel and his associates (Brown *et al.*, 1976; Lebleu *et al.*, 1976; Sen *et al.*, 1976) also found that extracts of interferon-treated mouse cells when mixed with ATP and double-stranded RNA, produced endonuclease activity and phosphorylation of a 67,000-dalton protein. Similar data were reported by Revel and his associates (Zilberstein *et al.*, 1976a, b). Roberts *et al.*, (1976) also found that in addition to two proteins being phosphorylated at about 60,000 and 30,000 daltons, a low-molecular weight translation inhibitor was phosphorylated. Thus interferon treatment induces a precursor which requires double-stranded RNA and ATP to activate it to produce a low molecular weight inhibitor of translation (LMWIT, see below). Revel *et al.* (1977) have proposed that the phosphorylated 67,000 dalton and 35,000 dalton proteins are M 1 and eIF 2 initiation factors, respectively.

Sen *et al.* (1976b) reported that when double-stranded RNA and ATP were added to interferon-treated cell saps, an endonuclease action was generated which degraded reovirus messenger RNA, larger messages being degraded faster than small messages. Two phosphorylated proteins were also generated during this reaction, at 64,000 and 37,000 daltons (Lebleu *et al.*, 1976). Galster and Lengyel (1976) reported that the reovirus subviral particle double-stranded RNAs isolated from interferon-treated cells were shorter than those from control infected cells, suggesting endonuclease lead to degradation. Reovirus double-stranded RNA was itself able to activate endonuclease in interferon cell saps in ATP (Lengyel *et al.*, 1978). Kerr *et al.* (1976) also found that cell saps from interferon treated cells showed enhanced capacity to degrade EMC viral RNA when reacted with double-stranded RNA.

Endonuclease generated from cell-saps of interferon-treated cells in the presence of double-stranded RNA and ATP were also able to degrade cellular RNAs. It seems worthwhile mentioning at this point that the interferon preparations used in these studies were purified to about 10^9 units/mg of protein and (in contrast to the earlier report from the same laboratories: Graziadie, Weidell, and Lengyel, 1973) this interferon was nuclease-free (Ratner et al., 1977). In regard to the relevance of this nuclease in vivo, it is interesting that SV 40 messenger RNA is found undegraded in interferon-treated cells (Yakobson et al., 1977a, b; Revel, 1977; Revel et al., 1977), though it does not associate with polyribosomes, and in interferon-treated cells, dimethylsulfoxide-induced globin synthesis is undiminished (Lieberman et al., 1974; Swetly and Ostertag, 1974) at least at doses of interferon sufficient to completely inhibit vesicular stomatitis virus, although it is inhibited by much higher interferon concentrations (Rossi et al., 1977a, b, c). However, the generation by ATP and double-stranded RNA of endonuclease activity in cell saps from interferon-treated HeLa cells was also reported, so this phenomenon is apparently not restricted to particular species (Shaila et al., 1977).

The low molecular weight inhibitor of translation (LMWIT) found to be generated in extracts from interferon-treated cells mixed with double-stranded RNA and ATP (Roberts et al., 1976b) could also be generated on a column to which double-stranded RNA was immobilized, when interferon-cell saps and ATP were provided. The LMWIT was not a polypeptide. It also appeared not to be directly inhibitory itself, as there was a lag period of about 15 minutes after its addition to a reticulocyte translating system before translation was inhibited. Thus LMWIT itself appeared to regulate formation of inhibitor(s) (Hovanessian, Brown, and Kerr, 1977).

Kerr, Brown, and Hovanessian (1977) reported that LMWIT is apparently synthesized by an enzyme present in extracts of interferon-treated cells which is activated by double-stranded RNA. ATP appeared to become incorporated into the LMWIT, which was sensitive to alkali, alkaline phosphatase, and snake venom phosphodiesterase, but was resistant to micrococcal nuclease and nucleleases P 1, T 2 and U 2. LMWIT appears to be an unusual oligonucleotide that is able at nanomolar concentrations to cause inhibition of translation. The structure of this material has recently been published (Kerr and Brown, 1978; Ball and White, 1978) and its formula is included in Fig. 17. An apparently identical substance is synthesized by enzymes from rabbit reticulocytes (Hovanessian and Kerr, 1978). The significance of this material will be greatly enhanced if it is demonstrated to exert selective (interferon-type) translation inhibition against viral RNA in intact cells. In view of the enhanced sensitivity of interferon treated cells to toxicity of double-stranded RNA (Stewart II et al., 1972) it will be interesting to determine the sensitivity of cells treated with LMWIT to the toxicity of double-stranded RNA, or the toxicity of LMWIT for interferon-treated cells. Recently, it has also been reported that the action of LMWIT is to activate an endonuclease (Clemens and Williams, 1978).

Clearly the involvement of interferon in generation of enzyme(s) which are activated by double-stranded RNA and which phosphorylate specific proteins and/or LMWIT is a reproducible and wide-spread phenomenon (Werenne and Rousseau, 1976b). Phosphorylations of such marker proteins have also been reported in cells treated with Type II interferons (Wietzerbin et al., 1977b) and have been observed in double-stranded RNA- and ATP-activated cell-saps from virus-resistant mutant mouse cells which presumably are spontaneously producing low levels of interferon (Jarvis and Colby, 1978). Recently, Slate *et al.* (1978) also found that human-mouse hybrids containing human chromosome 21, when treated with human interferon, produced extracts, which, when exposed to double-stranded RNA and ATP, phosphorylate the mouse 67,000-dalton protein marker, whereas the human protein phosphorylated in human cell extracts was reported to be somewhat larger (Lebleu *et al.*, 1976). Cooper and Farrell (1977) have also reported that a cytoplasmic extract of interferon-treated L cells, when activated with double-stranded RNA and ATP inhibited protein synthesis in the rabbit reticulocyte system, apparently through phosphorylation of met-tRNA binding factor, thus causing a defect in initiation of polypeptide chains; this report again demonstrates the lack of host-specificity of the antiviral mechanism components. These workers also reported that addition of initiation factor eIF-2 greatly reduced the translation inhibition. Thus *one* of the ways interferons may restrict translation is by phosphorylation of eIF-2, thereby preventing polypeptide chain initiation.

These data indicate that extracts of interferon-treated cells contain: 1) an enzyme precursor able to be converted to endonuclease; 2) an enzyme precursor able to be converted to a kinase; 3) an enzyme precursor able to be converted to a LMWIT-synthetase.

It is curious (and possibly more than coincidence) that the double-stranded RNA structure which is involved in induction of interferon is also the structure involved in activation of a number of actions of interferon.

iii) The tRNA Effect. A number of studies on the interferon-induced-block in ability of cell-free extracts to translate RNAs demonstrated that addition of tRNA to the reaction mix would reverse the restriction (Gupta, Sopori, and Lengyel, 1973, 1974; Content *et al.*, 1974, 1975; Hiller *et al.*, 1976; Weissenbach *et al.*, 1977). This effect could be detected with different minor tRNAs for viral messenger RNA and cellular messenger RNA (Content *et al.*, 1974; R. Falcoff *et al.*, 1976: Zilberstein *et al.*, 1976a; Mayr *et al.*, 1977). Falcoff and her associates (1976) reported that tRNA[leu] was responsible for reversion of inhibition of polyuridylic acid, whereas Mengovirus RNA translation inhibition was reversed by total yeast tRNA but only partially by tRNA[leu]. Interestingly, poly C translated *better* in extracts of interferon-treated cells than in those from normal cells. It was suggested that the tRNAs in cell-saps of interferon-treated cells were more labile than those from control cells (Sen *et al.*, 1976a; Lengyel *et al.*, 1978). Colby and his collaborators (1976) compared the tRNAs from control and interferon-treated mouse L cells and ascites cells and found that both had the same numbers of leucyl tRNA isoacceptors and both equally efficiently reversed interferon-mediated inhibition of reovirus messenger RNA translation in the cell-free system. Content *et al.* (1974) had also found no difference in tRNAs from normal and interferon-treated cells in this regard.

iv) Messenger RNA Methylation. Lengyel and his associates (Sen *et al.*, 1975, 1977; Shaila *et al.*, 1977), following the discovery that methylated, capped reovirus messenger RNAs were more efficiently translated than unmethylated, capped reovirus messages, compared the ability of extracts from interferon-treated cells to methylate these messages; indeed, as seems to be the case with any other testable parameter, methylation was impaired in such systems. An inhibitor of methylation was identified which could be inactivated during incubation. This inhibitor awaits, too, an assignment of significance.

v) Aminoacyl Discharge. Another potential antiviral mechanism acting at translation level is the finding that extracts from interferon-treated cells are able to discharge an amino acid previously esterified to a viral RNA, but failed to affect amino acylated transfer RNA (Sela *et al.*, 1976). As there are no known functional analogies in animal cells for such a situation it is so far difficult to realize the significance of these data.

4. Inhibition of Maturation and Release

If viruses have successfully avoided possibilities of being prevented from attaching to interferon-treated cells, penetrating into and uncoating within the interferon-treated cells, and if they are able to evade potential interferon-induced blocks at transcriptional and translational levels, their progeny can then gather their newly proliferated parts together and exit to look for new virus factories. Maybe not. Several pieces of evidence suggest that even should viruses be able to make their parts, interferon treatment may yet prevent them being put together or may even arrest release of assembled virions. Data on these effects have all appeared since 1974 and interpretations of mechanisms are still evolving with each new publication on this aspect of interferon action; however, the significance of these data are heightened all the more by the fact that this mechanism seems to involve the inhibition of tumorviruses.

Virtually all interferon antiviral mechanism studies have been aimed at finding the *earliest* possible site of action of interferon; thus little attention has previously been paid to late effects of interferon on virus replication. In fact, it was not until two separate laboratories independently observed accumulations of RNA tumor virus components in interferon-treated cells which liberated significantly less C-type particles than normal cells (Billiau *et al.*, 1974, 1975; Friedman and Ramseur, 1974; Friedman *et al.*, 1975) that attention has turned to the possibility that interferon might also inhibit viruses which apparently get past its earlier obstructions. This is not to imply that RNA tumorviruses are the only types of viruses restricted by this "novel" mechanism; rather, other viruses may be so effected.

Nor should it be presumed that this late arrest is the only mechanism whereby tumor-viruses are inhibited. Interferons have long been known to "conventionally" inhibit replication of several RNA and DNA tumorviruses (Bader, 1962; Oxman, Rowe, and Black, 1967; Gottlieb–Stematsky, Rotem, and Karby, 1966; Sarma *et al.*, 1969; Fitzgerald, 1969; Peries *et al.*, 1968; Van Griensven *et al.*, 1971; Birg and Meyer, 1975).

In evaluating data on effects of interferon on replication events in tumor-virus infections, a number of special circumstances must be considered. The virus genome is retrocopied and incorporated into the cell genome, and cells then become chronic provirus carriers which can either spontaneously produce virus or can be induced to do so. Thus interferon can act to prevent the primary infection, or can suppress chronic production, or it can inhibit activation of virus in latent carrier cultures.

When cultures are treated with interferon prior to infection with murine sarcoma virus and if interferon was maintained in the culture medium, it apparently inhibited transformation and virus production (Fitzgerald, 1969; Peries et al., 1968; Sarma et al., 1969), but if added after the virus it was ineffective. This effect was recently demonstrated by Pitha, Rowe, and Oxman (1976) to not decrease numbers of infectious centers, suggesting that interferon inhibited virus production but not synthesis and incorporation of proviral RNA.

In cells already infected with oncornaviruses but which are not producing virions, activation is possible with halogenated pyrimidines, cycloheximide and glucocorticoids. Interferon treatment can inhibit the amount of virions released in such induced cultures (Blaineau et al., 1975; Pitha, Rowe, and Oxman, 1976; Ramseur and Friedman, 1976; Wu et al., 1975; Wu, Schultz, and Gallo, 1976; Ramoni et al., 1976; Rossi et al., 1977a, b, c; Swetly and Ostertag, 1974; Lieberman et al., 1974). However, interferon had no effect on the amount of intracellular gs-antigen induced by iododeoxyuridine (Wu, Schultz, and Gallo, 1976), and as soon as interferon was removed from AKR cells infected with murine leukemia virus, virus production rapidly resumed. Thus interferon appears not to block activation steps of latent oncornavirus genome but instead blocks later step(s).

It may be pertinent to point out that many of these oncornavirus studies have been performed with unusual doses of interferons. One study seemingly used interferon at 50,000 units/ml (50 units/μl; Lieberman et al., 1974). Some workers find effects not seen by others, but use significantly higher interferon concentrations (several thousand reference units/ml; Rossi et al., 1977a, b). Some workers have reported a lack of effect of interferon on certain oncornavirus functions, but used a maximum dose of only four interferon units/ml (Aboud et al., 1978; Salzberg, Bakhanashvili, and Aboud, 1977). And while some have used interferon preparations purified to more than 10^8 units/mg of protein (Billiau et al., 1976a), others have used very crude preparations (3×10^3 units/mg of protein; Salzberg, Bakhanashvili, and Aboud, 1978). One study reports that the genome of vesicular stomatitis virus could be eliminated by prolonged treatment of cells with 100 units of interferon/ml, that herpesvirus genome could be eliminated by 1000 units/ml, but murine leukemia virus genome was not eliminated by interferon at 30 units/ml. One paper reports determining a concentration-dependent effect of interferon on rate of decay of the antitumorvirus activity and found no concentration effect: the high dose was 3.0 units of interferon/ml and the low dose was 1.5 units/ml. Clearly more considerations need to go into evaluating the effects than just looking at apparent results obtained. It is entirely possible that interferon activities are sequentially concentration-dependent, such that certain actions are activated in response to low levels of interferon whereas others require stronger stimuli. While it is not possible for me to detail all interferon doses, purities, and timings (partly because these are sometimes not even put in the publications, I do caution against acceptance of many of the interpretations presented by authors without first assessing reasonableness of these variables.

Interferon can also inhibit production of C-type particles when added to many cultures that are chronically producing such virions (Van Griensven et al., 1971; Allen et al., 1976; Billiau, Sobis, and DeSomer, 1973; Billiau et al., 1974; 1975, 1976a, b; Billiau, 1975, 1976; Peries et al., 1968; Pitha, Rowe, and Oxman, 1976; Ramseur and Friedman, 1976; Friedman, 1977; Friedman and Ramseur, 1974; Friedman et al., 1975, 1976, 1977; O'Saughnessy et al., 1974; Shapiro, Strand, and Billiau, 1977; Salzberg et al., 1977). Chany and Vignal (1970) first reported that the numbers of C-type viral particles associated with interferon-treated cultures was not decreased. Billiau, Sobis, and Desomer (1973) also found that cell-associated virions were not depressed in thin-section electron micrographs of murine sarcoma virus-infected cells treated with interferon; however, extracellular virus was markedly depressed. Radiolabelled C-type particle synthesis in cells was also uneffected by interferon, whereas extracellular labelled virions were inhibited (Billiau et al., 1974) and in fact, intracellular virions were increased (Billiau et al., 1976a, b; Friedman and Ramseur, 1974; Chang et al., 1977a). Thus interferon appeared to inhibit release of oncornavirions. It was suggested that this inhibition of release might result from a "thickening" of the mucopolysaccharide layer of the surface of interferon-treated cells (Billiau et al., 1977b).

The amount of murine leukemia viral protein p 30 and reverse transcriptase produced in interferon-treated cells is often undiminished or even increased (Friedman and Ramseur, 1974; Friedman et al., 1975; Pitha, Rowe, and Oxman, 1976; Shapiro, Strand, and Billiau, 1977). It was also reported that interferon failed to inhibit cleavage of several precursors for the major viral protein (Shapiro, Strand, and Shapiro, 1977; Pitha et al., 1977). From these data it is clear that interferon does not uniformly restrict viral translation but may be able to selectively depress particular proteins. Such selective translation blocks should not be surprising in view of the extremes in interferon-sensitivities seen with different challenge viruses (Table 14).

It has been interpreted that interferon-treated cells "trap"-C-type virus particles at their membranes (Billiau et al., 1976b). (In fact, it has even been suggested that interferon-treated cells "trap" vesicular stomatitis virus and herpes virus; Friedman et al., 1976.) And it was reasonable to speculate that C-type virions from interferon-treated cells were defective in some respects. Van Griensven et al. (1971) suggested that C-type virions from interferon-treated cells were defective in RNA content. However, Billiau, et al. (1976b) were unable to detect any physical deficiencies in interferon-treated cell culture-derived particles. On the other hand, Pitha, Rowe, and Oxman (1976) found that viral particles associated with interferon-treated cells were disproportionately high in transcriptase-to-infectivity ratios. Chang et al. (1977b) have reported that numbers of murine leukemia virus particles budding on surfaces of interferon-treated cells are greatly increased and while the level of extracellular virus was decreased 90 to 95%, levels of intracellular group specific antigens and reverse transcriptase were not inhibited; these authors suggested that interferon might inhibit a single virus protein needed for assembly, maturation, and or release.

More recently, Chang and Friedman (1977) reported that, while interferon apparently may not effect cleavage of Rauscher murine leukemia virus precursors (Shapiro, Strand, and Billiau, 1977), it seemed to do so in Moloney leukemia virus infected cells. Interferon-treated Moloney murine leukemia virus-infected cells produce virions with high particle/infectivity ratios (Wong *et al.*, 1977; Chang *et al.*, 1977a). Chang and Friedman (1977) reported that whereas cells infected with this virus contain only trace components of a large 85,000-dalton glycoprotein, interferon-treated cultures produced a large amount of this material; these workers suggest this may represent an uncleaved precursor to gp 67–71. Thus the late assembly-maturation-release block of oncornaviruses by interferon could result from interferon selectively inhibiting translation of genome (viral?) material coding for a cleavage enzyme. Or it could block release by altering cell membranes; or both; or more.

Even if interferon fails to prevent release of virions, and even if the interferon-induced antiviral mechanism has failed to completely prevent replication of the infecting virus, a partial reduction of infectious virus yields could mean that in some cases a proportion of the virions released are non-infectious or defective. Such defective virions could also be interferon-inducing particles (Stewart II, 1969), and such defective-interfering particles could play a role in limiting subsequent virus cycles (Section XII).

C. An Oversimplified Summation of Interferon-Induced Antiviral Actions

The mechanisms by which interferons make cells resistant to viruses (and, as will be described in Section X, alter the cells in other ways) have evaded attempts at unifying answers for many years; rather almost any function within eukaryotic cell processes that can be dissected can be implicated. Even if all phenomenon of interferon-induced virus restrictions are ultimately reconciled to occur through " translation-inhibition", that is small conciliation in view of the myriad possible mechanisms comprising translation processes (as described below). It seems possible that the interferon-induced mechanisms have diversified to allow the host cell multiple methods to manage various types of viruses.

The model in Fig. 17 was developed from the data described in this Section. Obviously, it is vastly over-simplified, but by following a virus through the mechanisms of its replication, it is possible to envision several possible sites of interferon's antiviral actions.

Attachment of viruses may not be effected in interferon-treated cells, though it seems premature to generalize this from available data. Penetration (or pinocytòsis) and uncoating are possibly not generally altered, but may be involved in inhibition of some virus.

If the infecting virus is a negative-strand RNA virus, it can directly attempt to translate into the proteins necessary to produce progeny; however, if the invader is double-stranded RNA or DNA or positive-strand RNA virus, it must first attempt to transcribe itself into a functional enzyme-producing RNA before it can undertake translation. This process of transcription could be inhibited by interferon-induced mechanisms that might inactivate the virions transcriptase, or even directly degrade the template. Transcription could also be arrested by inhibition of initiation or elongation which could in turn result from deficiencies in factors involved in these processes.

For the viruses whose replicative processes, either directly from uncoating or indirectly through transcription, achieve a messenger RNA to be translated, these must be able to avoid a great number of potential interferon-induced blocks in this "unifying" mechanism of interferon's action. Translation inhibition can be achieved by degradation of the template, or its modification such that it is unable to bind to ribosomes. Or ribosomes of interferon-treated cells may be altered such that they are unable to bind to the viral messenger RNA. If message is able to bind ribosomes to form polysomes, translation could be inhibited by interferon-induced initiation factor deficiencies or alterations, or polypeptide chain elongation could be arrested by deficiencies of elongation factors or of tRNAs. Also polypeptide chains could be prematurely terminated or released. It should also be remembered that many viruses have been shown to perform their translational processes on membrane-associated replication complexes, which themselves might be disrupted by interferon-induced membrane alterations.

Should a virus be able to perform its translation processes and begin to assemble its pieces, other interferon-induced antiviral mechanisms not yet called into play could then begin to act. As a response to signs of a virus' initial success (as evidenced by its forming the replicative-intermediate double-stranded RNA-type structure, the cell would "call in the cavalry" by investing some of its energy-pool of ATP to activation of a kinase and an enzyme to synthesize a low molecular weight inhibitor of translation (LMWIT), which itself activates an endonuclease which would then undertake to inhibit translation by degrading viral messages, inactivating initation factors, and likely other events, including prevention of methylation of the messages that get formed.

Additionally, the formation of double-stranded RNA in the interferon-treated cell could trigger the third line of defense which aborts the infectious cycle by the suicidal tendency of interferon-treated cells when confronted with this type of molecule (described in Section X).

However, should a virus be able to elude these translation-inhibition obstacles and produce at least most of its products, it might be inhibited by a deficiency of a minor product required to cleave a precursor protein to its mature components. Thus arrest of morphogenesis could be affected indirectly by partial restriction of translation.

And even if mature virions can be assembled, they might find their exit blocked by interferon-induced cell-surface alterations. Also, even in absence of prevention of release, it is possible that the interferon-induced cells might release virions which are largely defective. Such defective (interfering?) virions could play a role in the efficiencies of subsequent virus replication cycles, and thereby alter pathogenesis.

Thus, cells have apparently evolved an intricate network of ways to handle a virus invader when warned of its approach by the word "interferon", a signal sent from a less fortunate neighbor cell.

But it now appears that interferons are, in fact, telling cells something more than "the viruses are coming". In the following Section, a number of other alterations induced in cells by interferons are described, some of which appear to function by even more mysterious methods.

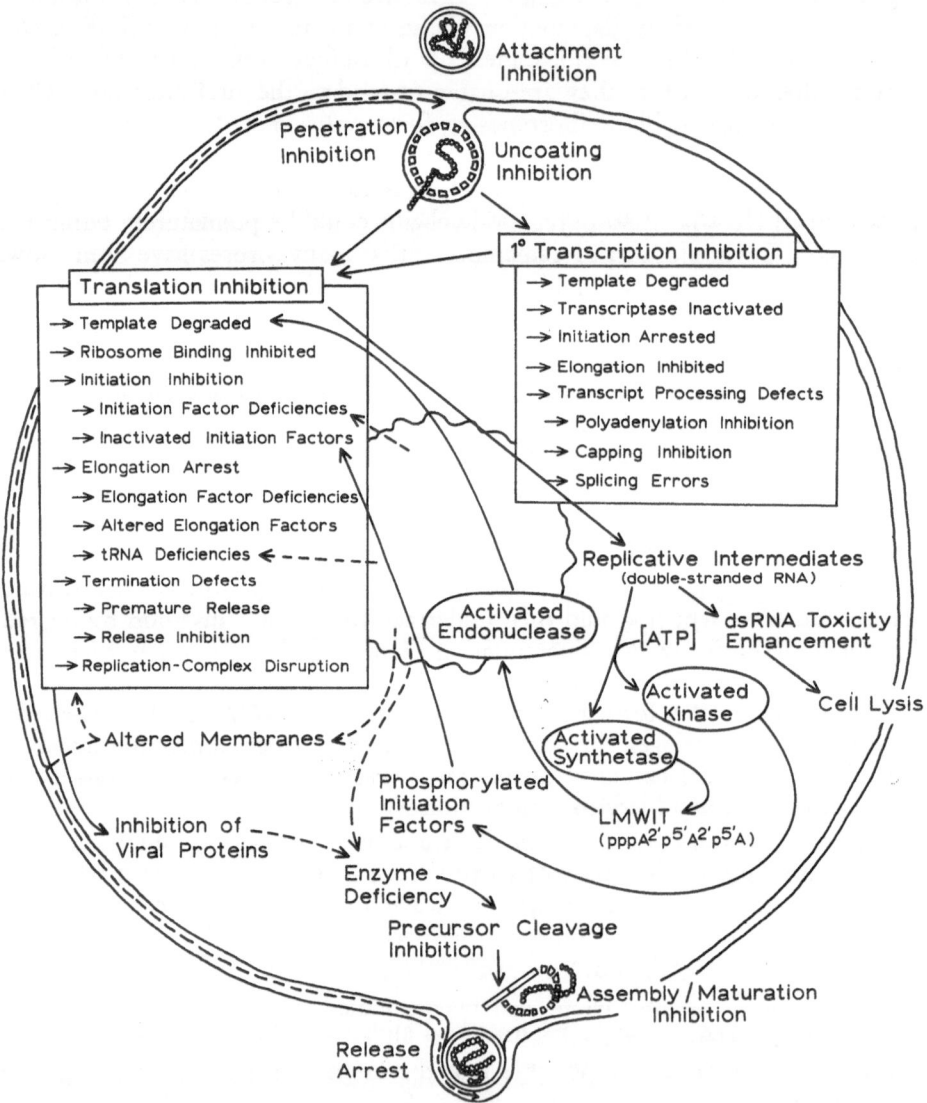

Fig. 17. A simplistic view of the antiviral action of interferon

X. Non-Antiviral Actions of Interferons

Interferons induce cells to inhibit virus replication, by an intricate system that can be described as a primary line of defense activated in cells by interferon which, by itself can likely handle translation processes of some viruses. However, if viruses are able to avoid being completely restricted by this mechanism and can begin to produce double-stranded RNA replicative forms, the cell responds more affirmatively by activating a number of more potent resistance mechanisms, such as kinases to phosphorylate (and thus inactivate) initiation factors, and an enzyme can also be activated that synthesizes a low molecular weight effector which then activates an endoribonuclease which degrades messenger RNAs. And if all else fails, the cell can abort the whole system by an interferon-induced self-destruct mechanism. It is possible that the severity of the cell's initial response may be determined by the concentration of interferon it is exposed to, and dimensions of its secondary or subsequent responses may be determined by interferon concentrations and ability of the viruses to form triggers for these reactions.

After a thorough consideration of the complex of altered reaction-sets manifested in cells by interferon treatment, it would be tempting to speculate that interferon-treated cells might be altered in their responses to substances other than viruses. For example, would the replication of other agents trying to replicate in interferon-treated cells be inhibited? Also, if one exposed interferon-treated cells to double-stranded RNA would there by cytotoxic effects not seen in cells not treated with interferon? Also, wouldn't such a series of translation obstacles and potential membrane modification be likely to alter the cells' ability to produce other products? And, would interferon-treated cells be able to carry on their own synthetic processes as well as normal cells? And if so, why wouldn't cells constitutively produce interferon so that they would be in a virus-resistant state at all times?

Interestingly, the answers to all the above questions, except the last two, are yes. The answer to the penultimate question is no, thus giving an answer to the last question. In fact these answers were revealed long before these questions were posed. It was demonstrated twenty years ago that interferons were able to alter cells in ways other than making them resistant to viruses, but, owing to the passion of the virologists who long "owned" interferon as a purely antiviral substance, it has only very recently become fashionable to recognize this reality. In this section, I shall describe several of the activities of interferons not associated with antivirus activities. The antitumor activities of interferon which possibly involve a composite of antiviral mechanisms and non-antiviral activities will be dealt with separately in Section XIII.

A. The Breadth of Interferon Action: The Expanding Realm of Interferonology

The coinage of the term "non-antiviral function of interferon" (Stewart II, Gosser, and Lockart, 1971a) had been preceded by repeated reports showing that interferons were not exclusively antiviral, but these were generally dismissed as artifacts, being due to impurities in the preparations, or at best, being somehow mediated by "the antiviral action". However, as it is now certain that interferons can induce a number of alterations in cells, the list of such non-antiviral activities grows at an accelerating pace. Many of the effects listed in Table 15 as interferon-induced cellular alterations are obviously related

Table 15. *Pleiotypic activities of interferons*

Activity	References
I. Antiviral	
Adenoviruses	Gallagher and Khoobyarian (1969, 1971, 1972); Barahona and Melendez (1971); Oxman, Rowe, and Black (1967)
Bovine Enterovirus	Finter (1968)
Bunyamwera	Ruiz-Gomez and Isaacs (1963 a); Isaacs, Porterfield, and Baron (1961); Baron *et al.* (1966 a); Hitchcock and Isaacs (1960)
Chikungunya	Ruiz-Gomez and Isaacs (1963 a); Friedman (1964); Gifford, Mussett, and Heller (1964)
Coronavirus	Stewart II and Desmyter (unpublished data)
Coxsackievirus	Marchenko, Povolotsky, and Krivokhatskaya (1976)
Cytomegalovirus	Glasgow *et al.* (1967); Rabson, Tyrrell, and Levy (1969); Postic and Dowling (1977)
Eastern Equine Encephalitis	Glasgow and Habel (1962 a); Vilcek and Rada (1962); Vilcek (1962)
Echo Virus	Ho and Enders (1959 a)
Encephalomyocarditis	Gresser *et al.* (1968 b); Schachter *et al.* (1970); Billiau and Schonne (1970)
Feline Leukemia	Rodgers *et al.* (1972)
Fowl Plague	Ruiz-Gomez and Isaacs (1963 a)
Fowl Pox	Asch and Gifford (1970)
Foamy Virus	Hooks *et al.* (1976)
Foot and Mouth Disease	Ahl and Rump (1976)
Friend Leukemia	Sarma *et al.* (1969); Gresser *et al.* (1967 a, b, c, d); Wheelock and Larke (1968)
GD-7	Oie *et al.* (1972 a)

Table 15 (continued)

Activity	References
Gross Leukemia	Gresser, Coppey, and Bourali (1969)
Herpesviruses	DeMaeyer and Desomer (1962); Ho and Enders (1959 a); Glasgow et al. (1967); Oh and Gill (1966); Vilcek (1962); Schachter et al. (1970); Billiau and Schonne (1970); Isaacs, Burke, and Fadeeva (1958); Fruitstone, Waddell, and Sigel (1964); Barahona and Melendez (1971)
Infectious Bovine Rhinotracheitis	Babiuk and Rouse (1976)
Influenza Viruses	Isaacs and Lindenmann (1957); Oh and Gill (1966); Burke and Isaacs (1960); Isaacs, Lindenmann and Valentine (1957); Riley, Toy and Gifford (1966); Portnoy and Merigan (1971)
Japanese Encephalitis	Stewart II, Scott and Sulkin (1969); Yamazaki (1968)
Mengo	Schachter et al. (1970); Billiau and Schonne (1970)
Middleburg	Bodo, Palese, and Lindner (1971)
Moloney Sarcoma/Leukemia	Sarma et al. (1969); Peries et al. (1968); Fitzgerald (1969); Berman (1970); Rhim and Huebner (1971); Declercq and Desomer (1971 a)
Newcastle Disease	Friedman (1964); Lampson et al. (1963); Grossberg and Scherer (1964); Isaacs, Klemperer, and Hitchcock (1961); Hallum, Thacore, and Youngner (1970)
O'Nyong-Nyong	Ruiz-Gomez and Isaacs (1963 a)
Parainfluenza-1	Balducci, Verani, and Balducci (1963); Burke and Isaacs (1960)
Parainfluenza-3 (Sendai)	Rosenquist and Loan (1967)
Poliovirus	Buckler, Wong, and Baron (1968)
Polyoma	Allison (1961); Oxman and Takemoto (1970); Dulbecco and Johnson (1970); Taylor-Papadimitriou and Stoker (1971); Atanasiu and Chany (1960)
Pseudorabies	Vilcek and Rada (1962); Vilcek (1962); Youngner, Thacore, and Kelly (1972)
Rabiesvirus	Stewart II and Sulkin (1968); Postic and Fenje (1971 a)
Radiation Leukemia	Lieberman, Merigan, and Kaplan (1971)
Rauscher Leukemia	Sarma et al. (1969); Gresser et al. (1968 a)
Reovirus	Vassef et al. (1974); Gauntt (1972)
Rhinoviruses	Fiala (1972)
Rous Sarcoma	Bader (1962); Strandstrom, Sandelin, and Oker-Blom (1962); Traub and Morgan (1967)
Rubella	Desmyter et al. (1967)
Semliki Forest	Stewart II, Scott, and Sulkin (1969); Stewart II and Lockart (1970); Buckler, Wong, and Baron (1968); Finter (1964 a, b, c, 1966 a, 1967 a, b, 1968)
Sindbis	Glasgow and Habel (1962 a); Stewart II, Scott, and Sulkin (1969); Stewart II and Lockart (1970); DeMaeyer and Desomer (1962); Ho and Enders (1959 b); Glasgow et al. (1967); Denys (1963)

Table 15 (continued)

Activity	References
St. Louis Encephalitis	Stewart II, Scott, and Sulkin (1969)
SV 40	Oxman and Takemoto (1970); Todaro and Baron (1965); Oxman and Black (1966); Todaro and Green (1967); Oxman, Rowe, and Black (1967); Oxman and Levin (1971)
Vaccinia	Glasgow and Habel (1962 b); Gallagher and Khoobyarian (1969); McCullough (1972); Armstrong and Merigan (1971)
Varicella-Zoster	Armstrong and Merigan (1971)
Vesicular Stomatitis	Glasgow and Habel (1962 a); Stewart II and Lockart (1970); Rosenquist and Loan (1967); Wagner *et al.* (1963); Rabson, Tyrrell and Levy (1969); Declercq and Desomer (1971 b); Declercq, Nuwer and Merigan (1970 b)
Venezuelan Equine Encephalitis	Jordan (1973); Jahrling, Navarro, and Scherer (1976)
West Nile	Ruiz-Gomez and Isaacs (1963 a)
Western Equine Encephalitis	Vilcek and Rada (1962); Brown (1966); Balducci, Verani, and Balducci (1963)
Yellow Fever	Ruiz-Gomez and Isaacs (1963 a); Finter (1970 a)

II. Antimicrobial

A. Chlamydiae

C. psittacosis	Sueltenfuss and Pollard (1963)
C. trachomatis	Hanna, Merigan, and Jawetz (1966, 1967); Jenkin and Lu (1967); Mordhorst, Reinicke, and Schonne (1968); Reinicke, Mordhorst, and Schonne (1967); Kazar, Krautwurst, and Gordon (1971); Kazar, Gillmore, and Gordon (1971)

B. Protozoa

Eperythrozoon coccoides	Suntharasamai and Rytel (1973)
Plasmodium berghei	Schultz, Huang, and Gordon (1968); Jahliel, Vilcek, and Nussenzweig (1970)
Toxoplasma gondii	Remington and Merigan (1968)

C. Rickettsiae

R. Akari	Kazar, Krautwurst, and Gordon (1971)

D. Bacteria

Shigella flexneri	Gober *et al.* (1972)

III. Interferon Priming

A. *Chicken Cells*

+ Influenza	Isaacs and Burke (1958)
+ Chikungunya	Friedman (1966 a); Levy, Buckler, and Baron (1966)
+ Venezuelan Encephalitis	Jordan (1973)
+ Polyoma	Ustacelebi and Williams (1973)
+ Adenovirus	Rosztoczy (1976 a)

Table 15 (continued)

The Breadth of Interferon Action

227

Activity	References

B. *Mouse L Cells*

+ Western Equine Encephalitis — Lockart (1963)

+ Newcastle Disease — Paucker and Boxaca (1967); Levy-Koenig, Golgher, and Paucker (1970 a); Stewart II, Gosser, and Lockart (1971 b, 1972); Stewart II *et al.* (1973 a); Rousset (1974); Margolis, Oie, and Levy (1972); Lobodzinska, Biernacka, and Skurska (1975)

+ MM — Giron (1969); Giron *et al.* (1971); Stewart II, Gosser, and Lockart (1971 a, 1972); Gauntt (1973); Knight (1974 b)

+ Mengo or Rhinoviruses — Stewart II, Gosser, and Lockart (1971 a)

+ poly rI·poly rC — Rosztoczy and Mecs (1970); Rosztoczy (1971, 1974, 1976 a, b, 1977); Stewart II, Gosser, and Lockart (1971 b, 1972); Stewart II *et al.* (1972, 1973 a); Stewart and Declercq (1974); Margolis, Oie, and Levy (1972); Rousset (1974); Ito and Kobayashi (1974); Ito, Suzuki, and Kobayashi (1975)

C. *Rabbit Kidney Cells*

+ Newcastle Disease — Margolis, Oie, and Levy (1972)

+ poly rI·poly rC — Barmak and Vilcek (1973); Stewart II and Declercq (1974)

D. *Monkey Cells*

+ MM, Mengo or Polio — Stewart II, Gosser, and Lockart (1971 a)

+ Newcastle Disease — Rousset (1974)

E. *Human Cells*

1. Human Leukocytes + ˆSendai — Tovell and Cantell (1971); Goore *et al.* (1973)

2. Human Fibroblasts — Babayants, Dyuisalieva, and Marchenko (1970)

+ MM, Mengo or Polio — Stewart II, Gosser, and Lockart (1971 a)

+ Influenza — Hahon (1974)

+ poly rI·poly rC — Stewart II *et al.* (1972); Mozes *et al.* (1974); Billiau *et al.* (1977 a); Billiau, Joniau, and Desomer (1972)

IV. Cell-Multiplication-Inhibition

A. *Mouse Cells*

L Cells — Paucker, Cantell, and Henle (1962); Paucker and Golgher (1970); Ohwaki and Kawade (1972); Knight (1973); Borecky *et al.* (1973); Broecky, Fuchsberger, and Hajnicka (1974); Matsuzawa and Kawade (1974); O'Shaughnessy *et al.* (1974); Billiau (1975); Fuchsberger, Hajnicka, and Borecky (1975); Stewart II *et al.* (1976)

L$_{1210}$ Leukemia Cell — Gresser *et al.* (1970 a, b, 1973); Maciera-Coelho *et al.* 1971); Gresser, Thomas, and Brouty-Boye (1971); Gresser, Thomas, Brouty-Boye, and Maciera-Coelho (1971); Gresser, Maury, and Brouty-Boye (1972); Fontaine-Brouty-Boye *et al.* (1969); Brouty-Boye *et al.* (1973 a, b); Gresser, Bandu, and Brouty-Boye (1974); Tovey, Brouty-Boye, and Gresser (1975); Stewart II *et al.* (1976)

Table 15 (continued)

Activity	References
Primary Mouse Embryo and Kidney	Lindahl-Magnusson, Leary, and Gresser (1971, 1972); Ohwaki and Kawade (1972)
Friend Cells	Rossi et al. (1975); Matarese and Rossi (1977)
3T3 Cells	Knight (1973); Sokowa et al. (1977); Ohwaki and Kawade (1972)
EMT6 Tumor Cells	Collyn d'Hooghe et al. (1977)
Granulocytic Precursor Cells	McNeill and Gresser (1973)
Regenerating Liver (in vivo)	Frayssinet et al (1973)
B. *Human Cells*	
Lymphoblastoid Cells	Hilfenhaus and Karges (1974); Adams, Strander, and Cantell (1975); Stewart II et al. (1976); Hilfenhaus et al. (1976); Block et al. (1977); Einhorn and Strander (1977); Hilfenhaus, Damm, and Johannsen (1977); Finter et al. (1976)
Human Transformed Cell Lines	Gaffney, Picciano, and Grant (1973)
HeLa Cells	Dahl and Degre (1975, 1976 b)
U-Amnion Cells	Dahl and Degre (1975, 1976 b)
RSa, RSb Transformed Fibroblasts	Fuse and Kuwata (1976); Finter et al. (1976); Kuwata, Fuse, and Morinaga (1976, 1977); Kuwata et al. (1976)
Osteosarcoma Cells	Strander and Einhorn (1977)
Human Diploid Fibroblasts	Lee et al. (1972); Dahl and Degre (1975, 1976 a); Knight (1976 b); Einhorn and Strander (1977)
Trisomic-21 Fibroblasts	Tan (1976)

V. Interferon-Blocking

A. *Chick Cells*

+ Tick-borne Encephalitis	Vilcek and Rada (1962)
+ Chikungunya	Friedman (1966 a)

B. *Mouse L Cells*

+ Western Equine Encephalitis	Lockart (1963)
+ Tick-borne Encephalitis	Stancek and Vilcek (1965)
+ Newcastle Disease	Cantell and Paucker (1963 a); Paucker (1965); Paucker and Boxaca (1967); Paucker and Golgher (1969); Golgher and Paucker (1973); Stewart II, Gosser and Lockart (1971 a, b); Margolis, Oie, and Levy (1972); Borden and Murphy (1971); Borden, Prochownik, and Carter (1975); Byrd et al. (1973); Chadha et al. (1974); Youngner and Hallum (1969); Rousset (1974); Lobodzinksa, Bienacka, and Skurska (1975)
+ poly rI·poly rC	Youngner and Hallum (1969); Stewart II, Gosser and Lockart (1971 b); Rousset (1974)
(1° Mouse Kidney Cells) + Newcastle Disease	Stewart II, Gosser, and Lockart (1971 b)

C. *Rabbit Kidney Cells*

+ poly rI·poly rC	Billiau (1970); Barmak and Vilcek (1973)

Table 15 (continued)

Activity	References
D. Monkey Cells	
+ Newcastle Disease	Rousset (1974)
E. Human Fibroblasts	
+ Newcastle Disease	Bausek and Merigan (1970 b); Mozes and Vilcek (1975)
VI. Toxicity Enhancement	
A. Vaccinia Virus	
Mouse L Cells	Joklik and Merigan (1966); Horak, Jungwirth, and Bodo (1971); Bodo et al. (1972); Jungwirth et al. (1972 a); Stewart II, Declercq, and Desomer (1973); Suh et al. (1974)
B. Double-Stranded RNA	
Mouse L Cells	Stewart II et al. (1972, 1973, 1975); Stewart II, Declercq and Desomer (1973); Stewart II and Declercq (1974); Declercq and Desomer (1975); Lackovic and Borecky (1976); Heremans et al. (1976)
Mouse Embryo Cells	Stewart II et al. (1972)
Human Fibroblasts	Stewart II et al. (1972); Declercq, Edy and Cassimans (1975)
C. Influenza Virus	
Human Conjunctival Cells	Green and Mowshowitz (1977)
D. Vesicular Stomatitis Virus	
Mouse L Cells	Katz, Lee, and Rozee (1974)
E. Others	
DEAE-Dextran, Protamine Sulfate; Methylated Albumin	Katz, Lee, and Rozee (1974)
Concanavalin A	Stewart II et al. (1975 b)
Arginine Starvation	Lee and Rozee (1975)
VII. Depression of Syntheses	
A. Uninduced Syntheses	
Protein Synthesis	Johnson, Lerner, and Lancz (1968); Falcoff et al. (1975)
DNA Synthesis or Thymidine Uptake	O'Shaughnessy, Lee, and Rozee (1972); Tovey, Brouty-Boye and Gresser (1975); Brouty-Boye and Tovey (1977); Fuse and Kuwata (1977); Balkwill and Oliver (1977)
B. Induced Syntheses	
Tyrosine Amino-Transferase (Induced in Rat HTC by Steroid)	Beck et al. (1974); Vassef et al. (1974)
Glycerol-3-Phosphate Dehydrogenase (Induced in Rat Glial Cells by Steroid)	Illinger et al. (1976)
Glutamine Synthetase (Induced in Chick Neural-Retina by Steroid)	Matsuno, Shirasawa, and Kohno (1976)

Table 15 (continued)

Activity	References
DNA Synthesis Induced by:	
a. Lectins	Lindahl-Magnusson *et al.* (1972); Rozee, Lee, and Ngan (1973); Blomgren, Strander, and Cantell (1974); Pacheco *et al.* (1976); Heine and Adler (1977)
b. Antigens	Thorbecke, Friedman-Kien, and Vilcek (1974); Cupples and Tan (1977)
c. Erythropoietin	Smith *et al.* (1976)
VIII. Enhanced Syntheses	
A. *Uninduced Products*	
Hyaluronic Acid	Yaron *et al.* (1976)
Prostaglandin E	Yaron *et al.* (1977); Karmazin *et al.* (1977)
B. *Induced Products*	
tRNA methylase	Rozee, Katz and McFarlane (1969)
Aryl Hydrocarbon Hydroxylase Induced by Benzanthracene	Nebert and Friedman (1973)
Histamine Induced by Ragweed Antigen E	Ida *et al.* (1977)
IX. Surface Alterations	
A. *Toxicity Depression*	Yabrov (1966, 1967); Moehring, Moehring, and Stinebring 1971); Boquet (1975)
B. *Surface Charge*	Knight and Korant (1977)
C. *Increased Concanavalin A Binding*	Huet *et al.* (1974)
D. *Increased Surface Antigen Expression*	Lindahl, Leary, and Gresser (1973, 1974); Lindahl *et al.* 1976 a, b); Killander *et al.* (1976); Skurkovich *et al.* (1976 a, b); Vignaux and Gresser (1977); Lonai and Steinman (1977)
E. *Enhanced Cytotoxicity of Lymphocytes for Target Cells*	
1. Specific	Lindahl, Leary, and Gresser (1972); Lindahl (1974)
2. Non-specific	Svet-Moldavsky and Chernyakovskaya (1967); Chernyakovskaya, Slavina, and Svet-Moldavsky (1974); Slavina and Svet-Moldavsky (1973); Borecky, Lackovic, and Waschake (1970)
F. *Enhanced Sensitivity of Target Cells to Cytotoxic Antibody*	Skurkovich, Klinova, and Eremkina (1976); Skurkovich *et al.* (1976 a)
G. *Enhanced Phagocytosis*	
Mouse Macrophages + Carbon	Huang *et al.* (1971); Donahoe and Huang (1973, 1976)
Human Monocytes + Latex	Imanishi *et al.* (1975)

Table 15 (continued)

Activity	References
H. *Macrophage „Activation"*	Khesin *et al.* (1973); Schultz, Papamatheakis, and Chirigos (1977)
I. *Reversible Metamorphosis of Human Amnion Cells*	Gresser (1961 c)
X. Toxicity of Interferons	
A. *In Vitro*	
Human Bone Marrow	Nissen *et al.* (1977)
Human Granylocytic Progenitor Cells	Greenberg and Mosny (1977)
B. *In Vivo*	
Lethality (Liver Degeneration in Newborn Mice)	Gresser *et al.* (1975)
Glomerulonephritis (in Mice)	Gresser *et al.* (1976 a)
Febrile Skin Toxicity (in Human)	Desomer, Edy, and Billiau (1977)
XI. Immunodepression	
A. *Antibody Production*	
1. In Vivo	Braun and Levy (1972); Brodeur and Merigan (1974); Chester, Paucker, and Merigan (1974); Merigan, Chester, and Paucker (1975)
2. In Vitro	Gisler, Lindahl, and Gresser (1974); Johnson, Smith, and Baron (1974, 1975); Johnson, Bukovic, and Baron (1975); Johnson and Baron (1976 a, b); Booth, Booth, and Marbrook (1976); Sonnenfeld, Mandel, and Merigan (1977)
B. *Delayed-Type Hypersensitivity*	DeMaeyer, DeMaeyer-Guignard, and Vandeputte (1975); DeMaeyer-Guignard, Cachard, and DeMaeyer (1975); DeMaeyer (1976)
C. *Heterologous Adaptive Cutaneous Anaphylaxis*	Ngna, Lee, and Kind (1976)
D. *Graft-vs-Host Reaction*	Hirsch *et al.* (1973, 1974); Hirsch, Black, and Proffitt (1977); Mobraaten, DeMaeyer, and DeMaeyer-Guignard (1973); DeMaeyer, Mobraaten, and DeMaeyer-Guignard (1973); Imanishi *et al.* (1977)
(Enhanced Graft-vs-Host Reaction)	Skurkovich *et al.* (1973 a, b); Chernyakhovskaya and Slavina (1972)
E. *Complement Fixation*	Strander *et al.* (1973, 1977); Aho *et al.* (1976)
XII. Antitumor Activity	(Section XIII and XIV)

phenomena, and some may prove to not be induced by interferons, as only a few have been ascertained with the most highly purified interferons. In this section, emphasis will be placed on proving whether these effects are due to interferons rather than to non-interferon materials in the preparations. It should soon be possible to determine how many types of alterations are induced by interferon preparations and how many of these are induced by pure interferons. Then we shall begin to decipher which effects mesh into the schemes of regulatory mechanisms involved in interferon-induced antiviral activity and which alterations are mechanistically unique. Then perhaps the "true" function(s) of interferons will begin to be more apparent.

B. Inhibition of Non-Viral Agents

Interferon preparations have been shown to inhibit the growth of several non-viral agents (Table 15) both in animals and in cell cultures. All are obligate intracellular parasites. Little information has accumulated on this aspect of interferon action since it was reviewed by Vilček and Jahiel (1970). However, with the availability of highly potent and purified interferon preparations, these activities should be further explored, and evaluation of the effect of antiserum to interferons on the replication of these agents *in vitro* and *in vivo* should be informative.

Where the sensitivities of these microorganisms have been compared to those of viruses, they have generally been found to be less sensitive (Kazar, Gillmore, and Gordon, 1971; Hanna, Merigan, and Jawetz, 1966; Kazar, Krautwurst, and Gordon, 1971; Remington and Merigan (1968), at least in relation to vesicular stomatitis virus. This has been interpreted to imply that these agents are less dependent on the host cell metabolism (Kazar, Gillmore, and Gordon, 1971; Kazar, Krautwurst, and Gordon, 1971). However, as illustrated in Table 14, many viruses can also be much less sensitive than vesicular stomatitis virus to interferon action, so such evaluations are mechanistically meaningless.

Interferon inducers have been reported to inhibit multiplication of *Klebsiella pneumoniae* (Weinstein, Weitz, and Came, 1970), *Pasteurella tularensis* or *Diplococcus pneumoniae* (Giron et al., 1972) and *Mycobacterium leprae* (Levy and Merigan, 1977); however, as interferon had no such effect itself, it is likely these actions are not mediated by interferons. Inducers of interferon have also been shown to enhance infections with fungi (Worthington and Hasenclever, 1972), *Trypanosoma cruzi* (Kumar et al., 1971) and *Listeria monocytogenes* (Gruenewald and Levine, 1976), again without reason to suspect interferon involvement.

Interferon did not seem to inhibit growth of *Coxiella burneti* (Kazar, 1969), and, whereas rabbit interferon was inhibitory for *Toxoplasma gondii* in rabbit cells, mouse interferon did not exert such an effect in mouse cells (Schmunis et al., 1973). Interference with replication of *Plasmodium gallinaceum* malaria in chickens was demonstrated, which presumably involved interferon (Herman, Shiroishu, and Buckler, 1973; Herman, 1972). And one study demonstrated inhibition of extracellular multiplication of *Shigella flexneri* by cell-free lysates prepared from mouse or human cells pretreated with interferons (Green, 1973).

C. Priming

Isaacs and Burke (1958) observed that chick cells treated with interferon were able to produce more interferon than untreated cells when exposed to influenza virus; they referred to this effect of interferon pretreatment as "priming". This phenomenon was subsequently observed in numerous other virus-cell systems (Table 15). Priming can also be demonstrated in a number of systems where cells are repeatedly exposed to interferon inducers (Burke and Isaacs, 1958; Ho and Breinig, 1962; Mahdy and Ho, 1964; Billiau, 1970; Goorha and Gifford, 1970a, b). The apparent explanation of this effect would be that interferon pretreatment inhibited viral functions in cells that prevented the virus from shutting off cellular functions involved in interferon synthesis, and there seemed to be support for this interpretation in the findings that treatment of cells with low concentrations of interferon enhanced their ability to make interferon when subsequently induced, while with pretreatment higher concentrations of interferon inhibited ("blocked") their ability to produce interferon (Lockart, 1963; Friedman, 1966a); the larger amounts of interferon presumably induced enough antiviral activity to not only prevent virus from shutting-off cellular synthesis (of interferon) but also prevented virus from producing the "inducer molecule" (Bausek and Merigan, 1970a, b).

However, on the basis that certain evidence cannot be satisfactorily rationalized into this comforting blanket of interferon acting solely as an antiviral, Stewart II, Gosser, and Lockart (1971a) reported priming to be a "non-antiviral function of interferon". It has been a consistent finding that interferon-treated cells are able to produce interferon more quickly, whether their total production is quantitatively enhanced or depressed ("blocked") by the interferon pretreatment (Fig. 18; Paucker and Boxaca, 1967; Stewart II, Gosser, and Lockart, 1971a, b; Rosztoczy and Mecs, 1970; Rosztoczy, 1971; Stewart II *et al.*, 1972; Ustacelibi and William, 1973; Friedman, 1966a; Levy, Buckler, and Baron, 1966; Stewart II and Declercq, 1973; Levy–Koenig, Golgher, and Paucker, 1970). It is difficult to imagine that the supposed viral replicative event requisite for interferon induction could occur more quickly in interferon-treated cells than in normal cells.

Also, it was found that interferon-treated cells produce more interferon than do normal cells when they are induced with poly rI·poly rC (Rosztoczy and Mecs, 1970; Stewart II, Gosser, and Lockart, 1971b; Table 15).

The requirments for cells to produce interferon after priming are similar to those of normal cells, requiring induction of RNA and protein. However, the interferon response of primed cells becomes resistant to inhibition by actinomycin D much sooner than the response of normal cells (Friedman, 1966a; Levy, Buckler, and Baron, 1966; Stewart II, Gosser, and Lockart, 1971a; Rosztoczy, 1976b), suggesting they produce interferon messenger RNA more quickly than do normal cells, though this has not been directly determined by messenger RNA isolations. Interferon treatment seemingly sensitizes cells to induction processes and shortens the induction process in those cells having a long induction lag-phase (Fig. 7), making these responses occur with kinetics similar to those already seen in cells with short lag-phase. In fact, cells with normally short induction lag-phases do not show quicker responses when primed (Stewart II, Gosser, and Lockart, 1971b; Tovell and Cantell, 1971; Barmak and Vilček, 1973). These data suggest that interferon priming removes some restriction on the induction process that normal cells with long induction-lags must perform before producing interferon messenger RNA (Stewart II, Gosser, and Lockart, 1972). A partial induction of a sequential induction process would also explain the quantitative and temporal aspects of priming. However, a more direct shunt-mechanism of interferon induction in primed cells can be envisioned, as interferon priming also removes the requirement of mouse cells for DEAE-dextran to be induced by poly rI·poly rC (Rosztoczy, 1971; Stewart II et al., 1972), suggesting a direct surface membrane alteration by interferon treatment.

Development of priming differs from development of antiviral activity in a number of respects. Priming can develop rapidly (less than one hour) in cells treated with high concentrations (100 to 1000 units/ml) of interferon, whereas development of antiviral activity is delayed (Giron et al., 1971; Stewart II,

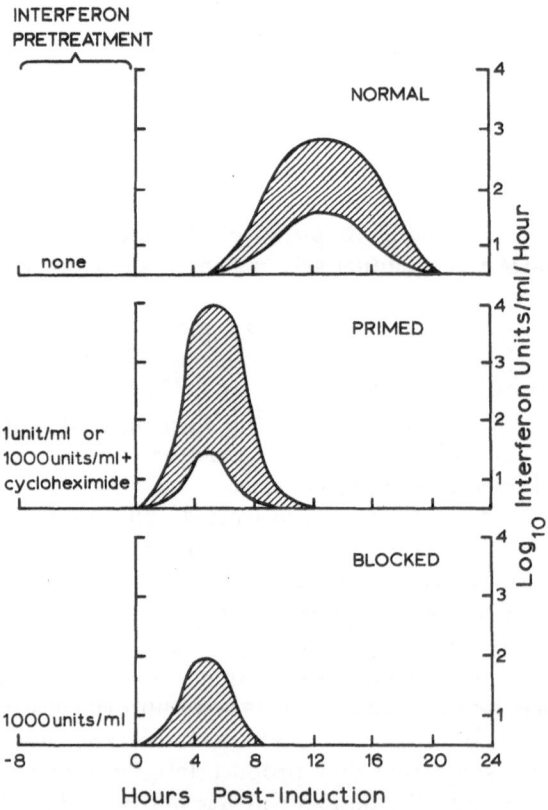

Fig. 18. Requirements for development of blocking and priming

Gosser, and Lockart, 1971a). Pretreatment for longer periods with high concentration of interferon can give both priming and blocking; that is, the total amount of interferon produced can be decreased but it will be made sooner than normal (Stewart II, Gosser, and Lockart, 1971b). The development of priming can also vary in different cell types (Havell and Vilček, 1972).

The major distinction between requirements for development of antiviral activity and priming is protein synthesis. Whereas protein synthesis is always required for cells to become resistant to viruses, it is not required for at least some cells to become primed. Friedman (1966a) reported that chick cells failed to become primed by treatment with interferon in the presence of protein synthesis inhibitors. However, Stewart II, Gosser, and Lockart (1971a) found that L cells treated with interferon in the presence of cycloheximide, puromycin or p-fluorophenylalanine developed no virus resistance yet became fully primed. This observation was confirmed in L cells by Knight (1974b) and Rosztoczy (1974) and in rabbit kidney cells by Barmak and Vilček (1973). Curiously, Ito, Suzuki, and Kobayashi (1975) claimed a requirement for newly synthesized protein for priming activity of interferon; their data do not, however, support this interpretation. In fact, they looked only at amounts of interferon made, not when it is made; even so, the amount of interferon produced by cells treated with interferon in cycloheximide was more than that made by normal cells, though slightly less than that made by cells primed with interferon alone, and no data indicate the efficiency of reversal of protein synthesis inhibition, which could diminish interferon production. Similar problems of interpretation are involved in the data of Saito and Kohno (1977), in which case interferon yields were enhanced in cells exposed to interferon and protein synthesis inhibitors, though less so than in cells exposed to interferon alone; however, complete reversal of the protein inhibition was not achieved, thereby further obscuring the results. Where these complications are considered, it is evident the protein synthesis inhibition during interferon treatment does not prevent priming.

It was reported by Rosztoczy (1974) that whereas antiviral activity induced by interferon decayed slowly over a period of over 72 hours, cells had reverted to the unprimed state within 24 hours after removal of interferon.

Priming is, as pointed out previously (Section VI. B. 3.), of considerable practical importance, as it can increase interferon yields significantly, and often exerts a cooperative enhancement with superproduction.

Studies on the mechanism of priming by determining the fate of polynucleotide inducers have added little to our understanding. Stewart II and DeClercq (1974) found that primed cells had the same molecular size requirements for poly rI·poly rC molecules to trigger interferon production. DeClercq, Stewart II and Desomer (1973c) and DeClercq and Stewart II (1974a) reported that priming did not alter the degradation of poly rI·poly rC by cells.

It is also important to note that while there are a number of substances that can enhance the ability of cells to produce interferons, none of these can be classified as able to prime cells, in terms of the cells' ability to make more interferon than normal and to make it sooner than normal. Rosztoczy (1977) was unable to prime cells by pretreatment with cyclic AMP, norepinephrine or

DEAE-dextran (though the latter can enhance the ability of cells to respond to induction with poly rI·poly rC) or ethanol. Similarly, the enhancement of interferon production in L cells induced with poly rI·poly rC after amphotericin B also did not alter the production kinetics (Borden, Booth, and Leonhardt, 1978).

In contrast to all the other non-antiviral actions of interferons, the interpretation that priming activity resides in interferon itself rather than in impurities in the interferon preparations has never been much doubted, perhaps because priming was initially interpreted as resulting from antiviral activity. Priming activity has been found in every species that has been tested, with each interferon preparation assayed. Priming activity exhibits the same defined host-range of activity as the antiviral activity, though often being a more sensitive assay system than induction of antiviral action (Levy–Koenig et al., 1970; Stewart II, Gosser, and Lockart, 1971a; Ito and Kobayashi, 1974; Rousset, 1974). Interferon was found to maintain constant ratios of antiviral unit/priming unit through more than a 1000-fold purification (Stewart II, Gosser, and Lockart, 1971a), and a 1,000,000-fold purification (Stewart II et al., 1973); it was also demonstrated that each of the distinct molecular species of mouse interferons were identical in this respect (Stewart II, 1975b; Fig. 13); and we have recently found that mouse interferon purified to 10^9 units/mg of protein is able to prime cells in the same ratio/antiviral unit as "crude" (10^4 units/mg protein), "semi-crude" (10^5 units/mg), "partially–purified" (10^6 units/mg), "purified" (10^7 units/mg) and "highly purified" (10^8 units/mg) preparations. Further, the low molecular weight mouse interferoid (Fig. 15) is identical in this respect to native mouse interferon (Stewart II, Lin, and Wiranowska–Stewart, 1978). The priming factor fulfills all the criteria for acceptance as an interferon.

Additionally, priming activity in human cells is, in spite of the claim to the contrary (DeClercq et al., 1975), apparently determined by chromosome 21 (Frankfort et al., 1978).

D. Blocking

As demonstrated in Fig. 18, pretreatment of cells with interferon can either increase interferon yields (priming), or it can diminish interferon responsiveness of cells (blocking). This blocking effect of interferon on interferon production was first reported by Vilček and Rada (1962), and has since been observed in many cell-interferon systems (Table 15). However, the early exclusively antiviral attitude of interferonologists dictated only two possible interpretations of this phenomenon:

1. The antiviral action induced by interferon prevented the virus from performing "the viral function responsible for initiation of interferon production" (Bausek and Merigan, 1970b); or,

2. Blocking was due to an impurity in interferon preparations (Baron and Levy, 1966).

The former interpretation was comfortable until it was reported that interferon responses induced by poly rI·poly rC were also blocked in interferon-treated cells (Youngner and Hallum, 1969; Stewart II, Gosser, and Lockart, 1971b; Golgher and Paucker, 1973; Rousset, 1974; Barmak and Vilček, 1973). These data make it difficult to rationalize blocking in terms of antiviral action. In fact, as illustrated in Fig. 18, when cells are blocked and not able to produce normal levels of interferon in response to inducers, the residual interferon they make is made earlier. For this to be interpretable as an antiviral manifestation it would be necessary to imagine that the production of the viral event necessary for interferon induction was performed sooner in interferon-treated cells. More likely the interferon-treated cells are primed by interferon (to produce interferon earlier) and blocked at a post-transcriptional step (to translate less of the induced interferon message). It could be imagined that the message translation obstacles imposed in interferon-treated cells as part of "the antiviral mechanism" could as well turn to the attack of newly induced interferon messenger RNA, thus restricting the production of new interferon in cells previously exposed to "enough" of it.

Whereas development of priming requires only brief exposure to low concentrations of interferon, during which time no protein synthesis is required (see above), development of blocking is in each case different: blocking requires several hours of exposure to relatively high concentrations of interferon (Paucker and Boxaca, 1967; Stewart II, Gosser, and Lockart, 1971b; Barmak and Vilček, 1973; Rousset, 1974; Lobodzinska, Biernacka, and Skurska, 1975), and during this exposure protein synthesis is required (Stewart II, Gosser, and Lockart, 1971b; Barmak and Vilček, 1973). In fact, if protein synthesis is arrested during prolonged exposure of cells to high concentrations of interferons, the cells not only do *not* become blocked, they become primed (Stewart II, Gosser, and Lockart, 1971b; Barmak and Vilcek, 1973). Thus blocking must develop under conditions allowing development of a pronounced antiviral state, perhaps even sufficient to activate the restrictions imposed on transcripts that avoid the first line of interferon-induced defenses. In this regard it should be recalled that Chany and Vignal (1968, 1970) reported an interferon-resistant cell line that did not develop hypo-responsiveness (blocking?) to repeated induction (Section VI. 3.).

Kleinschmidt (1972) offered an intriguingly elaborate explanation of blocking based on the formation of complexes of the monomeric interferon "subunits"; however, as the "subunit hypothesis" (Carter, 1970, 1971) has been debunked, so has this model (Section VII. A.).

There have been three papers on induction of cultures with virus and poly rI·poly rC in which the virus induced "late" interferon while the poly rI·poly rC induced "early" interferon (Bausek and Merigan, 1970a; Stewart II, Gosser, and Lockart, 1971b; Mozes and Vilček, 1975). In these systems the early interferon responses were not markedly inhibited by interferon pretreatment and could be repeatedly stimulated, whereas the late responses were quite sensitive to blocking and could not be restimulated. However, when these cultures were simultaneously induced with virus and double-stranded RNA, the "early" response did not restrict the "late" response.

So, again we have an effect that does not allow us to attribute it to restriction of virus replication (though it may reflect a similar altered cellular state).

Can it then be attributed to impurities in the interferon preparations? This interpretation was favored previously, as it was claimed that the antiviral component could be separated from the blocking component by chromatography (Paucker and Boxaca, 1967; Borden, Prochownik, and Carter, 1975), or that interferons collected at different intervals after inductions exhibited different degrees of blocking activity per antiviral unit (Borden and Murphy, 1971; Chadha et al., 1974). However, as described earlier (Section VI. A. 3.), all these claims seem to err in interpretation, the former claim of chromatographic separation having been withdrawn (Golgher and Paucker, 1973), and the claimed enrichments being insignificant. It is not possible to reliably distinguish between interferon responses that are blocked by about 95% and those blocked about 90% (Borden and Murphy, 1971), nor is it reasonable to rely on reports claiming assay differences of 5% (Chadha et al., 1974). Also, where more highly purified interferon preparations have been evaluated for ability to block, they have been found to do so (Stewart II, Gosser, and Lockart, 1971b; Golgher and Paucker, 1973), and recently we have found blocking activity in mouse interferon preparations purified to about 10^9 units/mg of protein and have found mouse interferoid (Fig. 15) to possess this property (Stewart II et al., 1978).

E. Cell-Multiplication-Inhibition

In this Section I shall discuss those phenomena which seem to relate to the ability of interferons to inhibit cell multiplication, those measured directly by cell counts, those inferred from reduced incorporation of precursors, and those repressing cell-stimulating effects or depression of syntheses of uninduced and induced cell products. The antitumor action of interferon which is likely, at least in part, to be attributable to this anti-proliferative effect will be discussed in Section XIII.

1. Evidence That Interferon Is the Active Component Inhibiting Cell-Multiplication

The controversy concerning the ability of interferons to inhibit or not to inhibit normal cell replicative events and cell-multiplication has been by far the most long-standing argument over the interferon system. Paucker, Cantell, and Henle (1962) first reported that interferon preparations restricted the growth of cells in culture, but Cocito, Schonne, and Desomer (1965), Baron, Merigan, and McKerlie (1966), and Levy and Merigan (1966) attributed this effect to "non-interferon" impurities in interferon preparations since they were unable to measure inhibitory activity on cell synthesis with partially-purified (i. e., somewhat less crude) interferon preparations. The intervening decade has seen constant confusion on the issue, with some investigators presenting evidence that interferon is itself the factor restricting replication (Fontaine–Brouty–Boye et al., 1969; Gresser et al., 1970b, c, 1973; Gresser, Bandu, and Brouty–Boye, 1974; Lindahl–Magnusson, Leary, and Gresser, 1971; Tovey, Brouty–Boye, and Gresser, 1975; Knight, 1973; Hilfenhaus and Karges, 1974; Adams, Strander, and Cantell, 1975; Tan, 1975; Gaffney, Picciano, and Grant, 1973; Hilfenhaus *et al.*, 1976; Lee *et al.*, 1972; O'Saughnessy, Lee, and Rozee, 1972; McNeill and Gresser, 1973; Kishida *et al.*, 1971, 1973; Ohwaki and Kawade, 1972), while others either failed to observe any inhibition or observed inconsistencies in the ratios of antiviral and cell-multiplication-inhibitory activity in given preparations (Baron and Isaacs, 1962; Marcus and Salb, 1966; Moehring and Stinebring, 1971; Kishida *et al.*, 1971; Borecky *et al.*, 1972; Fuchsberger, Hajnicka, and Borecky, 1975; Matsuzawa and Kawade, 1974).

The evidence for or against interferon exerting cell-multiplication-inhibitory activity has hinged on ability to accurately demonstrate cell-multiplication-inhibition and on the question of purity of interferon preparations.

The conditions for demonstration of interferon cell-restriction delineated by Lindahl–Magnusson, Leary, and Gresser (1971) have been helpful in reproducing this effect. Cultures must be initiated at sufficiently low density to allow several days of observations before control cell cultures have reached saturation (Fig. 19).

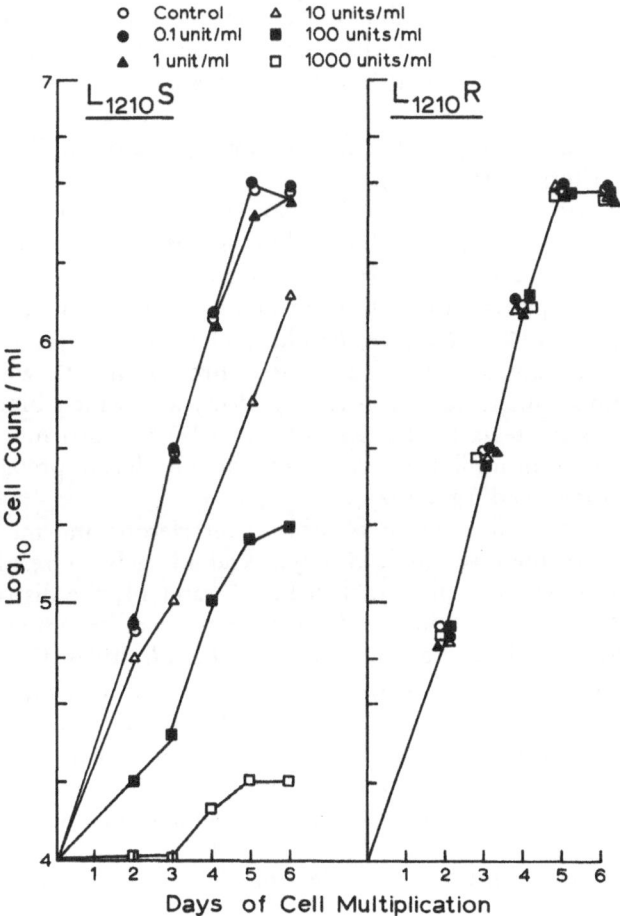

Fig. 19. Cell-multiplication-inhibitory activity of interferon. An assay of mouse interferon in mouse leukemia L1210S and L1210R cells. (Data courtesy of T. Chudzio and E. Chou)

The evidence for interferon involvement in this effect has evolved with each increase in interferon purification. Clearly this issue was decided mostly on emotional basis during the years of stagnation of interferon purification studies. For each claim there were counter-claims. The first demonstration of inhibition of cell growth (Paucker, Cantell, and Henle, 1962) being countered by claims that less crude preparation did not do so (Baron, Merigan, and McKerlie, 1966); some workers demonstrated inhibition with yet higher purity preparations (Paucker and Golgher, 1970; Gresser et al., 1970b, c) and others claimed separation of the activity from the antivirally active component (Borecky et al., 1972). More highly purified interferon seemed to have the activities at constant ratios (Gresser et al., 1973; Knight, 1973), but some interferon preparations were reported to be devoid of cell-multiplication-inhibitory action (Dahl and Degre, 1975; Dahl, 1977a, b; Dahl and Degre, 1976a, b).

The evidence now available is clearly overwhelmingly in favor of the interpretation that interferon inhibits cell multiplication:

a) Crude and purified interferon preparations, regardless of their cell sources or inducing agents, exhibit constant ratios of antiviral and cell-multiplication-inhibitory activity, and the defined host-range of the activities are identical (Gresser et al., 1970, 1971, 1973; Stewart II et al., 1976; Babiuk and Rouse, 1977).

b) The component responsible for cell-multiplication-inhibition fulfills all the interferon criteria (VII. A. 7.).

c) Mouse L1210 cells resistant to the antiviral action of interferon (Gresser et al., 1970a) and which are unable to bind interferon (Gresser, Bandu, and Brouty–Boye, 1974), are also resistant to the cell-multiplication-inhibitory action of interferon preparations (Gresser et al., 1970b; Lindahl–Magnusson, Leary, and Gresser, 1971; Gresser, Bandu, and Brouty–Boye, 1974). And the reverse situation, human cells trisomic for chromosome-21 which are more sensitive to human interferon (Tan et al., 1973) and which bind more interferon (Wiranowska–Stewart and Stewart II, 1977) are also more sensitive to the cell-multiplication-inhibitory effect of the interferon preparations (Tan, 1976, 1977; Cupples and Tan, 1977).

d) Both human (leukocyte or fibroblast) interferons and mouse interferon preparations electrophoresed in SDS-polyacrylamide gels are resolved into each of the profiles of activities presented in Fig. 13 and 14; the distribution of activities in these profiles are identical whether assayed for antiviral activity or cell-multiplication-inhibitory activity (Stewart II et al., 1976; Knight, 1976b).

e) Mouse interferon purified to about 10^9 units of antiviral activity/mg of protein (Gresser, 1977a; Stewart II, Lin, and Wiranowska-Stewart, 1978), human fibroblast interferon purified to apparent homogeneity (at least 2×10^8 units/mg of protein) (Knight, 1976b), and apparently pure human leukocyte interferon purified to a single spot in two-dimensional gel electrophoresis (Stewart II, Lin, and Wiranowska-Stewart, 1978) are equally as able to induce cell-multiplication-inhibition as crude interferon preparations of various specific activities.

f) Mouse interferoid (Fig. 15) purified to about 10^9 units/mg of protein is equally able to perform this function.

2. Cellular Systems Inhibited by Interferon

The interferon-induced cell-restriction is a reversible event (Gresser *et al.*, 1970b, c; Paucker, Cantell, and Henle, 1962; Gaffney, Picciano, and Grant, 1973; O'Shaughnessy *et al.*, 1974). When cells are washed free of interferon they return to their normal growth rate. As viruses can vary several hundred-fold in sensitivities to interferon restriction, cells also can so vary. The multiplication of mouse L1210 cells can be inhibited almost completely by 100 units/ml, and can be inhibited by about 90% by 10 antiviral unit/ml (Stewart II *et al.*, 1976; Gresser *et al.*, 1970b).

Certain human lymphoblastoid cell lines are very sensitive [Daudi cells being markedly inhibited by about one unit or less (Stewart *et al.*, 1976)], whereas others are resistant to several thousand units (Adam, Strander, and Cantell, 1975; Hilfenhaus, Damm, and Johannsen, 1977; Hilfenhaus and Karges, 1974). Primary cell cultures have usually been reported to be markedly less sensitive than established cultures (Lindahl–Magnusson, Leary, and Gresser, 1971, 1972; Knight, 1973; Lee, O'Shaughnessy, and Rozee, 1972). However, Ohwaki and Kawade (1972) found no difference in susceptibility of transformed or untransformed 3T3 cells and mouse embryo fibroblasts to cell-multiplication-inhibition. Strander and Einhorn (1977) found that several lines of osteosarcoma cells were all inhibited by human leukocyte interferon, and were more sensitive than non-tumor-derived lines. These authors (Einhorn and Strander, 1977) have also interpreted that osteosarcoma cells are more sensitive to human fibroblast interferons than to human leukocyte interferons, suggesting tissue specificities of interferons. However, the unusual method employed to gauge cell-multiplication-inhibition (cells grown in interferons and cultures split once/week × 2 to 4 weeks), the differences in specific activities of the interferon preparations, and the narrow margins of the differences reported, make the validity of this interpretation suspect.

These effects are not mediated by an overt cytotoxicity, as ratios of viable cell counts/total cell counts remain similar during inhibition, but interferon-treated cells often plateau at a lower saturation density than do normal cells (Gresser *et al.*, 1970b, c; Knight, 1973). Collyn d'Hooghe *et al.* (1977) have reported that the intermitotic time, as followed by time-lapse photomicrography, was markedly and progressively increased, rather than arrested. Sokawa *et al.* (1977) recently reported that interferon suppressed the transition of 3T3 cells from a quiescent to a growing state.

Interferons also inhibit the growth of normal and tumor cells *in vivo*. The latter of these effects will be discussed later (Section XIII). Interferon or its inducers can inhibit the multiplication of allogeneic and syngeneic bone marrow cells in irradiated mice (Cerottini *et al.*, 1973), and an inhibitor of hemopoietic colony-forming cells was reported in serum of mice, rabbits and hamsters inoculated with poly rI·poly rC (McNeill and Fleming, 1971; Fleming, McNeill, and Killen, 1972; McNeill, Fleming, and McCance, 1972). Interferon inducers (poly rI·poly rC, Newcastle disease virus and statolon) were reported to inhibit the mitotic response of liver cells to partial hepatectomy (Jahiel *et al.*, 1971) and subsequently interferon itself was found to inhibit the regeneration of mouse liver after partial hepatectomy (Frayssinet *et al.*, 1973).

Early experiments with repeated inoculations of interferon preparations into newborn mice (32,000 to 64,000 units/day), showed no effect on growth or development (Gresser and Bourali, 1970b). However, when more potent preparations (800,000 units) were injected daily into newborn mice for about one week, mice died with extensive liver damage (Gresser et al., 1975). If interferon treatment were stopped between days 6 and 9, liver damage appeared reversible and mice appeared to recover; however, in the next months several of these mice died from progressive glomerulonephritis (Gresser et al., 1976a). Interestingly, inoculation of newborn mice with lymphocytic choriomeningitis virus results in decreased weight gain, liver necrosis and death; when antiserum to mouse interferon was inoculated into such mice, virus levels increased more than 100-fold but the disease manifestations were inhibited (Riviere et al., 1977), suggesting that chronic virus-induced interferon leads to weight loss, liver disease and mortality. Also, Bekesi et al. (1976) have reported that repeated injections of high doses of interferon into AKR mice caused early death with marked signs of "wasting" (organ atrophy, small spleens and athymic), whereas lower doses prolonged survival.

3. Metabolic Alterations in Interferon-Treated Cells

The actual mechanism of the suppression of cell-multiplication is far from being approachable. As the antiviral mechanism seems to be related to a network of mechanisms to restrict translation, it could be envisioned that similar restrains might be imposed on at least certain classes of cellular messenger RNAs. In fact, in view of the wide range of sensitivities to insensitivities of viruses and their messenger RNAs to interferon-induced translation restrictions, it would be somewhat surprising to find that all classes of cellular messenger RNAs would be evenly sensitive or resistant to this restriction. Several early studies reported that crude interferon preparation exerted little, if any, effect on the metabolism of noninfected cells (Joklik and Merigan, 1966; Levy and Merigan, 1966; Merigan, Winget, and Dixon, 1965; Wagner, 1963b; Cocito, DeMaeyer, and Desomer, 1962b; Sonnabend, 1964; Friedman and Sonnabend, 1970), but again, these slight effects were readily related to impurities (Baron, Merigan, and McKerlie, 1966; Cocito, Schonne, and Desomer, 1965; Levy, Snellbaker, and Baron, 1963). Johnson, Lerner, and Lancz (1968) reported that mouse interferon preparations at about 800 units/ml inhibited amino acid incorporation in mouse L cells by 50%, but did not so effect heterologous cells. Falcoff and her associates (1975) reported that treatment of L cells with 1000 units/ml of mouse interferon consistently inhibited endogenous protein synthesis by 20 to 40%; this effect was obtained with several batches of interferon, some purified to 10^7 units/mg of protein. Inhibition paralleled kinetics of viral resistance.

Brouty–Boye et al. (1973a, b) reported that interferon in L_{1210} cells sensitive to interferon exerted a signicant decrease in synthesis of total cellular RNA and protein, but had no such effect in L_{1210} cells resistant to interferon action. O'Shaughnessy, Lee, and Rozee (1972) reported that interferon treatment of synchronized L cells delayed their thymidine uptake, and Fuse and Kuwata

(1976) found that DNA and protein synthesis are reduced in human RSa cells treated with interferon. Synchronized RSa cell cultures seemed to respond to interferon in the late G 1 phase by stopping DNA synthesis but did not do so when interferon was added in G 1/S boundary phase. However, Kariniemi (1977) reported that human leukocyte interferon did not depress DNA synthesis in human psoriatic epidermal cell cultures.

Tovey, Brouty–Boye, and Gresser (1975) and Brouty–Boye and Tovey (1977) have reported studies using the chemostat culture system developed in their laboratory (Tovey and Brouty–Boye, 1976). Mouse interferon preparations inhibited the multiplication of L1210 cells cultivated in steady-state conditions, and a rapid inhibition of incorporation of thymidine was detectable within two hours after interferon was added. Interferon did not inhibit the incorporation of amino acids or uridine. These investigators also reported that interferon reduced the uptake of thymidine but not of deoxyadenosine or deoxy-D-glucose (Brouty–Boye and Tovey, 1977), suggesting that interferon induced a specific alteration of cellular membranes. It seems worth noting that the interferon used in these studies was added continuously to maintain a rather high final concentration (24,000 mouse interferon reference units/ml).

4. Restraints Imposed by Interferon

Interferon treated cells are slowed from rapid proliferation and are also resistant to being stimulated to proliferate. Lindahl–Magnusson, Leary, and Gresser (1972) showed that interferon preparations inhibited DNA-synthesis induced in mouse splenic lymphocytes by phytohemagglutinin or allogeneic lymphocytes. Blomgren, Strander, and Cantell (1974) reported that human leukocyte interferon (at 10 units/ml) suppressed the proliferative response of human lymphocytes to the mitogens phytohemagglutinin, concanavalin A and PPD and to the mixed lymphocyte reactions. Interferon was also able to suppress cells *in vivo*. Pacheco *et al.* (1976) reported that spleen cells from mice inoculated with 10^5 units of interferon 18 hours before excision were resistant to stimulation of thymidine incorporation when exposed to lectin, phytohemagglutinin or concanavalin A, or to lipopolysaccharide. Cupples and Tan (1977) found that cells from Down's syndrome patients were inhibited in DNA synthesis to a greater degree than normal cells by interferon treatment prior to antigenic or mitogenic stimulation.

It has also been reported that induction of specific cellular products can be inhibited in interferon-treated cells. Beck *et al.* (1974) reported that mouse interferon, which had antiviral activity in rat cells, and rat interferon could significantly inhibit the ability of rat HTC cells to produce tyrosine amino-transferase (TAT) when exposed to dexamethasone. Vassef *et al.* (1974) also reported partial depression of TAT induction in interferon-treated rat HTC cells, but only with 200 to 700 times higher concentrations than those required to inhibit reovirus or vesicular stomatitis virus replication; however, some viruses can also be that much less sensitive to interferon than these viruses, so the argument for these results revealing a selectivity of interferon action for viral rather than cellular functions is not valid. Illinger *et al.* (1976) have reported that pretreatment of rat glial cells with rat interferon prior to induction with hydrocortisone hemisuccinate inhibits production of glycerol 3-phosphate dehydrogenase. Chicken interferon was reported to suppress the induction of glutamine synthetase in chick embryonic neural retina by hydrocortisone (Matsuno, Shirasawa, and Kohno, 1976); levels of lactate dehydrogenase, and acetylcholine esterase, were unaffected.

Recently, Smith and his associates (1976) reported, also, that interferon treatment prevented the proliferative response induced in normal erythroid precursor cells by erythropoietin.

These data all indicate a general restraint induced in cells by interferon which manifests itself as an anti-proliferative mechanism and limits several cellular syntheses. The recent reports that interferons can stimulate release of prostaglandin E (Yaron et al., 1977; Karmazyn et al., 1977) which is able to regulate cell replication, indicate the further complexity of evaluating the mechanism of interferon actions. Cortisol and indomethacin, which inhibit prostaglandin E production, reportedly prevented the inhibitory effect of interferon on synovial fibroblast growth (Yaron et al., 1977).

F. Toxicity Enhancement

Several studies have found direct correlations between the ability of polyribonucleotides to induce interferons and their toxicity (Niblack and McCreary, 1971; Declercq, Stewart II, and Desomer, 1972; Declercq and Stewart II, 1972; Stewart II and Declercq, 1974); in fact, there has been no convincing data reporting separability of these properties of double-stranded RNAs, though several such claims have been made (O'Malley et al., 1975a, b; Tso et al., 1976). Thus, the findings that interferon-treated (primed) cells could be induced to produce interferon by concentrations of poly rI·poly rC that were insufficient to stimulate interferon synthesis in unprimed cells (Rosztoczy, 1971; Stewart II et al., 1972) suggested two possibilities: either interferon-treated cells can be induced by less toxic levels of double-stranded RNA inducers, or the inducer double-stranded RNA is more toxic for interferon-treated cells than it is for normal cells. In fact, Stewart II et al. (1972) found that the latter was case: interferon-treated cells were markedly more sensitive than normal cells to toxicity of the double-stranded RNA, poly rI·poly rC. Normal L cells, human skin fibroblasts and mouse embryo cell cultures remained healthy after exposure to poly rI·poly rC, but interferon-treated cells lysed between 3 and 6 hours after exposure to this material (Fig. 20).

This enhanced sensitivity to toxicity was also found with several natural and synthetic double-stranded RNAs (Stewart II, Declercq, and Desomer, 1973), and correlated with the relative abilities of these polynucleotides to induce interferon and with required polynucleotide size for induction of both effects (Stewart II and Declercq, 1974). Toxicity enhancement was not seen with single-stranded RNAs, DNA, tilorone, endotoxin, COAM, cycloheximide, actinomycin D, DEAE-dextran, rattlesnake venom, diphtheria toxin or cholera toxin, and it was thus suggested that the enhancement of toxicity of interferon treated cells was specific for double-stranded RNAs.

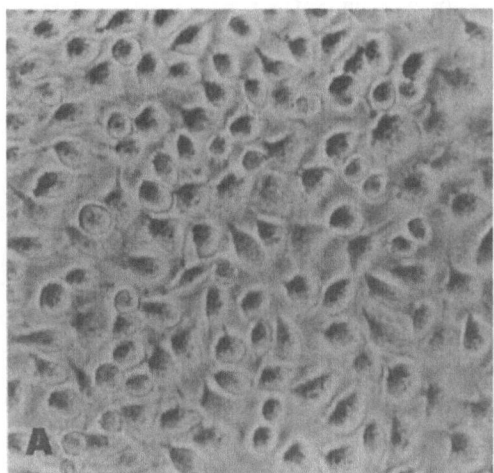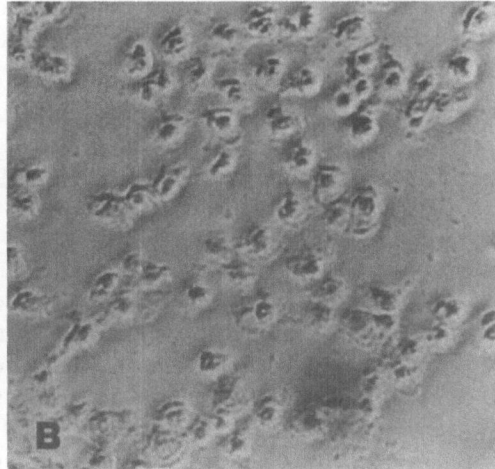

Fig. 20. Double-stranded RNA toxicity-enhancing activity of interferon. Cultures of L929 cells were incubated in growth medium *(A)* or growth medium containing 10 units of interferon/ml *(B)*. Both cultures were then exposed to 25 μg of poly rI·poly rC and photographed about 3 hours later. (Experiment courtesy of Sohan Gupta)

This interpretation of double-stranded RNA specificity of toxicity-enhancement was further supported by the observations that vaccinia virus infection caused an early disintegration of interferon-treated cells (Joklik and Merigan, 1966; Horak, Jungwirth, and Bodo, 1971; Jungwirth *et al.*, 1972a, b; Bodo *et al.*, 1972; Stewart II *et al.*, 1972). Joklik and Merigan (1966) first observed that interferon-treated L cells began to be converted to "ghosts" about 3 hours after infection with vaccinia virus and by 6 hours after infection practically all the cells had been lysed, while infected cells not previously exposed to interferon were all intact. Horak, Jungwirth, and Bodo (1971) found that a viral gene product must be synthesized for the lysis of vaccinia virus-infected interferon-treated cells, which in their L cells occurred between 4 and 8 hours after infection. Stewart II, Declercq, and Desomer (1973) also found that vaccinia virus was not lytic for interferon-treated cells if cells were treated with cycloheximide or actinomycin D when infected (however, these inhibitors did not prevent poly rI·poly rC from lysing interferon-treated cells). These data suggest that a viral gene product, not the input virus itself, is responsible for the lysis of interferon-treated cells. As doublestranded RNA was reported in vaccinia virus-infected cells (Colby and Duesberg, 1969), it is tempting to speculate that this type of toxicity enhancement is specific for double-stranded RNA.

This effect emphasizes the myriad mechanisms involved in the antiviral network of interferon-treated cells. As illustrated in Fig. 17, viruses which are able to avoid the early inhibitory actions of interferon-treated cells and which form sufficient double-stranded replicative structures can activate the kinase → phosphorylated initiation factor block and the LMWIT → endonuclease effect and then may push the cell to suicide, taking the premature "embryonic" virus with it.

Enhanced lysis of interferon-treated cells has also been reported with L cells infected with vesicular stomatitis virus (Katz, Lee, and Rozee, 1974) and with human conjunctival cells infected with influenza virus (Green and Mowshowitz, 1978); in the latter case it was also reported that a viral synthetic process in cells was required to produce lysis. Other have observed enhanced cytopathic effects in cells repeatedly exposed to poly rI·poly rC (Billiau, Van den Berghe, and Desomer, 1972; Martelly and Jullien, 1974), possibly owing to induced interferon priming cells for enhanced toxicity of the double-stranded RNA.

The amount of interferon required to induce this effect is similar to that required for measuring resistance to viruses, and the amount of destruction of the interferon-treated cells is dependent on both the amount of double-stranded RNA added to the cells and the concentration of interferon applied (Stewart II, Declercq, and Desomer, 1972a; Lackovic and Borecky, 1976); this relationship was used to develop a sensitive non-antiviral interferon assay for this effect. Toxicity enhancement with double-stranded RNA can be demonstrated in several lines of L cells; it can be demonstrated in mouse embryo cell cultures (Stewart II et al., 1972; J. Desmyter, personal communication, 1972). It is seen in mouse leukemia L1210S cells which are interferon sensitive, but not in the L1210R cells resistant to (and not binding) interferon (Werrene and Rousseau, 1976a; Gresser and Stewart II, unpublished data). I have observed a distinct toxicity-enhancement in 3 of 10 different human fibroblast cultures, a slight effect in 4 of 10 cultures and no detectable effect in 3 of these cultures. Nor have I seen this effect in rabbit kidney cell cultures (unpublished data). In view of the variable abilities of human fibroblasts to express this action, it would perhaps not be surprising that Declercq, Edy, and Cassiman (1975) were unable to correlate toxicity-enhancement to numbers of chromosome 21 in human fibroblast. In view of my experience with this effect, what was surprising with the study of Declercq et al., however, was their phenomenal luck in finding 5 out of 5 human fibroblasts that not only expressed the double-stranded RNA toxicity-enhancement but all expressed it very distinctly and to the same extent.

Several hours of treatment with interferon are required for cells to develop toxicity-enhancement, during which time protein synthesis is required (Stewart II, unpublished data). This suggests that while perhaps priming can develop through a direct membrane alteration effect, toxicity-enhancement like antiviral activity, requires cellular protein synthesis to develop, in contrast to the direct membrane alteration mechanism proposed by Declercq and Desomer (1975).

Double-stranded RNA toxicity-enhancement appears to lead to cell lysis within about three hours after addition of the double-stranded RNA; no damage is visible before that time and lysis is complete in those cells effected by no later than about 6 hours. Just prior to lysis it was possible, by use of cytochemical staining techniques, to detect intracellular injury to mitochondria, as evidenced by marked loss of succinic dehydrogenase, lysosomal injury, as suggested by diffuse acid phosphatase activity and nuclear swelling concurrent with lowered protein synthesis (Stewart II et al., 1975b). By using electron microscopy it was similarly revealed that mitochondrial and nuclear damage precede cell disruption (Heremans et al., 1976). As the mitochondrial distortions seen in these studies are common to numerous cellular toxicities, these studies only tell us the obvious, that the cells have been damaged somehow. Preliminary attempts to isolate various cell membranes from normal and interferon-treated cells and to mix these directly with double-stranded RNA and detect membrane disruptions by altered sedimentation patterns proved technically difficult (Stewart II, unpublished data) but should be interesting to attempt by improved membrane isolation methods. It would be tempting to relate the toxicity-enhancement directly to the shut-off of protein synthesis, as seen in cell-free protein synthetic systems derived from interferon-treated cells whose translating functions are arrested by addition of double-stranded RNA. However, in interferon-treated cells it is possible to completely arrest cellular RNA and/or protein synthetic processes by addition of various metabolic inhibitors, and in such cultures no lytic activity is detectable, even after 24 hours (Stewart II, unpublished data).

Interferon-treated L cells were also reported to be more sensitive to arginine starvation (Lee and Rozee, 1975) and to the toxicity of DEAE-dextran, protamine sulfate and methylated albumin (Katz, Lee, and Rozee, 1974); however, others did not find enhancement of sensitivity to DEAE-dextran (Stewart II, Declercq, and Desomer, 1973; M. Tovey, personal communication, 1972). However, Stewart II et al. (1975b) did observe an increased toxicity of concanavalin A in interferon-treated cells, but this toxicity was distinct from the lysis seen with vaccinia virus and double-stranded RNA; it was rather an increased vacuolation of the cytoplasm. It seems likely this increased toxicity of the lectin for interferon-treated cells relates to the increased binding reported with concanavalin A in interferon-treated cells (Huet et al., 1974).

It could be expected that toxicity enhancement plays a role in vivo as well as in cell cultures. The presence of interferon in virus infected patients might preclude the utility of double-stranded RNAs in treatment of such diseases. Stewart II et al. (1972) cautioned that safety assessments based on toxicity levels of poly rI·poly rC in normal individuals might not accurately reflect the therapeutic index of this inducer in virus-infected patients who might have infection-induced interferon levels. In fact, Declercq, Stewart II, and Desomer (1973a) reported that virus-infected mice were markedly more susceptible to the toxicity of double-stranded RNAs than were normal uninfected mice. Cantell, Pyhala, and Strander (1974) also observed that the combined administration of interferon and virus was dangerous to rabbits: none of more than 150 rabbits injected with a few million units of human leukocyte interferon died; likewise, none of several rabbits injected with Newcastle disease virus died; however, a significant number of the rabbits injected with both virus and interferon died, and most of the survivors were toxified to some extent. In a perhaps related effect, Huang and Landay (1969) reported that interferon inducers poly rI·poly rC and Newcastle disease virus enhanced the lethal effect of endotoxins in mice.

On the assumption that the antitumor activity of double-stranded RNA is related at least in part to its direct toxicity for tumor cells, and on the basis that a significant amount of intramuscularly inoculated interferon binds locally (Stewart II, unpublished data; Harmon and Janis, 1975), Stewart II *et al.* (1975c) attempted to take advantage of the toxicity-enhancing activity of interferon to attack Moloney sarcoma virus-induced tumors in mice. Mice developing autochthonous tumors were given injections of interferon or poly rI·poly rC, or interferon followed by poly rI·poly rC, all injections directly into the palpatable tumors. Whereas treatments with interferon alone were ineffective in prolonging life, and poly rI·poly rC alone was only marginally effective (Declercq and Stewart II, 1974b), sequential local treatment with interferon and poly rI·poly rC was, in this preliminary trial, markedly more effective in both prolonging life and inducing tumor regressions. Clearly this apparent *in vivo* application of double-stranded RNA toxicity-enhancement merits further investigations.

The toxicity-enhancing factor in interferon preparations has been shown to possess all the attributes of interferons (Section VII. A. 7.); it purified with interferon through more than 1000-fold (Stewart II *et al.*, 1972) and 1 million-fold (Stewart II *et al.*, 1973) increases in the specific activity. It was found to parallel the activity profiles of mouse and human interferons in SDS gels as seen in Fig. 13 and 14 (Stewart II, 1975b), and recently we have found identical ratios of antiviral/toxicity-enhancing activity in mouse interferon purified to 10^9 units/mg of protein (Stewart II, Lin, and Wiranowska-Stewart, 1978) and in mouse interferoid (paralleling the profile in Fig. 15) (Stewart II *et al.*, 1978).

Thus, toxicity enhancement, priming, blocking and cell-multiplication-inhibition are all cellular alterations induced by interferons. The subsequent activities described in this section are not so well characterized in terms of the proof that interferon is the factor inducing them, but present evidence at least strongly implicates interferons as the active component. Studies with pure interferons should soon clarify this involvement.

G. Enhanced Synthetic Activities

In addition to enhancing the ability of cells to produce interferon (priming), interferon can apparently also assist cells to make other products.

Yaron *et al.* (1976) reported that either poly rI·poly rC or human interferon could stimulate production of hyaluronic acid by rheumatoid and non-rheumatoid human synovial fibroblasts, and suggested a relationship between interferon production and pathology of accumulated joint fluid during virus infections. Yaron *et al.* (1977) also found that either poly rI·poly rC or human interferon (100 units/ml) could stimulate prostaglandin E production by these synovial cells or by foreskin fibroblasts. As prostaglandin E is a mediator of inflammatory processes, it is tempting to speculate that the "interferon fever" reported in skin wheals following inoculation with human fibroblast interferon (Desomer *et al.*, 1977) and the febrile response often observed with systemic administration of human leukocyte interferon (Section XIV) may be related to this activity.

Interferon can also enhance the amount of certain induced cell products.

Nebert and Friedman (1973) reported that mouse interferon pretreatment (100 units/ml) enhanced the amount of aryl hydrocarbon hydroxylase induced in cultures with benzanthracene. And Ida et al. (1977) found that either virus, poly rI·poly rC or human leukocyte interferon enhanced the ability of human leukocytes to release histamine when exposed to ragweed antigen E or anti-IgE. These authors suggest that interferon may, therefore, play a role in precipitating or potentiating attacks of bronchial asthma during viral infections. In this regard it is interesting that Skurkovich and Eremkina (1975) have suggested the role of interferon in allergy and have proposed use of anti-interferon immunoglobulins in the treatment of certain autoimmune diseases.

H. Surface Alterations Induced by Interferons

Interferon treatment has been repeatedly reported to increase the resistance of cultured cells to diphtheria toxin (Yabrov, 1966, 1967; Moehring, Moehring, and Stinebring, 1971; Boquet, 1975; Marchenko et al., 1976b). However, this effect could not be detected in some laboratories (Stewart II, Declercq, and Desomer, 1973), possibly because it is very slight. As interferon and cholera toxin can apparently interfere with receptor-interactions of one another (Kohn et al., 1976) it seems likely that interferon interferes with binding of the diphtheria toxin to cells, though Yabrov (1966, 1967, 1975, 1976) has interpreted that interferon acts by stabilizing cells against perturbations of protein syntheses.

Knight and Korant (1977) have provided direct evidence for a surface alteration of cells by interferon, though not a direct one resulting from binding (or priming), as it required several hours and protein synthesis for such an effect to develop. The interferon-treated cells then migrated in an electric field with a greater net negative charge than normal cells.

Huet et al. (1974) also reported that mouse interferon treatment induced an increase in binding of ^{63}Ni-labeled concanavalin A to interferon-sensitive L1210 cells but did not do so in interferon-resistant L1210 cells. The increased binding was slight at 24 hours but was greatest after 48 hours.

A number of workers have found that interferon treatment can increase the expression of surface antigens on cells. Lindahl, Leary, and Gresser (1973) demonstrated that mouse interferon preparations enhanced the expression of surface antigens of leukemia L1210 cells. Interferon treatment increased the cell-antibody-absorbing capacity of interferon-sensitive cells but not of interferon-resistant cells. About 100 units/ml for 24 hours enhanced the expression of histocompatibility antigens of thymocytes from mice of various ages, splenic lymphocytes from young mice and did not affect the expression of theta antigens (Lindahl, Leary, and Gresser, 1974). Killander et al. (1976) demonstrated further that interferon treatment of L1210 cells enhanced the expression of histocompatibility antigens similarly in all stages of the cell cycle, suggesting that the enhancement was not due to a concentration of cells in a particular phase of the cycle. Skurkovich et al. (1976b) demonstrated that interferon-treated L1210 cells exerted an enhanced cell-mediated immune response in mice. Lindahl et al. (1976a, b) also found that injection of interferon into young or mature mice enhanced the histocompatibility displays on the surfaces of their thymocytes and splenic lymphocytes.

The availability of restricted antisera against specific determinants of the H-2 complex allowed Vignaux and Gresser (1977) to determine that interferon-treated mouse splenic lymphocytes displayed increased amounts of H-2 K and H-2 D antigens (4- to 8-fold greater than normal), but did not express enhanced Ia antigens. In these studies cells were treated with high concentration of interferon of about 3000 units of interferon/ml (about 12,000 reference units), and in one experiment Ia antigen was increased slightly by treatment with 10^5 units/ml. This study again emphasized the dose-effect of interferon actions not being an "all-or-none phenomenon". These authors also found an enhanced H-2^k, H-2K^k and H-2D^k on splenic lymphocytes and thymocytes of mice injected with interferon (dosage: "mice injected i. p. four times with an interferon preparation titering 1×10^{-6}"; volume administered not specified). Lonai and Steinman (1977) reported that mouse interferon (4000 units/ml)[8] increased the H-2 antigens exposed on mouse T cells but did not enhance Ia antigen expression, and suggested that interferon influences suppressor or killer cells. In this regard it is interesting that interferon is released by immunocytes in response to antigens or target cells (Svet–Moldavsky et al., 1974), again relating the induction-action ends of the interferon system.

I. Enhanced Immunolysis

Svet–Moldavsky and Chernyakovskaya (1967) demonstrated that in the presence of crude mouse interferon preparations normal mouse lymphocytes acquired a killer activity on target mouse L cell, though it did not enhance the sticking of the lymphocytes to the L cells. Syngeneic lymphoid cells in interferon preparations also acquired the ability to exert an antitumor effect against sarcomas in mice inoculated with benzanthracene (Chernyakhovskaya and Slavina, 1972). Skurkovich and Aleksandrovskaya (1973) also reported stimulation of cytotoxic activity of lymphocytes of mice towards target cells following administration of crude interferon preparations in vivo. Svet–Moldavsky and his colleagues (1974) also demonstrated that lymphoid cells removed from mice at the peak of interferon production, which had been induced by injection of allogeneic cells, exhibited a strong cytotoxic effect on non-specific target L cells. This interesting study emphasized that interferon may play a role as a mediator molecule for initiations of various immune reactions.

Lindahl, Leary, and Gresser (1972) extended these findings by demonstrating that in the interferon-mediated sensitization of sensitized lymphocytes for leukemia L1210 cells, the enhanced specific cytotoxicity resulted from an effect of interferon on lymphocytes rather than from an effect on the target cells. She and her coworkers also provided evidence that interferon was the active agent in the preparations. In contrast to previous reports, however, these workers

---

[8] This report does not indicate interferon *reference* units, and as this preparation was provided by Gresser, who reports his units to equal 4 mouse reference units (Vignaux and Gresser, 1977), this dose may mean 16,000 reference units/ml. This again emphasizes the need for stating titers in reference units.

did not detect cytotoxicity with interferon-treated or normal lymphocytes of mice not specifically sensitized to target cells. Slavina and Svet–Moldavsky (1973) reported rather that interferon induced the sensitivity of L cells to the cytotoxic effects of lymphocytes. Thus, in the nonspecific system the alteration seems to be in the target cell, while in the specific system the alteration appears to be in the effector cells.

Recently, Heron, Berg, and Cantell (1976) found that the killer activity of human lymphocytes was enhanced by treatment with human leukocyte interferon. In related studies, Skurkovich et al. (1976a) reported that treatment of human lymphocytes with interferon enhanced their cytotoxicity toward cells of lymphoblastoid lines. These authors (Skurkovich et al., 1976b; Skurkovich, Klinova and Eremkina, 1976) also reported that L1210 cells incubated with interferon preparations were more sensitive to the action of cytotoxic antibodies.

J. Enhancement of Phagocytosis

Huang and his associates (1971) demonstrated that mouse peritoneal macrophages exposed to interferon preparations (50 units/ml) exhibited significantly (200 to 300%) enhanced phagocytic activity for colloidal carbon particles. These investigators demonstrated this effect with a variety of different mouse interferon preparations and showed that the enhancing effect of such preparations was neutralized by antiserum prepared against partially purified mouse interferon (Donahoe and Huang, 1973). It was also demonstrated that interferon preparations or an inducer, Newcastle disease virus, injected into mice enhanced phagocytic activity against the carbon particles injected intraperitoneally (Donahoe and Huang, 1976). Enhancement began after several hours and lasted for at least 60 hours.

Imanishi et al. (1975) also reported that human leukocyte interferon preparations enhanced the phagocytic activity of human peripheral monocytes for latex particles. At 4000 interferon units/ml the interferon preparations increased both the number of phagocytic cells and the degree of phagocytosis by individual cells. However, in this study no preincubation of cells with interferon was required for phagocytosis-enhancement to develop: latex and interferon added simultaneously gave the same enhancement.

It was suggested that interferon and its inducers could exert an antibacterial and anti-protozoal effect by stimulating phagocytosis (Donahoe and Huang, 1973). In fact, some studies have demonstrated that interferon inducers enhanced reticuloendothelial clearance of bacteria (Remington and Merigan, 1970) and protozoa (Herman and Baron, 1970). On the other hand, Kazar, Krautwurst, and Gordon (1971) did not find an increased uptake of Chlamydia trachomatis by interferon-treated mouse peritoneal cells. However, Gresser and Bourali (1970a) observed that macrophages of mice treated with interferon and then injected with RC19 leukemia cells exhibited greater phagocytosis of tumor cells than controls.

It could also be imagined that enhanced pinocytosis of virions could be induced in cells by interferons (perhaps not only in specialized motile phagocytic elements) and that this enhancing effect on uptake could obscure inhibitory effects on binding and penetration. Further studies on both these phenomena seem appropriate.

K. Macrophage "Activation"

Several interferon inducers administered to mice enhanced the spreading of peritoneal macrophages when these were then plated on glass (Rabinovitch *et al.*, 1977), and it was suggested that this "activation" of macrophages resulted from interferon action. Khesin *et al.* (1973) reported that by studies of comparative morphology, cytochemistry and biochemistry of peritoneal exudate macrophage of mice it was determined that macrophages from mice treated with interferon preparations were "activated". Schultz, Papamatheakis, and Chirigos (1977) reported that a number of interferon inducers, pyran copolymer, poly rI·poly rC, and dextran sulfate when injected into mice rendered their peritoneal macrophages cytotoxic for leukemia cells, and demonstrated that partially purified mouse interferon (2×10^7 units/mg of protein) at 1000 units/ml rendered macrophages cytotoxic for tumor cells. Interferon-treated macrophages showed enhanced spreading on plastic and had prominent cytoplasmic granulations; cytotoxicity appeared to result from direct activity as it was not transferred as a soluble factor, and did not result from enhanced phagocytosis. The effect was induced by as little as 100 units/ml, was maximal at 1000 units/ml. Human interferon was about 1 percent as effective, requiring at least 10^4 units/ml to "activate" the mouse macrophages.

These findings further implicate the interferon system as the determinants in yet another mechanism of "immune"-mediated antitumor activity.

L. Delayed-Type Hypersensitivity-Inhibition

The effect of interferon and interferon inducers in mice on the delayed-type hypersensitivity (DTH) response to picryl chloride or sheep red blood cells (SRBCs) was first investigated by DeMaeyer, DeMaeyer–Guignard, and Vandeputte (1975). Mice inoculated with Newcastle disease virus, Sendai virus, or statolon eight hours prior to challenge by picryl chloride painting of shaved ears showed decreased ear swelling at 24 hours. As a control for this study they used both If-1[1] and If-1[h] mice; the latter group, being better interferon producers with Newcastle disease virus (Section V. D. 1.), also showed better DTH inhibition with this inducer. Also, four doses of about 10^6 units of mouse interferon administered on the day before or the day of challenge also inhibited the reaction. Similarly, interferon inhibited foot-pad swelling in sensitized mice inoculated with SRBCs. The interferon used in these studies was purified to about 10^8 units/mg of protein.

These investigators (DeMaeyer–Guignard, Cachard, and DeMaeyer, 1975) also showed that the afferent arc of the DTH response (the primary sensitization) as well as the efferent arc, was inhibited by interferon. Mice treated with interferon 1 or 2 days before sensitization had decreased response to SRBCs. Similar results were obtained with both afferent and efferent arcs of the DTH response using a viral (Newcastle disease virus) immunogen (DeMaeyer, 1976).

Thus interferon can inhibit sensitization and expression of the DTH reactions to a hapten, a T-cell-dependent antigen or a virus.

These studies point up a paradox of interferon activities: interferon, an antiviral agent important in recovery from virus diseases and tumors, can inhibit cell-mediated immune reactions which are important in elimination of certain virus diseases and tumor cell destruction. It is possible that this effect of interferon explains the enhanced tumor growth reported in certain systems with interferon inducers and interferon (Gazdar, 1972; Gazdar *et al.*, 1972a, b, 1973).

It is also possible (as will be described below) that at different doses, and under different schedules, interferon might decrease immune response in one case, and increase it in another. Such effects on the cell-mediated immunity, DTH reaction, likely explain the following observation on graft survivals.

M. Graft-vs-Host Reactions: Effects of Interferon on Transplantation

The effects of interferon on graft survivals are quite conflicting. It was first reported by Chernyakhovskaya and Slavina (1972) that injection of an interferon preparation under allogeneic skin graft in mice accelerated the processes of necrosis. Similarly, Skurkovich *et al.* (1973a, b) reported that daily injections of mice with crude mouse interferon preparations intraperitoneally after they were grafted with allogeneic skin accelerated the rejection process, in association with an enhanced cytotoxic activity of their lymphocytes for target cells. Repeated transplantations to mice which were treated with interferon during the first grafting accelerated rejection of these second-set grafts. These workers concluded that interferon given after transplantation enhanced cell-mediated rejections.

Cerottini *et al.* (1973) also found that interferon-inducers or interferon preparations exerted inhibitory effects on the multiplication of transplanted allogeneic spleen cells and syngeneic bone marrow cells in irradiated mice. However, this effect was more likely a result of the cell-multiplication-inhibitory action than an immunomodulation. OReilly *et al.* (1976) reported that interferon did not suppress marrow engraftment in two bone marrow transplant patients given daily doses of 10^6 units of crude human leukocyte interferon.

Hirsch *et al.* (1973) also reported that interferon could inhibit the proliferative response of the graft-vs-host reaction in mice and could inhibit the activation of leukemia virus concomitant with this reaction. Mice injected with about 10^5 units daily of mouse interferon starting a day before the injection of spleen cells showed suppression of the graft-vs-host-response.

Mobraaten, DeMaeyer, and DeMaeyer–Guignard (1973) found also that injection of mice with Newcastle disease virus or statolon sufficient to give serum interferon levels of about 10^5 units/ml on the day of or after grafting significantly prolonged allograft survival. If given prior to grafting, the inducer was ineffective. Tilorone, orally, also prolonged allograft survivals. In other studies tilorone has been reported to prolong both skin and heart allografts in rats (Wildstein, Stevens, and Hashim, 1976) and kidney transplants in dogs (Wildstein *et al.*, 1976)[9].

---

[9] The presence of interferon in these experiments was not determined as the authors con-

DeMaeyer, Mobraaten, and DeMaeyer–Guignard (1973) also found that injections of mouse interferon preparations, intraperitoneally, delayed allograft rejections across an H-2 barrier in mice. These workers also showed that allografts on the If-1ʰ mice injected with Newcastle disease virus survived longer than on the If-1¹ mice so induced (DeMaeyer, Mobraaten, and DeMaeyer–Guignard, 1973).

Hirsch *et al.* (1974) reported that interferon treatment of mice twice daily from 1 day before grafting until graft rejection increased transplant survival by 2 days with A/J skin on Balb/c mice, by 4 days with DBZ/2 skin on Balb/c, indicating that minor loci as well as the major H 2ᵈ histocompatibility locus were involved in rejection. Hirsch, Black, and Proffitt (1977) also showed that about 10^5 units of crude mouse interferon daily reduced virus activation and the incidence of lymphomas following graft-vs-host reaction in mice and reduced the severity of the rejection reaction itself. These data suggest that interferon may prove useful in immune disorder, in viral infection, in neoplasia, and as an immunosuppressive with antiviral activity in organ transplant recipients, who are at high risk for both virus infection and neoplasia [10].

Imanishi *et al.* (1977) also reported that high doses of rabbit interferon, in eyedrops (2×10^6 units/ml; one drop/eye × twice daily) suppressed rejection of rabbit corneal xenograft. Interestingly, a low dose (2×10^3 units/ml) enhanced rejection. Thus this high dose-low dose response relationship proferred by the Japanese workers may reconcile the discrepancies between increased rejections seen by Eastern block workers and increased survivals reported by their Western counterparts. It seems that several more years of careful attention to timings, dosages and purities of interferon administrations will be necessary for sufficient data to accumulate to allow accurate analysis of these variables in regard to application for transplantation survival.

N. Effects of Interferon on Antibody Production

1. In vivo *Antibody Production*

Early experiments on the effects of interferon on antibody production in mice reported no effects (Anderson, 1965; Desomer, Billiau, and Declercq, 1967; Mazzur and Paucker, 1967; Mazzur, Ellsworth, and Paucker, 1967). The demonstration of an effect of interferon on antibody production was first reported by Braun and Levy (1972) who found that intraperitoneal injection of mouse interferon with SRBCs either enhanced or inhibited the plaque-forming-cell response measured 2 days later. Low doses (250 to 1500 units) enhanced antibody producers whereas high doses (5000 to 10,000 units) inhibited the production of plaques. Chester, Paucker, and Merigan (1973) reported that intravenous injection of about 10^5 units of interferon into mice two days prior to the antigen significantly suppressed their antibody response to SRBC. When

---

tended that "interferon assay is not well established in the canine species"; such a situation did not, however, deter Depoux (1965), or Aurelian and Roizman (1965); see Table 1.

[10] In view of the growing hopes for this substance and in light of its cell-multiplication-inhibitory activity, it seems surprising that no one has yet proposed using it to treat giantism!

poly rI·poly rC was used to induce interferon, however, a slight increase in antibody-producing cells was observed after SRBC challenge (Merigan, Chester, and Paucker, 1975). Brodeur and Merigan (1974) showed that both the primary and secondary hemolysin and agglutinin antibody responses were inhibited in mice injected intravenously with about 10^5 units of interferon 2 days before primary immunization with SRBC, and both IgM and IgG antibody synthesis was depressed, as revealed by sensitivity and resistance to mercaptoethanol.

Brodeur and Merigan (1975) also demonstrated that about 10^5 units of interferon inhibited the primary antibody response of mice to a thymus-independent antigen, *Salmonella typhimurium* lypopolysaccharide, and thus indicated a direct action of interferon on B lymphocytes.

Others have reported that intravenous injection of rabbits with about 10^6 units of rabbit interferon did not alter the ability of these animals to produce antibodies to SRBCs (Thorbecke, Friedman–Kien, and Vilček, 1974).

Ngan, Lee, and Kind (1976) reported that mouse interferon was able to strongly inhibit an heterologous adoptive cutaneous anaphylaxis (HACA) reaction. Sensitized mouse spleen cells which synthesized IgE caused HACA reaction in rat skin; when these cells were treated with 200 units of interferon/ml, the reaction was reduced about 50%; when treated with 600 units/ml, the reaction (i. e., IgE antibody production) was completely inhibited.

Virelizier, Virelizier, and Allison (1976) found that infection of mice with the coronavirus, murine hepatitis virus-3, modified their humoral response to SRBCs, and showed that the modification correlated with the circulating interferon levels: presence of interferon before antigen reduced antibody responses; its presence after antigen enhanced antibody response. These authors speculate that interferon induction may account for the many modifications of immune responses seen in man during virus diseases. Berencsi and Baladi (1977) reported that interferon induced in hamsters by Newcastle disease virus apparently suppressed both their primary and anamnestic responses to SRBCs.

2. In vitro *Antibody Production*

In the first report on effects of interferon on *in vitro* antibody response, Gisler, Lindahl, and Gresser (1974) showed that several thousand units (about 3000 "units"/ml; about 12,000 reference units/ml) were required to suppress the *in vitro* PFC response of Balb/c mouse spleen cells to SRBCs. When these workers treated spleen cells that were poor responders with lower doses of interferon (1000 to 2000 units/ml), antibody production was enhanced. These effects were seen when cells were treated with interferon 6 hours before antigen or up to 40 hours after it. Johnson, Smith, and Baron (1974, 1975) also found that the antibody response of mouse spleen cells to SRBCs was inhibited by interferon *in vitro*, by using C 57 Bl/6 mouse cells they were able to show a marked inhibition (90% or greater) with only 20 units of interferon and more than 90% inhibition with 40 units/ml. Reasons for this apparently large quantitative discrepancy are not clear. Booth et al. (1976) also found that the antibody response of mouse spleen cells to SRBC, inhibited by 80 units of interferon, was slightly enhanced by 0.8 unit/ml. Interferon treatment apparently did not inhibit the growth of spleen cultures (Booth, Booth, and Marbrook, 1976).

The *in vitro* antibody response to T cell- and macrophage-independent antigen, *E. coli* lipopolysaccharide, was also found to be sensitive to interferon, at about 100 units/ml (Johnson, Bukovic, and Baron, 1975; Johnson and Baron, 1976a, b, 1977).

It has also been shown that poly rI·poly rC is able to inhibit primary antibody response to SRBCs and *E. coli* lipopolysaccharide in mouse spleen cells (Johnson, Bukovic, and Smith, 1975). Concanavalin A and Staphylococcal enterotoxin (T-cell mitogens) were also able to inhibit the PFC response to SRBC or lipopolysaccharide (Johnson and Baron, 1976b, c). Interestingly, the antiviral activity induced by double-stranded RNA and the inhibitory effect of double-stranded RNA on antibody synthesis were both inhibited by antibody prepared against mouse type I interferon, whereas the interferon and the immunosuppression induced in these cultures by concanavalin A or Staphylococcal enterotoxin were not neutralized by this antiserum.

It has recently been suggested that type I and type II interferons are functionally distinct, in that the latter, often being a product of immune recognition reactions, or at least produced by immunocompetent cells, would have a greater predilection for cells of the immune system. It has even been reported that type II interferons have significantly more antitumor activity than type I interferon (Salvin *et al.*, 1975b). In this regard I should again point to the fact emphasized in Fig. 5: these suppositions are premature until type II interferons are significantly purified, and will be difficult to accept until demonstrated with pure type II interferons.

The demonstrations that interferons are able to induce a number of alterations in cells other than selective inhibition of virus replication has opened the interferon system to explorations by many fields of research. The applications of interferon to immunomodulations is particularly exciting, and is a fertile new field for rampant speculation: I shall resist rushing in.

Thus far we have followed the interferon system from its start, the descriptions of the inducers, to the interaction of these with cells, through the processes leading to production of interferons. We have purified and characterized these proteins and have examined what they can do at the molecular level to inhibit viruses and have examined their other actions and possible actions at the cellular level. Now we shall examine reports of what they do in the intact animal.

The remainder of this book will deal with the uses of interferons against virus diseases and tumors in animals and in the clinic.

XI. Pharmacokinetics of Interferons

Interferons are able to induce resistance to viruses, and are apparently able to induce a number of potentially useful modifications of immune mechanisms. So, we now begin to administer it to patients to achieve the effects desired. But how much do we need to administer to attain and maintain effective levels? In fact, what is the desired level? And how long must it be maintained? We have previously seen (Fig. 8) that even very high levels of circulating interferons induced in animals very rapidly disappeared within just a few hours. Where did this interferon go? And what happened to it? The answers to these questions are not yet known. Present applications of interferons are based on the limited information presented in this Section: interferon is usually administered on the basis of giving as much as possible, based on either availability or restrictions imposed by "side" effects (which have usually been presumed to be due to non-interferon impurities in the preparations). Much more work is required on the pharmacokinetics of interferons before clinical applications will be more rational. In view of some of the differences observed with high or low doses mentioned previously in cell cultures and some that will be mentioned later (Section XIII) it seems likely that more attention should be paid to this problem.

Clearly the rapid disappearance of interferon from the blood stream, as illustrated in Fig. 8, cannot be attributed to the intrinsic instability of the interferon, as its stability in tissue culture systems in which it is induced is markedly greater. Thus interferons must be rapidly bound to tissues, degraded or excreted, or all of these.

A. Distribution of Interferon

1. Circulating Interferon Levels

Interferons, whether induced by viruses, endotoxins, or synthetic inducers, rapidly disappear from both the blood and tissues of animals (Baron *et al.*, 1966a; Subrahmanyan and Mims, 1966; Finter, 1966a; Stewart II and Sulkin, 1966; Billiau, 1969). When interferons are administered exogenously, it also disappears in the animal, falling to less than 10% of the initial level within one hour in the mouse (Baron *et al.*, 1966a; Finter, 1966a). Subramanyan and Mims (1966) injected about 300 units of interferon intravenously into mice and recovered only trace levels about 5 to 10 minutes later and none after 6 hours. Gresser *et al.* (1967b) injected mice with about 10^4 units, recovered about 30% after 1 minute and less than 1% after 1 hour. Ho (1973) has calculated from these reported data that the half-life for mouse interferon *in vivo* was about 10 minutes. Ho and his colleagues (Ho and Postic, 1967; Ho, Postic, and Ke, 1967; Ho, 1967) found the half-life of rabbit interferon in rabbits to be about 11 minutes, virus-induced and endotoxin-induced interferons cleared at about the same rate. Bocci, Russi, and Rita (1967) found the half-life for rabbit interferon in rabbits to be only a couple of minutes; however, these workers injected interferon isolated from rabbit urine, which may be already processed for excretion.

At one time it seemed feasible that the rapidly cleared circulating interferon was stored to be released rapidly as "preformed" material (Baron and Levy, 1966). Declercq and his collaborators (Declercq, Nuwer, and Merigan, 1970b; Nuwer, Declercq, and Merigan, 1971) claimed that repeated injections of a few hundred units of interferon into mice every 2 hours saturated this supposed clearance mechanism, increasing the early half-time from 1 to 1½ minutes. These authors imagined that the interferon receptor sites in the body became saturated after 3 injections, and thus concluded that treatment of virus infection by passive interferon might be more feasible than previously thought. In a subsequent publication, these authors claimed that the previously cleared interferon could be released as "preformed" interferon by injection of cycloheximide (Chester *et al.*, 1972). These curious data are difficult to rationalize in view of present information on "preformed" interferon (see Section IV. A. 1), and should apparently be disregarded. Declercq (1977) has also claimed that intraperitoneally injected interferon *all* enters the blood and it all stays there several hours.

After the initial rapid fall of circulating interferon within 1 hour after intravenous injection, the clearance rate decreased. Cantell and Pyhala (1973) injected human leukocyte interferon into rabbits (in which it is active) and found the early clearance half-time was about 13 minutes, whereas the late halftime was about 1 hour and 13 minutes. Significantly, rabbit interferon gave similar results. No interferon was detectable after 6 hours. In contrast to Declercq and his colleagues (see above: Declercq, Nuwer, and Merigan, 1970b; Nuwer, Declercq, and Merigan, 1971) and in spite of several efforts, Cantell, and Pyhala (1973) found that repeated injections did not affect the clearance rate. They also found that *intramuscular* injections of interferon apparently prolonged serum interferon levels for 12 hours, and higher initial doses gave higher tailing-levels. When injected intramuscularly, it is likely the interferon binds locally and thus sets up a local interferon-pool which leaches into circulation over a prolonged period. Local binding of interferon at the site of its injection into muscle was found in hamster (Stewart II and Sulkin, unpublished data, 1965); also, Harmon and Janis (1975) found that poly rI·poly rC was protective against rabies in mice if injected into the same leg, but was ineffective if injected into the opposite leg: the locally injected muscle contained significantly more interferon at later times than did the non-injected leg muscle. A single injection of 30 million units of human interferon intramuscularly maintained detectable serum interferon for 48 hours, and subcutaneous injections seemed to give even longer persistence. Interferon (6 × 10⁶ units) administered orally was not detectable in the serum. Schafer *et al.* (1972) were also unable to detect interferon in circulation of adult mice administered mouse or rabbit interferon *per os*, but interferon was found in the blood of neonatal mice given oral doses of interferon. Skreko *et al.* (1973) also showed that clearance rates of human leukocyte interferon in the gibbon was the same as that seen in rabbits.

It is likely that the prolonged tailing-effect of circulating interferon in animals receiving interferon injections results from release of tissue bound interferon. To accurately determine how much of the injected interferon so "stored" can be eluted it would be necessary to devise experiments to periodically exchange blood volumes of the injected animal to see how much more interferon would continually leach into the new fluid to reach a new equilibrium. Such experiments have not been done.

Strander *et al.* (1973) reported administering about 5×10^5 units of human leukocyte interferon to a patient intravenously (7000 units/kg body weight). No immediate reaction was seen but after about $1\frac{1}{2}$ hours the patient became nauseated, had fever, increased blood pressure and pulse rate, began vomiting and shivering severely. Symptoms decreased with hydrocortisone injection and were normal 10 hours later. Serum interferon level was 200 units/ml 1 minute after injection, and 65 units/ml at 15 minutes. Since this interferon was tolerated after intramuscular injections in rabbits and since such inoculation route gave long-lasting blood interferon levels, all further patients were injected intramuscularly. The same patient was later given intramuscular interferon injections without side effects. Some patients given 3×10^6 units of human leukocyte interferon[11] complained of local pain, and temperatures increased with increasing interferon dose. After several treatments patients tended to tolerate injections of 3×10^6 units better than initially but always developed fever after injections.

In a subsequent study Ahstrom *et al.* (1974) reported administering 2.5×10^6 human leukocyte interferon units to 6 leukemic children (about 10^5 units/kg, intramuscularly daily). These children had peak serum interferon levels of about 60 units/ml. No serious toxic effects were recorded, except one child had fever, and one had joint pains.

Cantell, Pyhala, and Strander (1974) also compared serum interferon levels in guinea pigs, rabbits, sheep and man given different doses of human leukocyte interferon intramuscularly and got about the same results in each species, the level of interferon in the serum depending directly on the units/body weight injected. These studies indicate that about 3×10^5 units of human leukocyte interferon/kg body weight maintains serum interferon levels of about 100 units/ml for about 12 hours.

It was also mentioned that more purified interferon gave higher serum peaks but was cleared more rapidly (Cantell *et al.*, 1974). Using this dosage, Arvin, Yeager, and Merigan (1976) achieved serum interferon titers of about 500 units/ml in patients. Habif, Lipton, and Cantell (1975) also demonstrated similar clearance rate of human leukocyte interferon (30×10^6 units) in *Macaca sp.* monkey; rapid fall after intravenous, prolonged plateau after intramuscular inoculation.

---

[11] Human leukocyte interferon injections in all of these studies are at the purity of P-IF (about 10^5 to 10^6 units/mg of protein; see Fig. 11).

Finter (1973b) reported that mouse interferon injected intravenously into mice one day after interferon was induced in these animals by Newcastle disease virus or poly rI·poly rC was cleared more slowly than in control mice. Pyhala an Cantell (1974), however, found that the rate of clearance of human leukocyte in rabbits injected with or after Newcastle disease virus was not altered.

Jordan, Fried, and Merigan (1974) administered as much as 240 million units of human leukocyte interferon to a patient over a 3-day period. After slow intravenous infusion high serum levels were achieved, but prolonged levels of over 100 units/ml were obtained with intramuscular interferon injections, peaks rising after each daily dose. The only adverse effect observed was fever of 38 to 40° C after injections.

In one report (Emodi *et al.*, 1975a, b) 30×10^6 units of relatively crude human leukocyte interferon was inoculated intravenously into a patient and 6 hours later no serum interferon was detectable; however, intramuscular injection of 10^6 units reportedly gave a level of about 100 units/ml for about 6 hours, and low levels were detectable at 24 hours. Similar results were obtained after subcutaneous injections. While these authors report that no side reactions resulted from intramuscular or subcutaneous inoculations, shock occurred after intravenous application into a patient previously injected intramuscularly 20 times with 10^6 units.

Edy, Billiau, and Desomer (1975) presented preliminary data that human leukocyte and human fibroblast interferons had similar clearance rates in rabbits. Both cleared rapidly after injection into bloodstream and both survived longer after intramuscular dosages (Edy, Billiau, and Desomer, 1976b).

Desmyter and his collaborators (1976) reported that a patient with chronic hepatitis-B was injected with 10^7 units of human fibroblast interferon intramuscularly seven times in two weeks. Fever was the only side effect observed.

Cantell and Pyhala (1976) reported that whereas the purity of the human leukocyte interferon preparations influenced the rate at which interferon entered the bloodstream after intramuscular injection, it did not affect blood clearance of intravenously injected preparations. These workers also showed that circulating levels of interferons obtained by either intramuscular or intravenous injections cleared at similar rates.

Thus, as summarized in Fig. 21, human interferons are rapidly cleared from circulation following their intravenous injections into human beings, monkeys or rabbits. After intramuscular inoculations into these animals, interferon attains a slightly higher initial level than that reached at the same time after intravenous injection and then is cleared at a similar rate, but because of this initially higher peak, persists somewhat longer.

2. Clearance From the Cerebrospinal Fluid: The Blood-Brain-Barrier for Interferon

Little of the interferon introduced or produced in the bloodstream gets into the cerebrospinal fluid, and little of the interferon introduced into this com-

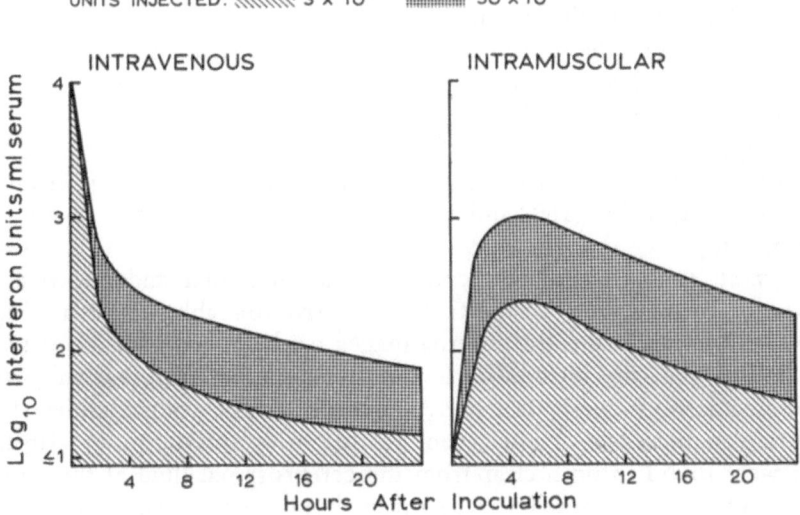

Fig. 21. Clearance rates of human interferons in man and other animals. Composites of data from the following references: Cantell and Pyhala (1973), Pyhala and Cantell (1974); Cantell *et al.* (1974); Mogensen *et al.* (1974); Edy *et al.* (1976b); Skreko *et al.* (1973); Cantell, Pyhala, and Strander (1974); Habif, Lipton, and Cantell (1975); Emodi *et al.* (1975a)

partment or produced in this location passes into circulation. Even in those inducers producing very high serum interferon levels, interferon in the cerebrospinal fluid or brain tissues remains relatively low. Thus Kono and Ho (1965) injected Sindbis virus intravenously in mice and obtained high titers of circulating interferon but little or no interferon in brain tissue. Poly rI·poly rC gave similar results in mice (Ho and Ke, 1970) and in rabbits (Cathala and Baron, 1970). Jameson, Schoenherr, and Grossberg (1970) reported that bluetongue virus inoculated intraperitoneally into rabbits induced about 10^5 units of interferon per ml of serum but only a few hundred units/gram was found in brain tissue.

On the other hand, when high levels of brain interferon are produced, serum interferon levels remain low. Thus Stewart II and Sulkin (1966) found high titers (3000 units/gram of tissue) of interferon in the brains of hamsters infected intramuscularly with rabies and little or no circulating interferon. Similarly intracerebral injections of West Nile virus induced high brain interferon titers (about 10^4 units/brain), but little or no interferon was detectable in blood (Stewart II, unpublished data). Cathala and Baron (1970) found that intrathecal inoculation of poly rI·poly rC gave lower levels of interferon in the blood stream than in the brain, and the brain levels were maintained longer. Allen and Cochran (1972) also found that brain interferon levels of mice injected intracerebrally with poly rI·poly rC or Sendai virus, though initially lower than those in blood, lasted significantly longer. Thus target-organ treatment with inducers or interferons may have advantages in certain situations. Luby, Sanders, and Sulkin (1971) found cerebrospinal fluid interferon in patients dying of Western equine encephalomyelitis virus infection, but no interferon was detectable in the serum.

Within the brain there also appears to be compartmentalization of interferon. Luby et al. (1969) found that patients dying from St. Louis encephalitis had interferon in frontal lobes, cerebellum and basal ganglia but not in brain stem. Luby, Sanders, and Sulkin (1971) also found marked differences in interferon content between certain areas of the brain in patients dying from Western equine encephalitis (1600 units/gram of basal ganglia vs ≤ 12 units/gram of cerebellum).

Ho et al. (1974) found that combined intramuscular and intravenous administration of interferon was partially protective for rabbits against rabies. Injections of interferon into the cisterna magna or the lateral ventricle maintained about 1 to 5% of the introduced levels after 24 hours. Intramuscular and intravenous injections were, however, more protective against rabies than intraventricular injections of interferon. In this study interferon and labelled albumin were found to both clear from the cerebrospinal fluid at the same rate. Habif, Lipton, and Cantell (1975) injected monkeys intramuscularly or intravenously with 30 million units of human leukocyte interferon and found that the level of interferon in the cerebrospinal fluid paralleled that in the bloodstream but at about $^1/_{30}$th the level in the serum. Interferon injected into the cerebrospinal fluid was also detectable in serum but at a level about $^1/_{30}$th that found in the cerebrospinal fluid, and both disappeared in parallel. Declercq et al. (1975) injected about 5 million units of crude human leukocyte interferon intrathecally into a newborn infant in 8 doses and found that 0.1 to 1% of the interferon injected could be recovered in the cerebrospinal fluid 12 or 24 hours after each injection, and significantly lower levels were detected in serum.

Hilfenhaus and his associates (1977) have administered human leukocyte interferon into the cerebrospinal fluid of monkeys after they were injected intramuscularly with rabiesvirus; these monkeys developed high antibody levels against rabiesvirus. Other monkeys were injected with interferon intramuscularly after virus infection and did not develop antibodies to rabiesvirus. Thus the virus appeared to replicate peripherally in the former monkeys but was arrested by interferon when it got to the central nervous system. Titers of interferon in cerebrospinal fluid of monkeys after intralumbar injection of 10^5 units were about 10^3 units/ml at 1 hour and 10^2 units/ml at 4 hours, with none detectable in serum. These authors interpret that the blood-brain-barrier prevents distribution to the whole body and thus allows high interferon levels to be achieved in the cerebrospinal fluid by lumbar-spinal injection.

3. Transplacental Passage and Other Barriers to Distribution of Interferon

A few studies have indicated that there are other compartment partitions restricting uniform interferon distributions within the body.

Ho, Postic, and Ke (1967) found that interferon injected into pregnant rabbits did not efficiently enter the blood of the embryo or the amniotic fluid. After inoculation with Newcastle disease virus the level of serum interferon in the maternal circulation was about 10^4 units/ml, the placenta contained about 10^3 units/ml, and the fetal blood contained about 10^2 units/ml. In view of the cell-multiplication-inhibitory effect of interferon, such a mother-fetus barrier may be important; in fact, it should be interesting to determine the effect of intrauterine or intraembryonic administration of interferon on growth and development of the fetus. Overall and Glasgow (1970) also found that high levels of interferon induced in the fetus by intrauterine inoculation of Newcastle disease virus did not enter the blood of the pregnant ewe. Korsantiya and Smorodintsev (1971) reported that induced maternal interferon seemed to cross the placenta to confer virus-resistance to mice shortly after birth. However, Schaefer et al. (1972) attributed this protection to interferon passed to sucklings via milk.

Interferon induced with endotoxin or poly rI·poly rC also may be restricted in migrating between the bloodstream and the aqueous and vitreous humor of the eye (Oh and Gill, 1966; Polikoff et al., 1970; Weissenbacher et al., 1970), in either direction. In one study, however, rabbits were injected subconjunctivally with poly rI·poly rC and high interferon levels were detected in the conjunctiva but only low levels were found in the cornea. Moderate levels of interferon were reported in the serum which apparently diffused into the conjunctiva of collateral eyes which showed presence of equal levels of interferon in the aqueous humor. Kobza et al. (1975) also reported that intramuscularly administered human leukocyte interferon (5×10^5 units) seemed to offer beneficial effect against herpes keratitis in a patient, suggesting passage from bloodstream to these tissues; as the serum levels themselves would be rather low in this situation, any effect would indicate rather unlimited passage.

B. Metabolism of Interferons

Distribution seems to account for only slight drops of interferon activities after its local production or injection. The possible role of renal clearance and tissue degradations have also been implicated.

1. Renal Clearance

Ho and Postic (1967) reported that interferon injected into rabbits was partially passed in urine, but this accounted for only about 1% of it. Ho (1967) calculated that renal clearance of virus-induced interferon and endotoxin-induced interferon occurred at somewhat different rates, presumably on basis of different molecular weights (Ke and Ho, 1967, 1968; Ho, 1973), the former being faster. Gresser et al. (1967b) detected injected interferon that was ejected in urine, and Bocci, Russi, and Rita (1967) found that about 2 to 20% of injected interferon was eliminated in this manner. Ho (1967) also reported that the collection of urine interferon was an important source of potent partially purified interferon preparations in his laboratory; fortunately we have since found better ways!

However, Waddell, Wilbur, and Merigan (1968) found that patients with mumps had high levels of serum interferon but little, if any, interferon in urine, and Bucknall, Finter, and Draper (1968) could not detect urine interferon in patients with various virus infections inducing serum interferon.

Human interferon inoculated intramuscularly into patients was also detectable (<10 units to 100 units/ml) in urine of most patients, but did not correlate with serum levels (Emodi et al., 1975a, b). Cesario and Tilles (1973) have reported that human interferon can be inactivated by urine; perhaps it is difficult therefore to account for appreciable losses by this route even if they occur. However, results in some of such studies suggest that losses of interferons through the kidneys or intestine are minimal (Bocci et al., 1968a, b; 1977a, b).

2. Catabolism of Interferon: Role of Carbohydrates

Early studies suggested that mouse and hamster interferons rapidly disappeared from isolated organs (Stewart II and Sulkin, 1966; Subrahmanyan and Mims, 1966). However, others have reported that rabbit interferon was not appreciably catabolized in this manner (Bocci et al., 1968b).

Bocci et al. (1968b) observed that the catabolic role of the perfused liver for rabbit interferon was initially slow and increased after about 90 minutes. As interferons are apparently glycoproteins this accelerated catabolism could suggest that terminal sialic acid residues were removed and the exposure of the penultimate galactose residues increased its hepatic clearance rate.

On such an assumption, Mogensen et al. (1974) attempted to modify the clearance of human leukocyte interferon in rabbits by treating it with neuraminidase. This experiment was, however, negative as the neuraminidase treatment did not alter the charge-heterogeneity of the interferon or its clearance rate; nor did presumably deglycosylating chemical treatments. These authors concluded that sialic acid did not contribute to pharmacokinetics of human leukocyte interferon. However, subsequent studies suggest otherwise. Stewart II et al. (1977) demonstrated that chemical modifications of carbohydrates altered the charge heterogeneity of human leukocyte interferons (Section VII. C. 1), and Bridgen et al. (1977) found similar effects of glycolytic enzymes on human lymphoblastoid interferon. Bose and Hickman (1977) found that human lymphoblastoid interferon injected intravenously into rats was cleared slightly more quickly after it was treated with neuraminidase. Similarly, Bocci et al. (1977a) found that removal of sialic acid of rabbit interferon by neuraminidase increased its clearance from perfusate of normal livers.

If this effect were due to increased exposure of the hepatic-recognized galactose residues, further deglycosylation of asialointerferons might remove this specific hepatic clearance and thus prolong circulating life of the interferon. In this regard, treatment of presumed asialointerferon with a mixture of glycosidases was recently reported to reverse its rapid clearance (Bose and Hickman, 1977).

These data suggest that interferons are glycoproteins that are cleared from circulation by removal of sialic acids and subsequent sequestration by hepatic recognition of the exposed galactose terminals. Confirmation of this effect is important. The apparently carbohydrate-free "interferoids" (Stewart II et al., 1978) or carbohydrate-free synthetic interferons (which are feasible to consider

because interferons can apparently still exert all their actions without carbohydrates; Stewart II *et al.*, 1978) may prove to have prolonged circulating
life-spans.

C. Effective Interferon Levels

Are prolonged circulating interferons desirable? We only assume so. But
perhaps it reflects interferon that is less effective, or defective, in binding *in
vivo.* Answers to these questions will only be available when sufficient
amounts of purified native interferon and interferoid are available to allow direct comparisons of their *in vivo* clearance rates, *in vivo* antiviral efficacies, antitumor actions and immunomodulatory activities.

It is difficult to evaluate the needed levels of interferon, and it is impossible
to extrapolate from circulating levels obtained with inducers how much exogenous interferon must be administered to achieve similar interferon effect.
Declercq (1977) has offered the untenable interpretation that the role of interferon induction in the mechanism of antitumor action of poly rI· poly rC can
be eliminated. This misinterpretation was based on the finding that administration of exogenous interferon in amounts "mimicking" the interferon blood
levels induced by endogenous poly rI·poly rC failed to duplicate the antitumor
effect of the inducer. Such studies fail to consider that circulating interferon
levels seen with inducers likely represent spillover interferon. And, importantly, they ignore the fact that, as was succinctly pointed out by Dianzani and
Baron (1975), the concentration of interferon occuring in the intercellular
spaces in tissue surrounding an interferon-producing cell *in vivo* are very much
higher than levels measured in circulation. Dianzani and Baron (1975) calculated that immediate environment of interferon surrounding producers could
be as high as 10^7 units/ml.

It is generally assumed that a maintained interferon-induced effect requires
maintained interferon levels, apparently because that is the situation with antibiotics. However, interferon induces an effect of some duration, during
which it may not be needed. The required doses to maintain "desired" levels
are presently purely guesses, and the present guess is: the more the better.
However, certain of the limitations presently imposed by suspected impurities
may prove to be an intrinsic property of interferon, and the benefits of main-
taining high levels of interferon may be offset by the adverse effects. It should
be considered that the interferons were designed for rapid clearance because
there are reasons for its rapid removal. In fact, the non-specific prodromal
symptoms of generalized virus diseases (headache, fever, anorexia, and malaise)
have regularly been encountered with inoculations of interferons. It is tempting
to speculate that interferon, which is the common denominator in such virus
diseases, is responsible for these symptoms. As indicated in Section X, it may
induce prostaglandin E, it may enhance histamine release, and it may induce
hyaluronic acid; it may induce "interferon fever" and it may account for
common prodrome in virus diseases. In fact, interferon may account for febrile
responses to endotoxin, an interferon inducer. It would be interesting to determine febrile responses of animals inoculated with anti-interferon antibodies
prior to injection with interferon inducers.

XII. Antiviral Actions of Interferons in Animals

Interferon production is usually a constant companion to virus replication during the course of virus infections (Stewart II and Sulkin, 1966; Luby, Sanders, and Sulkin, 1971; Luby et al., 1969; Vilček, 1969; Vilček and Stancek, 1963 a; Link et al., 1965), as opposed to the rapid rise and fall of interferon levels seen following large doses of intravenously injected virus, and the influence of interferon during virus infections is thus exerted at each stage of pathogenesis.

In this Section I shall describe the studies on involvement of interferon in the resistance to virus infections in non-human animals. This is not to imply that the role of interferon is different in man; rather all the studies on interferon in humans are for convenience of reference grouped in Section XIV. The studies on antitumor activities of interferons in animals are described in Section XIII, again for reference function, not to imply that these actions are distinct from those reviewed here.

In summary, this Section will show that interferon is a key determinant of resistance to initiation of virus infection, in determining severity of these infections, and in determining recovery from infections with viruses.

A. Natural Recovery Processes From Viral Infections

The ability of a normal animal to resist virus infection, or once infected to rid itself of the virus, is impressive. Most infections with potentially lethal viruses are eliminated even before they can cause symptoms. Only very few avoid early eradication and manage to establish infections and cause disease. And most of those that do are only briefly tolerated by the host animal which rapidly rids itself of the invader and continues as before. Thus the primary defense mechanisms are highly efficient, with only a very small failure rate, and the back-up defenses add several magnitudes of efficiency to this, such that of the total exposures to potentially lethal virus infections, only a statistically insignificant number produce disease, and of those animals developing disease an insignificant proportion fail to recover completely.

While it is beyond the scope of this text to comprehensively cover each of the host factors mediating resistance and recovery from virus infections, it is important to present an abbreviated analysis of the interplays of these mechanisms, so that the effects of augmentations of the interferon system can be evaluated.

It is important to have answers to these questions: What factors are involved in deciding susceptibility to viruses? When is the outcome of virus infection predestined? and, Can outcome be altered after virus infections are symptomatic? If interferon plays a crucial role only in early events (establishment of infection in target tissues), its application later would be wasted, and its role would be limited to prophylaxis. If outcome of generalized virus disease is determined prior to appearance of symptoms, interferon, or anything else, would be worthless as antiviral therapy. Indeed, the whole concept of antiviral *therapy* is based on the premise that the outcome of viral diseases can be altered by inhibiting further virus replication after symptoms in generalized virus infections have developed. Evidence for this, however, has been slight, and it is only with recent studies that it has even been possible to conclusively demonstrate the involvement of interferon in determining outcome of such virus infections.

It is possible to separately describe each of the factors involved in determining recovery from viral diseases; it is not possible, however, to assess their relative importance, which likely vary in different diseases as well as at different stages during the course of each disease.

It is possible that continued replication of virus in target tissues after it has reached its peak level and has produced symptoms is responsible for disease severity. In such cases late inhibition of this "tailing-effect" of virus would be advantageous. In other cases, it is possible that once symptoms occur virus replication is virtually finished, in which case antiviral treatment is worthless. Often the mechanisms by which the body eliminates the virus are the processes causing the disease.

It will also become apparent in these discussions that many of the factors work synergistically so that recovery is a composite effect.

1. Progression of Virus Infections

In this segment I shall briefly reconstruct various virus disease processes, to indicate steps at which outcome can be altered and shall indicate which defense mechanisms are involved at each step.

a) Localized Infections

Influenza viruses, parainfluenza viruses, adenoviruses, rhinoviruses and coronaviruses can all cause symptoms by local replication at the site of introduction into the host; such infections are usually referred to as "common colds", if they become symptomatic, which most don't (Bradburne and Tyrrell, 1971; Bradburne and Somerset, 1972). The symptoms are primarily caused by local cell damage by the replication of the virus, and the incubation period (between virus inoculation and symptoms) is usually only 1 to 3 days, just long enough for a few virus cycles to cause sufficient cellular involvement to be noticeable.

The restriction of infections with the coronaviruses and rhinoviruses to the upper respiratory tract may be because these viruses grow best at lower than body temperatures (Tyrrell, 1968; Bradburne, 1972). Recovery from these infections is usually complete within a few days, without residual effects.

Influenza virus can involve both the upper and lower respiratory tract. The neuraminidase produced at local infection foci facilitates involvement of large areas of the ciliated epithelial layer; with respiratory symptoms resulting from the ensuing desquamation. The constitutional disturbances reported in man likely also occur in animals, and the malaise, fever, and joint pains are not readily accountable in terms of virus replication. It has been proposed that viral replicative-product double-stranded RNA might account for such symptoms, but it is difficult to imagine serum survival of these molecules in primates in view of serum double-stranded ribonuclease levels (Levy et al., 1975). It is interesting that many of these symptoms also occur in patients injected with interferons (Section XI: fever, joint pain, malaise, anorexis). In fact, in view of the many non-antiviral actions described in Section X, such as the reported "interferon fevers", prostaglandin E induction, histamine release and hyaluronic acid production, it is tempting to speculate that serum interferon is not only the common denominator of virus infections, but is also the common denominator of many of the non-specific premonitory symptoms of virus diseases. In fact, these symptoms in man seem to parallel the serum interferon levels persisting after its inoculation (Fig. 21), and in virus infections with viremia may parallel induced serum interferon levels.

In some animals it has been demonstrated that influenza virus infection is localized for reasons of cell susceptibilities (Gould et al., 1972). It can also induce local interferon production both in man and animals (Isaacs and Hitchcock, 1960; Gresser and Dull, 1964; Link et al., 1965; Link, Blaskovic, and Raus, 1965) which could facilitate its arrest, and the cell damage due to viral replication may initiate chemotactic phagocytic infiltration (Snyderman, Wohlenberg, and Notkins, 1972). Also by the time infection has progressed to this stage, the mononuclear infiltration could have acquired immuno-enhanced interferon producing capacity (Glasgow, 1966; Green, Cooperband, and Kibrick, 1969; Epstein, Stevens, and Merigan, 1972). Also, cell-mediated immunity has been shown to develop in influenza virus infections (Rossen, Kasel and Couch, 1971), and the contribution of interferon would be amplified by serving both to sensitize infected target cells (Svet–Moldavsky, and Chernyakovskaya, 1967; Svet–Moldavsky et al., 1974) or effector cells (Lindahl, Leary, and Gresser, 1972). Also the sensitized lymphocyte could produce enhanced levels of interferons when interacting with the target cells (Svet–Moldavsky et al., 1974). And interferon could act by enhancing the ingestive appetite of infiltrating phagocytic elements (Huang et al., 1971; Donahoe and Huang, 1973, 1976; Imanishi et al., 1975).

Local infection with primary herpes-virus can occur in the eye or mucus membranes of the genitalia. It can also locally infect traumatized skin. The most common primary herpes virus infection, acute herpetic gingivostomatitis is usually self-limiting in 1 or 2 weeks. Primary herpesvirus infection of the eye can produce keratitis which is usually severe, often lasting several months and producing a dense vision-impairing scar. Mechanisms for this eventual limitation are not clear; the evidence for interferon involvement in pathogenesis of herpesvirus infection, both localized and systemic, will be described below.

Local infection of skin at site of inoculation can also occur with vaccinia virus. Several studies using rabbits have demonstrated the importance of cell-mediated immunity in arresting vaccinia progression and in eliminating the infectious focus (Flick and Pincus, 1963; Pincus and Flick, 1963) and in man similar mechanisms seem important (Freed, Duma, and Escobar, 1972; Douglas, Lynch, and Spira, 1972). However, the contention that interferon plays no significant role (Freed, Duma, and Escobar, 1972) does not consider that induced interferon can work interdependently with both humoral and cellular immune mechanisms, as described previously. Thus when one is defective the efficiency of the others is reduced and recovery, which is often a delicate balance of multiple factors, can be effected.

b) Generalized Infections

Disease with most virus infections is not produced at the portal of entry but results from virus passage to and replication in specific target tissues. This passage can be either through the bloodstream (viremic spread) or along nerves. All these virus infections have prolonged incubation periods. Characteristic late symptoms of the specific diseases are determined by the target tissues involved, the mechanisms involved in the replication of the virus and mechanisms of host defenses enlisted to eliminate the infection.

i) Nervous Spread: Rabies. Nervous spread from the portal of entry to the target tissue, the central nervous system is seen in rabies, herpesvirus and polio. As the latter two viruses are most commonly generalized by hematogenous routes these will be dealt with later. Rabiesvirus is usually inoculated into a bite wound (though oral and respiratory routes have been reported), from which site it migrates by peripheral nervous routes (though viremia may occur in some cases) to the central nervous system (CNS). Interruption of nerve paths between the site of inoculation will prevent spread of virus to the CNS and thus prevent disease (Stewart II, 1973). Virus does not "grow" up nerve paths but rather "flows" up them at a speed of about 2 to 3 mm per hour, apparently via conduit in the interspaces within nerve bundles.

The incubation period of rabies in man is variable between about 13 days to over 9 months. Though often believed to be dependent on the distance of the bite-wound (inoculation site) from the head, this relationship is likely to be because bites nearer the head are often more severe, thus more virus initially being inoculated. The locally inoculated virus apparently remains at or near the site of the wound for most of the incubation period, and only begins to migrate to the CNS at a relatively fixed interval of about 2 weeks before development of symptoms. Thus the length of the incubation period depends on the amount of virus introduced, with migration not initiated until local virus replication has reached levels "triggering" this migration. This temporary local arrest of virus at the site of inoculation has very important implications for the postexposure "therapy" of rabies, as local treatment of wounds with interferon or interferon inducers has been significantly more effective in prevention of rabies than treatment with interferon or inducers at other sites (Harmon and Janis, 1975).

After rabies virus reaches the CNS, it infects only specific neurons, the Purkinje's cells, in the gray matter (Johnson and Mims, 1968), but produces no evidence of neuronal cytopathology, inflammation or cell necrosis up until death (Campbell et al., 1968). However, cellular dysfunctioning becomes first evident, presumably as the virus replicates to disruptive levels within the infected (though intact) nerve cells. It is apparently important to reemphasize here, as before (Stewart II, 1973), that rabiesvirus – even up to death of the host – does not cause any detectable neuronal damage. Alarmingly, it has even recently been stated that this virus causes neuronal destruction even before neurologic symptoms develop (Carter et al., 1975). This would imply that antiviral therapy would be worthless in rabies. In fact, quite the contrary is likely, in view of the case of Matthew Winkler, which is discussed below.

Nerve cell dysfuntioning in rabies is first associated with non-specific symptoms of anorexia, headache, malaise, vomiting and fever. Subsequently, excessive salivation and biting are common in patients shortly after presentation, often with the classical signs of hydrophobia, extreme fear and anxiety and sensational abnormalities at the site of the wound, with paralysis in this locality common. Disease usually progresses to coma and death within a few days (from 1 to 20 days), resulting from respiratory or cardiac arrests.

However, some recent cases have been reported in which comatose disease lasted significantly longer (28 to more than 100 days), owing to intensive supportive therapy. And, in one case, that of Matthew Winkler (a 6-year-old boy bitten by a rabid bat), supportive therapy was sufficient to allow complete recovery from proven clinical rabies with no sequelae (Hattwick et al., 1972). This case shows that, rather than rabies being a futile disease to attempt antiviral therapy, it appears to be a prime candidate. Interferon treatment in cases of clinical rabies might aid in suppression and elimination of the virus from infected (but not destroyed) nervous tissues, and if patients can be maintained with intensive supportive therapy (such as tracheal suction and oxygen to reverse respiratory arrests and cardiac arryhthmias) recovery might be facilitated.

Rabiesvirus has been reported to be sensitive to dog interferon in dog kidney cells (Depoux, 1965), to hamster interferon in BHK 21 hamster cells (Stewart II and Sulkin, 1968), and to mouse interferon (Karakuyumchan and Bektemirova, 1968). Rabiesvirus is able to induce interferon (Stewart II and Sulkin, 1966; Vieuchange, 1967a, b). However, in both hamsters and mice interferon production only paralleled virus replication, suggesting that endogenously induced interferon was too little and too late to abort the establishment of infection (Stewart II and Sulkin, 1966; Karakuyumchan and Bektemirova, 1968; Campbell et al., 1968).

Rabies prophylaxis with interferon was early reported in guinea-pigs whose wounds were infiltrated with guinea-pig interferon (Kaplan et al., 1962), but the effect was slight, at best. Finter (1967b) reported that interferon administration failed to protect mice against rabies, but Vieuchange (1967b) reported that interferon protected rabbits; clearly in both cases interferon dosage was low. Induction of endogenous interferon by statolon gave also only slight protection in mice, though serum interferon levels were high (Soave, 1968). Exogenous interferon was reported to inhibit development of rabies in mice when given intramuscularly but not when interferon was inoculated intracerebrally (Karakuyumchan and Bektemirova, 1968). Nemes *et al.* (1969a, b) obtained moderate protection of mice against rabies by injections of poly rI·poly rC before virus, and Fenje and Postic (1970) reported that poly rI·poly rC, administered either before or up to 24 hours after injection of rabbits with rabiesvirus, protected most of the animals (Postic and Fenje, 1971b). These investigators also showed that interferon *per se*, at doses of about 10^6 units per rabbit, protected against rabies if given simultaneously with the virus, and prolonged the incubation period when given 24 hours after infection (Postic and Fenje, 1971a). In one study poly rI·poly rC alone protected mice against rabies, while chlorite-oxidized amylose (COAM) enhanced its mortality (Harmon, Janis, and Levy, 1974). Induction of endogenous interferon by orally administered tilorone hydrochloride completely protected mice against either subcutaneous or intracerebral challenge with low doses (<10 LD_{50}) of rabiesvirus and prolonged incubation periods with large challenge doses of 100 or 1000 LD_{50} (Fornosi *et al.*, 1971).

Stewart II and Sulkin (1966) suggested that the protective value of the Pasteur post-exposure anti-rabies prophyllaxis might be due to induction of interferon by the large doses of vaccine-virus. Wiktor and his colleagues (1972), in fact, found that rabies vaccine of tissue culture origin given shortly before or after rabies challenge protected hamsters against death, and the rabies vaccine stimulated circulating interferon. Rabies vaccines also induced interferons in rabbits and in human and rabbit cell cultures. Rabies vaccine in mice induced rapid induction of *both* circulating interferon and brain interferon, and it was suggested that the protective effect of this vaccine was mediated through interferon rather than antibodies (Wiktor *et al.*, 1972). Similarly, Baer and Cleary (1972) and Baer *et al.* (1977) speculated that the high levels of interferon induced by rabies vaccines that were effective in protecting mice might be responsible for the protection, rather than the antibodies induced later. Nozaki and Atanasiu (1975) also found that rabies vaccines with high protective indices induced high interferon titers in mice and hamsters, and suggested that the protection by these vaccines is double: non-specific (interferon) at early times, and specific (antibodies) at 4 to 5 days.

Ho *et al.* (1974) attempted prevention of rabies in rabbits by daily intraventricular injections of 10^6 units of interferon/day for up to 3 weeks. The outcome was less favorable than when 10^6 units were given in an intramuscular and intravenous dose at the time of challenge.

Baer and his associates (1977) recently reported that addition of interferon to ineffective rabiesvirus vaccines or local injection of the inducing complex of poly rI·poly rC·poly L·lysine and carboxymethylcellulose in rabies-infected mice dramatically reduced mortality. Similar results were obtained in rhesus monkeys.

Human interferon inoculated intramuscularly beginning 24 hours after infection of Cynomolgus monkeys with rabiesvirus was reported to protect them (Hilfenhaus *et al.*, 1975). Monkeys received from 10^5 to 10^6 units/day for about 10 days and virus was given in the neck. Interferon given in this manner starting at a time when clinical rabies had developed was without effect.

Janis and Habel (1972) demonstrated better protection of mice and rabbits if poly rI·poly rC was injected into the same site as rabiesvirus. Harmon and Janis (1975) also found that poly rI·poly rC was protective in mice if injected shortly after challenge into the same intramuscular site as the rabiesvirus; however, if injected in the opposite leg, it was not effective; the locally-injected muscle always contained 4 to 8 times more interferon than the noninjected muscle.

Wiktor and his collaborators (1976) found that Rhesus monkeys could be completely protected against rabies by a single dose of highly concentrated human diploid cell-derived rabiesvirus vaccine given several hours after rabiesvirus infection. Protection was related to ability of this vaccine to induce interferon; less concentrated vaccine was unable to induce interferon and was only partially protective; the level of virus-neutralizing antibody induced by the vaccines did not correlate with protection.

Recent studies have reported that 114 rabies-virus-infected Cynomologus monkeys were treated with human leukocyte interferon, intramuscularly and/or intralumbarly (Hilfenhaus et al., 1977; Majer, Weinmann, and Hilfenhaus, 1977). With dosages of about 10^6 units/day intramuscularly beginning 24 hours after virus, about 50% protection was achieved. When interferon was given into the cerebrospinal fluid, it was possible to achieve similar protection even when treatment was delayed until 11 days after infection. However, no effect was observed if clinical rabies had developed before treatment; of course no physical supportive therapy was given along with the interferon, and animals died within 1 to 3 days after developing symptoms. In human rabies, however, death usually does not result for several days after symptoms occur, so that interferon and supportive therapy would have greater chance of success.

These studies clearly indicate that interferon is a primary determinant in prevention of development of rabies; they do not indicate what mechanisms might be effective in arresting the virus-induced brain misfunctioning after symptoms have developed. If rabies nervous disease can, in fact, be completely reversed, as suggested by the Winkler case, the recovery mechanism must be non-cytocidal and not involve extensive cell-mediated immunity, suggesting that interferon is directly involved.

ii) Viremic Spread. The vast majority of virus diseases result from virus infections which spread from the portal of entry (respiratory tract, GI tract, or insect bite) to the target tissue (liver, skin or brain) by the bloodstream (Fig. 22). However, this viremic spread is not direct, but first requires an asymptomatic replication phase at a secondary site at or near the initial entry point. From this focus of infection virus spills into the bloodstream (primary viremia: low virus titers) to relocate at secondary foci in internal organs. After extensive replication in these tissues, the virus bursts into a sustained and substantial secondary viremia which allows it to seed the "target" tissue. This pattern can consume several days, and the similarities of this process in numerous virus infections explains many of their common premonitory symptoms. The interferon induced by the secondary viremia, also being common to virtually all these infections, may also explain the similarities of the non-specific signs of these infections in advance of the viruses localizing in specific target tissues.

The severity of disease is related to the level of the secondary viremia in two ways:

a) The level of secondary viremia is determined by the extent of systemic multiplication: this can sometimes be the major cause of disease, due to damage to these tissue (e. g. giving rise to the liver damage and hence the jaundice of yellow fever).

b) Higher and more prolonged viremia makes it more likely that inoculation of the target tissue will succeed.

The interferon induced by the secondary viremia may in fact cause the febrile, non-specific premonitory symptoms, but it can also confer some virus resistance to the target tissue, provided the barriers between the blood and the target are passable, which may depend on the level of the interferonemia.

Thus an "avirulent" virus might be one that had identical invasive properties to a more virulent strain, was able to replicate to the same extent locally in primary and in secondary foci and which produced the same level of secondary viremia, yet induced higher levels of interferon during the secondary viremia, thus more effectively preventing subsequent target-tissue replication. If this relation indeed exists it would be tempting to speculate that there would be an inverse correlation between severity of prodromal symptoms (possibly determined by interferon levels) and outcome of disease. Such "data" are available only in the old-wives tales relating strong fevers to strong recoveries.

Recovery can also depend on control of virus growth in the secondary foci, thus avoiding both severity-possibilities 1 and 2, above. Usually replication at the secondary foci produces no symptoms or only minor illness, the only prodrome often being the fever, malaise, etc., accompanying the second viremia (and interferonemia).

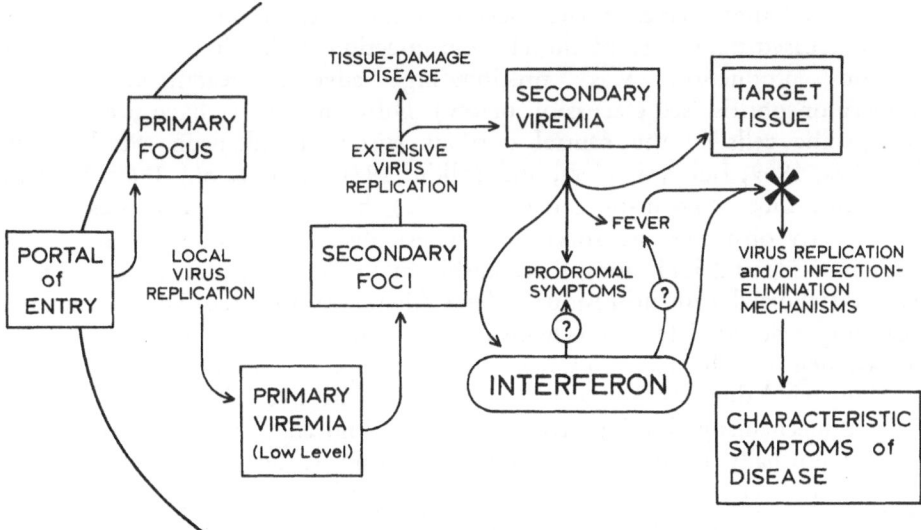

Fig. 22. Possible involvements of interferon in generalized viral diseases

The second viremia often initiates "target tissue" infections in the skin and mucous membranes which lead to developments of pathonomonic rashes due to types of cells effected and mechanisms of formation. This apparent predilection for the body surface may reflect the fact that the viremia-induced (interferon-induced?) febrile response often elevates body temperatures above those allowing virus growth. Thus, while poxvirus cannot grow above a temperature of 38.5° C, body temperature due to viremia often may exceed 39° C (Bedson and Dumbell, 1961), as they do with interferon injections (Strander et al., 1974). Consequently, virus replication occurs only at external surfaces. The importance of the febrile response has long been recognized as an important determinant of virus infections, and the intriguing possibility that interferon is the factor triggering this response significantly expands the potential role of interferon in altering the pathogenesis of virus disease. If the second viremia fails to seed the central nervous system, the pathology is limited and recovery is assured by the time these distinguishing symptoms of virus infection have appeared. Antiviral therapy at this point would have no effect on the disease.

However, if the viremia has established central nervous system infection, antiviral therapy would be advantagous. Within the nervous tissue, damage can result from virus replication causing cell destruction (as in polio or lymphocytic choriomeningitis virus in adult mice) or cellular dysfunction (as in rabies). However, virus replication in the brain does not necessarily cause acute disease. In chronic lymphocytic choriomeningitis virus infection of mice, virus brain levels can be as high as those acutely infected; in the former the infection is immunologically tolerated; and in the latter it is immunologically recognized, thus precipitating cell-mediated attack and destruction of infected brain tissue (Gilden et al., 1972).

The role of interferon in chronic lymphocytic choriomeningitis has been clearly demonstrated by Riviere et al. (1977) by use of antibodies to interferon, in which case virus levels increase significantly. However, this important study also showed that increased virus levels in the tolerant mice were associated with decreased pathology of the chronic infection, indicating that chronic interferon production was precipitating adverse reactions: runting, glomerulonephritis (see discussion below). Different viruses have predilections for specific cells in the central nervous system (Nathanson, Stolley, and Boolukas, 1969; Luby, Sanders, and Sulkin, 1971; Luby et al., 1969; Nathanson et al., 1966; Nathanson and Cole, 1970). Even with those viruses passing all the early obstacles and succeeding in establishing infections in the central nervous tissue and replicating there sufficient to cause disease, most infections are soon aborted with no residual effects (therefore no extensive cell damage), indicating that the defense mechanisms have not surrendered the fight even at the last step. On this late resistence hangs the hope of antiviral therapy.

Many viral diseases that seem to have been effectively handled by host resistance mechanisms develop sequelae. Thus, children who appear to have recovered normally from measles months to years earlier develop slow mental deterioration characterized as subacute sclerosing panencephalitis (SSPE). Measles virus isolates are identifiable in these tissues (Connolly et al., 1967; Chen et al., 1969; Katz, Oyanagi, and Koprowski, 1969; ter Meulen, et al.,

1972 a, b). Thus, it appears that viruses are not always efficiently eliminated by defense mechanisms, but rather defensive mechanism can alter the pathologic processes. It has been suggested that mice also develop "slow virus" diseases following infection with and apparent recovery from arbovirus infections (Zlotnick et al., 1972). Gresser et al. (1976b) have demonstrated that antiserum to interferon can alter the pathologic process with encephalitic virus, accelerating fatality and involving tissues not normally affected. Perhaps it is not premature to consider that artifical augmentation of host resistance mechanisms (e. g. exogenous interferon late in encephalitic infections) might have the opposite effect: thus converting acute virus disease to subacute (slow) virus infections. Katz and Koprowski (1968) have shown that interferon was not effective at low dose against the slowvirus Scrapie. However, it would be more interesting to see if antiserum to interferon would accelerate the pathogenesis of slowvirus diseases.

2. Factors Modifying Pathogenesis: Interactions With Interferon Mechanism

As the virus races to establish infection, spread and proliferate, the host responds to restrict the invader. The efficacy of these responses depends on a multiple of non-specific "predisposing" factors such as the physiological well-being of the host. These non-specific factors likely operate in regard to their interaction with the interferon system and the immune system. The relative significance of any of these is difficult to ascertain, as recovery is clearly a composite of their effects. It is possible, however, to show that each is important, as either immunodepressions or interferonodepressions can enhance virus susceptibilities (Gresser et al., 1976b, c).

a) Restriction of Establishment of Infections

i) Primary Infections. The entry of virus into the body initiates the protective reaction mechanisms of interferon, cell-mediated immunity, antibody and non-specific reaction. In primary exposures to the particular virus these reactions are probably all too little and too late to prevent establishment of infection locally and, thus, most first-time infections are initially successful.

Interferon is probably not produced in sufficient amounts to prevent primary portal of entry infections, as the first cycle of virus will likely be nearly complete before interferon is produced, which usually requires several hours (Fig. 6). Also the interferon produced by the single or few, initially infected cells would likely not be sufficient to protect all the neighboring cells invaded by the primary progeny. And the interferon produced in response to the initial invader must then induce antiviral resistance in the cells it contacts, again a process requiring several hours (Fig. 16), and this may not have become developed before the second or third generation virions can partially arrest its progression by destroying such cells. Thus, the ability of the virus in establishing at the portal of entry or primary focus is likely related to its ability to induce interferon and to its sensitivity to the interferon. In some cases, this inhibition could arrest infections by totally blocking virus production as the early stages (Fig. 17), or interferon could cause the cells to produce progeny

18*

which are "enriched" for defective virions (the role of defective-interfering particles in pathogenesis will be discussed below).

The viruses' initial success could also depend on such factors as the type of cells infected initially (site of entry). It has been demonstrated, for example, that route of infection can determine recovery in smallpox, the dermal route related to benignity, the respiratory route being virulent (Wheelock, 1964). Also, it is possible that the type of tissue infected can influence the defectiveness of the progeny. The speed of the virus replication cycle and its ability to inhibit cellular synthesis (thus shutting off interferon production and/or action) can also influence early success of infections. That input virus is initially able to avoid the interferon system is clearly demonstrable in cell cultures: viruses which are able to induce interferon and which are sensitive to the interferon induced are able to form plaques in such cells; apparently the interferon restriction eventually takes hold after a few virus cycles, as the plaques are size-limited. However, the addition of antiserum against interferon to such cultures allows the virus to produce significantly larger plaques (Fauconnier, 1970) and increases virus yields (Vilček, Yamazaki, and Havell, 1977).

Antibody production is clearly too slow to prevent initial primary infection at the entry site. The entering virus must usually multiply many times before it constitutes sufficient antigenic mass to even trigger antibody production (Fenner, 1965). However, the specious argument often proffered that antibody, appearing later than interferon, plays no important role in protection against or recovery from primary viral infection, is untenable. Even though antibody appears too late to prevent establishment of primary infections, it can modify later stages of the process, even in primary infections, as will be discussed below.

Lymphocytes migrating into the primary infection focus will interact with infected cells to initiate the cell-mediated immunolytic mechanisms and attracted phagocytic elements can ingest and digest virus-infected cells (see Stewart II, 1973, for Refs.). These processes are initially too low level to be effective at the initial stages but can probably play a role later to help restrict the infection to this locale. As was previously indicated (Section X), interferon may increase the level of the cell-mediated reaction and the phagocytic activity.

The local inflammatory reaction consisting of local leukocyte accumulation, acidity, fever, and hypoxia has been attributed to tissue damage caused by the virus replication, but may result from immune-mediated interactions of cells (Synderman, Wohlenberg, and Notkins, 1972), which may in turn be related to the release of interferon in the area, indirectly through its enhancing of histamine release (Ida et al., 1977) or induction of prostaglandin E (Yaron et al., 1977). It should again be recalled that injection of interferon preparations have been reported to cause this local febrile reaction (Desomer, Edy, and Billiau, 1977). Thus each of these conditions can serve as an adjunct to the resistance process and each in turn may be augmented by the interferon response. Thus each of these manifestations of infection resistance can be considered as part of the in vivo interferon system.

It has been repeatedly demonstrated that elevated hormone levels can increase the susceptibilities of animals to virus infections, and this has been related partly to the interferon inhibitory influences of hormone (Kilbourne, Smart, and Pikorny, 1961; DeMaeyer and DeMaeyer, 1963; Smart and Kilbourne, 1966; Rytel and Kilbourne, 1966; Talas and Stoger, 1972).

It has occasionally been reported that increased temperature is correlated with decreased susceptibility to virus and increased interferon responsiveness (Ruiz–Gomez and Sosa–Martinez, 1965; Stancek, 1965); suggesting that contribution of fever to interferon production causes elimination of infection. However, this correlation is inconsistent (Section V. D. 2).

Hyperthermia may also be protective against viruses by decreasing viral replicase activity or by activating cellular ribonucleases (Lwoff, 1969)[11a].

In the absence of a specific block for interferon action it was only possible for many years to speculate on the role of endogenous interferon in resistance to virus infections in animals. Many early studies demonstrated that correlations could occasionally be found between the abilities of animals to produce interferons in response to certain virus and their abilities to resist these infections (Isaacs and Baron, 1960; Baron and Isaacs, 1962; Sawicki, 1961; Heineberg, Gold, and Robbins, 1964; Rytel and Kilbourne, 1971); but on the other hand most studies failed to support this correlation, increased susceptibility often even being associated with greater interferon production, likely as a consequence of better replication of virus providing more inducer, thus more interferon detectable (Vilček, 1964 b; Craighead, 1966).

However, recently the involvement of endogenous interferon in the natural resistance to virus diseases has been clearly demonstrated. Fauconnier (1971) demonstrated that inoculation of antibodies prepared against mouse interferon into mice injected with Semliki Forest virus lead to both earlier onset of disease and increased mortality. Gresser and his colleagues (1976 b, c) employed a highly potent antiserum to mouse interferon and demonstrated convincingly the key role of interferon in the early response to several virus infections. This antiserum, which was capable of neutralizing about 10 units of interferon at a dilution of about 2×10^{-6} (Table 10), caused rapid evolution of encephalomyocarditis virus-disease in mice. It is also noteworthy that the pathogenesis was entirely different from the disease developing in normal mice: the mice died of visceral damage (enhanced virus replication at secondary foci) and showed no signs of central nervous system disease (the normal target tissue). Thus production of interferon early in disease restricts visceral replication, but still may not always be sufficient to spare the animal from target-tissue infection.

These workers (Gresser et al., 1976 c) also studied the role of interferon in infections with herpes simplex, Moloney sarcoma, vesicular stomatitis, Newcastle disease and influenza virus infections by inoculating mice with anti-interferon. Herpes simplex virus disease was accelerated, and the infectivity of this virus was increased by several hundred-fold in lethal dose/ml of virus stock. The antibodies also caused earlier appearance of Moloney Sarcoma virus tumors, which became much larger and were present longer than in control

---

[11a] In this regard, it would be interesting to see if the nuclease activated in interferon-treated cell-free systems by LMWIT (Fig. 17) can be thermally activated.

mice. Importantly, the tumor-inducing efficiency of the virus was 100-fold greater in antiserum-treated mice. The antiserum also shortened the incubation period in mice inoculated intranasally with vesicular stomatitis virus. However, the antiserum did not alter influenza virus infection in mice, even when the antiserum was injected intranasally, perhaps because the anti-interferon did not diffuse to the tracheobronchial epithelium. These data clearly demonstrate the early role of endogenous interferon responses in virus resistance to primary virus disease. Apparently, the interferon system is able to protect animals against virus infections *without antibody* involvement; it would be interesting to determine the role of interferon in immunized animals; by use of anti-interferon serum it would be possible to see if antibodies are sufficient for protection in such infections *without interferon* involvement.

Thus, if present at the time of infections, interferon can prevent the establishment of virus infections. Cell-mediated or humoral immunity can also prevent establishment of virus if present at the start of infections. However, at early stages of primary infection, these latter factors are likely present in insufficient amounts. Their roles must be re-evaluated later in the infectious process and during reinfections in the immune animal, when they appear earlier and are quantitatively, and qualitatively, more efficient.

ii) Reinfections. Since the ability to resist establishment of infections is directly related to the speed with which the host can react to the virus, most *re*infections are not successful in becoming established.

The ability of the cells to produce interferon is specifically enhanced in lymphocytes from immune animals (Glasgow, 1966; Green, Cooperband, and Kibrick, 1969). This enhancement is also extended to substances that would not previously have been interferon inducers in the unsensitized animal (Epstein, Stevens, and Merigan, 1972).

Antibody production on the memory-basis is also quicker and quantitatively enhanced, and the anamnestic antibodies have higher avidity than early (primary) response antibodies (Fenner, 1965). Several studies have reported correlations between virus resistance and the speed with which animals can produce antibodies (Subrahmanyan, 1968; Schell, 1960). However, early and/or already present antibodies do not always prevent repeat virus-invaders from reestablishing. Reinfection-associated rise in antibody is often found following second exposures to measles virus (Stokes *et al.*, 1961), suggesting that the infection proceeded past initial entry but the infection process was limited to subclinical levels. Some arboviruses have been shown to replicate for the first 24 hours in immune animals to the same level as in primary infections (Stewart II, 1973), suggesting that these reinfections are not prevented from reestablishing, but that the pathogenesis is altered subsequent to primary foci proliferation.

Localized viral re-infections of the respiratory tract are possibly prevented in part by local secretory antibodies (Rossen *et al.*, 1966; Chanock, 1970; Mills *et al.*, 1971), but in many of these infections neither secretory nor serum antibodies develop, and resistance may be mediated by specific-recognition type enhanced interferon responsiveness, and specific cell-mediated immunity likely plays a role in resisting reinfections with viruses invading at these sites (Stewart II, 1973).

Those viruses that are able to reestablish in the host previously infected with the same virus are often eliminated by immune-mediated cell-destroying mechanisms, either antibody- or cell-mediated immune lysis. This type of intruder-arrest can prevent secondary infections from becoming established, and it can also act to eliminate primary infections later after they have become established. Thus sensitized cells or specific antibodies, in the presence of complement, can combine to destroy a wide variety of virus-infected cells (Stewart II, 1973), and recall that the cytotoxicity of both antibodies (Skurkovich, Klinova, and Eremkina, 1976) and lymphocytes (Svet–Moldavsky and Chernyakovskaya, 1967; Lindahl, Leary, and Gresser, 1972) have been reported to be increased in the presence of interferon (Section X. I), and the phagocytic "clean-up crew" called into the area by chemotatic responses to the immunolytic events can also be enhanced by interferon (Huang et al., 1971) whose production will be triggered not only by the invading virus, but possibly also by many of the immune-reactions of the lymphocytes (Section III. B. 5).

Thus, it is necessary to consider the role of interferon not only in regard to its antiviral action, but also to assess its interactions with immune mechanisms. It has often been reported that interferon production did not correlate with infection outcome in virus infections of immunodeficient animals (Subrahmanyan, 1968; Vilček, 1964b; Craighead, 1966). It should be considered that in these cases infection outcome could be determined by interferon not only acting alone but also as an adjunct to immune mechanisms. Such considerations could also explain the findings that in vitro interferon-sensitivities of a virus to interferon (antiviral) action does not necessarily correlate with apparent in vivo sensitivities of the virus to interferon action(s). Thus, vaccinia virus has been demonstrated to be quite resistant to interferon action in rabbit cell cultures (Stewart II, Scott, and Sulkin, 1969; Youngner, Thacore, and Kelly, 1972), but rabbit interferon has been reported to be effective against vaccinia virus in rabbit skin (Isaacs and Westwood, 1959b) and eyes (Cantell and Tommila, 1960; Oh and Yoneda, 1969). Herpesviruses are quite refractory to interferon (antiviral) action in many in vitro systems (Table 14), but appears to be very sensitive in the eye (Section XIV). Also, Mayer and Krueger (1970) found a reversed order of sensitivities of viruses to interferon inducers Statolon and poly rI·poly rC in vivo as compared to their sensitivities to interferons in vitro. These observations support the interpretation that interferon's actions in vivo are not restricted to the solitary system measured in cell cultures as "the (in vitro) antiviral action" of interferon. These multiple interactions may also partially explain the efficacy of interferons in vivo against tumors (Section XIII).

b) Elimination of Established Infections

Infection foci of those viruses avoiding elimination by primary defenses at the portal of entry can establish at a number of locations in the body. And in each of these secondary foci they soon begin to encounter similar resistance mechanisms to those encountered at the primary focus. Again, disease is going to be determined by the swiftness with which the virus can replicate sufficient to form a high level and sustained secondary viremia, and recovery is going to result and disease severity restricted if host forces answer the challenge rapidly and with effective intensity. The magnitude of the secondary viremia determines prognosis, both as it reflects extent of secondary foci replication (and possible pathology) and allows target tissue seeding. Limitation of the secondary viremia can be accomplished either by limitation of secondary foci virus replication or by inactivation of virus during viremic spread.

Cell-mediated immunity can restrict virus and eliminate infectious foci; it was previously pointed out (Stewart II, 1973) that it was not possible to conclude that cell-mediated immunity could act effectively alone unless interferon response were somehow selectively blocked. Indeed, interferon produced locally apparently also exerts antiviral action directly and it clearly enhances the cell-mediated eradication mechanism: the altered secondary foci multiplication of encephalomyocarditis virus and failure of cell-mediated immunity to arrest the virus in anti-interferon-treated mice (Gresser et al., 1976b) proves the importance of interferon as well as the cell-mediated control. It has been demonstrated that lymphoid cells infiltrating infection foci begin to attack cells in the foci when "activated" to do so by "factors" generated by the immune interactions; interferon involvements are obvious.

Thus, in elimination of infection foci, interferon antiviral mechanism may not be the determinant of recovery, but interferon can be the determinant of recovery through another mechanism (Lodmell and Notkins, 1974).

Importantly, a delay of cell-mediated responses can allow virus to infect a critical number of cells so that destruction of these by the subsequent cell-mediated response can be the cause of disease (see below). Often this type of over-involvement of tissues with viruses can be prevented by the development of antibody, thus allowing modest cell-mediated immunity, working with interferon, to eliminate infection foci. The efficacy of exogenous antibody in such infections has been reported (Worthington, Rabson, and Baron, 1972; Murphy and Glasgow, 1966).

Secondary viremia can be cleared by phagocytic elements, and the rate of this clearance has been correlated inversely with virulence (Johnson and Mims, 1968; Campbell, Buera, and Tobias, 1970). Interferon induced by the viremia or spilling-over into circulation from the secondary foci, can presumably enhance this phagocytic clearance. Thus interferonemia can possibly be protective by: 1. circulating to target tissues to confer virus resistance (Baron et al., 1966a, b); 2. inducing febrile mechanisms (Yaron et al., 1977); 3. enhancing phagocytic clearance of viremia. Clearance can also be facilitated by antibodies which can both enhance ingestion and clearance of viremia and neutralize circulating viruses (Nathanson and Cole, 1970).

Once virus reaches the target tissue by this sequential 1° focus → viremia → 2° focus→ viremia→ target route, it finds that the environment has been alerted of its coming. Evidence for this is that many viruses are lethal when injected intracerebrally but are immunizing if injected parenterally, yet both reach the central nervous system and begin to replicate (Webb et al., 1968; Stewart II,

1973). Circulating interferon produced during the secondary viremia may have conferred some restrictive ability to the target tissue, and the elevated temperature produced by the secondary viremia (interferonemia?) may restrict virus replication.

Also, by the time the circuitous route of entry to the target tissue has been completed the hosts immune responses have been marshalled. If these processes are functional soon enough and if target seeding is not too extensive, the cell-destructive immune mechanisms can force the virus from these final foci before enough cells have become involved to cause disease, or for their destruction to cause disease. However, if many target cells become infected before the immuno-removal begins to function, immunolysis can, especially in the central nervous system, cause damage and disease. This is best illustrated by lymphocytic choriomeningitis (LCM) viral infections of mice. When inoculated intracerebrally into immunocompetent mice this virus produces fatal disease with lesions in the central nervous system; in neonatal mice or immunosuppressed mice it produces a persistent infection with chronic syndrome of runting and liver necrosis. In both cases virus replicates to similar levels in the brain (see Stewart II, 1973 for references). Thus elimination of virus can sometimes be detrimental in infections with non-cyticidal virus. On the other hand, its persistence can also be detrimental, though not necessarily because of *virus*-induced damage: Riviere *et al.* (1977) have reported that injection of antibodies to mouse interferon in mice inhibited the runting, liver necrosis and death resulting from chronic LCM virus infection, and concluded that the chronic production of interferon causes this disease.

The immunolytic elimination of viruses having skin as their target-tissues is probably the cause of the rashes produced in these infections (Fenner, 1968), and removal of target cells likely causes the characteristic symptoms complicating mumps (Speel, Osborn, and Walker, 1968). Interestingly, in the absence of cellular immunity, measles virus has been reported to develop persistent central nervous system disease in animals (Schumacher, Albrecht, and Taurasa, 1972). This suggests that factors impeding such responses during recovery from measles could produce "slow-type" measles infections.

On the other hand, infections involving cytolytic viruses show increased target tissue destruction in the immunosuppressed host (Hirsch and Murphy, 1967; Zlotnick *et al.*, 1972).

An additional contribution to disease development, besides immunity or interferon, is the role of defective-interfering (DI) viral particles in pathogenesis (Huang and Baltimore, 1970). These particles have been demonstrated in many virus-cell systems (Huang, 1977), and arise spontaneously during infection cycles in different types of cells. DI particles replicate at the expense of infectious virions, but are dependent on the standard virus, thus their accumulation is progressive but self-limiting. Early production of DI particles in the pathogenic process could slow virus progression and reduce levels of infective virus, thus allowing host defenses to gain the temporal advantage needed to arrest and eliminate the virus. The production of DI particles (and, as we have seen, the outcome of infection) can be determined by the particular cell-type infected (e. g., portal of entry), as some cells produce little if any DI particles and others produce many (Huang, 1977). Such variables as age, hormone levels, fever and other factors shown to influence recovery from viruses may do so at least in part because they effect production of DI particles. Also, the conversion from acute to chronic, or slow-virus diseases may be attributable to this phenomenon. It has been demonstrated that interferon treatment can cause cells that are producing infective particles to start producing defective, noninfective particles (IX. B. 4). Thus interferon may have yet another antiviral function in pathogenesis of virus disease.

Fig. 23 summarizes the possible central involvement of interferons in host recovery mechanisms against virus infections, as indicated by the literature reviewed in this Section. Many of these mechanisms are obviously interdependent and are potentially effective at each stage in the virus disease process.

B. Antiviral Studies With Interferons and Interferon Inducers in Animals

The interposition of interferon at various stages of the pathogenesis of virus infections immediately seemed worth attempting when it was demonstrated that it was active against a wide variety of viruses *in vitro* and was not overtly toxic in animals, even in the crude preparations employed. The variables in these studies have been numerous: interferon doses have ranged from a few to a few million units; doses of virus challenge have been very high and very low; time of interferon relative to virus infection has ranged from pretreatment with interferon before virus-inoculation to treatment in late stages of target-tissue symptoms; both route of virus and route of interferon inoculations have varied; and each of these variables has been reported in several animal species. The general conclusion from all the studies listed in Table 16 is that interferons are effective against a variety of virus infections in all animals tested, usually being more effective the earlier administered; and the higher the interferon dose, the better the protection, so far.

Induction of endogenous interferon in animals has usually been found to be more effective than exogenous interferon, likely because the total amounts of interferon formed are larger than those that can be injected. In the following Sections, the literature on the *in vivo* antiviral effects of exogenously applied

Table 16. *Antiviral activities of exogenous interferons in animals*

Animal	Virus	References
Rabbit	Vaccinia (skin)	Lindenmann, Burke, and Isaacs (1957); Isaacs and Westwood (1959 b); Pinto et al. (1970)
	Vaccinia (eye)	Cantell and Tommila (1969); Oh and Yoneda (1969)
	Vaccinia (generalized)	Arakawa, Sawa, and Fujiwara (1965)
	Newcastle disease (eye)	Oh and Gill (1966)
	Herpes simplex (eye)	Ermolieva and Furer (1968); Finter (1970 a)
	Rabbies	Vieuchange (1967); Postic and Fenje (1971 b); Ho et al. (1974)

Table 16 (continued)

Animal	Virus	References
Mouse	Vaccinia	Baron *et al.* (1966 b)
	Vesicular stomatitis	Baron *et al.* (1966 b); Declercq and Desomer (1968, 1971 b); Glasgow (1970); Gresser, Tovey, and Maury (1975)
	Bunyamwera	Hitchcock and Isaacs (1960)
	Influenza	Pollikoff, Donikian and Liu (1961); Takano, Jensen, and Warren (1963); Link, Blaskovic, and Raus (1963)
	Semliki forest	Finter (1964 a, c; 1966 a; 1967 b); Worthington, Levy, and Rice (1973)
	Encephalomyocarditis	Finter (1964 a); Baron *et al.* (1966 b); Gresser *et al.* (1968 b); Olsen *et al.* (1976)
	Herpes simplex	Declercq (1975)
	Friend leukemia	Gresser *et al.* (1967 a, b, c, d); Wheelock and Larke (1968)
	Rauscher leukemia	Gresser *et al.* (1968 a)
	Radiation leukemia	Lieberman, Merigan, and Kaplan (1971)
	Gross leukemia	Gresser, Coppey, and Bourali (1969)
	Moloney sarcoma	Berman (1970); Rhim and Huebner (1971); Declercq and Desomer (1971 a)
	Rabies	Karakuyumchan and Bektimerova (1968); Baer *et al.* (1977)
Rat	Sindbis	Denys (1963)
Hamster	Polyoma	Atanasiu and Chany (1960)
Guinea-pig	Rabies	Kaplan *et al.* (1962)
Chicken	Newcastle disease	Lampson *et al.* (1963)
	Rous sarcoma	Lampson *et al.* (1963)
	Polio RNA	Youngner and Kelley (1965)
Monkey	Vaccinia (skin)	Pinto *et al.* (1970)
	Vaccinia (eye)	Neumann-Haefelin *et al.* (1975)
	Vaccinia (generalized)	Neumann-Haefelin, Shrestha, and Manthey (1976)
	Herpesvirus (eye)	Sugar, Kaufman, and Varnell (1973); Neumann-Haefelin *et al.* (1975, 1977)
	Herpesvirus (generalized)	Neumann-Haefelin, Shrestha, and Manthey (1976)
	Yellow fever	Scientific Committee on Interferon (1970)
	Rabies	Hilfenhaus *et al.* (1975, 1977); Majer, Weinmann, and Hilfenhaus (1977)
	Hepatitis-B	Desmyter *et al.* (1976)

interferon will be described in relation to the different types of virus diseases. In addition, studies with inducers will be appended to each Section for comparative purposes.

1. Localized Infections

a) Effects of Exogenous Interferons

The first demonstration of effect of interferon as an antiviral *in vivo* was the protection of rabbit skin against vaccinia virus (Lindenmann, Burke, and Isaacs, 1957). Interferon preparations were then shown to delay and suppress the symptoms of vaccinial infections in rabbit eyes when given for four days following corneal inoculation of virus. This treatment did not affect herpes simplex infection of rabbit eyes. However, others have observed protection against herpes simplex with interferon eyedrops (Ermolieva and Furer, 1968; Finter, 1970a). Oh and his associates (Oh and Gill, 1966; Oh and Yoneda, 1969) also reported that interferon injected into the eyes of rabbits protected them against Newcastle disease virus and vaccinia virus injected a few hours later.

Human leukocyte interferon has also been shown to be topically effective against both vaccinia and herpes viruses in eyes of monkeys when given prophylactically, and therapeutic administration moderated the course of the keratitis and shortened the period of virus shedding (Sugar, Kaufman, and Varnell, 1973; Sundmacher, Neumann–Haefelin, and Shrestha, 1975; Neumann–Haefelin *et al.*, 1975).

Recently, Neumann–Haefelin *et al.* (1977) demonstrated that both human leukocyte interferon and human fibroblast interferon were effective in prevention of herpes simplex virus keratitis in monkeys when administered at about 2×10^6 units/ml but were ineffective at 2×10^3 units/ml; 2×10^4 units/ml of either interferon was marginally effective.

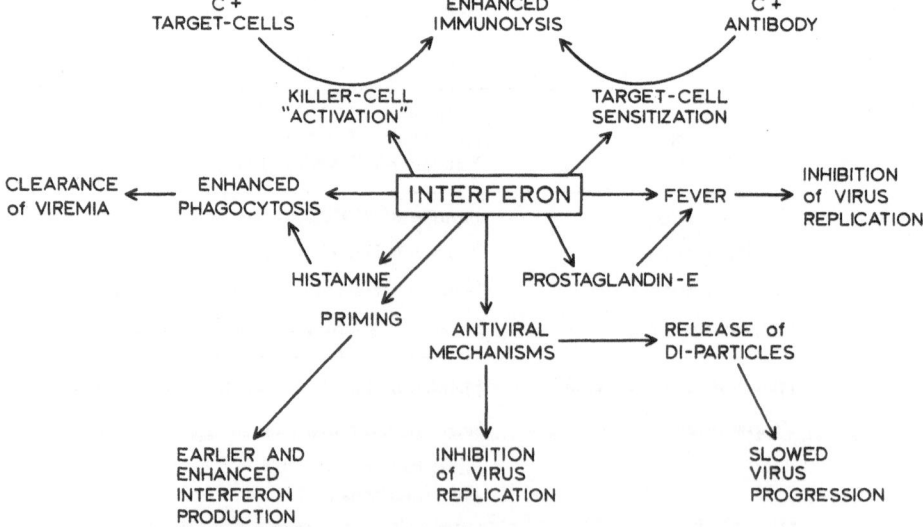

Fig. 23. Involvement of interferon in host defense mechanisms

The injection of human leukocyte interferon intravenously into monkeys reduced the ability of vaccinia virus to replicate in the skin (Pinto *et al.*, 1970); similar results were obtained with the human leukocyte interferon in rabbits.

Local infections with aerosolized influenza virus were found not to be inhibited in mice when interferon was inoculated intramuscularly or intravenously in amounts sufficient to protect against intraperitoneal infection with Semliki forest virus (Finter, 1966a, 1967b), though high levels of interferon were detectable in the blood. Others have reported that aerosolized interferon preparations or interferon preparation nose-drops were effective against influenza in mice (Pollikoff, Donikian, and Liu, 1961; Takano, Jensen and Warren, 1963; Link, Blaskovic, and Raus, 1963), but Finter (1973b) has argued that these effects were not due to the interferon in the preparations.

b) Effects of Inducers of Endogenous Interferons

Interferon inducers of a large variety have also been shown to inhibit development of localized virus infections in animals.

Influenza virus has been used to induce interferon in eyes of rabbits, which protected them against herpes simplex infection (Tommila and Penttinen, 1962).

Endotoxin and typhoid vaccine were used to induce interferon in the aqueous humor which induced resistance to Newcastle disease virus and vaccinia virus (Oh and Gill, 1966; Oh and Yoneda, 1969) and herpesvirus (Pollikoff *et al.*, 1968) in the eyes of rabbits.

Poly rI·poly rC has been shown to induce interferon in the aqueous and vitreous humor when injected into the eyeball of rabbits (Pollikoff *et al.*, 1970; Weissenbacher *et al.*, 1970), and eyedrops of poly rI·poly rC induced interferon in rabbit tears (Centifanto, Goohra, and Kaufman, 1970). By either route of administration the inducer was protective against herpes simplex keratitis infections of the eyes (Park and Baron, 1968; Park *et al.*, 1969; Pollikoff *et al.*, 1970; Kaufman, Ellison, and Waltman, 1969).

A number of interferon inducers have been demonstrated to be protective against respiratory viral infections when the inducers were given intranasally, and it is presumed that the mechanism of protection is via interferon production (Finter, 1973b).

Inactivated influenza will protect against the live virus intranasally (Denys, Desomer, and Prinzie, 1961; Schulman and Kilbourne, 1963). Endotoxin was shown to protect mice against pneumonia virus (Nemes and Hilleman, 1962). Pyran copolymer intranasally protected mice against intranasal inoculation with vesicular stomatitis virus; Statolon, intranasally protected mice against influenza virus (Kleinschmidt, 1970). And poly rI·poly rC when administered intranasally protected against a challenge by this route with influenza virus (Hill, Baron, and Chanock, 1969; Lindh *et al.*, 1969; Nemes *et al.*, 1969a), vaccinia (Lindh *et al.*, 1969) or vesicular stomatitis virus (Declercq and Merigan, 1969b).

2. Generalized Infections

Many early studies were unable to demonstrate an effect of exogenous interferons against systemic viral infections, likely because the doses of interferons were too low and often because the doses of challenge virus were overwhelming. However, once it became possible to inject larger doses of exogenous interferon, against doses of challenge virus in the range of what could be considered natural exposure levels (Finter, 1967b), positive results were obtained.

a) Effects of Exogenous Interferons

The first demonstration of interferon effectiveness against generalized virus infections was reported by Glasgow and Habel (1962a) who injected virus-induced leukocytes into mice to protect against intracerebral challenge with vesicular stomatitis virus.

Most studies report that interferon given prior to virus is effective, whereas when given after infection interferon becomes increasingly less effective with time (Denys, 1963; Declercq and Desomer, 1968). However this ineffectiveness of later administration of interferon can sometimes be overcome by increasing the interferon dose. Thus, Finter (1967b) protected mice against Semliki forest virus by injecting interferon 24 hours after virus, but this effect required about 20 times more interferon than needed when interferon was given before the virus. Also, repeated administration of interferon has been found to be more effective than a single injection (Gresser et al., 1967a, 1968b).

In one study interferon treatment (about 5000 units/mouse) was effective against arbovirus encephalitis in mice when given after infection, at a time determined by the authors to constitute "late therapy" rather than prophylaxis (Worthington, Levy, and Rice, 1973). This distinction between viral prophylaxis and therapy is often confused. Glasgow (1970) claimed therapeutic value of interferon in mice showing central nervous symptoms at the time of treatment. Declercq and Desomer (1971b) reported that mice could be protected if treatment was begun at any time before onset of symptoms. Catalano et al. (1972) claimed that endogenous interferon was protective in mice if induced even when an occasional mouse in the experimental group was showing central nervous symptoms of illness; it was not stated whether any of these occasional animals were in the surviving fraction. If not, only prophylaxis can be claimed, rather than therapy (Lefkowitz and Baron, 1974).

In an important analysis, Gresser, Tovey, and Maury (1975) showed that initiation of treatment of mice with interferon as late as 4 days after intranasal inoculation of vesicular stomatitits virus, resulted in marked survival. By the time interferon (about 6×10^6 units) was given, the virus had already multiplied to high titers in the target tissue, the brain. These results demonstrate that even late in the cycle illustrated in Fig. 22, exogenous interferon can alter the disease outcome. Thus interferon therapy as well as prophylaxis in such systemic diseases may be realizable. Declercq (1975) claimed that a single dose of 10^5 units of mouse interferon given intramuscularly, intraperitoneally or subcutaneously was significantly protective against intranasal inoculation of herpesvirus; however, when given after virus it was ineffective. This author interprets from these data that parenteral interferon therapy may be possible in herpetic encephalitis if interferon is administered early in the disease; the data in fact argue to the contrary.

Recently, human leukocyte interferon has been found to protect monkeys against vaccinia virus or herpes virus (Neumann–Haefelin, Shrestha, and Manthey, 1976). At 5×10^5 units/day, starting one day before or 3 days after infection, interferon was able to avert disease completely. Therapy initiated at the first lesions prevented enlargement and generalization of herpetic lesions in all of the monkeys, suggesting therapy can be effected.

As previously indicated, rabiesvirus could also apparently be arrested at the target tissue stage (Section XII. A. 1): intralumbar injection of interferon into monkeys did not prevent peripheral replication of virus but prevented the disease (Hilfenhaus et al., 1977).

b) Combined Effects of Interferons and Other Agents

A few recent reports have suggested that interferon can work synergistically in combination with other antiviral agents in animals.

Werner, Jasmin, and Chermann (1976) reported that ammonium 5-tungsto-2-antimoniate (HPA 23) partially protected mice against encephalomyocarditis virus or vesicular stomatitis virus. When mice were injected with 75,000 units of interferon prior to HPA 23, and both were given prior to virus, protection was complete.

Since it had been reported that adenine arabinoside (ARA-A) and interferon worked synergistically in cell cultures against herpesvirus (Lerner and Bailey, 1974), Lefkowitz et al. (1976) investigated this possibility in mice but found no such effect.

Chany and Cerutti (1977 a, b) recently found that the antiviral effect of interferon in mice against encephalomyocarditis virus was enhanced by isoprinosine, provided that both interferon and virus were inoculated intraperitoneally and that isoprinosine injection preceded interferon and virus by several hours.

c) Effect of Inducers of Endogenous Interferons

A much greater number of studies have been reported using inducers of interferon in generalized virus infections than using interferons per se, primarily because the interferons are difficult to obtain in sufficient quantities for many such studies. Some of these studies have used interferon-inducing viruses. Avirulent influenza virus was used by Hitchcock and Isaacs (1960) to induce circulating interferon in mice which protected them from subsequent challenge with Bunyamwera virus. Baron et al. (1964a, 1966b) used intravenously injected Newcastle disease virus to induce interferon in mice, which protected them from encephalomycarditis virus when challenged 24 hours later, but not when challenged at only 2 or 5 hours. The attenuated American BT-8 strain of bluetongue virus which was recently found to be a very good inducer of interferon in mice, is also very effective in protecting mice against otherwise lethal infection with encephalomyocarditis virus (Jameson, Schoenherr, and Grossberg, 1977).

Like interfering viruses, endotoxins were known to induce virus resistance in animals long before they were known to induce interferons in them (Gledhill, 1964; Wagner et al., 1959). It has been repeatedly demonstrated that endotoxins induce interferon, and it has been assumed that this interferon accounts for the virus resistances observed (Borecky, Lackovic, and Russ, 1969; Declercq and Desomer, 1969; Furer et al., 1968).

Brucella abortus, which induced interferon in mice and made them resistant to vaccinia virus (Desomer et al., 1970), may act partially by induction of interferon. However, heat-killed brucellae were found to be good inducers of interferon, but not of protection in this system. And rabbits injected with the live organisms did not produce interferon yet became resistant to vaccinia. On the other hand BRU-PEL shows a good correlation between ability to induce virus resistance and interferon in mice (Feingold, Keleti, and Youngner, 1976). Mice were also reported to be protected against vaccinia virus by prior injection with *Proteus rettgeri* or *E. coli* (Declercq and Desomer, 1969), and *Listeria monocytogenes* induced interferon and protection against Mengo virus in mice (Remington and Merigan, 1969). These latter workers also found that *Toxoplasma gondii*, which induced interferon in mice, protected them against Mengo virus.

Pyran copolymer and a number of related anionic polymers induce interferons in animals and protect against a variety of viruses (Regelson, 1967; Merigan and Finkelstein, 1968; Declercq and Merigan, 1969b; Miner and Koehler, 1969; Richmond, 1971). However, the fact that this protective activity against virus lasts months rather than a few days, as seen with interferons, suggests that interferon does not account for its activity.

Polyacrylic acid also induced interferon and virus resistance in mice (Desomer et al., 1968a, b; Leunen, Desmyter, and Desomer, 1971; Niblack, McCreary, and Stone, 1970; Declercq and Desomer, 1968; Billiau, Desmyter, and Desomer, 1970). Again, this compound's ability to induce interferons did not correlate with its antiviral activity in various animals (Desomer, 1970)., suggesting its action was not attributable to interferon.

Chlorite-oxidized amylose (COAM) induced both virus resistance and interferon in mice and rabbits (Claus et al., 1970; Billiau, Desmyter, and Desomer, 1970; Billiau, Muyembe, and Desomer, 1971a, b; 1972). Again, this compound apparently does not act solely via interferon. It worked much more effectively against Mengo virus when given at the same intraperitoneal location, and its activity seems to last too long to be rationalized as an interferon action.

Statolon and helenine also induce virus resistance and interferons in animals (Kleinschmidt and Murphy, 1967; Schmidt and Pindak, 1968; Pindak and Schmidt, 1967; Wheelock and Larke, 1968; Pindak et al., 1971). The protective effect is likely a composite of interferon induction (short-term protection) and immunological (long-term protection) mechanisms (Wheelock, Caroline, and Moore, 1969; Wheelock, 1970).

Tilorone, which induced interferon in mice, rats and rabbits after oral administration also protected the animals against challenge with several viruses given either intracranially, intraperitoneally or subcutaneously (Krueger and Mayer, 1970; Krueger *et al.*, 1971; Declercq and Merigan, 1971a; Hoffmann and Kunz, 1972; Giron, Schmidt, and Pindak, 1972). Some evidence has also been offered that interferon is only part of the antiviral mechanism of tilorone (Giron, Schmidt, and Pindak, 1972; Declercq, 1974). Stringfellow, Overall, and Glasgow (1974a, b) found that tilorone was protective against encephalomyocarditis virus when given prophylactically by completely preventing the viremic phase but was ineffective if target organs became infected. Tilorone and its analogues were also prophylactic against Venezuelan equine encephalitis virus in mice, when given orally, but not peritoneally (Kuehne, Pannier, and Stephen, 1977).

Polyribonucleotides, especially poly rI·poly rC, have been shown to induce interferon and virus resistance in a large number of animal-virus combinations (Hilleman, 1970). In addition to the local effects against herpetic keratitis and influenza referred to previously, these inducers have shown activity when applied prophylactically against herpesvirus encephalitis (Lindh *et al.*, 1969; Catalano and Baron, 1970; Catalano *et al.*, 1972), numerous arbovirus encephalidites (Finter, 1970a; Worthington and Baron, 1971a, b; Postic and Sather, 1970; Haahr, 1971; Kunz and Hoffman, 1969), enteroviral encephalidites (Lindh *et al.*, 1969; Nemes *et al.*, 1969; Catalano and Baron, 1970; Gresser *et al.*, 1969), rhabdoviral infections of the central nervous system (Declercq and Merigan, 1969b, 1970; Declercq, Nuwer, and Merigan, 1970a, b; Declercq and Desomer, 1971b; Declercq 1972; Richmond and Hamilton, 1969), including rabies (Fenje and Postic, 1970; Janis and Habel, 1972; Harmon and Janis, 1975) and generalized vaccinia (Lindh *et al.*, 1969; Nemes *et al.*, 1969). This inducer is also active in protecting mice against leukemia-sarcoma viruses (Sarma *et al.*, 1969, 1971; Pearson *et al.*, 1969; Weinstein *et al.*, 1971; Rhim, Greenawalt, and Huebner, 1969; Declercq and Merigan, 1971b; Larson *et al.*, 1969a; Slamon, 1973, 1975; SectionXIII).

The extent of work on these inducers has paralleled the hopes for their utilization in man. Early studies demonstrating that they were active in microgram quantities spurred exhaustive testings, but reports of toxicities (discussed below) and hyporesponsiveness to repeated inductions and inactivity in primates, including man, have diminished intensity of these efforts.

Repeated doses of poly rI·poly rC, as with the other inducers *in vivo*, induces less interferon after second or subsequent doses (Section VI. B. 2; Buckler, *et al.*, 1971; DuBuy *et al.*, 1970; Stringfellow and Glasgow, 1972a; Finter, 1973b). However, a prolonged resistance to virus during interferon hyporesponsiveness to poly rI·poly rC has been reported by Sharpe, Birch, and Planterose (1971) and by Worthington and Baron (1971b). Tazulakhova, Novokhatsky, and Yershov (1973) found that, whereas a single injection of 100 μg of poly rI·poly rC in mice was not sufficient to protect them against Venezuelan equine encephalomyelitis virus, repeated injections were effective. Multiple doses of poly rI·poly rC were also reported to be more effective than single injections in protecting mice against encephalomyocarditis virus (Stringfellow, Overall, and Glasgow, 1974b). Repeated injection of poly rI·poly rC every 24 hours was also more effective in prolonging the decrease of viremia in mice infected with lactic dehydrogenase virus (Johnson and DuBuy, 1975), but repeated injections every 12 hours did not further increase this protective effect. At present there is no satisfying explanation for the discrepancy between refractoriness and prolonged protection, but they suggest again that high spillover-levels of circulating interferon are not accurate measures of local interferon and tissue resistance to virus infections.

Levy, Duenwald, and Buckler (1973) found that COAM potentiated the interferon response to poly rI·poly rC; however this combination of drugs was not found to increase the protection of mice against rabies infection above that obtained with poly rI·poly rC alone.

The complex of poly rI·poly rC-poly-L-lysine in carboxymethylcellulose was more effective than poly rI·poly rC against encephalomyocarditis virus in mice; the former complex also inducing more interferon (Olsen et al., 1976): Protection was associated with prevention of viremia and, consequently, of seeding of target organs.

The nuclease-resistant poly rI·poly rC-poly L-lysine complex was also found to protect monkeys against hemorrhagic fever (Levy et al., 1976). Whereas poly rI·poly rC induced no or only modest levels of interferon in primates or man, poly rI·poly rC-poly-L-lysine induced high levels (Levy et al., 1975). This inducer was also reported to modify several markers of infection with hepatitis-B virus in chimpanzees (Purcell et al., 1976).

3. Unifying Speculation on Inducer Toxicities

All interferon inducers have basically the same common drawbacks. These are best documented with poly rI·poly rC, apparently because this inducer has been most studied for toxicity. Most, if not all, interferon inducers have demonstrated a characteristic spectrum of toxic effects in animals. Principle among these are pyrogenicity. It has been suggested that poly rI·poly rC, endotoxin and pyran, and other inducers damage cell membranes and thus release pyrogens along with interferons and other lymphokines (Braun, 1969). Absher and Stinebring (1969) pointed out the "endotoxin-like" effects of poly rI·poly rC. Declercq and Stewart II (1972) reviewed the activities of poly rI·poly rC which are reminiscent of the *in vivo* biologic effects of endotoxin. Among these were: 1. Interferon induction and virus resistance; 2. Pyrogenicity; 3. Stimulation of phagocytic activity; 4. Toxic effects on certain cell populations.

Pyrogenicity of poly rI·poly rC has been observed in rabbits (Lindsay et al., 1969; Hilleman, 1970), calves (Rosenquist, 1971) and man (Hill et al., 1971). It has been reported to inhibit liver regeneration after partial hepatectomy (Jahiel et al., 1971). It has also been shown to be embryotoxic and to damage nervous tissue (Adamson and Fabro, 1969; Young et al., 1970). It enhanced cell-mediated immune mechanisms and induced runting in mice (Leonard, Eccleston, and Jones, 1969). Interferon *per se* apparently does these things (Section X).

It is tempting to speculate that many of the toxic manifestations and side effects attributed to inducers and which are common for all the inducers in proportion to the interferon-inducing potentials, may be mediated by the interferon they induce. It will not be possible to verify this assumption until sufficient quantities of purified interferon preparations are available. However, many adverse effects seen with administration of interferons to date closely resemble those seen with the inducers. To date it has not usually been possible to administer exogenous interferon in amounts sufficient to match those maintained for several hours by inducers, and exogenous interferon is rapidly cleared from circulation. However, when high levels of interferon have been administered for prolonged periods, it has been toxic, or lethal (Gresser et al., 1975, 1976a), and caused wasting (Bekesi et al., 1976). Interferon preparations have been reported to be cytotoxic for certain cells (Nissen et al., 1977; Greenberg and Mosny, 1977).

While these data must for now be considered preliminary, and interferon involvement only presumptive, it would seem appropriate to keep these analogies of inducer-interferon toxicities in mind when clinical trials attempt to continually increase interferon dosage to maintain higher circulating interferon levels for longer periods. Again, it seems likely that there are reasons for interferons being inducible rather than constitutive.

XIII. Antitumor Activities of Interferons in Animals

In view of the pleiotypic alterations induced in cells by interferons and the multifaceted modulations of host defenses, it would really be surprising if interferon were inactive against tumors. This action could be mediated by its antiviral activity, its cell-multiplication-inhibitory activity or its immunomodulatory actions. But, in fact, the antitumor activities of interferon preparations were described several years before it became accepted that this represented more than merely a measure of its antiviral activity. And, again, when this argument was unconvincing, it was assumed that the impurities in the interferon preparations employed accounted for antitumor actions. Now it is clear that interferons are able to induce antitumor activities in many animals with many types of tumors (Table 17). In this Section these tumor system studies with interferons and its inducers are described and proposed mechanisms of antitumor activities are discussed.

It should be emphasized that it has only been with recent evolution of techniques for large-scale production of interferons and developments on purification of these interferons that it has become possible to undertake experiments to more carefully evaluate the antitumor effects of interferons. Studies with inducers of interferon provide less than satisfactory evidence for interferon's role in the antitumor effects.

A. Activities Against Virally-Induced Tumors

1. Antitumor Effects of Exogenous Interferons

The first demonstration of interferon activity inhibiting virally-induced tumors was provided by Atanasiu and Chany (1960) who found that pretreatment of hamsters with a low titered, crude interferon preparation inhibited the appearance of polyoma virus tumors and increased survival. Strandstrom, Sandelin, and Oker–Blum (1962) and Lampson et al. (1963) also reported that

Table 17. *Antitumor activities of exogenous interferons in animals*

Animal	Tumor	References
A. *Oncogenic virus-induced tumors*		
Hamster	Polyoma	Atanasiu and Chany (1960)
Chicken	Rous sarcoma	Strandstrom, Sandelin, and Oker-Blum (1962)

Table 17 (continued)

Animal	Tumor	References
Mouse	Friend leukemia	Gresser et al. (1966, 1967 a, b, c, d); Wheelock and Larke (1968)
	Rauscher leukemia	Glasgow and Friedman (1969); Toth, Vaczi, and Berencsi (1971 a, b)
	Harvey sarcoma	Berman (1970)
	Moloney sarcoma	Rhim and Huebner (1971); Declercq and Desomer (1971 a)
	Graft-induced Malignant Lymphoma	Hirsch et al. (1973)
	Spontaneous AKR leukemia	Gresser et al. (1968 b, 1969 a); Graff, Kassel, and Kastner (1970); Bekesi et al. (1976); Gresser, Maury, and Tovey (1976)
	Spontaneous Mammary Carcinoma	Came and Moore (1971, 1972)
Monkey	Herpesvirus Saimari Malignant Lymphoma	Laufs et al. (1974); Rabin et al. (1976)

B. *Transplantable tumors*

Animal	Tumor	References
Mouse	Polyoma tumor cells	Corragio et al. (1965)
	Ehrlich Ascites	Gresser et al. (1969 b, c); Ferris, Padnos, and Malomut (1971); Gresser et al. (1970 a)
	RC 19 Ascites	Gresser et al. (1969 b)
	EL 4 Ascites	Gresser et al. (1969 b); Gresser and Boulari (1969, 1970 a)
	Lewis lung carcinoma	Gresser and Bourali (1972)
	Lstra leukemia [a]	Chirigos and Pearson (1973)
	Friend leukemia Cells	Rossi et al. (1975)
	Sarcoma MC-36 [b]	Salvin et al. (1975 b)
	Sarcoma 180	Yokota et al. (1976)
	HeLa Cells [c]	Yokota et al. (1976)
Rabbit	Brown-Pearce Carcinoma	Pudov (1971)
Rat	256 Walker carcinosarcoma	Babbar, Singh, and Bajpai (1973)

C. *Chemically- and radiation-induced tumors*

Animal	Tumor	References
Mouse	Methylcholanthrene-induced Fibrosarcomas and Lung Adenomas	Kishida et al. (1971); Salerna et al. (1972)
	Radiation-induced Lymphosarcoma	Lieberman et al. (1971)

a Interferon used in combination with BCNU
b Type II interferon preparation
c Human interferon in nude mice

chicken interferon preparations were protective against Rous sarcoma virus in chick embryos but only if given before the virus.

Gresser and his associates (Gresser *et al.*, 1966, 1967a, b, c, d) studied the effect of repeated interferon injections on the development of Friend virus leukemia in mice. These workers found that interferon was effective in inhibiting splenomegaly of Friend disease in Swiss mice when treatment was initiated 2 days or 1 week after virus inoculation, when symptoms had already developed, provided treatment was repeated daily for the duration of the experiment; if interferon was given for only a few days it was ineffective (Gresser *et al.*, 1967a). Similar treatment inhibited Rauscher leukemia in Balb/c mice and prolonged survival (Gresser *et al.*, 1968a).

On the other hand, Vandeputte *et al.* (1967) failed to demonstrate an effect of low-titered interferon preparations on Rauscher leukemia in mice. Wheelock (1967a) was also unable to prevent development of Friend virus leukemia in mice, but later reported that daily injections of interferon prolonged survival in this disease even when begun a month after infection (Wheelock and Larke, 1968). Others found that only a single injection of interferon along with Rauscher leukemia virus, or a day or two after it, could prolong survival of newborn mice (Glasgow and Friedman, 1969). Toth, Vaczi, and Berencsi (1971a, b) reported that daily injections of interferon preparations of low titer slightly prolonged life of Rauscher virus-infected mice; these workers (Toth, Vaczi, and Balogh, 1974) also reported a relationship between interferon and antibody production in resistance to this virus.

Chany and Robbe-Maridor (1969) reported that interferon injections did not inhibit Moloney murine sarcoma virus tumors. Similar findings were reported by Weinstein *et al.* (1971) and Rhim and Huebner (1971). However, Berman (1970) found that daily injections of interferon[12] delayed mortality in mice inoculated with Harvey strain of murine sarcoma virus. Rhim and Huebner (1971) found that small doses (about 10^3 units) were ineffective, or only very slightly so, against Moloney sarcoma, but Declercq and Desomer (1971a) claimed that injection of interferon "administered in amounts mimicking the interferon blood levels obtained endogenously with poly rI·poly rC" were inhibitory to the development of Moloney murine sarcomas[13].

Hirsch *et al.* (1973a, b) found that repeated injections of interferon into mice reduced endogenous C-type virus-activation seen following transfer of spleen cells and prevented development of malignant lymphomas. About 10^5 units of interferon/mouse were given each day for 28 days. However, in a subsequent study, skin homograft activation of C-type viruses was not inhibited by interferon treatment (Hirsch, Black, and Proffitt, 1977).

The malignant lymphomas induced by herpesvirus saimari in marmoset monkeys was not prevented by intraperitoneally injected human leukocyte in-

---

[12] Again, the amount of interferon employed here is unclear, as the titer was quoted at 8,000 to 16,000 units/0.2 ml.

[13] This blood-level of interferon was supposedly achieved by injections of only 200 units of interferon per mouse given at 12, 8 and 4 hours before virus challenge. These authors also claimed that the total intraperitoneally injected interferon entered the blood and remained there several hours.

terferon, about 10^4 units/2 days from just before infection, but survival time was increased significantly (Laufs et al., 1974). However, Rabin et al. (1976) have reported that herpesvirus saimiri-induced lymphoma in owl monkey responded to interferon given in doses of about 3×10^5 units of human leukocyte interferon/day over a period of about 2 weeks. All animals were treated at a time when leukemia was established, and 2 or 5 monkeys showed lymphocyte counts temporarily returned to normal and restored competency to mitogens.

Gresser and his colleagues (1968, 1969b) have studied carefully the effects of interferon on the spontaneous lymphoid leukemia appearing in AKR mice presumably caused by vertically transmitted Gross virus. Daily interferon treatment for the first 3 months of life reduced occurence of leukemia and increased survival in male mice but not in female mice. When daily interferon treatment was extended for 1 year, both sexes survived significantly longer than controls (Gresser et al., 1969b). Other workers also reported that interferon delayed appearance of leukemia in older AKR mice (Graff, Kassel, and Kastner, 1970). Bekesi et al. (1976) reported that the median life-span of AKR control mice was 36 weeks, whereas AKR mice treated with 5 doses of interferon (5×10^4 units/dose) had markedly decreased Gross virus titers (greater than decreases seen with combination of cytoreductive therapy with Virazole or immunotherapy) and 45% of the mice were still alive at 54 weeks. Interestingly, most mice given doses of 5×10^5 units of interferon died with wasting disease rather than from leukemia.

Most drugs that are effective against malignancy are relatively ineffective in treatment of AKR leukemia after diagnosis (reviewed by Gresser, 1977b). Graff and his associates (Graff, Kassel, and Kastner, 1970) and Kassel and his associates (Kassel, 1970; Kassel, Pascal, and Vas, 1972) claimed that large doses of crude interferon injected daily into AKR mice with advanced leukemia induced rapid "carcinolytic" activity which greatly prolonged lifespans. It now seems likely that this "interferon" effect was mediated by another serum lymphokine (Kassel et al., 1973), possibly a "tumor-necrosis factor" (Hoffman et al.; Kassel et al., 1977) or lymphotoxin. On the other hand, Gresser, Maury and Tovey (1976), using potent mouse interferon purified to about 10^6 units/mg of protein, showed that daily injections of about 6×10^6 units begun after clinical diagnosis of lymphoma in AKR mice significantly delayed the evolution of the lymphomas and increased survival about 100%. It did not, however, induce tumor regression.

Interferon was also reported to inhibit the development of spontaneous mouse mammary carcinoma (Came and Moore, 1971). One injection per week of about 1000 units of mouse serum interferon intraperitoneally begun at 6 weeks of age was continued for 35–42 weeks in this study. Came and Moore (1972) also claimed an effect with mouse brain interferon preparations against mouse mammary tumors.

One report has appeared in which interferon treatment *enhanced* tumors produced by oncogenic virus: local interferon as site of virus inoculation the day before virus accelerated murine sacroma virus-induced tumors; systemically injected interferon had no such effect (Gazdar et al., 1972a). This effect possibly relates to the immunomodulations described previously (Section X).

2. Antitumor Effects of Inducers of Endogenous Interferons Against Virally-Induced Tumors

Several studies have demonstrated the ability of viruses to interfere with tumor development by oncogenic viruses. In many of these cases it is probable that interferon induction is involved in the tumor interference, in other cases it seems unlikely.

Herpesvirus infection of hamsters has been reported to inhibit polyoma virus tumors (Barski, 1963). Similarly, lymphocytic choriomeningitis virus (which can induce chronic interferon production; Rivieri et al., 1977) was reported to significantly prolong survival of guinea pigs with leukemia (Jungeblut and Kodza, 1962), and it markedly delayed mortality of mice inoculated with Rauscher leukemia virus (Barski and Youn, 1964; Youn and Barski, 1966). West Nile virus was reported to inhibit Rous sarcoma in chickens (Shirodkar, 1965), as was rabiesvirus vaccine (Kravchenko, Voronin, and Kosmiadi, 1967) and coccal virus was reported to inhibit Friend leukemia in mice (Stim, 1970), presumably by inducing interferon.

Sendai virus was able to protect mice against Friend leukemia even when injected several weeks before the friend virus inoculation, but other interferon-inducing viruses did not induce protection (Wheelock, 1966b, 1967a). Thus the effect of Sendai virus is likely not mediated by interferon.

Statolon was shown to prevent Friend virus disease if injected intraperitoneally into mice before or after infection (Regelson and Foltyn, 1966; Wheelock, 1967a; Wheelock and Lark, 1968; Wheelock, Caroline, and Moore, 1969). Presumably this effect was related to immunologic mechanisms (-Wheelock, 1970; Wheelock, Caroline, and Moore, 1971; Wheelock et al., 1972; Levy and Wheelock, 1975), with interferon helping to inhibit viremia (Toy, Weislow, and Wheelock, 1973). The potential of statolon to protect against Friend disease was increased by inoculation with COAM (Weislow and Wheelock, 1975b). Rhim and Huebner (1969) also found that statolon was able to provide protection to mice against murine sarcoma virus.

Pyran copolymer also protected mice against Friend and Rauscher viruses (Regelson and Foltyn, 1966; Regelson, 1967; Chirigos et al., 1969; Schuller, Morahan, and Snodgrass, 1975; Morahan et al., 1974, 1976, 1977a, b). Presumably this effect, and its anti-Rauscher AKR leukemia activity, are attributable in part to macrophage "activation" and enhanced phagocytosis (Hirsch et al., 1970, 1972, 1973b). Pyran also inhibited polyoma-induced tumors in mice (Hirsch et al., 1972), and COAM inhibited Moloney murine sarcoma development (Claes et al., 1970; Declercq and Desomer, 1972b).

Tilorone has also been reported to inhibit Friend virus disease in mice (Barker, Rheins, and Wilson, 1971; Rana, Pinkerton, and Rankin, 1975).

The antitumor effect of poly rI·poly rC against oncogenic virus-induced tumors has been extensively studied. It has been demonstrated to be active against development of Rauscher disease (Youn, Barski, and Huppert, 1968) in mice, and Friend leukemia (Larson et al., 1969; Sarma, Neubauer, and Rabstein, 1971). Rats were also found to be protected against erythroblastosis when infected with Kirsten-murine erythroblastosis virus (Slamon, 1973), thus circumventing the hemolytic disease syndrome (Slamon, 1975).

Poly rI·poly rC also protected chickens against Rous sarcoma (Nemes et al., 1969a), hamsters against adenovirus-induced (Larson, Clark, and Hilleman, 1969) or SV 40-induced (Larson, Panteleakis, and Hilleman, 1970) tumors and rats against polyoma (Vandeputte et al., 1970).

The activity of poly rI·poly rC against murine sarcoma virus-induced tumors has been shown effective even when the polynucleotides were administered several days after the virus (Sarma et al., 1969, 1971; Pearson et al., 1969; Baron et al., 1970; Declercq and Merigan, 1971b; Kende and Glynn, 1971; Weinstein et al., 1971; Rhim and Huebner, 1971). Some investigators found that murine sarcoma was inhibited in neonatally infected mice by repeated doses of poly rI·poly rC (Declercq and Desomer, 1971a). In one study it was found that repeated injections of poly rI·poly rC induced regression of established murine sarcoma virus-induced tumors (Declercq and Stewart II, 1974b). To my knowledge, this is the only report to date of regression of virally-induced tumor with either interferon or an inducer.

In addition to the many reports of inhibition of virus-induced tumors by interferon inducers, a few studies have demonstrated enhancement of oncogenesis with viral inducers (Turner, Chirigos, and Scott, 1968; Steeves et al., 1969; Rheins, Barker, and Wilson, 1971) or poly rI·poly rC (Larson et al., 1969). Declercq and Merigan (1971b) reported that poly rI·poly rC inhibited murine sarcoma virus-induced tumors in 4- to 6-day-old mice but enhanced them in 3-week-old mice. Gazdar and Ikawa (1972) found that poly rI·poly rC, pyran or tilorone could enhance tumor development in mice infected with murine sarcoma virus. Schuller, Morahan, and Snodgrass (1975) and Morahan et al. (1977b) observed both tumor inhibition and enhancement with pyran in mice, depending on the route of its administration. Likely, these paradoxical tumor-enhancing activities relate to the depressive effects of induced interferons on immune mechanisms.

3. Combined Antitumor Efficacies of Interferon and Other Antitumor Agents

Very few studies have been reported in which another antitumor agent has been administered in conjunction with interferon to determine additive, synergistic or conflicting effects.

Barker, Rheins, and Wilson (1971) found that poly rI·poly rC, statolon tilorone and Sendai virus increased survival time in mice with Friend virus disease when these inducers were used one after another.

Chirigos and Pearson (1973) reported that interferon was ineffective against murine leukemia when host tumor load is large. However, after tumor cells were first reduced by treatment with 1,3- bis (2-chloroethyl)-1-nitrosourea (BCNU), interferon treatment then led to a significant number of cures, suggesting that the combination of BCNU and interferon exerted a synergistic antitumor effect.

Stewart II *et al.* (1975c) treated autochthonous Moloney murine sarcoma virus-induced tumors with direct local injections of interferon followed by poly rI·poly rC after several hours, to take advantage of the toxicity-enhancing effect of interferon for double-stranded RNA (Section X. F.). This scheme was significantly more effective than either agent separately, suggesting synergy.

Recently, Gresser, Maury, and Tovey (1978) reported that combined treatment with interferon and cyclophosphamide was effective therapeutically after diagnosis of lymphoma in AKR mice. While a single injection of cyclophosphamide increased survival after diagnosis from 17 to 29 days, cyclophosphamide treatment followed by daily injections of about 3×10^6 units of interferon increased survival by about 200%, to about 53 days. These data suggest at least an additive effect of cyclophosphamide and interferon, the former agent reducing the tumor load so that the interferon can act more effectively.

B. Activities Against Transplantable Tumors

1. Antitumor Effects of Exogenous Interferons

The antitumor effects of interferon against the oncogenic virus-induced tumors has generally been interpreted as a consequence of inhibition of virus multiplication. Corragio *et al.* (1965) observed an inhibition by interferon of growth of transplanted polyoma-induced sarcoma in mice, and interpreted this effect as virus suppression. It has also been considered that this antitumor activity could result from host mediated defense mechanisms or inhibition of tumor cell multiplication (Gresser *et al.*, 1967c, d).

Gresser and his associates (1969a; Gresser and Bourali, 1969, 1970a) studied the effect of interferon on the growth of a number of transplantable ascetic tumors in several strains of mice, and found that daily intraperitoneal or intramuscular inoculations of about 4×10^4 units of interferon inhibited tumor growth and prolonged survival of the animals. When mice were inoculated with both tumor cells and interferon intraperitoneally, effect was marked: with RC 19 tumors cells about 96% of the control animals died before 3 weeks, while 98% of the interferon-treated group survived beyond this time.

In each case interferon pretreatment of mice was without effect, and only prolonged treatment after tumor inoculation was beneficial (Gresser *et al.*, 1969b, 1970a; Gresser and Bourali, 1970a). These studies also demonstrated that interferon antitumor activity was dependent on the tumor load.

Interferon injections were also demonstrated to inhibit Ehrlich carcinoma and subcutaneously transplanted carcinogen-induced lymphatic leukemia in mice (Ferris, Padnos, and Molomut, 1971). Pudov (1971) reported that human leukocyte interferon inhibited the metastases of Brown-Pearce carcinoma transplanted in rabbits.

Gresser and Bourali (1972) found that interferon treatment, begun 6 days after subcutaneous implantation of Lewis Lung carcinoma in mice, was effective in preventing development of primary tumors and in inhibiting development of pulmonary metastases.

Interferon was also effective (Section XIII. A. 3.) in combination with

BCNU, in inhibition of transplantable LSTRA murine leukemia (Chirigos and Pearson, 1973).

Babbar, Singh, and Bajpai (1973) reported that rat interferon could block tumor-forming ability of Walker carcinosarcoma 256 cells in rats; however, only 600 units/day were injected, and the crudity of the preparation and the type of results obtained suggest the effects reported were not interferon-mediated.

Takeyama et al. (1975) reported that interferon treatment prolonged survival of mice inoculated with either L1210 leukemia cells or Ehrlich ascites cells. Rossi et al. (1975) also found that transplantable Friend leukemia in irradiated mice was inhibited by daily injections of interferon. Yokota et al. (1976) reported that mouse interferon (25,000 units/mice, twice/week × 3 weeks, intraperitoneally, starting when tumor nodules became palpable) was significantly inhibitory of the growth of Sarcoma 180 cells transplanted subcutaneously in normal or nude mice, but human interferon was not effective. However, when human HeLa cells were transplanted in nude mice, their growth was inhibited by *human* interferon, suggesting interferon was acting directly on the tumor rather than the host.

Declercq (1977) recently claimed that he injected 40 nude mice intraperitoneally with about 10^3 units of interferon/mouse, 3 time/week for several weeks after their injection with L929 cells, and obtained no tumor inhibition; he did, however, achieve antitumor effect by repeated injections of poly rI·poly rC. His interpretation from these observations was the "the role of interferon induction in the mechanism of antitumor actions of poly rI·poly rC can be eliminated". A more likely interpretation is that intraperitoneal injections of 10^3 units of interferon/mouse 3 times/week would not even approximately mimick endogenous interferon levels induced by poly rI·poly rC. Indeed, it is surprising that after injecting 10^3 units intraperitoneally into a mouse Declercq was able to detect 10^3 units/ml in the serum even 24 hours later. Clearly such data do not conform to the majority of data on interferon clearance (Section XI.) and should be regarded cautiously until confirmed in another laboratory. In fact, Gresser and his associates (1978) recently concluded that the antitumor activity of poly rI·poly rC *is* mediated by interferon, as it was nullified when mice were injected with anti-interferon globulin.

Only one report has appeared on the antitumor activity of Type II interferon preparations. Salvin et al. (1975b) reported that daily injections of sera containing Type II interferon directly into the tumor sites of mice implanted with sarcoma MC-36 markedly suppressed tumor growth. The total interferon dose injected/day was only about 300 units, and this amount of Type I interferon was ineffective. It could be interpreted from these data that Type II interferon had much higher antitumor activity than Type I interferon, but again to emphasize the point illustrated in Fig. 5, it seems premature to assign such activities to any single one of the many lymphokines present in such preparations.

2. Antitumor Effects of Inducers of Endogenous Interferons Against
Transplantable Tumors

The literature on abilities of viruses to inhibit transplantable tumors is enormous and mostly of historical value only (reviewed by Gresser, 1972); in many instances large doses of viruses now known to induce interferon were found to be effective. Molomut and Padnos (1965) injected mice with M-P virus and found that it induced interferon and inhibited spontaneous AKR leukemia, mammary carcinoma and several transplantable tumors. Newcastle disease virus was used to protect mice against RC 19 tumors (Gresser *et al.*, 1967b, c; Gresser and Bourali, 1969) and Ehrlich ascites (Rhim and Huebner, 1971). Rossi *et al.* (1975) also found that Newcastle disease virus, as well as interferon *per se*, inhibited multiplication of transplanted Friend leukemia cells in mice.

Pyran copolymer induced interferon and inhibited the growth of Sarcoma 180 tumors (Regelson, 1967, 1968); it also was effective against B-16 melanoma and Lewis lung carcinoma (Morahan *et al.*, 1974; Snodgrass, Morahan, and Kaplan, 1975; Morahan and Kaplan, 1976). Most data suggest that interferon plays a minor role in the antitumor effect of pyran, the major role likely taken by "activated" macrophages (Morahan *et al.*, 1977a).

Tilorone has been reported to be ineffective against L_{1210} leukemia (Adamson, 1971a) but was inhibitory to Walker carcinosarcoma 256 (Adamson, 1971b). It was also reported to enhance Lewis lung carcinoma and B-16 melanoma cells in mice when given prior to tumor cells (Morahan *et al.*, 1974).

Keleti, Feingold, and Youngner (1977) reported that BRU-PEL, the aqueous ether-extract of *Brucella abortus*, significantly inhibited development of sarcoma-180 tumors in mice, when injected 7 days before or 7 days after tumor cells.

Poly rI·poly rC has been shown to inhibit a number of transplantable tumors. It increases survival of mice inoculated with L_{1210} cells, presumably by inducing interferon (Zeleznick and Bhuyan, 1969). Repeated injections of poly rI·poly rC were reported to induce regression of reticulum cell sarcoma, apparently by causing tumor necrosis (Levy, Law, and Rabson, 1969; Levy *et al.*, 1970).

Poly rI·poly rC inhibited the growth of murine B 16 malignant melanoma (Bart and Kopf, 1969), leading to apparent cures in some mice (Bart *et al.*, 1971). In these mice there was a correlation between serum interferon levels and tumor inhibition (Bart *et al.*, 1973), and the inducer was also effective in thymectomized, irradiated, leukopenic mice (Bart *et al.*, 1975), suggesting the role of interferon in the antitumor effect.

Declercq (1977) reported that poly rI·poly rC inhibited tumors in nude mice developing at the site of inoculation of L_{929} cells, and since this effect was not matched by injection of low levels of exogenous interferon (though higher levels of exogenous interferon were effective), he deduced that interferon was not involved, and as the mice were athymic he concluded that thymus-dependent immunity can be eliminated, and attributed the effect of poly rI·poly rC to its direct cytotoxicity. Such interpretation seems premature. Clearly it is an important point to resolve whether interferon is involved in the antitumor mechanism of poly rI·poly rC, and resolution of its involvement has required a specific interferon block, such as those experiments showing involvement of interferon in recovery from virus infections by blocking interferon action with antiserum to interferon (Section XII. A. 2.) Thus, Gresser *et al.* (1978) demonstrated that injection of anti-interferon antibodies into mice together with poly rI·poly rC eliminated its antitumor effect. Such studies should enlighten us on the involvement of interferon in the antitumor action of other inducers as well.

C. Activities Against Chemically- and Radiation-Induced Tumors

1. Antitumor Effects of Exogenous Interferons

Interferon injections were reported to be highly effective in inhibiting the development of chemically-induced tumors in mice inoculated subcutaneously with 3-methylcholanthrene (Salerno *et al.*, 1972). Mice were first injected intraperitoneally with 2,500 units/day, 5 days/week for 1 month, then 2 such doses/day, one subcutaneously and one intraperitoneally, for 1 month; after the second month, dosage was doubled (10^4 units/day) for 2 months, after which interferon treatment was stopped. None of the treated mice developed tumors while 11/18 controls did. In another study interferon treatment only delayed tumor development in 20-methylcholanthrene injected mice (Kishida *et al.*, 1971).

Lieberman, Merigan, and Kaplan (1971) reported that interferon, injected intraperitoneally in low doses (about 300 units) immediately after X-irradiation of mice and continued 3 times/week throughout the experiment (3 months), significantly decreased the incidence of lymphomas. Considering the amount of interferon applied, these results are intriguing, and if reproducible, this effect deserves more study.

2. Antitumor Effect of Inducers of Endogenous Interferons Against Chemically- and Radiation-Induced Tumors

Poly rI·poly rC has been reported to inhibit chemical carcinogenesis in mice treated with 9, 10-dimethylbenzanthracene (Gelboin and Levy, 1970), or methylcholanthrene (Kreibich *et al.*, 1970). Repeated poly rI·poly rC injections also inhibited 3-methyl-cholanthrene induced tumors if given during early stage of tumor promotion (Elgjo and Degre, 1973). Others have found that while poly rI·poly rC reduced incidence of radiation-induced lymphomas in neonatal mice, it enhanced the incidence of thymic lymphomas induced by dimethyl-benzanthracene (Ball and McCarter, 1971), and Lieberman, Merigan, and Kaplan (1971) reported that poly rI·poly rC slightly increased lymphomas in X-irradiated mice.

Glaz (1972) reported that statolon was unable to inhibit methylcholanthrene-induced tumors in mice. However, he found that tilorone, administered continually in water, significantly retarded the appearance of tumors induced by methylcholanthrene.

In summary, it appears clear that administration of exogenous interferon in animals can reduce the incidence and development of tumors, even after they are well-advanced, but it has not yet been demonstrated that interferon can cure tumors. Clearly the phenomena of antitumor activities of interferons are often phenomenal in terms of effects reported by injecting even extremely low doses of interferons; if these effects are reproducible, interferons should hold hopes for clinical applications as antitumor agents. The development of large-scale production methods for interferons and the purification of these interferons should now allow many of these preliminary studies (often performed with terribly crude and low-titered interferon preparations) to be reinvestigated.

The interferon-inducers seem to hold little promise as tools to study interferon-mediated antitumor activities in animals, as their activities are closely allied with their toxicities, they induce hyporesponsiveness, and their activities are often not associated with induction of interferon. However, polyribonucleotides likely owe their antitumor activities primarily to their abilities to induce interferons, and these inducers may prove worthwhile in combination with other antineoplastic drugs.

The antitumor activities of interferons in combination with other tumor-load-reducing agents should, with the availability of highly potent and purified interferon preparations, provide exciting literature to follow in the near future. Hopefully, the word "cure" will soon reenter the realm of antitumor terminology.

D. Mechanisms of Antitumor Activities of Interferons

The mechanism of antitumor activities of interferons apparently depends on the type of tumor involved, the time of administration of interferon, and possibly the amount of interferon used. Inhibition of each type of tumor will thus be considered separately.

1. Virus-Induced Tumors

The tumorigenic potentials of virally-induced neoplasms relates directly to the viral inoculum dose, and the virus proliferative potential in the host. In many of the interferon-induced tumor inhibitions described above for virus-induced tumors, pretreatment with interferon was necessary prior to infection, probably resulting in induction of antiviral resistance in the animals. This seems likely in the case of inhibition of the oncogenicity of polyoma virus (Atanasiu and Chany, 1960) and Rous sarcoma virus (Strandstorm, Sandelin, and Oker-Blom, 1962; Lampson et al., 1963).

In other cases, it was necessary to continue interferon treatment after infection to achieve inhibition, as in the cases of Friend virus and Rauscher virus leukemias (Gresser et al., 1967a, b, c, d, 1968a; Wheelock and Larke, 1968), in which case continued virus suppression would account for the effect. In studies on the effects of interferon in Friend disease, Gresser et al. (1967c, d, 1968a) reported that spleens of interferon-treated mice had reduced amounts of Friend-virus compared to control infected mice. However, Rossi et al. (1975) found that interferon treatment also inhibited the multiplication of transplantable Friend cells in mice. Others have suggested that the activity of interferon against Rauscher leukemia is mediated by immunologic enhancement (Toth, Vaczi, and Berencsi, 1971a, b). On the other hand, Furmanski *et al.* (1975) discounted the role of interferon altogether in spontaneous regressions of Friend leukemia because they could not achieve regressions with interferon inducers.

Rather than an "either-or" choice of these effects, I think a composite of "each-and" is more likely. Gresser and his associates (1976c) clearly demonstrated the importance of endogenous interferon production in resistance of mice to Moloney sarcoma virus by injecting mice with antiserum to mouse interferon. In such mice, tumors appeared earlier and were much larger than in mice not injected with antiserum. Also, the tumor-inducing potential of Moloney sarcoma virus in anti-interferon treated mice was 100-times greater than in normal mice. Recently, Inglot, and Chudzio (1977) also reported that prolonged administration of antiserum against mouse interferon markedly potentiated Rauscher leukemia in mice. These data suggest that low-level endogenous interferon plays an essential role in controlling infections with oncogenic viruses. And, in spite of protestations that "the role of interferon induction in the mechanism of antitumor action of poly rI·poly rC can be eliminated" (Declercq, 1977), Gresser and his colleagues (1978) recently found that antiserum to mouse interferon eliminated the antitumor activity of poly rI·poly rC in mice.

2. Transplantable Tumors

In the tumors developing from transplanted cells, it appears that tumor progression may not lead to continued transformation of host cells by tumor viruses. In such cases the antitumor action of interferons can be less gratifyingly explained in terms of antiviral activities.

Rather, the resistance mechanisms would appear to involve a direct cell-multiplication-inhibitory effect or enhancements of host-mediated defense mechanisms involved in tumor limitation and eliminations. These would likely be similar to those described for elimination of infections in virus diseases (Section XII. A. 2.), and would involve similar interferon modulations.

Gresser and Bourali (1970a) suggested that interferon-induced antitumor activity in mice infected with Ehrlich ascites cells resulted from cell-multiplication-inhibition similar to that seen *in vitro* (Section X. E.). Murine L1210 leukemia cells incubated 24 hours with interferon were much less tumorigenic in mice than control L1210 leukemia cells (Gresser, Thomas, and Brouty-Boye, 1971), likely owing partly to inhibition of their ability to multiply and partly by enhancing exposure of host-recognized surface antigens (Lindahl, Leary, and Gresser, 1973, 1974; Huet *et al.*, 1974; Lindahl *et al.*, 1976a, b), thereby infuriating the reactionary host. However, *in vitro* treatment of cells with interferon required several hours contact with interferon to inhibit cell multiplication (Gresser *et al.*, 1970c) or to expose its "hidden parts", and as injected interferon is rapidly cleared from circulation (Section XI), it seems more likely that host mechanisms are "activated" by interferon to enhance their basic resentment and hostilities to the presence of the tumor cells, rather than some alteration of the tumor cells themselves by interferon treatment.

To test these alternatives, Gresser and his associates (1972) injected mice with leukemia L1210 cells which were sensitive to interferon (L1210-S) and L1210 cells resistant to interferon (L1210-R) [in terms of antiviral and cell-multiplication-inhibitory (Gresser et al., 1970c) and double-stranded RNA toxicity-enhancement (Gresser and Stewart II, unpublished data, 1975) and which did not bind interferon (Gresser, Bandu, and Brouty-Boye, 1974)]. Interferon treatment increased survival of mice inoculated with L1210-S cells *and* increased survival of mice inoculated with the L1210-R cells, suggesting that the interferon acted on *host* defense mechanisms rather than directly on the cells.

In some cases, however, antitumor activity of interferon in transplanted tumors may also be directed against the cells rather than the host. Thus, Yokota et al. (1976) reported that human interferon was active against human (HeLa) cells transplanted in nude mice, but this interferon was not effective against transplanted mouse tumor cells, and mouse interferon, which was active against mouse tumor cells, was not effective against the HeLa cells in mice. Also, Gresser et al. (1972) found that while L1210-R leukemia cells were sensitive to interferon effects in mice, L1210-S cells were more sensitive.

It has been clearly demonstrated that, as first reported by Svet–Moldavsky, and Chernyakhovskaya (1967), interferon can render lymphocytes cytotoxic for tumor cells (Section X. I.). Thus, interferon treatment of animals could activate this killer-instinct against tumors. However, Gresser, and Bourali-Maury (1972) reported that injection of antilymphocytic sera into mice did not diminish the antitumor activity of interferon, suggesting that more than lymphocyte cytotoxicity was involved in tumor inhibitory action of interferons. Also, several reports have suggested that the antitumor effect of poly rI·poly rC is not mediated via lymphocytes (Potmesil and Goldfeder, 1972; Fisher, Cooperband, and Mannick, 1972; Kreider and Benjamin, 1972).

Tumors have been reported to secrete a variety of factors that apparently enable them to escape host resistance mechanism (reviewed by Gresser, 1977b) and it has been speculated that interferon may somehow counteract certain of these tumor products (Gresser, 1977b).

Clearly we have only just begun to probe the involvement of interferon in host defenses against tumors. In tumor-bearing animals the difference between death and survival is likely determined by a fine balance between these forces. It seems likely that the interferon system plays a key role in the maintenance of this balance.

XIV. Interferon in the Clinic

Two decades of research in the interferon system have demonstrated that interferons are cellular proteins whose production can be induced by a wide variety of agents and whose activities are as diverse as those events inducing their synthesis. Interferons can inhibit viruses and tumors in animals and can modulate several immune functions.

As soon as interferon was discovered speculation began as to its clinical potential and such musing has not subsided since. The chronic curiosity and skepticism about interferon application to man can perhaps best be evidenced by the titles of recurring reviews of this topic by the "closet-hopefuls":

"Interferon – the Prospects" (Isaacs, 1959a)

"Interferon's Promise in Clinical Medicine: Fact or Fancy?" (Merigan, 1967c)

"Will Interferon be Clinically Useful?" (Finter, 1970b)

"Can Interferon Be Applied to Clinical Medicine?" (Kishida, 1975)

"Interferon Therapy: Obvious and Not so Obvious Applications" (Gresser, 1975)

"Prospects for the Clinical Use of Exogenous Interferon" (Cantell, 1977)

"Interferon, An Antiviral Drug for Use in Man" (Galasso and Dunnick, 1977)

"Interferons: Anti-Neoplastic Drugs?" (Strander, 1977a)

However, it has only been in the last few years that amounts of human interferon sufficient for even small preliminary trials have been available. Nearly all of this has been provided by Dr. Kari Cantell and the Finnish Red Cross (Section VI. C. 2). Yet even these limited trials of interferon have demonstrated its potential in treatment of a variety of diseases in man, and with continued trials it seems imminent that the promise of interferon in the clinic will be fulfilled.

In this Section the clinical trials with interferons and its inducer will be described according to the type of disease treated. It should be kept in mind that, largely owing to the limited availability of interferons, many of the studies have been with only a few individuals in open trials; such results must be considered preliminary until controlled double-blind trials are completed. Several such trials are presently being conducted.

A. Preliminary Testing of Interferons: Therapeutic-Index of Interferon?

How much interferon should be administered to a patient? And how often? And by what route? These questions are presently unanswerable without considerable extrapolation from very limited data.

Primarily, interferon is administered on the rationale of injecting as much as possible. This has been limited by the tolerance of the patient to the relatively crude material being administered (usually injected in the form of "P-IF"; Fig. 11). Often relatively crude interferon is given and is replaced by P-IF if patients develop "troublesome" side effects (Adamson *et al.*, 1977). As previously described, most patients will tolerate injections of a few million units of this interferon every day or two (Section XI. A. 1). The common adverse reaction is a transient fever lasting a few hours. It has been suggested that these are due to impurities, as more purified interferon was less noxious (Strander and Cantell, 1974); this may not be the case entirely (Adamson *et al.*, 1970). It is interesting that when five different samples of P-IF of different purity (5 to 10-fold differences) were tested for pyrogenicity in rabbits, all the samples started to show pyrogenicity at a dose of about 200,000 units/kg (approximately those given to man). Importantly, the pyrogenicity did *not* correlate with the purity of the interferon preparation, suggesting the interferon itself could be pyrogenic (Kauppinen, Myllyla, and Cantell, 1977). Recall that interferon, at levels similar to those in bloodstream after injections, has been reported to induce prostaglandin E and histamine release *in vitro* (Section X. G.). Strander (1977) reports that it has never been necessary to discontinue P-IF-treatment of a patient for any side effects, though he has treated some 70 patients with interferon intramuscularly, some receiving multiple injections each week for years on an ambulatory basis.

It has been reported that patients with hepatitis B developed thrombocytopenia and granulocytopenia (Greenberg *et al.*, 1976) after interferon treatment. It is perhaps noteworthy in this regard that interferon at levels similar to those in patients' blood was also found to be cytotoxic for human granulocytic progenitor cells (Greenberg and Mosny, 1977) and bone marrow cells (Nissen *et al.*, 1977) *in vitro*. Interferon-treated patients have also been reported to develop an inhibitor in their serum which decreased complement-fixing reaction (Strander *et al.*, 1973; Aho *et al.*, 1976).

Limited trials with human fibroblast interferon injections have conflicted. Desomer, Edy, and Billiau (1977) reported that injections of such interferon purified to $10^{6.5}$ units/mg of protein intramuscularly induced high fever about 6 to 12 hours later, sometimes necessitating withdrawal of therapy. All patients repeatedly reacted to each injection of about 50,000 units/kg. When 200,000 units of this interferon was injected intracutaneously, it (and human leukocyte interferon) induced inflammatory skin reactions. These authors caution that skin-test injections of 30,000 units of interferon should precede its intramuscular use, as some patients may be more reactive (allergic). Recall again that interferons have been reported to induce prostaglandin E and enhance histamine release (Section X. G). However, Scott *et al.* (1977a) reported that while human fibroblast interferon induced local inflammation when injected intradermally, neither of two patients treated with 10^7 units of this interferon intramuscularly developed fever or significant hematological alterations.

The frequency of administration has generally been extrapolated from its survival in the circulation. Thus, as interferon is rapidly cleared following either intramuscular or intravenous injections (Fig. 21), it has been assumed it is necessary to maintain as high level as possible by daily or 2-day schedules of "boosters". In some trials several millions of units/day/patient for extended periods have been injected. Clearly a lot of interferon (by present production standards) is required for only a few patients. The level of circulating interferon is likely to be directly related to efficacy in those diseases in which target tissues have a barrier between them and the blood; higher serum interferon levels being needed to breach the barrier.

Intramuscular dosage is routinely used in those circumstances in which sustained blood interferon seems desirable, as this route gives somewhat higher levels over a somewhat longer time than intravenously injected interferon (Fig. 21), and, also, early experiences with intravenously injected interferons were rather unpleasant, inducing vomiting, chills and fever (Strander et al., 1973) or shock (Emodi et al., 1975a).

Clearly, cautious long-term evaluation of interferon-treated patients seems warranted. The injection of relatively large quantities of products of human origin into patients for prolonged periods is a novel form of therapy. Each P-IF preparation is obtained from pooled buffy coats from numerous donors (Section V. C. 2). It was recently suggested that the acid-inactivation of virus inducer would perhaps not destroy certain agents, such as slow-viruses, which have been suggested to be transferred in human tissue transplants (Wadell, 1977).

The development of new techniques for purification of interferons will make it possible soon to determine which of the adverse effects so far described are due to interferon, and continued clinical testings will continue to provide more information about best dosages and routes of administration of the interferons, but it could be many years before full safety assessments of administering such a substance will be possible.

B. Antiviral Activities of Interferons in Man

The trials with interferon in man (listed in Table 18) have been both prophylactic and therapeutic. It has been administered in volunteers to determine whether interferon could prevent viruses from becoming established; all such tests have been against localized virus infections. Such trials determine only portal-of-entry efficacy (Section XII. A. 1). It has been tested in patients with various viral diseases to see if it could alter disease processes after target tissue infection; such tests have included both local and generalized viral diseases. Possibly the strongest evidence that interferon is effective in man in prophylaxis against viral diseases comes from the observations on its administration to cancer patients: such patients have shown few signs of manifest viral diseases, which are normally common complications in such patients (Strander et al., 1973; Ahstrom et al., 1974).

1. Localized Infections

a) Prophylaxis With Interferon

The first reported effect of exogenous interferon in man was against vaccinia virus inoculation in the skin (Scientific Committee on Interferon, 1962).

Table 18. *Clinical trials with interferons*

Disease	Treatment[a]	Effect[b] demon-strated	References
A. *Antiviral studies*			
1. *Localized infections*			
a) *Prophylaxis*			
Vaccinia	$\sim$200 unit (monkey) (id)	+	Scientific Committee on Interferon (1962)
Vaccinia	5×10^4 units (human leukocyte or fibroblast) (id)	+	Scott *et al.* (1977 b, c)
Rhinovirus, parainfluenza-1, coxsackie A-21	$\sim 10^4$ units (monkey) (in)	−	Scientific Comittee on Interferon (1965)
Rhinovirus	10^5 units (human leukocyte) (in)	−	Tyrrell and Reed (1973)
Rhinovirus	10^7 units (human leukocyte) (in)	+	Merigan *et al.* (1973 a)
Influenza	$\sim 10^4$ to 10^5 units (human leukocyte) (in)	+	Soloviev (1967, 1969)
Influenza	10^6 units (human leukocyte) (in)	±	Merigan *et al.* (1973 a)
b) *Therapy*			
Vaccinia gangrenosa	? (monkey) (sc)	−	Connolly, Dick, and Field (1962)
Post-vaccinial skin lesions c	4000 units/gm (ointment) (human leukocyte)	+	Soos *et al.* (1972)
Vaccinial keratitis	? (monkey) (eyedrops)	+	Jones, Galbraith, and Al-Hussaini (1962)
Herpes keratitis	? hourly (human amnion) (eyedrops)	±	Tommila (1063)
Herpes kreatitis c	10^5 units $\times$ 5/day (human leukocyte) (Eyedrops)	+	Kobza *et al.* (1975)
Herpes keratitis	10^7 units/ml daily $\times$ 7 days (human leukocyte)	+	Jones *et al.* (1976)
Herpes keratitis	2 to 6×10^4 units/ml $\times$ 2/day (human leukocyte) (Eyedrops)	−	Kaufman *et al.* (1976)
Herpes keratitis	6×10^4 units/ml 3 times/day (human leukocyte) (eyedrops)	±	Sundmacher *et al.* (1976c)
Herpes keratitis c	6×10^6 units/ml 3 times/day (human leukocyte) (eyedrops)	+	Pallin, Lundmark, and Brege (1976)

Disease		Treatment[a]	Effect[b] demon-strated	References
Herpes keratitis		3×10^6 units/ml 2 drops, 2 times/day (human leukocyte) (eyedrops)	+	Sundmacher, Neumann–Haefelin, and Cantell (1976 a, b)
Genital herpesvirus lesions		4000 units/GM (human leukocyte) (ointment)	+	Ikic et al. (1974; 1975 c)
Genital warts (condylomata acuminata)		4000 units/GM (human leukocyte) (ointment)	+	Ikic et al. (1975 a, b)

2. Generalized infections

Disease		Treatment[a]	Effect[b] demon-strated	References
Herpesvirus zoster		1 to 3×10^6 units 3 times/week (human leukocyte) (im)	+	Strander et al. (1973)
Herpesvirus zoster		3×10^7 units/day 2–5 days (human leukocyte) (im)	+	Jordan, Fried, and Merigan (1974); Merigan et al. (1977)
Herpesvirus zoster		10^6 units/day 5–8 days (human leukocyte) (im)	+	Emodi et al. (1975 b)
Disseminated herpes simplex	c	5×10^5 units/day $\times$ 7 days + 10^6 units/day X 14 days (human leukocyte) (im)	+	Kobza et al. (1975)
Disseminated herpes simplex	c	12×10^5 units/day $\times$ 2 days + 6×10^5 units/day $\times$ 4 days (human leukocyte) (intrathecal)	−	Declercq et al. (1975)
Cytomegalovirus inclusion disease	c	5×10^4 unit/day $\times$ 2 weeks (human leukocyte and amnion) (iv)	±	Falcoff et al. (1966)
Cytomegalovirus inclusion disease	c	10^5 to 10^6 units/ml 8–10 days (human leukocyte) (im)	+	Emodi et al. (1976)
Cytomegalovirus inclusion disease	c	$2–4 \times 10^5$ units/kg/day $\times$ 10–14 days (human leukocyte) (im)	±	Arvin, Yeager, and Merigan (1976)
Cytomegalovirus inclusion disease	c	30×10^6 units/kg (human leukocyte) (im)	+	Merigan et al (1977)
Cytomegalovirus complicating bone marrow transplantation		10^6 units/day $\times$ 5 days (human leukocyte) (im)	±	O'Reilly et al. (1976)
Chronic hepatitis-B		6×10^3 to 17×10^4 units/kg/daily (human leukocyte) (im)	+	Greenberg et al. (1976); Merigan et al. (1977)
Chronic hepatitis-B	c	$15–20 \times 10^4$ units/kg/day	+	Desmyter et al. (1976)

Table 18 (continued)

Disease		Treatment[a]	Effect[b] demonstrated	References
		7 times/2 weeks (human fibroblast)		
Chronic hepatitis-B	c	10^7 units/day × 14 days (human fibroblast) (im)	+	Kingham et al. (1977)
Congenital rubella Syndrome	c	3 × 110^6 units/day × 2 weeks (human leukocyte) (im)	+	Larsson et al. (1976)
Marburg virus	c	3 × 10^6 units/day × 2 weeks (human leukocyte) (im)	+	Anonymous (1977)

B. Antitumor studies

Disease		Treatment[a]	Effect[b] demonstrated	References
Acute leukemia		$\sim10^3$ units/ml, repeatedly (human leukocyte) (iv)	±	Falcoff et al. (1966)
Acute leukemia		1.25–2.5 × 10^6 units/day 1 to 12 month (human leukocyte) (im)	?	Ahstrom et al. (1974)
Hodgkin's disease (stage IVB)	c	5 × 10^6 units/day × 1½ month 7 × 10^6 units/day × 5½ months (human leukocyte) (im)	+	Blomgren et al. (1976)
Multiple myeloma	c	6 × 10^6 units/day (human leukocyte) (im)	+	Strander (1977 a, c)
Juvenile larynx papilloma	c	? (human leukocyte) (im)	+	Strander (1977 a, c)
Osteosarcoma		3 × 10^6 units/day × 1 month + 3 × 10^6 units, 3 times/week × 17 months	+	Strander et al. (1974, 1975, 1976, 1977) Strander (1977 a, b, c) Adamson et al. (1977)

a Indicated route of inoculation: id = intradermal; in = intranasal; sc = subcutaneous; iv = intravenous; im = intramuscular
b Effect demonstrated: – = no evidence of effect; ± = suggestive effect; + = effectiveness reported.
c Uncontrolled trial with only one or two patients.

Volunteers were injected intradermally with 0.1 ml of a preparation of monkey interferon titrating about 2000 units/ml, and vaccinia virus was scarified into the area the next day. A highly significant protection was reported. In more recent trials human fibroblast interferon was also found to be effective in preventing vaccinia "takes" (Scott et al., 1977c) and crude human fibroblast and human leukocyte interferon preparations seemed of similar efficacy (Scott et al., 1977b).

A large trial for prophylaxis against influenza was reported by Soloviev (1967) in which volunteers were treated with low-titered human interferon aerosol intranasally 24 hours prior to virus by the same route. Prophylaxis was apparent from lowered virus isolations 3 days later. In a field trial involving several thousand people during an influenza epidemic, such interferon treatment was reported to be successful (Soloviev, 1969). These surprising successes may be attributable to the interferon treatment priming the local tissues to produce interferon in response to subsequent infection, or perhaps residual inducer was also being applied. In any event, human leukocyte interferon preparations are commercially available in the USSR and are widely used for prophylaxis and therapy of a wide variety of diseases (Merigan, Jordan and Fried, 1975; G. Svet–Moldavsky, personal communication, 1978).

Interferon prophylaxis against influenza and "common colds" has been considerably less impressive in the Western countries. An initial trial against rhinoviruses by intranasally sprayed monkey interferon (about 10^4 units) was without apparent effect (Scientific Committee on Interferon, 1965). A followup study, using human interferon (about 10^5 units) against lower dose of rhinovirus challenge was also unsuccessful (Tyrrell, 1976). However, Merigan *et al.* (1973) reported that by using about 100 times more interferon intranasally both 1 day before and 3 days after virus it was possible to statistically-significantly prevent symptoms and virus shedding. But the effect obtained with a 10-fold lower dose of interferon against influenza B virus in volunteers was slight, only delaying development of symptoms about 1 day.

b) Therapy of Localized Infections

Locally injected monkey interferon into a lesion of vaccinia gangrenosa was ineffective (Connolly, Dick, and Field, 1962), perhaps because the interferon was low-titered. In Yugoslavia in 1972 a smallpox epidemic lead to mass vaccinia inoculations with a number of resultant postvaccinal complications on the skin. Soos *et al.* (1972) reported that application of an ointment of human leukocyte interferon (1 gm of ointment contained 4000 units), 5 times/day resulted in quicker healing of lesions.

Vaccinial keratitis was first treated with monkey interferon (Jones, Galbraith and Al-Hussaini, 1962). This interferon, of low titer, was applied in eyedrops each half-hour during the day, and in all cases the granular opacification of the epithelium resolved within 1 day, healing proceeding at about the same rate as seen after mechanical removal of the diseased tissues, within 1 to 4 days. However, stromal edema and diffuse infiltration developed subsequently in both debrided and interferon-treated patients.

Herpetic keratitis was also treated with low-titered human interferon, given hourly (Tommila, 1963). While lesions regressed more quickly than in control patients treated by iodine cauterization, they recurred at the same rates.

More than 10 years passed before interferon was again attempted in herpes infections of the eye. Kobza *et al.* (1975) reported that, as a last resort, a patient with severe herpetic keratitis (having persisted for 70 days despite locally applied idoxuridine, intravenous cytosine arabinoside and prednisone) was treated with topical human leukocyte interferon eyedrops (about 10^5 units 4 times/day)[14]. These authors report that the long-persisting burning pains

---

[14] The *concentration* of the interferon was not specified.

diminished rapidly and 8 days after initiation of interferon therapy only a small infiltration on the eye remained; it was reported that keratitis did not recur during the following year. Importantly in a randomized, placebo-controlled trial of human leukocyte interferon in human herpetic keratitis it was also found that daily interferon eyedrops for 7 days prevented recrudescence of epithelial herpetic lesions after minimal wiping-debridements (Jones et al., 1976); this treatment should likely be considered prophylaxis as interferon was apparently ineffective in inducing cure of established lesions.

Kaufman et al. (1976) reported an ongoing trial on patients with herpetic keratitis, employing human leukocyte interferon (at about 6×10^4 units/ml). Recurrences had occurred with the same frequency in interferon-treated and control groups in 18 months, possibly because the concentration of interferon was too low. Sundmacher et al. (1976c) reported preliminary results of a trial of interferon in 55 herpetic keratitis patients divided into three groups: one treated with interferon eyedrops alone, one with thermocautery alone and one with interferon and thermocautery. Interferon (at about 6×10^4 units/ml, 3 drops 3 time/day) was not effective alone but may have been of value in addition to thermocautery.

Pallin, Lundmark, and Brege (1976) reported a single case of herpetic keratitis, which was seemingly refractive to other therapeutic measures; this infant showed rapid improvement within 1 day and healing after treatment with human leukocyte interferon at 6×10^6 units/ml. Treatment was stopped after 2 weeks and the patient remained free of symptoms.

Sundmacher, Neumann–Haefelin, and Cantell (1976a, b), on the assumption that earlier partial effect of interferon was related to low concentration of the interferon used, applied interferon at 3×10^6 units/ml in virologically confirmed cases of dendritic keratitis in a randomized, double-blind placebo-controlled study, after thermodebridement of the corneal epithelium and after local anesthesia of the cul-de-sac. All interferon treated corneas healed within 8 days, healing was significantly faster with interferon, and herpesvirus shedding was stopped earlier. It was concluded that interferon was the most important factor in this combined therapy. These studies raise hopes that interferon therapy will also inhibit recurrent herpes by local application.

Ikic and his associates (1974, 1975c) have reported that interferon-ointment is useful in treatment of labial and genital herpes lesions. The genital warts, Condylomata acuminata, was also reported to rapidly regress when treated with the interferon cream (Ikic et al., 1975a, b).

Thus in all the local applications of interferon, effectiveness has increased in direct proportion to the concentration of interferon applied to the infected area.

2. Systemic Viral Infections

Interferon has been administered therapeutically in a few systemic virus diseases. These studies require much larger investments of interferon than the topical applications described above just to achieve general distribution of low levels of interferon, and it has been virtually impossible to achieve interferon concentrations at the sites of virus replication similar to the levels shown to be most effective in localized infections. Hopefully with availability of highly purified and potent interferon preparations it will soon be possible to enhance the modest effect so far observed in generalized virus diseases.

a) Disseminated Herpesvirus: Varicella-Zoster

Herpesviruses have often been reported to be resistant to interferons *in vitro* (Table 14), and it has thus been assumed that interferon treatment would be of little use in such infections. Such interpretation would presume that interferon action *in vivo* is restricted to the antiviral mechanisms measurable in cell cultures. Clearly the cell-mediated immune responses are important in control of such diseases *in vivo* with the viruses that can effectively avoid neutralizing serum antibodies (Jordan and Merigan, 1974; Rasmussen *et al.*, 1974); interferon might act by enhancing this infection erradication mechanism. Interferon is found in vesicle fluids of patients with chicken pox and zoster (Armstrong *et al.*, 1970). Often inability of leukocytes to produce interferon has correlated with susceptibility to recurrent herpes lesions (Rasmussen *et al.*, 1974), and it was reported that recovery from herpes zoster correlated only with time of appearance of interferon in vesicle fluid, which predicted lesion crusting and healing (Stevens and Merigan, 1972).

Strander *et al.* (1973) reported that 3 cancer patients with disseminated herpes zoster showed complete clinical recovery from the virus infection within 10 days after initiation of intramuscular injections of human leukocyte interferon ($1-3 \times 10^6$ units, 3 times/week).

Merigan and his associates (Jordan, Fried, and Merigan, 1974) injected interferon into 9 patients with malignancies complicated with disseminated zoster, some receiving as much as 80×10^6 units/day, intramuscularly. The only adverse effect seemed to be a fever of up to 40° C after injections. In these patients there was less frequent involvement of visceral organs, pain abatement was also apparent, and severity of post-herpetic neuralgia was lessened (Merigan *et al.*, 1977).

Another study on the effect of interferon (10^6 units/day for 5–8 days, intramuscularly) on disseminated herpesvirus infection was reported by Emodi *et al.* (1975b) in which the duration of pain was diminished and lesion crusting was enhanced. High interferon levels were recovered from vesicle fluid after injection of interferon. These workers (Kobza *et al.*, 1975) also reported a single case of disseminated herpes simplex that was treated with human leukocyte interferon injected intravenously and intramuscularly. Response was encouraging: the patient reportedly "is leading an active sexual life". Viva interferon.

b) Cytomegalovirus Infections

Infections with cytomegalovirus (CMV) are normally of little consequence, but in the fetus or in immunosuppressed patients it can cause severe disease. It is a major cause of infant death and mental retardation. CMV can be activated following transplantation, causing interstitial pneumonia and leukopenia, hepatitis and graft rejection.

In view of the known antiviral effect of interferons and their apparent ability to prolong graft rejections, it would seem that this substance would be ideally suited for administration to transplant recipients undergoing immunosuppressive therapy. Also congenitally infected infants have been reported to be defective in ability to produce interferon, in which case exogenous interferon might be beneficial (Emodi and Just, 1974 b).

However, the argument that was applied for herpesvirus not being a good virus for interferon trials, based on its *in vitro* resistance to interferon action, could as well apply to CMV (Table 14), assuming that the *in vivo* virus restraints are limited to those seen *in vitro*. Again, this is not likely the case considering all the other virus-restrictive possibilities with interferon in animals (Chapter XII).

Falcoff *et al.* (1966) were the first to report treating a CMV-infected patient with interferon. Three newborns with cytomegalic inclusion disease (congenital CMV infection) were given large injections of crude low titered ($\sim 10^3$ units/ml) leukocyte and amnion cell interferon intravenously.

Emodi and his collaborators (1976) injected human leukocyte interferon into 9 patients with either acquired or congenital CMV infections, and found that viruria was completely inhibited. In 5 patients virus in urine was only transiently suppressed, but in some patients it was reported to be negative even 6 months after treatment. Viremia was apparently unaltered. Repeated courses of interferon therapy gave similar transient effects.

Arvin *et al.* (1976) treated 5 infants having symptomatic cytomegalic inclusion disease and persistent viruria with doses of about $2-4 \times 10^5$ units of human leukocyte interferon/kg/day for 1 to 2 weeks. One infant showed a transient suppression of viruria in the first coarse of interferon but not on 5 further coarses of treatment. One child with hepatits became asymptimatic after 3 months, and one child showing no effect on first treatment showed suppressed urine viral titers during the second coarse at slightly higher dose ($\sim$ 2-fold increase).

O'Reilly and his associates (1976) reported on two patients that developed CMV infections following allogeneic bone marrow transplantation and that were injected intramuscularly with daily injections of 10^6 units of human leukocyte interferon prepared by Dr. Emodi. In one patient with graft-vs-host disease and hepatitis, interferon therapy was associated with significant clinical improvement and suppression of viremia. No suppression of bone marrow engraftment was observed. One patient injected with a separate interferon preparation failed to respond to a second course of therapy and died, though she had responded well previously. It was subsequently determined that this lot of interferon apparently had lost more than 90% of its original activity such that, instead of the usual 100 units/ml level obtained with the first interferon, only about 10 units/ml were achieved.

Recently, Merigan *et al.* (1977) have reported that human leukocyte interferon at a dosage of 35 million units/kg was required to diminish viruria in a newborn excreting CMV, and this effect was transient, with virus excretion returning to previous levels when interferon was stopped.

Cheeseman, Rinaldo, and Hirsch (1977) have concluded that so far the evidence for usefulness of interferon in CMV infections is unclear. It seems clear that it will require a lot of interferon to achieve an effect, and it will require double-blind placebo-controlled studies to demonstrate it. Such studies on a *prophylactic* basis of interferon against CMV in transplant recipients, both marrow and renal, are currently underway.

c) Hepatitis B Virus Infections

Interferon production is apparently deficient in hepatitis B infections (Taylor and Zuckerman, 1968; Wheelock, Schenker, and Combes, 1968; Hill, Walsh, and Purcell, 1971), and it has been reported that lymphocytes from children with chronic hepatitis B have decreased ability to produce interferon when stimulated *in vitro* (Tolentino et al., 1975). This would suggest that exogenous interferon would not be superfluous and might be worthwhile in hepatitis B infections. Clearly, any hope of treatment for this widespread disabilitating and often fatal disease would be worth exploring. It has been estimated that more than 200 million people are infected with this agent (Desmyter, 1977).

An advantage to studies on chronic hepatitis B is that the patients normally have stable levels of viral antigens in both blood and liver and any alteration would be evidence of effect even if not sufficient for clinical improvement. In 1976 two reports demonstrated that human interferons might have therapeutic value in this disease (Desmyter et al., 1976; Greenberg et al., 1976).

In one study (Greenberg et al., 1976) 4 patients with chronic active hepatitis B were injected daily with human leukocyte interferon, in doses ranging from only 6,000 to 170,000 units/kg. Three of the patients had circulating Dane-particle markers (Dane particle-associated DNA and DNA polymerase activity and hepatitis B core antigen) that had been consistently high. After interferon injections all these markers fell to low levels. When interferon injections were given for only 10 days or less the suppression of these markers was transient, but when administered for a month or more it appeared that their inhibition was more permanent. Liver function tests were apparently not restored to normal.

With prolonged treatment with interferon for more than a year, one patient maintained Dane particle surface antigens, though becoming negative for Dane particles, but one patient was reported to become negative for all the hepatitis B viral antigens and liver function improvement was noted (Merigan et al., 1977).

Desmyter and his associates (1976) treated one patient suffering chronic active hepatitis B with 7 intramuscular injections of 10^7 units of human fibroblast interferon over a 2-week period. Two chimpanzees carrying hepatitis B surface antigen were similarly treated. The patient showed depression of hepatitis B virus core antigen in the liver, but no significant changes were seen in circulating antigen levels or in liver pathology in man or monkeys.

These studies clearly demonstrated that exogenous interferon can exert an effect on viral markers of hepatitis B. Another report has recently appeared on the effect of human fibroblast interferon in 2 patients with chronic active hepatitis B (Kingham *et al.*, 1977). In this study both patients showed a marked fall in titer of antibody to hepatitis B core antigen.

The mechanism of the activity of interferon against hepatitis B infection is not known. However, an effect of interferon on immune mechanisms associated with cytotoxicity of lymphocytes for target cells (Vladutiu, 1977), as well as its *in vitro*-type antiviral effect, can be envisioned.

d) Interferon Therapy in Other Viral Diseases

Interferon was administered to a 14 month old baby suffering from congenital rubella syndrome who had developed a long-standing cutaneous eruption. Daily injection of 3×10^6 units of human leukocyte interferon for 2 weeks produced a marked regression of the cutaneous symptoms and healing was complete within 2 months. Rubella virus, which had been isolated in urine and blood, disappeared from the blood but persisted in the urine (Larsson *et al.*, 1976). This suggests that interferon treatment had suppressed the infection possibly by preventing infection of new cells, but it did not completely cure cells already infected.

Interferon was also administered in a patient infected with Marburg virus in a laboratory accident. The patient was injected with 3×10^6 units twice/day for 14 days starting within 48 hours of a rise in his temperature 5 days after infection. There was a rapid fall of viremia within 24 hours of treatment, nausea and vomiting declined on the 12th day and the patient recovered (Anonymous, 1977). While it is impossible to ascertain that interferon was responsible for this recovery from disease caused by a highly infectious agent with a high mortality rate, it certainly recommends interferon as one of the few options available for possible therapy in such accidents.

3. Antiviral Effects of Interferon Inducers in Man

Interferon inducers have repeatedly been shown to have antiviral activities in man, but clinical applications of this effect have usually been limited by the problems of inducer toxicities and the problem of hyporesponsiveness.

a) Virus Interference in Man

It has been observed that certain live virus vaccines given together or sequentially can interfere with development of antibody responses to one another, presumably because the virus must replicate to provide enough antigenic mass for immunization, and induced interferon would prevent the necessary virus growth. It has also been demonstrated that concurrent infections with measles and chickenpox can modify the disease manifestation of one or the other infection (Merigan *et al.*, 1968). Also, children inoculated with live measles vaccine were found to be refractory to anti-smallpox vaccination several days later, at a time when measles vaccine-induced serum interferon levels were elevated (Petrali, Merigan, and Wilbur, 1965a). Interference between viruses, possibly mediated by interferon, has also been suggested to control epidemics of influenza in populations being immunized on a large-scale with oral poliovirus vaccine (Hale et al., 1959) or measles vaccine virus (Byrne et al., 1967).

Inactivated influenza virus, introduced intranasally, was also reported to protect against experimental influenza infections and epidemic influenza (Balezina et al., 1966; Soloviev, 1967). Inactivated ZEW-4-virus was also claimed to induce interferon and provide therapeutic effect in herpetic keratitis (Tkacheva, Gvozdilova, and Smorodintsev, 1971).

b) Poly rI·poly rC in the Clinic

Hill et al. (1971, 1972) initiated trials on effectiveness of poly rI·polyrC in prophylaxis against rhinovirus and influenza. Given intranasally the day before rhinovirus 13 virus, 7 mg of poly rI·poly rC in 14 hourly doses, was not significantly effective, though symptoms may have been decreased. In a similar study against influenza A 2 Hong Kong virus, the inducer was also ineffective in reducing incidence of illness or virus shedding. Interferon was detectable in nasal washings after application of the inducer and no toxicity was observed.

Centifanto, Goohra, and Kaufman (1970) reported that poly rI·poly rC induced interferon in human eyes, and Guerra et al. (1970) reported on a double-blind study of poly rI·poly rC used therapeutically as eyedrops (1 mg/ml) against herpes keratitis; some effectiveness was suggested. Galin, Chow-chiweck, and Kronenberg (1976) also used poly rI·poly rC eyedrops in patients with herpes simplex keratitis and claimed some therapeutic benefits, without toxic effects at a dose of 1 mg/ml, 14 drops/day for 7 days.

When poly rI·poly rC was administered intravenously into one infant with herpes encephalitis at a daily dose of 0.10 mg/kg for 11 days liver-function parameters were elevated, but returned to normal after the treatment was stopped; also, cancer patients injected intravenously with poly rI·poly rC for 20 days and patients with subacute sclerosing panencephalitis (SSPE) injected for 10 days all had circulating interferon and fever. No benefits from these treatments were reported.

Recently, Guggenheim, and Baron (1977) reported a study conducted between 1969 and 1972 in which 15 children were infused intravenously with poly rI·poly rC. All these children had serious neurologic disease likely related to virus infections, 6 with SSPE, 7 with Reye's syndrome, one with congenital rubella and one with polio-dystrophy. No benefit to these children was evident. In each patient, serum interferon, 8 to 500 units/ml was detected after primary doses of 0.1 to 1.0 mg/kg, but persisted less than 24 hours, and hyporesponsiveness persisted for 7 days. If the protective effect is diminished during the hyporesponsive period, it would seem that maintenance of the antiviral activity would require inoculations of exogenous interferon during this refractory stage.

Twenty-four cancer patients suffering herpesvirus hominis or zoster infections were treated with poly rI·poly rC at doses of 3 to 12 mg/kg (Freeman et al., 1977). Toxicity, considered to be "acceptable", consisted of fever of up to 40.7° C, elevated liver enzymes, and coagulation abnormalities. Interferon was detectable in sera in the first day; peak responses were, however, very low, ranging from <3 units/ml to 128 units/ml. No benefit to the patients was apparent, though a slight effect was suggested on duration of disease. The numbers of patients were not great enough to clarify the significance of these effects. With the levels of interferon produced and with the reported toxicity, it would seem doubtful that further such tests would be worthwhile. However, on the basis of these data Freeman et al. (1977) report that they have initiated a randomized double-blind study to determine whether poly rI·poly rC is actually ineffective in the treatment of herpes zoster.

Borecky (1977) reports an instance where double-stranded RNA was injected into a patient with rabies, 10 mg/day for 6 days. This patient and 5 others with advanced cancer reportedly "tolerated" the injections. However, in view of their other problems it was difficult to evaluate what sort of alterations were tue to the inducer. Borecky (1977) emphasizes the problems of evaluating the toxicity and effectiveness of these drugs in patients with overlying diseases or combined diseases, such as cancer and herpesviruses, and mainly on the basis of these toxicological considerations he advocates limiting studies with this type of inducer to localized viral infections with topical administration of the inducer. Surely diseased patients hardly seem to need the further compromise of drug toxicities offering no obvious benefits.

Borecky (1977) reports several instances of apparently successful treatment of eye infections with the F 2 bacteriophage double-stranded RNA, and it was reported also to be effective for treating warts. An ointment containing this inducer was apparently topically effective when applied to genital herpesvirus lesions, shortening the duration of illness and causing a rapid feeling of relief. This type of therapy may be the appropriate application of the double-stranded RNA-type inducers in man. It seems, however, that the ribonuclease resistant poly rI·poly rC·poly-L-lysine in carboxymethylcellulose (PICLC) will undergo a trial period against local and systemic virus diseases (Galasso and Dunnick, 1977).

c) Propanediamine and Its Vehicle

The first trial on the effect of the low molecular weight interferon inducer propanediamine reported by Jackson and his associates (Gatmaitan, Stanley, and Jackson, 1973), suggested that the drug induced low levels of nasal interferon, but that the slight prophylactic beneficial effect against rhinovirus, if any was measurable at all, appeared not to be related to the interferon. Similar data were provided by Douglas and Betts (1974) and Douglas et al. (1975). Subsequently Jackson and his collaborators (Panusarn et al., 1974) claimed that a statistically significant drug-related and interferon-related protection against rhinovirus illness was offered by prophylaxis with the propanediamine in a "modified" preparation. Supposedly the same drug in small particle sizes was more effective, and the microtized preparation could then prevent symptoms and virus shedding in volunteers in association with production of nasal interferon.

The apparent success of this drug seemed to offer new hope for applicability of interferon inducers. Curiously, Jackson and his associates (Stanley et al., 1976) later found that the vehicle for the drug was itself an inducer of interferon in the nasal tissues and reduced the rate of infections. The vehicle, an emulsion of polysorbate-80 and glycerol, and the drug were both found to induce interferon, but the beneficial effect on symptoms did not appear to depend on suppression of virus. The authors conclude that these data emphasize the need to include proper placebo controls.

In summary, it seems that benefits from interferon inducers in man have not been as clearly demonstrated as the benefits of exogenous interferons, this in spite of the abundance of the former and scarcity of the latter.

C. Cancer Therapy With Interferon

In the previous Sections on effects of interferon and inducers in virus diseases in animals and in man, I first described the effects found with interferons and then described the effects found with the inducers. In this Section, I shall reverse this order, to end on a more positive note.

1. Antitumor Activity of Interferon Inducers in Man

The first application of an interferon inducer for cancer therapy might have been the report by Coley (1894) who reported that bacterial toxins could provide benefit to patients, and the modern equivalent of the phenomenon could be the widespread use of bacillus-Calmette-Guerin (BCG) therapy in cancer (Mathe, 1971). It is, of course, only speculation that interferon is involved in these effects, but this form of therapy also exerts antiviral activity (Old et al., 1963), and in combination with the other lymphokines induced by such treatment, interferon may prove more effective than when acting alone.

Viruses which induce interferons have also been used to treat cancer patients, with negligible results (Southam, 1960; Southam and Moore, 1952; Wheelock, 1970). Wheelock and Dingel (1964) injected a variety of interferon-inducing viruses into a patient with acute myelogenous leukemia and observed a transient improvement after each injection.

Pyran copolymers have been used in cancer patients with marked toxic effects and little beneficial effects; it also seems unlikely that these agents exert their action through interferon mechanisms (Regelson, 1973).

Poly rI·poly rC has been repeatedly studied for antineoplastic effects in man. Mathe et al. (1970) presented preliminary indications that it induced remission in patients with acute lymphoblastic leukemia (it was clearly a more defined therapy than BCG treatment), and other early evidence was promising (Young, 1971; DeVita et al., 1970). In one report, a group of patients with cervical carcinomas were inoculated with poly rI·poly rC and live measles vaccine directly into the lesion. The reported complete disappearance of neoplastic cells needs confirmation (Ayre, Narvaez, and LoGerfo, 1973).

Cornell et al. (1977) reported a preliminary study on the effects of poly rI·poly rC in 22 cancer patients. Patients developed a flu-like illness with fever and nausea when given poly rI·poly rC at 1 mg/kg intravenously. Mean interferon titers with one lot of inducer was 85 units/ml. Importantly, they found that one lot of poly rI·poly rC did not induce interferon. This unreliability of a definite synthetic molecule is worrisome. In a follow-up study on poly rI·poly rC in adjunct to remission maintenance therapy of acute myelogenous leukemia (McIntyre *et al.*, 1977), it was reported that the results of a nonrandom trial could not be compared with a control group because of differences in the chemotherapeutic programs employed; it was reported that the duration of remission and survival data for the poly rI·poly rC group showed no influence on these parameters, but "at the very least, the treatment had not been harmful".

2. Effects of Interferon

The first report of interferon administered to patients with cancer was several years before it was realized that enormous unitages of interferon would be required for an effect to be measured. Thus Falcoff and his colleague (1966) repeatedly injected a few thousand units of human leukocyte interferon into patients with acute leukemia for prolonged periods and reported that average survival appeared to be increased.

Ahstrom *et al.* (1974) reported treating 6 children with acute lymphoblastic or myelogenous leukemias with human leukocyte interferon, about 1 to 3×10^6 units/day for from one month to more than a year. The results did not permit any conclusion about the efficacy of interferon in regard to the leukemia, but the authors were impressed that no virus diseases ever developed in any of the patients during the treatment, though these diseases usually predispose to such infections.

Interferon treatment of a case of Hodgkins disease (lymphocyte predominance, stage IV. B) with human leukocyte interferon was reported by Blomgren et al (1976). Daily injections of 5×10^6 units, intramuscularly for $1^1/_2$ months, induced a remission, as measured by decrease in the size of peripheral glands, and decreased pulmonary infiltration; B symptoms disappeared completely, laboratory values normalized, and the patient's lymphocytes exhibited mitogenic responsiveness. As regression slowed after $1^1/_2$ months, daily dose was increased slightly to 7×10^6 units, without further improvement. After over 10^9 units of interferon had been injected, tumor began progressing and interferon treatment was replaced with cytostatic courses, which gave partial remission after 6 months.

Strander (1977a, c) also reported that a patient with advanced multiple myeloma responded similarly to the experience with Hodgkins disease. He has also demonstrated dramatic repeated tumor regressions in 2 children with larynx papilloma which regrows after each treatment course is stopped (Strander, 1977a, c).

Cantell (1977) reports that more interferon has been used for the treatment of osteosarcoma than for any other diseases. On the basis of the grave prognosis of this tumor, even despite early amputation and irradiation, he and Dr. Strander undertook an extended trial on this disease. This trial, initiated in 1971 at the Karolinska Hospital in Stockholm, has now been running for 7 years and has increased in numbers of patients and the results, which have been extensively and repeatedly analyzed by pathologists and clinicians, become more interesting with each successive report (Strander *et al.*, 1974; 1975; 1976; 1977; Adamson *et al.*, 1977; Strander, 1977a, b, c).

Patients with osteosarcoma of the long bones (as of the end of 1977, numbered 28 in the interferon-treated group) and who had no detectable metastases on admission are treated with 3×10^6 units of human leukocyte daily for 1 month as adjuvant therapy after removal of the primary tumor (either by exarticulation, amputation or resection; 30% have been resections). After 1 month interferon is injected 3 times per week on an ambulatory basis for another 17 months. Additionally it should be emphasized that whereas many of the present cancer treatments leave patients highly susceptible to often fatal virus infections, interferon has added value of apparently rendering the patient virus-resistant.

Survival without metastases has been compared to 2 different control groups, one of 35 historical cases treated at the Karolinska Hospital between 1952 and 1971, and one current control group of 23 cases from other Swedish hospitals from 1971 to 1974. At the end of a $2^{1}/_{2}$ year period of comparative studies, life-table analysis reveals 64% of the interferon-treated patients were free from metastases while only 30% of the concurrent control group and 10% of the historical control group were free of metastases (Strander, 1977a). Of the interferon-treated group, 73% have survived to date, compared to 35% in the concurrent control group.

Thus interferon appears to provide marked protection against metastasis in osteosarcoma. These results will continue to be evaluated in terms of other modalities of cancer chemotherpy. It should, therefore, also be emphasized that while many of the cytostatic-cytotoxic treatments are quite toxic, requiring hospitalization, interferon is virtually free of side effects, most patients administering their own dosages at home. Thus, even with the labor and expense of large-scale production of interferon, such out-patient treatment was cheaper than the high level methotrexate (in-patient) treatment (Strander, 1977 a, b, c).

The apparent success of these limited trials with interferon, though still not numerically large enough to be statistically significant, have encouraged a number of other ventures in this area of interferon therapy. Trials in patients with osteosarcoma and neuroblastoma were recently reported to be underway, using human fibroblast interferon (Desomer, 1977), and human lymphoblastoid interferon is being tested in osteosarcoma (G. Bodo, personal communication). A study in non-Hodgin's lymphoma patients who failed standard therapy is presently underway (Merigan et al., 1977). A trial of human leukocyte interferon to prevent metastases in patients who have lung removal for adenocarcinoma will soon begin (H. Oettgen, personal communication), and a study is presently underway to evaluate interferon in the therapy of breast cancer (Habif, personal communication; J. Gutterman, personal communication).

To meet the needs for part of the interferon required for further clinical trials, the Memorial Sloan-Kettering Cancer Center, New York, has recently established a production facility for human leukocyte interferon in Switzerland (a site chosen largely for availability of large numbers of hepatitis-B-free blood donors). Many more such facilities are already required to meet the demands for expanded clinical trials with interferon.

XV. Prelude to the Interferon System

The Interferon System has now been actively explored for 21 years since Alick Isaacs discovered it, and research on the System seems to have matured with the normal amount of growing pains and struggle for recognition. Ten years ago, Jan Vilček (1969) concluded his Monograph on Interferon with a reflection by a fellow scientist's teasing "do you *really* think interferon exists?" It now appears that it does.

After reviewing all the work that has so far been invested in studies on The Interferon System, it looks as though most of the labor is ahead. Clearly the past work has provided much information on how to produce interferon and how to purify it. These efforts have recorded several of its activities, and have begun probing a few of its mechanisms. The reports to date have described several of its potentials as antiviral and antitumor agents. These studies have, thus, cumulatively provided a good beginning.

The preview of things to come looks exciting:

1. Studies on the mechanisms controlling the transcription and translation of interferons will likely soon enable better artificial regulation of these mechanisms, to provide sufficient interferon messenger RNA to allow its retrocopy into prokaryotic cells from which clones interferon can become truly abundant.

2. Purification, sequencing and artificial synthesis of interferons, long considered next to ridiculous to even speculate on, now seems a likelihood in the near future. Work presently underway will likely provide small active cores of the second-generation of interferons – the interferoids – which should facilitate chemical synthesis, and mass availability.

3. With pure interferons it will be possible to define the breadth of interferon actions, which will likely encompass a number of antiviral-related, immune-related and physiological alterations. Extensive work remains to define the effective dosages of interferons required to achieve the effect desired, both in cell cultures and *in vivo*.

4. An abundance of pure interferons will enable its use in sufficient clinical trials to first define its therapeutic potential and subsequently to realize it.

5. Analyses of the actions and interactions of interferons and other lymphokines will likely reveal even more methods for potential physiological manipulations. This last point deserves emphasis. Interferon is only one of a large number of products by which cells communicate. It is as though we have learned only one of their words and pretend to speak their language. Some of these other lymphokines may in fact act by modifying interferon effects, or

vice versa; some may be induced by interferons, or vice versa; some may act synergistically with interferons, and others may be independent of interferon altogether. Thus, studies on this aspect of the Interferon System will require defining these various lymphokines, some of which are only measurable as rather obscure activities in preparations in which they are only trace components (rather reminiscent of interferons not so long ago).

In regard to Jan Vilček's Epilogue about 10 years ago, in which he related being tormented by an associate as to whether he really thought interferons existed, it is ironical that after listening to a Fellow working next door to my laboratories expound about some other lymphokine he works with, I found myself tempted to say "That's very interesting, but do you *really* think that it exists?".

Acknowledgements

The author thanks Marzenna Wiranowska–Stewart for her valuable assistance in translations of Russian literature and in preparation of this manuscript, and Dr. Leo S. Lin for help in designing the Figures. Work from the author's laboratory was supported by NIH Grant CA-20863 and Sloan-Kettering Institute Core Grant CA-08748, both from the National Cancer Institute. The author was supported by U. S. Public Health Service Research Career Development Award AI-00219 from the National Institute of Allergy and Infectious Disease.

References

Aboud, M., Shoor, R., Salzberg, S.: Effect of interferon on exogenous murine leukemia virus infection. Virology 84, 134–141 (1978).

Aboud, M., Weiss, O., Salzberg, S.: Rapid quantitation of interferon with chronically oncornavirus producing cells. Infect. Immun. 13, 1626–1630 (1976).

Absher, M., Stinebring, W. R.: Endotoxin-like properties of poly I·poly C an interferon stimulator. Nature 223, 715–718 (1969).

Acton, J. D.: The lymphoreticular system and interferon production. J. Reticuloendothel. Soc. 14, 449–461 (1973).

Acton, J. D., Myrvik, Q. N.: Production of interferon by alveolar macrophages. J. Bacteriol. 91, 2300–2304 (1966).

Adams, A., Lidin, B., Strander, H., Cantell, K.: Spontaneous interferon production and Epstein-Barr virus expression in human lymphoid cell lines. J. Gen. Virol. 28, 219–225 (1975).

Adams, A., Strander, H., Cantell, K.: Sensitivity of Epstein-Barr virus transformed human lymphoid cell lines to interferon. J. Gen. Virol. 28, 207–214 (1975).

Adamson, R. H.: Antitumor activity of tilorone hydrochloride against some rodent tumors: Preliminary report. J. Natl. Cancer Inst. 46, 431–433 (1971 a).

Adamson, R. H.: Antitumor activity of two antiviral drugs-rifampicin and tilorone. The Lancet 1, 398–400 (1971 b).

Adamson, R. H., Fabro, S.: Embryotoxic effect of poly I·poly C. Nature (London) 223, 718–720 (1969).

Adamson, R. H., Fabro, S., Homan, E. R., O'Garo, R. W., Zevzian, R. P.: Pharmacology of polyriboinosinic: polyribocytidylic acid, a new antiviral and antitumor agent. Antimicrob. Agents Chemotherapy 4, 148–152 (1969).

Adamson, U., Aparisi, T., Brostrom, L. A., Cantell, K., Einhorn, S., Hall, K., Ingimarsson, S., Nilsonne, U., Strander, H., Soderberg, G.: The role of non-specific immunity in treatment of cancer. Study Week of the Pontifical Acad. Sci. Vatican City, 17–21 October 1977. Interferon treatment of human osteosarcoma (1977).

Ahl, R., Rump, A.: Assay of bovine interferons in cultures of the porcine cell line IB-RS-2. Infect. Immun. 14, 603–610 (1976).

Aho, K., Strander, H., Leikola, J., Kleemola, M., Carlstrom, G., Cantell, K.: An inhibitor of the complement-fixation reaction associated with interferon treatment. Clin. Immunol. Immunopath. 5, 399–403 (1976).

Ahstrom, L., Dohlwitz, A., Strander, M., Carlstrom, G., Cantell, K.: Interferon in acute leukemia in children. Lancet 1, 166–167 (1974).

Aksenov, O. A., Golovin, B. P., Smorodintsev, A.: Antiviral action of the yeast RNA derivatives and the effect of polycations thereon. Vopr. Virusol. 27, 51–53 (1970). (In Russian.)

Allen, L. B., Cochran, K. W.: Target-organ treatment of neurotropic virus disease with interferon inducers. Infect. Immun. 6, 819–823 (1972).

Allen, L. B., Eagle, N. C., Huffman, J. M., Shuman, D. A., Mayer, R. B., jr., Sidwell, R. A.: Enhancement of interferon antiviral action in L-cells by cyclic nucleotides. Proc. Soc. Exp. Biol. Med. 146, 580–584 (1974).

Allen, P. T., Giron, D. J.: Rapid sensitive assay for interferons based on the inhibition of MM virus nucleic acid synthesis. Appl. Microbiol. 20, 317–322 (1970).

Allen, P. T., Schellekens, H., Van Griensven, L. J. L. D., Billiau, A.: Differential sensitivity of Rauscher Murine Leukemia Virus (MuLV-R) to interferons in two interferon-responsive cell lines. J. Gen Virol. 31, 429–435 (1976).

Allen, P. T., Stewart II, W. E.: Evidence that detergent-reactivated interferon is not renatured. J. Gen. Virol. **32**, 133–136 (1976).

Allison, A. C.: Interference with, and interferon production by, polyoma virus. Virology **15**, 47–51 (1961).

Anderson, C. D., Atherton, J. G.: Effect of Actinomycin D on measles virus growth and interferon production. Nature **117**, 671–673 (1964).

Anderson, S. G.: The production of antibody in the presence of interferon. Australian J. Exp. Biol. Med. Sci. **43**, 345–350 (1965).

Andrews, R. D.: Specificity of interferon. British Med. J. i, 1728–1730 (1961).

Anfinsen, C. B., Bose, S., Corley, L., Gurari–Rotman, A.: Partial purification of human interferon by affinity chromatography. Proc. Natl. Acad. Sci. U. S. A. **71**, 3139–3142 (1974).

Ankel, H., Chany, C., Galliot, B., Chevalier, M. J., Robert, M.: Antiviral effect of interferon covalently bound to sepharose. Proc. Natl. Acad. Sci. U. S. A. **70**, 2360–2363 (1973).

Anonymous: Interferon options. Br. Med. J. **1**, 64 (1977).

Anonymous: Exploiting interferon. Lancet **2**, 761–762 (1974).

Arakawa, J., Sawa, I., Fujiwara, K.: Influence du facteur inhibiteur du virus sur la multiplication du virus vaccinal dans des viscères du lapin. C. R. Acad. Sci. (Paris) **159**, 786–789 (1965).

Archer, D. L., Young, B. G.: Control of interferon, migration inhibitory factor, and expression of viral capsid antigens in Burkitts lymphoma derived cell lines: role of L-arginine. Infect. Immun. **9**, 684–689 (1974).

Arimura, H.: Correlation between molecular weight and interferon inducing activity of poly I·C. Acta Virol. **19**, 457 (1975).

Armstrong, D., Paucker, K.: Effect of mycoplasma on interferon production and interferon assay in cell cultures. J. Bacteriol. **92**, 97–101 (1966).

Armstrong, J. A.: Semi-micro, dye-binding assay for rabbit interferon. Applied. Microbiol. **21**, 723–726 (1971).

Armstrong, J. A., Ke, Y-H., Breinig, M. C., Ople, L.: Virus resistance in rabbit kidney cell cultures contaminated by a protozoan resembling *Encephalitozoan cuniculi*. Proc. Soc. Exp. Bioc. Med. **142**, 1205–1209 (1973).

Armstrong, R. W., Merigan, T. C.: Varicella zoster virus: interferon production and comparative interferon sensitivity in human cell cultures. J. Gen. Virol. **12**, 53–54 (1971).

Armstrong, R. W., Gurwith, M. J., Waddell, D., T. C.: Cutaneous interferon production in patients with Hodgkins disease and other cancers infected with varicella or vaccinia. N. Engl. J. Med. **283**, 1182–1184 (1970).

Arvin, A. M., Yeager, A. S., Merigan, T. C.: Effect of leukocyte interferon on urinary excretion of cytomegalovirus by infants. J. Infect. Dis. **133**, A 205–A 212 (1976).

Asch, B. B., Gifford, G. E.: Fowlpox virus: interferon production and sensitivity. Proc. Soc. Exp. Biol. Med. **135**, 177–179 (1970).

Ash, R. J., Bubel, H. C.: Temporal relationship of interferon production and resistance to experimentally induced virus infection. J. Infect. Dis. **116**, 1–7 (1966).

Atanasiu, P., Chany, C.: Action d'un interferon provenant de cellules malignes sur l'infection expérimentale du Hamster nouveau-né par le virus du polyome. C. R. Acad. Sci. (Paris) **251**, 1687–1689 (1960).

Atkins, G. J., Johnston, M. D., Westmacott, L. M., Burke, D. C.: Induction of interferon in chick cells by temperature-sensitive mutants of Sindbis virus. J. Gen. Virol. **25**, 381–384 (1974).

Atkins, G. J., Lancashire, C. L.: The induction of interferon by temperature-sensitive mutants of Sindbis virus: its relationship to double-stranded RNA synthesis and cytopathic effect. J. Gen. Virol. **30**, 157–161 (1976).

Aurelian, L., Roizman, B.: Abortive infection of canine cells by Herpes simplex virus. II. alternative suppression of synthesis of interferon and viral constituents. J. Mol. Biol. **11**, 539–548 (1965).

Ayre, J. E., Narvaez, R., Logerfo, J. J.: Effects of induced interferon upon cells of cervical carcinoma in situ. Oncology **27**, 108–117 (1973).

Azuma, M.: Participation of cytophilic antibody in enhancement of interferon production in macrophages by under-neutralized NDV. Arch. Ges. Virusforsch. **41**, 11–19 (1973).

Azuma, M.: Viral factors required for interferon induction by Newcastle Disease virus in mouse macrophages and chicken embryo cells. J. Gen. Virol. **30**, 51–57 (1976).

Azuma, M., Yamada, M., Nishioka, R.: Relationship between immunity and interferon production in macrophages. II. Molecular weight of interferon produced in macrophage cultures. Jap. J. Microbiol. **14**, 319–323 (1970a).
Azuma, M., Yamada, M., Nishioka, R.: Relationship between immunity and interferon production in macrophages. III. Enhancement of interferon production by antiserum. Japan. J. Microbiol. **14**, 325–331 (1970b).

Babayants, A. A., Dyuisalieva, R. G., Marchenko, V. I.: Investigation of the mechanism of interferogenesis stimulation in cell pretreated with interferon. Vopr. Virusol. **4**, 432–436 (1970) (In Russian.).
Babbar, O. P., Singh, D. P., Bajpai, S. K.: Effect of interferon on tumor forming ability of Walker carcinosarcoma 256 cells and secretion of exo-toxin by the Bacillus, *Clostridium welchii* (type C). Indian J. Exp. Biol. **11**, 199–206 (1973).
Babbar, O. P., Singh, D. P., Bajpai, S. K.: Studies on nature of inhibition of tumor-forming ability of Walker carcino-sarcoma cells in rats by chick interferon. Indian J. Med. Res. **64**, 730–737 (1976).
Babbar, O. P., Singh, D. P., Khan, S. K.: Production and defensive role of interferon. Indian J. Exp. Biol. **11**, 194–198 (1973).
Babiuk, L. A., Rouse, B. T.: Immune interferon production by lympoid cells: Role in the inhibition of Herpes virus. Infect. Immun. **13**, 1567–1569 (1976).
Babiuk, L. A., Rouse, B. T.: Bovine type II interferon: activity in heterologous cells. Intervirology **8**, 250–256 (1977).
Bachner, L., De Clercq, E., Thang, M. N.: Sepharose-bound poly (I)·poly (C): Interaction with cells and interferon production. Biochem. Biophys. Res. Comm. **63**, 476–479 (1975).
Bader, J. P.: Production of interferon by chick embryo cells exposed to Rous sarcoma virus. Virology **16**, 436–443 (1962).
Baer, G. M., Cleary, W. F. A.: A model in mice for the pathogenesis and treatment of rabies. J. Infect. Dis. **125**, 520–528 (1972).
Baer, G. M., Shaddock, J. H., Moore, V. A., Yager, P. A., Baron, S. S., Levy, H. B.: Successful prophylaxis against rabies in mice and Rhesus monkeys: the interferon system and vaccine. J. Infect. Dis. **136**, 286–294 (1977).
Bailey, M. D., DeMaeyer–Guignard, J.: Molecular weight of serum interferon induced by the Newcastle Disease virus in high and low producer mice. Ann. Inst. Pasteur (Paris) **123**, 835–848 (1972).
Bakay, M.: Interferon induction by gal virus in chick embryo cells. Acta Virol. **13**, 340–342 (1969).
Bakay, M., Burke, D. C.: The production of interferon in chick cells infected with DNA viruses: A search for double-stranded RNA. J. Gen. Virol. **16**, 399–403 (1972).
Balducci, M., Verani, P., Balducci, D.: Assay of interferon activity. Appl. Microbiol. **11**, 310–318 (1963).
Balezina, T. L., Borisov, Yu, V., Ermolieva, Z. V., Zalmanzon, E. S., Korabelnikova, N. I., Pilatskaya, E. P.: On a possibility of influenza prophylaxis by stimulation of the production of endogenous interferon. Vop. Virusol. **11**, 235–238 (1966). (In Russian.)
Balkwill, F. R., Oliver, R. T. D.: Growth inhibitory effects of interferon on normal and malignant human haemopoetic cells. Internatl. J. Cancer **20**, 500–505 (1977).
Ball, J. K., McCarter, J. A.: Effect of polyinosinic-polycytidylic acid on induction of primary or transplanted tumors by chemical carcinogen or irradiation. J. Natl. Cancer Inst. **46**, 1009–1011 (1971).
Ball, L. A., White, C. N.: Oligonucleotide inhibitor of protein synthesis made in extracts of interferon-treated chick cells: comparison with the mouse low molecular weight inhibitor. Proc. Nat. Acad. Sci. **75**, 1167–1171 (1978).
Baluda, M. A.: Homologous interference by ultraviolet-inactivated Newcastle disease virus. Virology **4**, 72–96 (1957).
Baluda, M. A.: Loss of viral receptors in homologous interference by ultraviolet-irradiated Newcastle disease virus. Virology **7**, 315–327 (1959).

Banatvala, J. E. Potter, J. E. Best, J. M.: Interferon response to Sendai and Rubella viruses in human foetal cultures, leucocytes and placental cultures. J. Gen. Virol. **13**, 193–201 (1971).

Banks, G. T., Buck, K. W., Chain, E. B., Darbyshire, J. E., Himmelweit, F.: *Penicillium cyaneofulvium* virus and interferon stimulation. Nature **223**, 155–157 (1969).

Banks, G. T., Buck, K. W., Chain, E. B., Darbyshire, J. E., Himmelweit, F., Ratti, G., Sharpe, J., Planterose, D. N.: Antiviral activity of double-stranded RNA from a virus isolated from *Aspergillus foetidus*. Nature **227**, 505–507 (1970).

Banks, G. T., Buck, K. W., Chain, E. B., Himmelweit, P., Marks, J. E., Tyler, J. M., Hollings, M., Last, F. T., Stone, O. W.: Viruses in fungi and interferon. Nature **218**, 542–545 (1968).

Barahona, H. H., Melendez, L. V.: Herpes virus Saimiri: *in vitro* sensitivity to virus-induced interferon and to polyriboinosinic acid: polyribocytidylic acid. Proc. Soc. Exp. Biol. Med. **136**, 1163–1166 (1971).

Barban, S., Baron, S.: Differential inhibitory effects of interferon on deoxythymidine kinase induction of vaccinia-infected cell cultures. Proc. Soc. Exp. Biol. Med. **127**, 160–164 (1968).

Barbosa, L. H., London, W. T., Hamilton, R., Buckler, C.: Interferon response of the fetal Rhesus monkey after viral infection. Proc. Soc. Exp. Biol. Med. **146**, 398–400 (1974).

Bárdoš, V., Šefčovićová, A.: On the interferon production inducing capacity of Tahyua virus. Acta Virol. **10**, 80 (1966).

Barker, A. D., Rheins, M. S., Wilson, H. E.: Amelioration of Friend virus leukemia by sequential administration of viral and non-viral interferon inducers. Proc. Soc. Exp. Biol. Med. **137**, 98–985 (1971).

Barmak, S. L., Vilček, J.: Altered cellular responses to interferon induction by poly I-poly C: Priming and hyporesponsiveness in cells treated with interferon preparations. Arch. Gesamte Virusforsch. **43**, 273–283 (1973).

Baron, S., Barban, S., Buckler, C. E.: Host cell species specificity of mouse and chicken interferons. Science **145**, 814–815 (1964).

Baron, S., Bogomolova, N. N., Billiau, A., Levy, H. B., Buckler, C. E., Stern, R., Naylor, R.: Induction of interferon by preparations of synthetic single-stranded RNA. Proc. Natl. Acad. Sci. **64**, 67–74 (1969).

Baron, S., Buckler, C. E.: Circulating interferon in mice after intravenous injection of virus. Science **141**, 1061–1063 (1963).

Baron, S., Buckler, C. E., Dianzani, F.: Some determinants of the interferon induced antiviral state. In: Interferon (Wolstenholme G. E. W., O'Connor M., eds.), p. 186. London: J. & A. Churchill (1968).

Baron, S., Buckler, C. E., Friedman, R. M., McCloskey, R. V.: Role of interferon during viremia. II. Protective action of circulating interferon. J. Immunol. **96**, 17–24 (1966 a).

Baron, S., Buckler, C. E., Levy, H. B., Friedman, R. M.: Some factors affecting the interferon-induced antiviral state. Proc. Soc. Exp. Biol. Med. **123**, 1320–1326 (1967).

Baron, S., Buckler, C. E., McCloskey, R. V. Kirschstein, R. L.: Role of interferon during viremia. I. Production of circulating interferon. J. Immunol. **96**, 12–17 (1966 b).

Baron, S., du Buy, H., Buckler, C. E., Johnson, M. L., Park, J., Billiau, A., Sarma, P., Huebner, R. J.: Induction of interferon and viral resistance in animals by polynucleotides. Ann. N. Y. Acad. Sci. **173**, 568–572 (1970).

Baron, S., Isaacs, A.: Absence of interferon in lungs from fatal cases of influenza. Brit. Med. J. **56**, 18–20 (1962).

Baron, S., Levy, H. B.: Interferon. Ann. Rev. Microbiol. **20**, 291–318 (1966).

Baron, S., Merigan, T. C., McKerlie, M. L.: Effect of crude and purified interferons on the growth of uninfected cells in culture. Proc. Soc. Exp. Biol. Med. **121**, 50–52 (1966).

Barski, G.: Interference entre les virus d'herpes et de polyome chez le Hamster adulte *in vivo*. C. R. Acad. Sci. **263**, 5459–5463 (1963).

Barski, G., Youn, J. K.: Interférence entre la chorioméningite lymphocytaire et la leucémie de Soucis de Rauscher. C. R. Acad. Sci. Paris **259**, 4191–4193 (1964).

Bart, R. S., Kopf, A. W.: Inhibition of the growth of murine malignant melanoma with synthetic double-stranded ribonucleic acid. Nature **224**, 372–373 (1969).

Bart, R. S., Kopf, A. W., Silagi, S.: J. Investigative Dermatology **56**, 33–36 (1971).

Bart, R. S., Kopf, A. W., Vilček, J., Lam, S.: Role of interferon in the anti-melanoma effects of poly (I)·poly (C) and Newcastle disease virus. Nature New Biol. **245**, 229–230 (1973).

Bart, R. S., Lam, S., Cooper, J. S., Kopf, A. W.: Retention of antimelanoma effect of polyinosinic-polycytidytic acid in neonatally thymectomized, irradiated, leukopenic mice. J. Investigative Dermatology **65**, 285–288 (1975).

Barth, R. F., Friedman, R. M., Malmgren: Depression of interferon production in mice after treatment with anti-lymphocyte serum. Lancet ii, 723–724 (1969).

Bausek, G. H., Merigan, T. C.: Cell interaction with a synthetic polynucleotide and interferon production *in vitro*. Virology **39**, 491–498 (1969).

Bausek, G. H., Merigan, T. C.: Simultaneous viral and non-viral interferon production in human cell cultures. Proc. Soc. Exp. Biol. Med. **133**, 982–985 (1970a).

Bausek, G. H., Merigan, T. C.: Two mechanisms of cell resistance to repeated stimulation of interferon. Proc. Soc. Exp. Biol. Med. **134**, 672–676 (1970b).

Baxt, B., Sonnabend, J. A., Bablanian, R.: Effects of interferon on vesicular stomatitis virus transcription and translation. J. Gen. Virol. **35**, 325–329 (1977).

Beasley, A. R., Sigel, M. M., Clem, L. W.: Latent infection in marine fish cell tissue cultures. Proc. Soc. Exp. Biol. Med. **121**, 1169–1174 (1966).

Beck, G., Poindron, P., Illinger, D., Beck, J. P., Ebel, J. P., Falcoff, R.: Inhibition of steroid inducible tyrosine aminotransferase by mouse and rat interferon in hepatoma tissue culture cells. FEBS Letters **48**, 297–299 (1974).

Bedson, H. S., Dumbell, K. R.: The affect of temperature on the growth of poxviruses in the chick embryo. J. Hyg. **59**, 457–464 (1961).

Bekesi, J. G., Roboz, J. P., Zimmerman, E., Holland, J. F.: Treatment of spontaneous leukemia in AKR mice with chemotherapy, immunotherapy or interferon. Cancer Res. **36**, 631–636 (1976).

Beladi, I., Bakay, M., Pusztai, R., Hidasi, G.: Induction of interferon in chick cells by Adenoviruses of different origin. J. Gen. Virol. **8**, 143–144 (1970).

Beladi, I., Pusztai, R.: Interferon-like substance produced in chick fibroblast cells inoculated with human Adenovirus. J. Naturforschg. **226**, 165–169 (1967).

Beladi, I., Pusztai, R. Szepessy, G., Molnar, J., Bakay, M.: Electron microscopic study of human adenoviruses with different interferon inducing ability. Acta Microbiol. Acad. Sci. Hung. **21**, 273–288 (1974).

Berencsi, K., Beladi, I.: Suppressive effect of NDV on the primary and secondary immune response of hamsters. Acta Virol. **21**, 296–300 (1977).

Berencsi, K., Beladi, I., Juhasz, A.: Interferon production and immunosuppression in NDV infected hamsters. Z. Immunitaetsforsch. **147**, 441–448 (1974).

Berg, K.: Sequential antibody affinity chromatography of human leukocyte interferon. Scand. J. Immunol. **6**, 77–86 (1977).

Berg, K., Ogburn, C. A., Paucker, K., Mogensen, K. E., Cantell, K.: Affinity chromatography of human leukocyte and diploid cell interferons on sepharose-bound antibodies. J. Immunol. **114**, 640–644 (1975).

Berman, B., Vilček, J.: Cellular binding characteristics of human interferon. Virology **57**, 378–386 (1974).

Berman, L. D.: Inhibition of oncogenicity of murine sarcoma virus (Harvey) in mice by interferon. Nature **227**, 1349–1350 (1970).

Besancon, F., Ankel, H.: Inhibition of interferon action by plant lectins. Nature **250**, 784–786 (1974a).

Besancon, F., Ankel, H.: Binding of interferon to gangliosides. Nature **252**, 478–480 (1974b).

Besancon, F., Ankel, H.: Inhibition of interferon action by glycoprotein hormones. C. R. Acad. Sci. D. **283**, 1807–1869 (1976).

Besancon, F., Ankel, H., Basu, S.: Specificity and reversibility of interferon ganglioside interaction. Nature **259**, 576–578 (1976).

Besancon, F., Basu, S., Ankel, H.: Interaction of interferon with gangliosides. Hoppe-Seyer's Z. Physiol. Chem. **357**, 251–255 (1976).

Besancon, F., Bourgeade, M. F.: Affinity of murine and human interferon for concanavalin A. J. Immunol. **113**, 1061–1063 (1974).

Bialy, H. S., Colby, C.: Inhibition of early vaccinia virus ribonucleic acid synthesis in interferon treated chicken embryo fibroblasts. J. Virol. **9**, 286–289 (1972).

Biernacka, I., Lobodzinska, M.: Rat interferon. II. Induction and properties of an interferon-like inhibitor from rat embryonic cell cultures. Arch. Immunol. Ther. Exp. (Warsz.) **21**, 471–475 (1973).

Billiau, A.: Systemic induction of interferon. Thesis, University of Leuven, Belgium (1969).

Billiau, A.: The refractory state after induction of interferon with double-stranded RNA. J. Gen. Virol. **7**, 225–232 (1970).

Billiau, A.: Sensitivity of oncornavirus-carrier lines to the antiviral and growth-inhibitory properties of interferon. Proc. Symp. Clin. Use of Interferon, Zagreb, Yugoslavia, p. 105 (1975).

Billiau, A.: Effect of interferon on RNA tumor viruses. Tex. Rep. Biol. Med. **35**, 406–419 (1977).

Billiau, A., Buckler, C. E.: Production and assay of rat interferon. Symp. Ser. Immunobiol. Stand. (Karger, Basel) **14**, 37–40 (1970).

Billiau, A., Buckler, C. E., Dianzani, F., Uhlendorf, C., Baron, S.: Induction of the interferon mechanism by single-stranded RNA: potentiation by polybasic substances. Proc. Soc. Exp. Biol. Med. **132**, 790–796 (1969).

Billiau, A., Buckler, C. E., Dianzani, F., Uhlendorf, C., Baron, S.: Influence of basic substances on the induction of the interferon mechanism. Ann. New York Acad. Sci. **173**, 657–667 (1970).

Billiau, A., Desmyter, J., Desomer, P.: Antiviral activity of a chlorite-oxidized oxyamylase, a polyacetal carboxylic acid. J. Virol. **5**, 321–328 (1970).

Billiau, A., Edy, V. G., DeClercq, E. Heremans, H., Desomer, P.: Influence of interferon on the synthesis of virus-particle in oncornavirus carrier cell lines. III. Survey of effects on A-, B- and C-type oncornaviruses. International J. Cancer **15**, 947–950 (1975).

Billiau, A., Edy, V. G., Heremans, H., Van Damms, J., Desmyter, J., Georgiades, J. A., Desomer, P.: Human interferon: Mass production in a newly established cell line, MG 63. Antimicrobiol. Agts. Chemother. **12**, 11–14 (1977 a).

Billiau, A., Edy, V. G., Sobis, H., Desomer, P.: Influence of interferon on virus particle synthesis in oncornavirus-carrier lines. II. Evidence for a direct effect on particle release. Int. J. Cancer **14**, 335–340 (1974).

Billiau, A., Heremans, H., Allen, P. T., Baron, S., Desomer, P.: Interferon inhibits C-type virus at a posttranscriptional prerelease step. Arch. Virol. **57**, 205–220 (1977 b).

Billiau, A., Heremans, H., Allen, P. T., DeMaeyer–Guignard, J., Desomer, P.: Trapping of oncornavirus particles at the surface of interferon treated cells. Virology **73**, 537 (1976 a).

Billiau, A., Heremans, H., Allen, P. T., Desomer, P.: Influence of interferon on the synthesis of virus particles in oncornavirus carrier cell lines. IV. Relevance to the potential application of interferon in natural infectious diseases. J. Infect. Disease **133**, A 51–A 57 (1976 b).

Billiau, A., Joniau, M., Desomer, P.: Production of crude human interferon with high specific activity. Proc. Soc. Exp. Biol. Med. **140**, 485–491 (1972).

Billiau, A., Joniau, M., Desomer, P.: Mass production of human interferon in diploid cells stimulated by poly I C. J. Gen. Virol. **19**, 1–8 (1973).

Billiau, A., Muyembe, J. J., Desomer, P.: Effect of chlorite-oxidized oxylamylose on influenza virus infection in mice. Applied Microbiol. **21**, 580–585 (1971 a).

Billiau, A., Muyembe, J. J., Desomer, P.: Mechanism of antiviral activity *in vivo* of polycarboxylates which induce interferon production. Nature New Biol. **232**, 183–186 (1971 b).

Billiau, A., Muyembe, J. J., Desomer, P.: Interferon-inducing polycarboxylates. Mechanism of protection against vaccinia virus infection in mice. Infect. Immun. **5**, 854–857 (1972).

Billiau, A., Schonne, E.: Induction of the interferon mechanism by natural RNA. Life Sci. **9**, 69–78 (1970).

Billiau, A., Sobis, H., Desomer, P.: Influence of interferon on virus particle formation in different oncornavirus carrier cell lines. Int. J. Cancer **12**, 646–653 (1973).

Billiau, A., Van den Berghe, H., Desomer, P.: Increased interferon release and morphological alteration in human cells by repeated exposure to double-stranded RNA. J. Gen. Virol. **14**, 25–31 (1972).

Birg, F., Meyer, G.: Effect of interferon on induction of S antigen by polyoma virus in BHK 21 cells. J. Gen. Virol. **26**, 201–204 (1975).

Blach-Olszewska, Z., Halasa, J., Cembrzynska–Nowak, M.: Why Hela cells do not produce interferon. Arch. Immunol. Ther. Exp. **25**, 435–444 (1977).

Blach–Olszewska, Z., Skurska, Z.: Tolerance of mouse tissues to stimulation of interferon. Arch. Immunol. Ther. Exp. (Warsz.) **22**, 435–444 (1974).

Black, D. B., Eckstein, F., Hobbs, J. B., Sternbach, H. Merigan, T. C.: The antiviral activity of certain thiophosphate and 2-chloro substituted polynucleotide homopolymer duplexes. Virology **48**, 537–542 (1972).

Blaineau, C., Kishida, T., Salle, M., Péries, J.: Inhibitory effect of interferon preparations on the induction of endogenous mouse type-C viruses by iododeoxyuridine. IRCS Medical Science **3**, 258–263 (1975).

Blalock, J. E., Baron, S.: Interferon-induced transfer of viral resistance between animal cells. Nature **269**, 422–425 (1977).

Blalock, J. E., Gifford, G. E.: Effect of aquasol A, vitamin A, and TWEEN 80 on vesicular stomatitis virus plaque formation and on interferon action. Arch. Ges. Virusforsch. **45**, 161–164 (1974).

Blalock, J. E., Gifford, G. E.: Inhibition of interferon action by vitamin A. J. Gen. Virol. **29**, 315–319 (1975).

Blalock, J. E., Gifford, G. E.: Suppression of interferon production by vitamin A. J. Gen. Virol. **32**, 143–146 (1976a).

Blalock, J. E., Gifford, G. E.: Comparison of the suppression of IF production and inhibition of its action by vitamin A and related compounds. Proc. Soc. Exp. Biol. Med. **153**, 298–301 (1976b).

Blalock, J. E., Gifford, G. E.: Retinoic acid (vitamin A) induced transcriptional control of interferon production. Proc. Nat. Acad. Sci. U. S. A. **74**, 5382–5386 (1977).

Blanden, R. V.: Mechanism of recovery from generalized virus infection. J. Exp. Med. **132**, 1035–1045 (1970).

Block, L. H., Cantell, K., Jamberger, S., Ruhevstroth–Bauer, G., Strander, H.: Lack of correspondence between human leukocyte type I interferon and human migration inhibitory factor (MIF). Arch. Virol. **56**, 341–344 (1978).

Blomgren, H., Cantell, K., Johansson, B., Lagergren, C., Ringborg, U., Strander, H.: Interferon therapy in Hodgkin's disease. Acta Med. Scand. **199**, 527–532 (1976).

Blomgren, H., Strander, H., Cantell, K.: Effect of human leukocyte interferon on the response of lymphocytes to mitogenic stimuli *in vitro*. Scand. J. Immunol. **3**, 697–673 (1974).

Bobst, A. M., Torrence, P. F., Kovidov, S., Witkop, B.: Dependence of interferon induction on nucleic acid conformation. Proc. Natl. Acad. Sci. USA. **73**, 3788–3792 (1976).

Bocci, V., Pacini, A., Pessina, G. P., Bargigli, V., Russi, M.: Role of sialic acid in determining survival of circulating interferon. Experientia **33**, 164–167 (1977a).

Bocci, V., Pacini, A., Pessina, G. P., Bargigli, V., Russi, M.: Metabolism of interferon: hepatic clearance of natural and desialylated interferon. J. Gen. Virol. **35**, 525–526 (1977b).

Bocci, V., Russi, M., Rita, G.: Recovery and identification of interferon in the rabbit urine. Experientia **23**, 309–310 (1967).

Bocci, V., Russi–Sorce, M., Cirri, G., Rita, G.: Role of liver in the inactivation of interferon. Proc. Soc. Exp. Biol. Med. **129**, 62–65 (1968a).

Bocci, V., Russi–Sorce, M., Cirri, G., Rita, G.: Virus-induced interferon in the rabbit: distribution, fate, and characterization of urinary interferon, in: The Interferons (Rita, G., ed.), p. 37. New York: Academic Press (1968b).

Bocci, V., Vita, A., Russi, M., Rita, G.: Isoelectric fractionation of desialyzed interferon. Experientia **27**, 1160–1161 (1971).

Bodo, G., Jungwirth, C.: Effect of interferon on deoxyribonuclease induction in chick fibroblast cultures infected with cow pox virus. J. Virol. **1**, 466–471 (1967).

Bodo, G., Palese, P. Lindner, J.: Activity of mouse interferon in human cells. Proc. Soc. Exp. Biol. Med. **137**, 1392–1395 (1971).

Bodo, G., Scheirer, W., Suh, M., Schultze, B., Horak, I., Jungwirth, C. Protein synthesis in pox-infected cells treated with interferon. Virology **50**, 140–147 (1972).

Booth, B. W., Borden, E. C.: Increase by calcium in production of poly rI·poly rC induced interferon by L929 cells. J. Gen. Virol. **40**, 485–488 (1978).

Booth, R. J., Booth, J. M. Marbrook, J.: Immune conservation – possible consequence of mechanism of interferon-induced antibody suppression. Europ. J. Immunol. **6**, 769 (1976).

Booth, R. J., Rastrick, J. M., Bellamy, A. R., Marbrook, J.: Modulating effects of interferon preparations on an antibody response *in vitro*. Austral. J. Exp. Biol. Med. Sci. **54**, 11–16 (1976).

Boquet, P.: Modification of the response of diphtheria treated hybrid mouse-monkey cells by interferon, in: Effects of Interferon on Cells, Viruses and the Immune System (Geraldes, A., ed.), pp. 482–492. London: Academic Press (1975).

Borden, E. C., Booth, B. W., Leonhardt, P. H.: Mechanistic studies of polyene enhancement of interferon production by poly (I)·poly (C). Antimicrobial Agts. Chemother. 13, 159–164 (1978).

Borden, E. C., Leonhardt, P. H.: Enhancement of rIn·rCn-induced interferon production by amphotericin B. Antimicrob. Agents Chemother. 9, 551–555 (1976).

Borden, E. C., Leonhardt, P. H.: A quantitative semi-micro, semiautomated colorimetric assay for interferon. J. Lab. Clin. Med. 89, 1036–1043 (1977).

Borden, E. C., Murphy, F. A.: The interferon refractory state: in vivo and in vitro studies of its mechanism. J. Immunol. 106, 134–138 (1971).

Borden, E. C., Murphy, F. A., Gary, G. W.: Interferon induction in mice treated with antilymphocytic serum. Proc. Soc. Exp. Biol. Med. 132, 865–868 (1970).

Borden, E. C., Prochownik, E. V., Carter, W. A.: The interferon refractory state. II. Biologic characterization of a refractoriness-inducing protein. J. Immunol. 114, 752–755 (1975).

Borecky, L.: Use of bacteriophage nucleic acid inducers of interferon in man. Tex. Rep. Biol. Med. 35, 535–540 (1977).

Borecky, L., Doskocil, J., Lackovic, V., Buchvald, J., Maly, E., Gruntova, Z., Obrucnik, M., Zuffa, A.: Double-stranded RNA of Czechoslovak production in the therapy of viral skin- and eye-diseases. Proc. Symp. Clin. Use of Interferon, Zagreb, Yugoslavia, pp. 149–158 (1975).

Borecky, L., Fuchsberger, N., Hajnicka, V.: Electrophoretic profiles and activities of human interferon in heterologous cells. Intervirology 3, 369–377 (1974).

Borecky, L., Fuchsberger, N., Hajnicka, V., Lackoui, C. V.: Antiviral and cell-growth inhibitory effect of interferon. Biomedicine Express 19, 281–286 (1973).

Borecky, L., Fuchsberger, N., Hajnicka, V., Stancek, D., Zemla, J.: Distribution of antiviral and cell-inhibitory activity in interferon preparations. Acta Virol. 16, 356–358 (1972).

Borecky, L. Fuchsberger, N., Zemla, J., Lackovic, V.: Properties of the interferon-like inhibitor released during interaction of mouse sensitized lymphocyges with their target cells. Europ. J. Immunol. 2, 213–216 (1971).

Borecky, L., Lackovic, V.: Partial heterologous tolerance to interferon production in mice infected with B. pertussis. Acta Virol. 10, 271–272 (1966).

Borecky, L., Lackovic, V.: The cellular background of interferon production in vivo. Comparison of interferon induction by Newcastle disease virus and Bordetella pertussis. Acta Virol. 11, 150–158 (1967).

Borecky, L., Lackovic, V., Blaskovic, D., Masler, L., Sikl, D.: An interferon-like substance induced by mannans. Acta Virol. 11, 264–266 (1967).

Borecky, L., Lackovic, V., Fuchsberger, N.: Comparison on interferon production in mouse leukocytes by statolon and complexed polyribonucleotide (poly I·C). Acta Virol. 14, 329–336 (1970).

Borecky, L., Lackovic, V., Russ, G.: Interferon production in leukocytes and the antiviral protection of mice treated with endotoxin. Ann. N. Y. Acad. Sci. 173, 320–324 (1969).

Borecky, L., Lackovic, V., Russ, G.: Interferon release from leukocytes during contact with target cells. Intnatl. Cong. Microbiol. X. (1970).

Borecky, L., Lackovic, V., Waschke, K.: Immunological implications of interferon production in leukocytes. Colloq. Interferon, INSERM, Paris, 37–52 (1970).

Bose, S., Gurari–Rotman, D., Ruegg, V. T., Corley, L., Anfinsen, C. B.: Apparent dispensability of the carbohydrate moiety of human interferon for antiviral activity. J. Biol. Chem. 251, 1659–1662 (1976).

Bose, S., Hickman, J.: Role of the carbohydrate moiety in determining the survival of interferon in the circulation. J. Biol. Chem. 252, 8336–8337 (1977).

Bostandzhyan, M. G., Bikbulatov, R. W.: Study on the dynamics of interferon formation in experimental herpes infection. Acta Virol. 11, 159–160 (1967).

Bourgeade, M. F.: Interferon cell species specificity: role of cell membrane receptors. Proc. Soc. Exp. Biol. Med. 146, 820–824 (1974).

Bourgeade, M. F., Besancon, F.: Affinity of murine interferon for concanavalin A. C. R. Acad. Sci. (Paris) D 277, 2833–2835 (1974).

Bourgeade, M. F., Chany, C.: Inhibition of interferon action by cytochalasin B, colchicine and vinblastine. Proc. Soc. Exp. Biol. Med. **153**, 486–488 (1976).

Bousquet, C., Ramuz, M., Serre, J. C., Roux, J.: Characterization of the interferon induced in mice following infection with *Brucella melitensis*. Ann. Microbiol. (Paris) **127** (1), 71–82 (1973).

Boxaca, M., Guerrero, L. B., Savy, V. L.: The occurrence of virus, interferon, and circulating antibodies in mice after experimental infection with Junin virus. Arch. Ges. Virusforsch. **40**, 10–20 (1973).

Boxaca, M., Paucker, K.: Neutralization of different murine interferons by antibody. J. Immunol. **98**, 1130–1135 (1967).

Bradburne, A. F.: An investigation of the replication of coronaviruses in suspension cultures of L1312 cells. Arch. Gesamte Virusforsch. **37**, 297–300 (1972).

Bradburne, A. F., Sommerset, B. A.: Coronavirus antibody titers in sera of healthy adults and experimentally infected volunteers. J. Hyg. **70**, 235–238 (1972).

Bradburne, A. F., Tyrrell, D. A. J.: Coronaviruses of man. Prog. Med. Virol. **13**, 373–378 (1971).

Bradish, C. J., Allner, K.: The production of mouse interferon in rolling monolayers of L cells. Symp. Ser. Immunobiol. Stand. (Karger, Basel) **14**, 35–38 (1970).

Brailovsky, C., Chany, C.: Un facteur produit par l'adénovirus 12 en culture cellulaire, stimulant le multiplication du virus K du rat. C. R. acad. Sci. Paris **260**, 2634–2637 (1965).

Braun, W.: Relationships between the effects of poly I·poly C and endotoxin. Nature **224**, 1024–1025 (1969).

Braun, W., Levy, M. B.: Interferon preparations as modifiers of immune responses. Proc. Soc. Exp. Biol. Med. **141**, 769–773 (1972).

Bray, D.: Actin plural. Nature **263**, 721–723 (1976).

Breinig, M. C., Armstrong, J. A., Ho, M.: Rapid onset of hyporesponsiveness to interferon induction on reexposure to polyribonucleotides. J. Gen. Virol. **26**, 149–158 (1975).

Brezina, R., Kazar, J., Schramek, S.: Induction of interferon activity in mouse spleen by phase 1 *Coxiella burnetti*. Acta Virol. **12**, 382–383 (1968).

Bridgen, P. J., Anfinsen, C. B., Corley, L., Bose, S., Zoon, K. C., Ruegg, V. T., Buckler, C. E.: Human lymphoblastoid interferon: large scale production and partial purification. J. Biol. Chem. **252**, 6585–6587 (1977).

Brodeur, B., Legar, E. C., Brailovsky, C. A.: Anti-interferon activity of extracts of cells transformed by SV 40 virus. Can. J. Microbiol. **19**, 7–14 (1973).

Brodeur, B. R., Merigan, T. C.: Suppressive effect of interferon on the humoral immune response to sheep red blood cells in mice. J. Immunol. **113** (4), 1319–1325 (1974).

Brodeur, B. R., Merigan, T. C.: Mechanism of the suppressive effect of interferon on antibody synthesis *in vivo*. J. Immunol. **114**, 1323–1330 (1975).

Brouty–Boye, D.: High sensitivity of a C3H mouse embryo-derived cell line to the antiviral action of interferon. Proc. Soc. Exp. Biol. Med. **155**, 438–439 (1977).

Brouty–Boye, D., Fiszman, M., Maciera–Cuelho, A., Gresser, I.: Effect of interferon on RNA, protein, and polyribosome synthesis in murine L1210 leukemia cells. C. R. Acad. Sci. D. **276**, 1793–1795 (1973 a).

Brouty–Boye, D., Little, J. G.: Enhancement of X-ray-induced transformation in C3H/10. Tl/2 cells by interferon. Cancer Res. **37**, 2714–2716 (1977).

Brouty–Boye, D., Maciera–Cuelho, A., Fiszman, M., Gresser, I.: Effect of interferon on macromolecular synthesis in L1210 cells *in vitro*. Int. J. Cancer **12**, 250–258 (1973 b).

Brouty–Boye, D., Tovey, M. G.: Inhibition by interferon of thymidine uptake in chemostat cultures of L1210 cells. Intervirology **9**, 243–252 (1977).

Brown, G. E., Lebleu, B., Kawakita, M., Shaila, S., Sev., G. C., Lengyel, P.: Increased endonuclease activity in an extract from mouse Ehrlich ascites tumor cells which had been treated with a partially purified interferon preparation: dependence on double-stranded RNA. Biochem. Biophys. Res. Commun. **69**, 114–116 (1976).

Brown, P., Besancon, F.: Effect of acid pH on induction of an antiviral resistance condition by interferon. C. R. Acad. Sci. D **275**, 2275–2278 (1972).

Brown, P., Besancon, F., Chany, C.: The effects of an acid pH upon the induction of antiviral resistance *in vitro* by interferon. Proc. Soc. Exp. Biol. Med. **142**, 1195–1198 (1973).

Brown, R. McK.: A quantitative study of inhibition of herpes simplex virus by interferon. Thesis, University of Texas (1966).

Buchvald, J., Borecky, L., Doskocil, J.: Möglichkeiten der Ausnutzung des Interferon-induktions-stoffes in der Therapie der Virusdermatosen. Z. Hautkr. 50, 909–911 (1975).

Buck, K. W., Chain, E. B., Himmelwett, F.: Comparison of interferon induction in mice by purified *Penicillium chrysogenum* virus and derived double-stranded RNA. J. Gen. Virol. 12, 131–139.

Buckler, C. E., Baron, S.: Antiviral activity of mouse interferon in heterologous cells. J. Bact. 91, 231–233 (1966).

Buckler, C. E., Baron, S., Levy, H. B.: Interferon: lack of detectable uptake by cells. Science 152, 80–82 (1966).

Buckler, C., DuBuy, M. C., Johnson, M. L., Baron, S.: Kinetics of serum interferon response in mice after single and multiple injections of poly I·poly C. Proc. Soc. Exp. Biol. Med. 136, 394–396 (1971).

Buckler, C. E., Wong, K. T., Baron, S.: Induction of the interferon system by various inducers. Proc. Soc., Exp. Biol. Med. 127, 1258–1263 (1968).

Bucknall, R. A.: Species specificity of interferons: a misnomer? Nature 216, 1022–1023 (1967).

Bucknall, R. A.: The assay of human interferon. Symp. Ser. Immunobiol. Stand. (Karger, Basel) 14, 97–100 (1970).

Bucknall, R. A., Finter, N. B., Draper, C. C.: Failure to detect interferon in the urine of persons with virus infection. Nature 217, 462–464 (1968).

Buimovici–Klein, E., Weiss, K. E., Cooper, L. Z.: Interferon production in lymphocyte cultures after rubella infection in humans. J. Infect. Dis. 135, 380–385 (1977).

Burke, D. C.: The purification of interferon. Biochem J. 78, 556–563 (1961).

Burke, D. C.: The role of nucleic acid in interferon production. Biochem J. 94, 2 P–3 P (1965).

Burke, D. C.: The assay of chick interferon. Sym. Ser. Immunobiol. Stand. (Karger, Basel) 14, 113–117 (1970).

Burke, D. C.: The mechanisms of interferon formation, in: Interferons and Interferon Inducers (Finter, N. B., ed.), pp. 107–134. Amsterdam: North Holland Publ. Co. (1973).

Burke, D. C.: The status of interferon. Scientific Amer. 236, 42–48 (1977).

Burke, D. C., Buchan, A.: Interferon production in chick embryo cells. I. Production by ultraviolet-inactivated virus. Virology 26, 28–35 (1965).

Burke, D. C., Isaacs, A.: Further studies on interferon. Brit. J. Exp. Path. 39, 78–84 (1958a).

Burke, D. C., Isaacs, A.: Some factors affecting the production of interferon. Brit. J. Exp. Path. 39, 452–458 (1958b).

Burke, D. C., Isaacs, A.: Interferon: relation to heterologous interference and lack of antigenicity. Acta Virol. 4, 215–219 (1960).

Burke, D. C., Morrison, J. M.: Interferon production in chick embryo cells. II. The role of DNA. Virology 27, 108–114 (1965).

Burke, D. C., Skehel, J. J., Low, M.: Interferon production and viral ribonucleic acid synthesis in chick embryo cells. J. Gen. Virol. 1, 235–237 (1967).

Burke, D. C., Veomett, G.: Enucleation and reconstruction of interferon producing cells. Proc. Natl. Acad. Sci. U. S. A. 74, 3391–3395 (1977).

Burke, D. C., Walters, S.: Search for an interferon messenger ribonucleic acid. Biochemical J. 101, 25 P–26 P (1966).

Burnet, F. M., Fraser, K. B.: Studies on recombination with influenza viruses in the chick embryo by influenza viruses. Aust. J. Exp. Biol. Med. 30, 447–458 (1952).

Byrne, E. B., Rosenstein, B. J., Jaworski, A. A., Jaworski, R. A.: A statewide mass measles immunization program. J. Am Med. Ass. 199, 113–117 (1967).

Came, P. E., Lieberman, M., Pascale, A., Shimonski, G.: Antiviral activity of an interferon-inducing synthetic polymer. Proc. Soc. Exp. Biol. Med. 131, 443–446 (1969).

Came, P. E., Moore, D. H.: Inhibition of spontaneous mammary carcinoma of mice by treatment with interferon and poly I·C. Proc. Soc. Exp. Biol. Med. 137, 304–305 (1971).

Came, P. E., Moore, D. H.: Effect of exogenous interferon treatment on mouse mammary tumors. J. Natl. Cancer Inst. 48, 1151–1154 (1972).

Came, P. E., Schafer, T. W., Silver, G. H.: Sensitivity of Rhinoviruses to human leucocyte and fibroblast interferons. J. Infect. Dis. 133, Suppl., A 136–A 138 (1976).

334 References

Campbell, J. B., Buera, J. G., Tobias, T. M.: Influence of blood clearance rates on interferon production and virulence of Mengo virus plaque mutants in mice. Canad. J. Microbiol. 16, 821–826 (1970).

Campbell, J. B., Colter, J. S.: Sensitivity to and production of interferon by three variants of Mengo virus. Can. J. Microbiol. 13, 931–937 (1967).

Campbell, J. B., Kaplan, M. M., Koprowski, H., Kuwert, E., Sokol, F., Wiktor, T. J.: Present trends and the future in rabies research. Bull. WHO 38, 373–380 (1968).

Cantell, K.: Production and action of interferon in Hela cells. Arch. Ges. Virusforsch. 10, 510–521 (1961).

Cantell, K.: Enhancement of animal virus growth by another virus, in: Medical and Applied Virology (Sanders, M., Lennette, E. H., eds.), pp. 31–40. St. Louis: W. H. Green (1968).

Cantell, K.: Prospects for the clinical use of exogenous interferon. Med. Biol. 55, 69–73 (1977).

Cantell, K., Hirvonen, S.: Preparation of human leukocyte interferon for clinical use. Tex. Rep. Biol. Med. 35, 138–144 (1977).

Cantell, K., Hirvonen, S., Mogensen, K. E., Pyhala, L.: Human leukocyte interferons: Production, purification, stability and animal experiments. The production and use of interferon for the treatment of human virus infections. In: In Vitro Monograph 3, 35–38 (1974).

Cantell, K., Paucker, K.: Quantitative studies on viral interference in suspended L cells. IV. Production and assay of interferon. Virology 21, 11–21 (1963a).

Cantell, K., Paucker, K.: Studies on viral interference in two lines of Hela Cells. Virology 19, 81–87 (1963b).

Cantell, K., Pyhala, L.: Circulating interferon in rabbits after administration of human interferon by different routes. J. Gen. Virol. 20, 97–104 (1973).

Cantell, K., Pyhala, L.: Pharmacokinetics of human leukocyte interferon. J. Infect. Dis. 133, A6–A8 (1976).

Cantell, K., Pyhala, L., Strander, H.: Circulating human interferon after intramuscular injection into animals and man. J. Gen. Virol. 25, 453–458 (1974).

Cantell, K., Strander, H., Hadhazy, G. Y., Nevanlinna, H. R.: How much interferon can be prepared in human leucocyte suspensions, in: The Interferons (Rita, G., ed.), p. 223. New York: Academic Press (1968a).

Cantell, K., Strander, H., Saxen, L., Meyer, B.: Interferon response of human leucocytes during intrauterine and post-natal life. J. Immunol. 100, 1304–1308 (1968b).

Cantell, K., Tommila, V.: Effect of interferon on experimental vaccinia and herpes-simples virus infections in rabbits eyes. The Lancet, 11, 682–684 (1960).

Cantell, K., Valle, M.: The ability of Sendai virus to overcome cellular resistance to vesicular stomatitis virus. II. Ann. Med. Exp. Fenn. 43, 61–64 (1965).

Cantell, K., Valle, M., Schakir, R., Saukkonen, J. J., Uroma, E.: Observation on production, assay and purification of chick embryo interferon. Ann. Med. Exp. Biol. Fenn. 43, 125–131 (1965).

Carter, W. A.: Interferon: evidence for subunit structure. Proc. Natl. Acad. Sci. U. S. A. 67, 620–628 (1970).

Carter, W. A.: Purification of mouse and human interferons and detection of subunit structure. Prep. Biochem. 1, 55–75 (1971).

Carter, W. A.: Workshop on Purification and Production of Interferons, N.I.H., Bethesda, Maryland, March 1977.

Carter, W. A., Hande, K. R., Essien, B., Prochownik, E., Kaback, M. M.: Comparative production of interferon by human fetal, neonatal, and maternal cells. Infect. Immun. 3, 671–677 (1971).

Carter, W. A., Levy, H. B.: Ribosomes: Effect of interferon on their interaction with rapidly labeled cellular and viral RNA's Science 155, 1254–1257 (1967a).

Carter, W. A., Levy, H. B.: Interaction of mammalian ribosomes with cellular and viral RNA's. Arch. Biochem. Biophys. 120, 563–567 (1967b).

Carter, W. A., Levy, H. B.: The recognition of viral RNA by mammalian ribosomes an effect of interferon. Biochem. Biophys. Acta 155, 437–443 (1968).

Carter, W. A., O'Malley, J. A., Horoszewiez, J. S., Huang, J.: Selective use of antiviral inhibitors: interferon, its inducers, and blockade of viral-reverse transcriptase, in: Cancer and Transplantation (Murphy, G. P., ed.), pp. 131–135. New York: Grune and Stratton (1975a).

Carter, W. A., O'Malley, J. A., Horoszewiez, J. S., Huang, J.: Selective use of antiviral inhibitors: interferon, its inducers, and blockade of viral-reverse transcriptase. Transplant. Proc. 7, 269–273 (1975b).

Carter, W. A., Pitha, P. M.: Structural requirements of ribopolymers for induction of human interferon: Evidence for interferon subunits. In: Biological Effects of Polynucleotides (Beers, R. F., jr., Brown, W. N., ed.), pp. 89–105. Berlin–Heidelberg–New York: Springer (1971).

Carter, W. A., Pitha, P. M., Marshall, L. W., Tazawa, I., Tazawa, S., Ts'O, P. O. P.: Structural requirements of the rI·rC complex for induction of human interferon. J. Mol. Biol. 70, 567–575 (1972).

Cartwright, T., Senussi, O., Grady, M. D.: The stabilization of fibroblast interferon for clinical use. Proc. Symp. Clin. Use of Interferon, Yugoslav Acad. Sci. and Arts, Zagreb, pp. 69–78 (1975).

Cartwright, T., Senussi, O., Grady, M. D.: The mechanism of the interaction of human fibroblast interferon by mechanical stress. J. Gen. Virol. 36, 317–321 (1977a).

Cartwright, T., Senussi, O., Grady, M. D.: Reagents which inhibit disulfide bond formation stabilize human fibroblast interferon. J. Gen. Virol. 36, 323–327 (1977b).

Carver, D. H., Marcus, P. I.: Enhanced interferon production from chick embryo cells aged in in vitro. Virology 32, 247–257 (1967).

Carver, D. H., Seto, D. S. Y., Migeon, B. R.: Interferon production and action in mouse, hamster and somatic hybrid mouse-hamster cells. Science 160, 558–564 (1968).

Cassingena, R., Chany, C., Vignal, M., Suarez, H., Estrada, S., Lazar, P.: Use of monkey-mouse hybrid cells for the study of the cellular regulation of interferon production and action. Proc. Nat. Acad. Sci. U. S. A. 68, 580–584 (1971).

Catalano, L. W., jr., Baron, S.: Protection against herpes virus and encephalomyocarditis virus encephalitis with a double-stranded RNA inducer of interferon. Proc. Soc. Exp. Biol. Med. 133, 684–688 (1970).

Catalano, L. W., London, W. T., Rice, J. M., Sever, J. L.: Prophylactic and therapeutic use of poly rI·poly rC [·poly-D-lysine] against herpes virus encephalitis in mice. Proc. Soc. Exp. Biol. Med. 140, 66–71 (1972).

Cate, T. R., Douglas, R. G., Couch, R. B.: Interferon and the common cold. Clin. Res. 16, 84–91 (1968).

Cathala, F., Baron, S.: Interferon in rabbit brain, cerebrospinal fluid and serum following administration of polyinosinic-polycytidylic acid. J. Virol. 14, 1355–1358 (1970).

Cavalieri, R. L., Havell, E. A., Vilček, J., Pestka, S.: Induction and decay of human fibroblast interferon messenger RNA. Proc. Natl. Acad. Sci. U. S. A. 74, 4415–4419 (1977a).

Cavalieri, R. L., Havell, E. A., Vilček, J., Pestka, S.: Synthesis of human interferon by Xenopus laevis oöcytes: two structural genes for interferons in human cells. Proc. Nat. Acad. Sci. U. S. A. 74, 3287–3291 (1977b).

Cembrzynska–Nowak, M.: Inhibitor of interferon activity from mouse embryo tissues: its physiochemcial characteristics. Arch. Immunol. Ther. Exp. 25, 663–668 (1977).

Centifanto, Y. M., Goorha, R. M., Kaufman, H. E.: Interferon induction in rabbit and human tears. Amer. J. Ophthalmol. 60, 1006–1010 (1970).

Cerottini, J. C., Brunner, K. T., Lindahl, P., Gresser, I.: Inhibitory effect of interferon preparations and inducers on the multiplication of transplanted allogenic spleen cells and syngenic bone marrow cells. Nature New Biol. 242 (118), 152–153 (1973).

Cesario, T. C.: The effect of body fluids on polynucleotide-induced fibroblast interferon and virus-induced leukocyte interferon. Proc. Soc. Exp. Biol. Med. 155, 583–588 (1977).

Cesario, T. C., Mandell, A., Tilles, J. G.: Inactivation of human interferon by body fluids. Proc. Soc. Exp. Biol. Med. 144, 1030–1032 (1973).

Cesario, T. C., Schryer, P., Mandel, A., Tilles, J. G.: Affinity of human fibroblast interferon for blue dextran. P. S. E. B. M. 153, 486–489 (1976).

Cesario, T. C., Schryer, P. J., Tilles, J. G.: Relationship between the physicochemical nature of human interferon, the cell induced, and the inducing agent. Antimicrobiol. Agts. Chemother. 11, 291–298 (1977).

Cesario, T. C., Tilles, J. G.: Inactivation of human interferon by urine. J. Infect. Dis. 127, 331–314 (1973).

Chadha, K. C., Davey, M. W., Byrd, D. M., Carter, W. A.: Differential production of interferon and refractoriness inducing principle in L cells. Infect. Immun. 10, 1057–1061 (1974).

Chang, E. H., Friedman, R. M.: A large glycoprotein of Moloney leukemia virus derived from interferon-treated cells. Biochem. Biophys. Res. Comm. 77, 392–398 (1977).

Chang, E. H., Mims, S. J., Triche, T. J., Friedman, R. M.: Interferon inhibits mouse leukemia virus release: an electron microscope study. J. Gen. Virol. 34, 363–371 (1977a).

Chang, E. H., Myers, M. W., Wong, P. K. Y., Friedman, R. M.: The inhibitory effect of interferon on a temperature-sensitive mutant of Moloney murine leukemia virus. Virology 77, 625–636 (1977b).

Chang, S. S., Rasmussen, A. F., Jr.: Stress-induced suppression of interferon production in virus-infected mice. Nature 205, 623–624 (1965).

Chanock, R. M.: Control of acute mycoplasmal and viral respiratory tract disease. Science 169, 248–250 (1970).

Chany, C.: Un facteur inhibiteur de la multiplication intracellulaire des virus rappelant l'interféron, provenant de cellules cancéreuses le phénomène d'autoinhibition. C. R. Acad. Sci. (Paris) 263, 3903–3905 (1960).

Chany, C.: An interferon-like inhibitor of viral multiplication from malignant cells (the viral autoinhibition phenomenon. Virology 13, 485–492 (1961).

Chany, C.: Membrane-bound interferon specific cell receptor system: role in the establishment and amplification of the antiviral state. Biomedicine 24, 148–160 (1976).

Chany, C., Ankel, H., Bourgeade, M. F.: Interferon cell receptor interactions (Perspectives in Virology 9) (Pollard, M., ed.), p. 269. Academic Press (1975).

Chany, C., Ankel, H., Galliot, B., Chevalier, M. J., Gregoire, A.: Mode of action and biological properties of insoluble interferon. Proc. Soc. Exp. Biol. Med. 147, 293–299 (1974).

Chany, C., Brailovsky, C.: Les stimulons facteurs antagonistes de l'interferon favorisant la multiplication intracellulaire des virus. C. R. Acad. Sci. (Paris) 261, 4282–4285 (1965).

Chany, C., Brailovsky, C.: Stimulating interaction between viruses (stimulons). Proc. Natl. Acad. Sci. 57, 87–94 (1967).

Chany, C., Cerutti, I.: Effet stimulant de l'isoprinosine sur l'action antivirale de l'interféron. C. R. Acad. Sci. D. 284, 499–501 (1977a).

Chany, C., Cerutti, I.: Enhancement of antiviral protection against encephalomyocarditis virus by a combination of isoprinosine and interferon. Arch. Virol. 55, 225–232 (1977b).

Chany, C., Fournier, F., Rousset, S.: Potentiation of the antiviral activity of interferon by Actinomycin D. Nature New Biol. 230, 113–114 (1971).

Chany, C., Gregoire, A., Vignal, M., Lemaitre–Moncuit, J., Brown, P., Besancon, F., Suarez, H., Cassingena, R.: Mechanism of interferon uptake in parental and somatic monkey-mouse hybrid cells. Proc. Natl. Acad. Sci. U. S. A. 70, 557–561 (1973).

Chany, C., Lemaitre, J., Gregoire, A.: Facteurs antagonistes de l'action antivirale dans des extraits d'interféron provenant de différents sarcomes humains. C. R. Acad. Sci. (Paris) 269, 2628–2631 (1969).

Chany, C., Robbe–Maridor, F.: Enhancing effect of the murine sarcoma virus (MSV) on the replication of the mouse hepatitis virus (MHV) in vitro. Proc. Soc. Exp. Biol. Med. 131, 30–33 (1969).

Chany, C., Vignal, M.: Etude du mécanisme de l'état réfractoire des cellules à la production d'interféron après inductions répétées. C. R. Acad. Sci. (Paris) D 267, 798–1800 (1968).

Chany, C., Vignal, M.: Effect of prolonged interferon treatment on mouse embryonic fibroblasts transformed by murine sarcoma virus. J. Gen. Virol. 7, 203–210. (1970).

Chany, C., Vignal, M., Covillin, P., Van Cong, N., Bové, J., Boye, A.: Chromosomal localization of human genes governing the interferon-induced antiviral state. Proc. Natl. Acad. Sci. U. S. A. 72, 3129–3134 (1975).

Chany–Fournier, F., Pauloin, A., Chany, C.: Tissue antagonist of interferon (TAI): isolation of a mammalian lectin-like substance. C. R. Acad. Sci. D 285, 941–945 (1977).

Cheeseman, S. H., Rinaldo, C. R., jr., Hirsch, M. S.: Use of interferon in cytomegalovirus infections in man. Texas Rep. Biol. Med. 35, 523–527 (1977).

Chen, J. K., Jankowski, W. J., O'Malley, J. A., Sulkowski, E., Carter, W. A.: Nature of the molecular heterogeneity of human leukocyte interferon. J. Virology 19, 425–434 (1976).

Chen, T. T., Watanabe, I., Zeman, W., Wealy, J.: Subacute sclerosing panencephalitis: Propagation of measles virus from brain biopsy in tissue culture. Science 163, 1193–1195 (1969).

Chernyakhovskaya, I., Slavina, E.: Lymphocyte activation by interferon. Vopr. Virusol. 4, 329–333 (1972).

Chernyakhovskaya, I. Yu., Slavina, E. G., Svet–Moldavsky, G. J.: Antitumor effect of lymphoid cells activated by interferon. Nature 228, 71–72 (1970).

Chester, T. J., Declercq, E., Merigan, T. C.: Effect of separate and combined injections of poly rI:poly RC and endotoxin on reticuloendothelial activity, interferon and antibody production in the mouse. Infect. Immun. 3, 516–520 (1971).

Chester, T. J., Declercq, E., Nuwer, M. R., Merigan, T. C.: In vivo release of previously cleared interferon by cycloheximide. Infect. Immun. 5 (3), 383–388 (1972).

Chester, T. J., Paucker, K., Merigan, T. C.: Suppression of mouse antibody producing spleen cells by various interferon preparations. Nature 246, 92–94 (1973).

Chirigos, M. A., Turner, W., Pearson, J., Griffin, W.: Effective antiviral therapy of two murine leukemias with an interferon-inducing synthetic carboxylate polymer. Int. J. Cancer 4, 267–269 (1969).

Claes, P., Billiau, A., Declercq, E., Desmyter, J., Schonne, E., Vanderhaeghe, H., Desomer, P.: Polyacetal carboxylic acids: a new group of antiviral polyanions. J. Virol. 5, 313–320 (1970).

Clavell, L. A., Bratt, M. A.: Relationship between the ribonucleic acid synthesizing capacity of ultraviolet-irradiated Newcastle disease virus and its ability to induce interferon. J. Virol. 8, 500–508 (1971).

Clemens, M. J., Williams, B. R. G.: Inhibition of cell-free protein synthesis by ppp A$^{2'}$ p$^{5'}$ A$^{2'}$ p$^{5'}$A: A novel oligonucleotide synthesized by extracts from interferon treated L cells. Cell 13, 565–572 (1978).

Clinton, B. A., Magoc, T. J., Aspinall, A., Rapoza, N. T.: The influence upon mitogenic and cellular immunologic reactive systems in vitro by poly IC and BCG-murine interferons induced in vivo. Cell Immunol. 27, 60–70 (1976).

Cocito, D., DeMaeyer, E., Desomer, P.: The action of interferon on the synthesis of RNA in fibroblasts infected with an RNA virus. Life Sciences 12, 753–758 (1962 a).

Cocito, D., DeMaeyer, E., Desomer, P.: Synthesis of mRNA in neoplastic cells treated with interferon. Life Sciences 12, 759–764 (1962 b).

Cocito, C., Schonne, E., Desomer, P.: Metabolism of nucleic acids in uninfected fibroblasts incubated in vitro with rat interferon. Life Sci. 4, 1253–1262 (1965).

Cogniaux–Leclerc, J., Levy, A. M., Wagner, R. R.: Evidence from UV inactivation kinetics for discrete cellular sites that code for interferon synthesis. Virology 28, 497–499 (1966).

Colby, C.: The induction of interferon by natural and synthetic polynucleotides. Prog. Nucleic Acid Res. Mol. Biol. 11, 1–32 (1971).

Colby, C., Chamberlin, M. J.: The specificity of interferon induction in chick embryo cells by Helical RNA. Biochemistry 63, 160–167 (1969).

Colby, C., Chamberlin, M. J., Duesberg, P. M., Simon, M. I.: The specificity of interferon induction. In: Biological Effects of Polynucleotides (Beers, R. F., jr., Brown, W., eds.), pp. 79–87. Berlin–Heidelberg–New York: Springer (1971).

Colby, C., Duesberg, P. M.: Double-stranded RNA in vaccinia virus infected cells. Nature 222, 940–944 (1969).

Colby, C., Morgan, M. J.: Interferon induction and action. Ann. Rev. Microbiol. 25, 333–360 (1971).

Colby, C., Penhoet, E. E., Samuel, C. E.: A comparison of transfer RNA from untreated and interferon-treated murine cells. Virology 74, 262–264 (1976).

Cole, B. C., Overall, J. C., Lombardi, P. S., Glasgow, L. A.: Mycoplasma-mediated hyporeactivity to various interferon inducers. Infect. Immun. 12, 1349–1360 (1975).

Cole, B. C., Overall, J. C., jr., Lombardi, P. S., Glasgow, L. A.: Induction of interferon in ovine and human lymphocyte cultures by mycoplasmas. Infect. Immun. 14, 88–94 (1976).

Coley, W. B.: Treatment of inoperable malignant tumors with the toxines of erysipelas and the bacillus prodigiosus. Trans. Am. Surg. Assoc. 12, 183–188 (1894).

Collyn d'Hooghe, M., Brouty–Boye, D., Malaise, E. F., Gresser, I.: Interferon and cell division. XII. Prolongation by interferon of the intermitotic time of mouse mammary tumor cells in vitro. Microcinematographic analysis. Exp. Cell Res. 105, 73–76 (1977).

Connolly, J. H., Allen, I. V., Hurwitz, L. J., Millar, J. H. D.: Measles virus antibody and antigen in subacute sclerosing panencephalitis. Lancet 1, 542–547 (1967).

Connolly, J. H., Dick, G. W. A., Field, C. M. B.: A fatal case of progressive vaccinia. Brit. Med. J. i, 1315–1317 (1962).

Considine, R. G., Starr, T. J.: Role of the reticuloendothelial system in interferon tolerance. J. Retic. Soc. **4**, 315–318 (1967).

Content, J., Lebleu, B., Nudel, V., Zilberstein, A., Berissi, H., Revel, M.: Blocks in elongation and initiation of protein synthesis induced by interferon treatment in mouse L cells. Europ. J. Biochem. **54**, 1–5 (1975).

Content, J. Lebleu, B., Zilberstein, A., Berissi, H., Revel, M.: Mechanism of the interferon-induced block of mRNA translation in mouse L cells: Reversal of the block by transfer RNA. FEBS Lett. **41** (1), 125–130 (1974).

Cooper, J. A., Farrell, P. J.: Extracts of interferon-treated cells can inhibit reticulocyte lysate protein synthesis. Biochem. Biophys. Rzs. Comm. **77**, 124–131 (1977).

Cooper, P. D., Bellett, J. D.: A transmissible interfering component of vesicular stomatitis virus preparation. J. Gen. Microbiol. **21**, 485–490 (1959).

Coraggio, F., Coto, V., Fantoni, V., Galeota, C. A., Lavegas, E.: Azione di un interferon, proveniente da culture *in vitro* di cellule embrionali di topo infettate col virus del polioma, su un tumore trapiantabile nel topo (ceppo C 57). Boll. Ist. Sieroter. Milanese **44**, 64–68 (1965).

Coraggio, F., Coto, V., Galeota, C. A., Georgiades, J.: Effeto dell'idiocortisone sulla produzione di interferon nel coniglio inoculato con endotossina baterica o con virus. Boll. Ist. Sieroter, Milan **47**, 308–310 (1968).

Cornell, J. C., jr., Smith, K. A., Cornwell, G. G. III, Burke, G. P., McIntyre, O. R.: The systemic effects of intravenous polyriboinosinic: polyribocytidilic acid in man. J. Nat. Cancer Inst. **57**, 1211–1213 (1977).

Craighead, J. E.: Growth of parainfluenza type 3 virus and interferon production in infant and adult mice. Brit. J. Exp. Path. **XLII**, 235–241 (1966).

Creagan, R. P., Tan, Y. H., Chen, S., Ruddle, F. H.: Somatic cell genetic analysis of the interferon system. Fed. Proc. **34**, 222–226 (1975).

Crenshaw, R. R., Luke, G. M., Simonoff, P.: Interferon inducing activities of derivatives of 1,3-dimethyl-4-(3-dimethylaminopropylamino)-1 H-pyrazoco-[3, 4-6] quinoline. J. Med. Chem. **19**, 262–266 (1976).

Crowell, R. L., Syverton, J. T.: The mammalian cell-virus relationship. VI. Sustained infection of Hela cells by coxsackie B-3 virus and effect of superinfection. J. Exp. Med. **113**, 419–435 (1961).

Cupples, C. G., Tan, Y. H.: Effect of human interferon preparations on lymphoblastogenesis in Down's syndrome. Nature **267**, 165–167 (1977).

Dahl, H.: A micro assay for mouse and human interferon. II. Dose-response in different cell-virus systems. Acta Pathol. Microbiol. Scand. **B 81**, 359–364 (1973).

Dahl, H.: Human interferon and cell growth inhibition. II. Biological and physico-chemical properties of the growth inhibitory component. Acta Path. Microbiol. Scand. **B 5979**, 1–4 (1977a).

Dahl, H.: Differentiation between antiviral and anticellular effects of interferon. Tex. Rep. Biol. Med. **35**, 381–387 (1977b).

Dahl, H., Degre, M.: A micro assay for mouse and human interferon. Acta Path. Microbiol. Scand. **B 80**, 863 (1972).

Dahl, H., Degre, M.: Separation of antiviral activity of human interferon from cell growth inhibitory effect. Nature **257**, 799–801 (1975).

Dahl, H., Degre, M.: The effect of ascorbic acid on production of human interferon and the antiviral activity *in vitro*. Acta Pathol. Microbiol. Scand. **B 84**, 280–285 (1976a).

Dahl, H., Degre, M.: Human interferon and cell growth inhibition. I. Inhibitory effect of human interferon on the growth rate of cultured human cells. Acta Pathol. Microbiol. Scand. **B 84**, 285–289 (1976b).

Danielescu, G., Barbu, C., Sorodoc, Y., Cajal, N., Sarateanu, D., Petrescu, A., Motas, C., Ganea, E.: The presence of interferon and type A immunoglobulins in the nasopharyngeal secretions of volunteers immunized with an inactivated influenza vaccine. Acta Virol. **19**, 245 (1975).

Davey, M. W., Huang, J. W., Sulkowski, E., Carter, W. A.: Hydrophobic interaction of human interferon with concanavalin A-agarose. J. Biol. Chem. **249**, 6354–6355 (1974).

Davey, M. W., Huang, J. W., Sulkowski, E., Carter, W. A.: Hydrophobic binding sites on human interferon. J. Biol. Chem. **250**, 348–356 (1975).

Davey, M. W., Sulkowski, E., Carter, W. A.: Purification and characterization of mouse interferon with novel affinity sorbents. J. Virol. **17**, 439–445 (1976a).

Davey, M. W., Sulkowski, E., Carter, W. A.: Hydrophobic interaction of human, mouse and rabbit interferons with immobilized hydrocarbons. J. Biol. Chem. **251**, 7620–7624 (1976b).

Davey, M. W., Sulkowski, E., Carter, W. A.: Binding of human fibroblast interferon to concanavalin A-agarose. Involvement of carbohydrate recognition and hydrophobic interaction. Biochem. **15**, 704–710 (1976c).

Davies, A.: Some properties of calf interferon. Biochem. J. **95**, 20–21 (1965).

DeClercq, E.: Mechanism of the antiviral activity of synthetic polyanions. Thesis, University of Leuven, Belgium (1971).

DeClercq, E.: Hyporeactivity to interferon production by ds RNA associated with hyporeactivity to antiviral protection and hyporeactivity to toxicity. Proc. Soc. Exp. Biol. Med. **141**, 340–345 (1972).

DeClercq, E.: Synthetic interferon inducers, in: Topics in Current Chemistry **52**, p. 173. Berlin–Heidelberg–New York: Springer (1974).

DeClercq, E.: Encephalitis induced upon intranasal challenge of mice with herpes simplex virus. Proc. Symp. Clinc. Use of Interferon, Zagreb, Yugoslavia, pp. 129–139 (1975).

DeClercq, E.: Effect of mouse interferon and poly I·C on L-cell tumor growth in nude mice. Cancer Res. **37**, 1502–1508 (1977).

DeClercq, E., Desomer, P.: Protective effect of interferon and polyacrylic acid in newborn mice infected with a lethal dose of vesicular stomatitis virus. Life Sci. **7**, 925–930 (1968).

DeClercq, E., Desomer, P.: Prolonged antiviral protection by interferon inducers. Proc. Soc. Exp. Biol. Med. **132**, 699–703 (1969).

DeClercq, E., Desomer, P.: Role of interferon in the protective effect of the double-stranded polyribonucleotide against murine tumors induced by moloney sarcoma virus. J. Natl. Cancer Inst. **47**, 1345–1355 (1971a).

DeClercq, E., Desomer, P.: Comparative study of the efficacy of different forms of interferon therapy in the treatment of mice challenged intranasally with VSV. Proc. Soc. Exp. Biol. Med. **138**, 301–307 (1971b).

DeClercq, E., Desomer, P.: Effect of chlorite-oxidized oxylamylase on moloney sarcoma virus-induced tumor formation in mice. Europ. J. Cancer **8**, 535–538 (1972b).

DeClercq, E., Desomer, P.: Relationship between cell-interaction and antiviral activity of polyriboinosinic acid-polyribocytidylic acid in different cell cultures. J. Gen. Virol. **19**, 113–118 (1973a).

DeClercq, E., Desomer, P.: Interferon production in rabbit kidney cell cultures exposed to poly C adsorbed to rabbit red blood cells. J. Gen. Virol. **22**, 271–275 (1974).

DeClercq, E., Desomer, P.: Are cytotoxicity and interferon-inducing activity of poly I·poly C invariably linked in interferon-treated L cells? J. Gen. Virol. **27**, 35–39 (1975).

DeClercq, E., Eckstein, F., Merigan, T. C.: Interferon induction increased through chemical modification of a synthetic polyribonucleotide. Science **165**, 1137–1139 (1969).

DeClercq, E., Eckstein, F., Steinbach, H., Merigan, T. C.: Interferon induction by and ribonuclease sensitivity of thiophosphate-substituted polyribonucleotides. Antimicrob. Agnts. Chemoth. **9**, 187–192 (1969).

DeClercq, E., Eckstein, F., Steinbach, H., Merigan, T. C.: The antiviral activity of thiophosphate-substituted polyribonucleotides *in vitro* and *in vivo*. Virology **42**, 421–428 (1970).

DeClercq, E., Edy, V. G., Cassiman, J. J.: Non-antiviral activities of interferon are not controlled by chromosome 21. Nature **256**, 132–134 (1975).

DeClercq, E., Edy, V. G., Cassiman, J. J.: Chromosome 21 does not code for an interferon receptor. Nature **264**, 249–251 (1976).

DeClercq, E., Edy, V. G., Devlieger, H., Eeckels, R., Desmyter, J.: Intrathecal administration of interferon in neonatal herpes. J. Pediat. **86**, 736–739 (1975).

DeClercq, E., Janik, B.: Antiviral activity of polynucleotides: poly (2' fluoro-2'-deoxyuridylic acid). Biochimica et Biophysica Acta **324**, 50–53 (1973).

DeClercq, E., Janik, B., Sommer, R. G.: Biological, biochemical and physicochemical evidence

22*

for the existence of the poly A·poly U·poly-2-fluore-2'-deoxyuridylate triple-stranded complex. Chem. Biol. Interactions 14, 113–118 (1976).

DeClercq, E., Luczak, M.: Antiviral activity of carbopol, a cross-linked polycarboxylate. Arch. Virol. 52, 151–158 (1977).

DeClercq, E., Merigan, T. C.: An active interferon inducer obtained from *Hemophilus influenzae* type B. J. Immunol. 103, 899–906 (1969 a).

DeClercq, E., Merigan, T. C.: Local and systemic protection by synthetic polyanionic interferon inducers in mice against vesicular stomatitis virus. J. Gen. Virol. 5, 359–367 (1969 b).

DeClercq, E., Merigan, T. C.: Requirement of a stable secondary structure for the antiviral activity of polynucleotides. Nature 222, 1148–1152 (1969 c).

DeClercq, E., Merigan, T. C.: Current concepts of interferon and interferon induction. Ann. Rev. Med. 21, 17–33 (1970 a).

DeClercq, E., Merigan, T. C.: Induction of interferon by nonviral agents. Arch. Intern. Med. 126, 94–98 (1970 b).

DeClercq, E., Merigan, T. C.: Bis-DEAE-Fluorenone: Mechanism of antiviral protection and stimulation of interferon production in the mouse. J. Infect. Dis. 123, 190–199 (1971 a).

DeClercq, E., Merigan, T. C.: Moloney sarcoma virus-induced tumors in mice: Inhibition or stimulation by (poly-I)·(poly-C). Proc. Soc. Exp. Biol. Med. 137, 590–594 (1971 b).

DeClercq, E., Merigan, T. C.: Thermal activation of the antiviral activity of synthetic polyribonucleotides: influence of DEAE-dextran in various cell cultures. J. Gen. Virol. 10, 125–130 (1971 c).

DeClercq, E., Nuwer, M. R., Merigan, T. C.: Potentiating effects of Freund's adjuvant on interferon production by endotoxin or poly rI·poly rC. Infect. Immun. 2, 69–76 (1970 a).

DeClercq, E., Nuwer, M. R., Merigan, T. C.: The role of interferon in the protective effect of a synthetic double-stranded polyribonucleotide against intranasal vesicular stomatitis virus challenge in mice. J. Clin. Invest. 49, 1565–1577 (1970 b).

DeClercq, E., Rottman, F. M., Shugar, D.: Antiviral activity of polynucleotides: poly 2'-O-ethyladenylic acid and poly 2'-O-ethyluridylic acid. FEBS Lett. 42, 331–334 (1974).

DeClercq, E., Stewart II, W. E.: Utilization of poly (rI)·poly (rC) for controlling virus diseases and tumors still in abeyance. Medikon 1, 331–345 (1972).

DeClercq, E., Stewart II, W. E.: The breadth of interferon action, in: Selective Inhibitors of Viral Functions (Carter, W. C., ed.), pp. 80–106. Cleveland, Ohio: CRC Press, Inc. (1973).

DeClercq, E., Stewart II, W. E.: Integrity of cell-bound poly (I)·poly (C). J. Gen. Virol. 24, 201–209 (1974 a).

DeClercq, E., Stewart, II. W. E.: Regression of autochthonous Moloney sarcoma virus-induced tumors in mice treated with polyriboinosinic acid polyribocytidylic acid. J. Nat. Cancer Inst. 52, 591–595 (1974 b).

DeClercq, E., Stewart II, W. E., Desomer, P.: Interferon production linked to toxicity of polyriboinosinic acid-polyribocytidylic acid. Infect. Immun. 6 (3), 344–347 (1972).

DeClercq, E., Stewart II, W. E., Desomer, P.: Increased toxicity of double-stranded ribonucleic acid in virus-infected animals. Infect. Immun. 7, 167–172 (1973 a).

DeClercq, E., Stewart II, W. E., Desomer, P.: Poly (rI) more important than poly (rC) in the interferon induction process by poly (rI)·poly (rC). Virology 54, 278–282 (1973 b).

DeClercq, E., Stewart II, W. E., Desomer, P.: Studies on the mechanism of the priming effect of interferon on interferon production by cell cultures exposed to poly (rI)·poly (rC). Infect. Immun. 8, 309–316 (1973 c).

DeClercq, E., Torrence, P. F.: Comparative study of various double-stranded RNAs as inducers of human interferon. J. Gen. Virol. 37, 619–624 (1977).

DeClercq, E., Torrence, P. F., Witkop, B.: Polynucleotide displacement reactions: detection by interferon induction. Biochem 15, 717–722 (1976).

DeClercq, E., Torrence, P. F., Witkop, B., Stewart II, W. E., Desomer, P.: Interferon induction: tool for establishing interactions among homopolyribonucleotides. Science 186, 835–837 (1974 a).

DeClercq, E., Torrence, P. F., Witkop, B., Desomer, P., Stewart II, W. E.: Previously unrecognized interactions among synthetic polynucleotides and their complexes reveled by interferon induction studies. Arch. Intern. Physiol. Biochim. 82, 769–772 (1974 b).

DeClercq, E., Wells, R. D., Grant, R. C., Merigan, T.: Thermal activation of the antiviral activity of synthetic double-stranded polyribonucleotides. J. Mol. Biol. 56, 83–100 (1971).

DeClercq, E., Wells, R. D., Merigan, T. C.: Increase in antiviral activity of polynucleotides by thermal activation. Nature **226**, 364–366 (1970).

DeClercq, E., Wells, R. D., Merigan, T. C.: Studies on the antiviral activity and cell interaction of synthetic double-stranded polyribo- and polydeoxyribonucleotides. Virology **47**, 405–411 (1972).

DeClercq, E., Zmudzka, B., Shugar, D.: Antiviral activity of polynucleotides: role of the 2-hydroxyl and a pyrimidine 5-methyl. FEBS Lett. **24**, 137–140 (1972).

Degre, M., Dahl, H.: Production of an interferon-like agent following inoculation with bacterial vaccine. Proc. Soc. Exp. Biol. Med. **137**, 233–236 (1971).

Degre, M., Dahl, H.: Interferon production and prevention of viral infections in mice by components of a mixed bacterial vaccine. Acta Pathol. Microbiol. Scand. **82**, 904–910 (1974).

Degre, M., Dahl, H., Vandvik, B.: Interferon in the serum and cerebrospinal fluid in patients with multiple sclerosis and other neurological disorders. Acta Neurol. Scand. **53**, 152–156 (1976).

Degre, M., Glaz, E. T.: Interferon induction in human cellcultures by small molecular inducers. Acta Path. Microbiol. Scand. **B 85**, 189–194 (1977).

Deinhardt, F., Burnside, J.: Spontaneous interferon production in cultures of a cell line from a human myeloblastic leukemia. J. Natl. Cancer Inst. **39**, 681–683 (1967).

DeMaeyer, E.: Interferon and delayed-type hypersensitivity to a viral antigen. J. Infect. Disease **133**, A 63–A 66 (1976).

DeMaeyer, E., DeMaeyer, J.: Two-sided effect of steroids on interferon in tissue culture. Nature **197**, 724–725 (1963).

DeMaeyer, E., DeMaeyer–Guignard, J.: Inhibition by 20-methylcholanthrene of interferon production in rat cells. Virology **20**, 536–539 (1963).

DeMaeyer, E., DeMaeyer–Guignard, J.: Effects of polycyclic aromatic carcinogens on viral replication similarity to actinomycin D. Science **146**, 650–651 (1964a).

DeMaeyer, E., DeMaeyer–Guignard, J.: Inhibition by 3-methylcholanthrene of interferon formation in rat embryo cells infected with Sindbis virus. J. Natl. Cancer Inst. **32**, 1317–1319 (1964b).

DeMaeyer, E., DeMaeyer–Guignard, J.: Inhibition of interferon synthesis by triethylenemelamine and 4-nitroquinoline-N-oxide. Arch. Ges. Virusforsch. **22**, 62–68 (1967).

DeMaeyer, E., DeMaeyer–Guignard, J.: Influence of animal genotype and age on the amount of circulating interferon induced by Newcastle disease virus. J. Gen. Virol. **2**, 445–451 (1968).

DeMaeyer, E., DeMaeyer–Guignard, J.: A gene with quantitative effect on circulating interferon induction – further studies. Ann. N. Y. Acad. Sci. **173**, 228–236 (1969).

DeMaeyer, E., DeMaeyer–Guignard, J., Bailey, D. W.: Effect of mouse genotype on interferon production. Lines cogenic at the If-1 locus. Immunogenetics **1**, 438–441 (1975).

DeMaeyer, E., DeMaeyer–Guignard, J., Hall, W. T., Bailey, D. W.: A locus affecting circulating interferon levels induced by mouse mamary tumor virus. J. Gen. Virol. **23**, 209–211 (1974).

DeMaeyer, E., DeMaeyer-Guignard, J., Jullien, P.: Circulating interferon production in the mouse: Origin and nature of cells involved and influence of animal genotype. J. Gen. Physiol. **56**, 43 S–47 S (1970).

DeMaeyer, E., DeMaeyer–Guignard, J., Montagnier, L.: Doublestranded RNA from rat liver induces interferon in rat cells. Nature New Biol. **229**, 109–110 (1971).

DeMaeyer, E., DeMaeyer–Guignard, J., Vandeputte, M.: Inhibition by interferon of delayed-type hypersensitivity in the mouse. Proc. Nat. Acad. Sci. U. S. A. **72**, 1753–1758 (1975).

DeMaeyer, E., Desomer, P.: Influence of pH on interferon production and activity. Nature **194**, 1252–1254 (1962).

DeMaeyer, E., Enders, J. F.: An interferon appearing in cell cultures infected with measles virus. Proc. Soc. Exp. Biol. Med. **107**, 573–578 (1961).

DeMaeyer, E., Fauve, R. M., DeMaeyer–Guignard, J.: Production d'interferon au niveau du macrophage. Annales de L'institut Pasteur **120**, 438–446 (1971).

DeMaeyer, E., Jullien, P., DeMaeyer–Guignard, J.: Interferon synthesis in X-irradiated animals. II. Restoration by bone-marrow transplantation of circulating interferon production in lethally-irradiated mice. Int. J. Radiat. Biol. **13**, 417–420 (1967).

DeMaeyer, E., Jullien, P., DeMaeyer–Guignard, J., Demant, P.: Effect of mouse genotype on interferon production. II. Distribution of IF-1 alleles among inbred strains and transfer of phenotype by grafting bone marrow cells. Immunogenetics **2**, 151–155 (1975).

DeMaeyer, E., Mobraaten, L., DeMaeyer–Guignard, J.: Prolongation by interferon of the survival of skin grafts in the mouse. CR Acad. Sci. (Paris) **D 277**, 2101–2103 (1973).

DeMaeyer–Guignard, J.: Mouse leukemia: Depression of serum interferon production. Science **177**, 797–799 (1972).

DeMaeyer–Guignard, J., Cachard, A., DeMaeyer, E.: Delayed-type hypersensitivity to sheep red blood cells: inhibition of sensitization by interferon. Science **190**, 574–578 (1975).

DeMaeyer–Guignard, J., DeMaeyer, E.: Effect of carcinogenic and noncarcinogenic hydrocarbons on interferon synthesis and virus plaque development. J. Natl. Cancer Institut. **34**, 265–276 (1965 a).

DeMaeyer–Guignard, J., DeMaeyer, E.: Inhibition of interferon synthesis and stimulation of virus plaque development in mammalian cell cultures after ultraviolet irradiation. Nature **205**, 985–988 (1965 b).

DeMaeyer–Guignard, J., DeMaeyer, E.: Depression of circulating interferon response in Balb/C mice after urethan treatment. Science **155**, 482–484 (1967).

DeMaeyer–Guignard, J., DeMaeyer, E.: Effect of antilymphocytic serum on circulating interferon in mice as a funtion of the inducer. Nature New Biol. **229**, 212–214 (1971).

DeMaeyer–Guignard, J., DeMaeyer, E.: The chromophore of blue dextran: a potent ligand for the purification of interferon by affinity chromatography. CR Acad. Sci. **283**, 709–711 (1976).

DeMaeyer–Guignard, J., DeMaeyer, E., Montagnier, L.: Interferon messenger RNA: Translation in heterologous cells. Proc. Natl. Acad. Sci. U. S. A. **69**, 1203–1207 (1972).

DeMaeyer–Guignard, J., Thang, M. N., DeMaeyer, E.: Binding of mouse interferon to polynucleotides. Proc. Natl. Acad. Sci. U. S. A. **74**, 3787–3790 (1977).

Dennis, A. J., Wilson, H. E., Barker, A. D., Rheins, M. S.: Interferon induction in normal and leukemic human lymphocyte cultures by tilorone hydrochloride. Proc. Soc. Exp. Biol. Med. **141**, 782–785 (1972).

Denys, P.: Protective effect of interferon in rats infected with Sindbis virus. Lancet **ii**, 174–176 (1963).

Denys, P., Desomer, P., Prinzie, A.: Protective effect of interferon in influenza-infected mice. Antonie van Leeuwenhoek J. Microbiol. Serol. **27**, 261–263 (1961).

DePoux, R.: Fixed rabies virus and interferon. C. R. Acad. Sc. (Paris) **260**, 354–356 (1965).

DeSena, J., Rio, G. J.: Partial purification and characterization of RTG-2 fish cell interferon. Infect. Immun. **11**, 815–822 (1975).

Desmyter, J.: The use of interferon in viral hepatitis B. Tex. Rep. Biol. Med. **35**, 516–522 (1977).

Desmyter, J., Rawls, W. E., Melnick, J. L.: A human interferon that crosses the species line. Proc. Natl. Acad. Sci. U. S. A. **59**, 69–76 (1968).

Desmyter, J., Rawls, W. E., Melnick, J. L.: Sensitivity of rabbit cells to primate interferons. Ann. New York, Acad. Sci. **173**, 492–504 (1970).

Desmyter, J., Rawls, W. E., Melnick, J. L., Yow, M. D., Barrett, F. F.: Interferon in congenital Rubella: response to live attenuated measles vaccine. J. Immunol. **99**, 771–777 (1967).

Desmyter, J., Ray, M. B., DeGroote, J., Bradburne, A. F., Desmet, V. J., Edy, V. G., Billiau, A., De Somer, P., Mortelmans, J.: Administration of human fibroblast interferon in chronic hepatitis B infection. Lancet **ii**, 645–648 (1976).

Desmyter, J., Stewart II, W. E.: Molecular modification of interferon: Attainment of human interferon in a conformation active on cat cells but inactive on human cells. Virology **70**, 451–458 (1976).

Desomer, P.: Clinical trials with human fibroblast interferon. Fifth Aharon Katzir-Katchalsky Conference, Rehovot, Israel (1977).

Desomer, P.: Polyacrylic and polymethacrylic acids as antiviral agents. In: Colloque No. 6 Institute National de la Santé et de la Recherche Médicale, p. 29 (1970).

Desomer, P., Billiau, A.: Interferon production by the spleen of rats after intravenous injection of Sindbis virus or heat-killed *Escherichia coli*. Arch. gesamte Virusforsch. **19**, 143–154 (1966).

Desomer, P., Billiau, A., DeClercq, E.: Inhibition of antibody production in rats and mice by intravenous injection of interferon-inducing amounts of Sindbis virus or E. coli. Arch. gesamte Virusforsch. **20**, 205–214 (1967).

Desomer, P., Billiau, A., DeClercq, E.: Influence of N-methylacetamide on interferon production *in vivo* in rat, in: The Interferons (Rita, G., ed.), pp. 65–81. New York: Academic Press (1968).

Desomer, P., DeClercq, E., Billiau, A., Schonne, E., Clausen, M.: Antiviral activity of polyacrylic and polymethacrylic acids. I. Mode of action *in vitro*. J. Virol. **2**, 878–885 (1968a).

Desomer, P., DeClercq, E., Billiau, A., Schonne, E., Clausen, M.: Antiviral activity of polyacrylic and polymethacrylic acids. II. Mode of action *in vivo*. J. Virol. **2**, 886–890 (1968b).

Desomer, P., DeClercq, E., Cocito, C., Billiau, A.: The interferon inducer from Brucella. Ann. N. Y. Acad. Sci. **173**, 274–278 (1970).

Desomer, P., Edy, V. G., Billiau, A.: Interferon-induced skin reactivity in man. Lancet ii, 47–50 (1977).

Desomer, P., Prinzie, A., Denys, P., Schonne, E.: Mechanism of action of interferon. I. Relationship with viral RNA. Virology **16**, 63–70 (1962).

Desomer, P., Stewart II, W. E.: The broadening concept of interferon activities: non-antiviral cellular alterations. Proceedings of the 1st International Congress of the International Associations for Microbiology, Tokyo, Japan (1975).

De Vita, V., Canellas, G., Carbone, P., Baron, S., Hevy, H., Gralnick, H.: Clinical trials with the interferon inducer poly rI·poly rC. Proc. Amer. Assoc. Cancer Res. **11**, 21–30 (1970).

Dianzani, F., Baron, S.: Unexpectedly rapid action of human interferon in physiological conditions. Nature **257**, 682–684 (1975).

Dianzani, F., Baron, S.: The continued presence of interferon is not required for activation of cells by interferon. P. S. E. B. M. **155**, 562–566 (1977).

Dianzani, F., Baron, S., Buckler, C. E. Mechanisms of DEAE-dextran enhancement of polynucleotide induction of interferon. Proc. Soc. Exp. Biol. Med. **136**, 1111–1114 (1971).

Dianzani, F., Baron, S., Levy, H. B., Gullino, P., Viano, I., Zucca, M.: Studies on the action of human interferon under physiologic conditions. Proc. Symp. Clin. Use of Interferon, Yugoslav Acad. Sci. and Arts, Zagreb, pp. 93–104 (1975).

Dianzani, F., Cantagalli, P., Gagnoni, S., Rita, G.: Effects of DEAE-dextran on production of interferon induced by synthetic double-stranded RNA in L cell cultures. Proc. Soc. Exp. Biol. Med. **128**, 708–710 (1968).

Dianzani, F., Gagnoni, R., Buckler, C. E., Baron, S.: Studies of the induction of interferon system by nonreplicating Newcastle Disease virus. Prod. Soc. Exp. Biol. Med. **133**, 324–328 (1970).

Dianzani, F., Gagnoni, S., Cantagalli, P.: Studies on the potentiating effect of DEAE-dextran on interferon production by double-stranded synthetic polynucleotides, Ann. N. Y. Acad. Sci. **173**, 727–730 (1970).

Dianzani, F., Levy, H. B., Berg, S., Baron, S.: Kinetics of the rapid action of interferon. Proc. Soc. Exp. Biol. Med. **152**, 593–596 (1976).

Dianzani, F., Neri, P., Zucca, M.: Effect of dibutyryl cyclic AMP on interferon production by cells treated with viral or nonviral inducers. Proc. Soc. Exp. Biol. Med. **140** (4), 1375–1378 (1972).

Dianzani, F., Pugliese, A., Baron, S.: Induction of interferon by nonreplicating single-stranded RNA virus. Proc. Soc. Exp. Biol. Med. **145**, 428–433 (1974).

Dianzani, F., Pugliese, A., Baron, S.: Induction of interferon by a nonreplicating single-stranded RNA virus, in: Effects of Interferon on Cells, Viruses and the Immune System (Geraldes, A., ed.), p. 249. New York: Academic Press (1975).

Dianzani, p., Viano, I., Santiano, M., Zucca, M., Baron, S.: Effect of cell density on development of the antiviral state in interferon-producing cells: A possible model of *in vivo* conditions. P. S. E. B. M. **153**, 460–463 (1977).

Diderholm, H., Dinter, Z.: Interference between strains of bovine virus diarrhea virus and their capacity to suppress interferon of a heterologous virus. Proc. Soc. Exp. Biol. Med. **121**, 976–980 (1966).

Diederich, J., Lodemann, E., Wacker, A.: New type of interferon inducer. Naturwissenschaften **59**, 172–173 (1972).

Diederich, J., Lodemann, E., Wacker, A.: Basic dyes as inducers of interferon-like activity in mice. Arch. Ges. Virusforsch. **40**, 82–85 (1973).

Diderholm, H.: Production of interferon by monkey kidney cells infected with simian virus 40. Arch. Ges. Virusforsch. **14**, 39–43 (1963).

Dima, V. F., Petrovici, A., Szabados, J., Vasilesco, T., Pop, A., Rudesco, K.: Modifications enzymatiques et morphologiques chez Brucella suis traitée par l'interférone. Canad. J. Microbiol. **13**, 721–727 (1967).

Dinter, Z.: An inhibitor of viral activity in cell cultures infected with the virus of foot-and-mouth disease. Acta Pathol. Microbiol. Scand. 49, 270–275 (1960).

Donahoe, R. M., Huang, K.-Y.: Neutralization of the phagocytosis-enhancing activity of interferon preparations by anti-interferon serum. Infect. Immun. 7 (3), 501–503 (1973).

Donahoe, R. M., Huang, K.-Y.: Interferon preparations enhance phagocytosis in vivo. Infect. Immun. 13, 1250–1253 (1976).

Dorner, F., Scriba, M., Weil, R.: Interferon: Evidence for its glycoprotein nature. Proc. Natl. Acad. Sci. U. S. A. 70 (7), 1981–1985 (1973).

Doskocil, J., Fuchsberger, N., Vetrak, J., Lackovic, V., Borecky, L.: Double-stranded F 2 phage RNA as interferon inducer. Acta Virol. 15, 523–525 (1971).

Douglas, R. G., jr., Betts, R. F.: Effect of induced interferon in experimental rhinovirus infections in volunteers. Infect. Immun. 9, 506–510 (1974).

Douglas, R. G., Betts, R. F., Simons, R. L., Hogan, P. W., Roth, F. K.: Evaluation of a topical interferon inducer in experimental influenza infection in volunteers. Antimicrob. Agents Chemother. 8, 684–689 (1975).

Douglas, R. G., Lynch, E. C., Spira, M.: Treatment of progressive vaccinia. Arch. Intern. Med. 129, 980–986 (1972).

Dubovi, E. J., Akers, T. G.: Interferon induction by Colorado tick fever virus, a dsRNA virus. Proc. Soc. Exp. Biol. Med. 139, 123–127 (1972).

Dubuy, H., Baron, S., Uhlendorf, C., Johnson, M. L.: Role of interferon in murine lactic dehydrogenase virus infection in vivo and in vitro, Infect. Immun. 8, 977–984 (1973).

Dubuy, H. G., Johnson, M. L., Buckler, C. E., Baron, S.: Relationship between dose size and dose interval of polyinosinic-polycytidylic acid and interferon hyporesponsiveness in mice. Proc. Soc. Exp. Biol. Med. 135, 340–344 (1970).

Duc-Goiran, P., Galliot, B., Chany, C.: Studies on virus-induced interferons produced by the human amniotic membrane and white blood cells. Arch. Ges. Virusforsch. 34, 232–243 (1971).

Dulbecco, R., Johnson, T.: Interferon sensitivity of the enhanced incorporation of thymidine into cellular DNA induced by polyoma virus. Virology 42, 368–383 (1970).

Edelman, R., Wheelock, E. F.: Vesicular stomatitis replication in human leukocyte cultures: Enhancement by phytohemagglutinin. Science 154, 1053–1055 (1966).

Edy, V. G., Braude, I. A., Declercq, E., Billiau, A., Desomer, P.: Purification of human fibroblast interferon by glass. J. Gen. Virol. 33, 517–521 (1976).

Edy, V. G., Billiau, A., Desomer, P.: Enhancement of interferon production in mouse cell line: a high-yielding source of mouse interferon. Appld. Microbiol. 26, 434–436 (1973).

Edy, V. G., Billiau, A., Desomer, P.: Pharmokinetics of human fibroblast interferon. Symp. Antivirals with Clinical Potential, Stanford, Calif. (1975).

Edy, V. G., Billiau, A., Desomer, P.: Human fibroblast and leukocyte interferons show different dose-response curves in assay of cell protection. J. Gen. Virol. 31, 251–255 (1976a).

Edy, V. G., Billiau, A., Desomer, P.: Comparison of rates of clearance of human fibroblast and leukocyte interferon from the circulatory system of rabbits. J. Infec. Diseas. 133, A 18–A 20 (1976b).

Edy, V. G., Billiau, A., Desomer, P.: Purification of human fibroblast interferon by zinc chelate affinity chromatography. J. Biol. Chem. 252, 5934–5936 (1977).

Edy, V. G., Billiau, A., Joniau, M., Desomer, P.: Stabilization of mouse and human interferons by acid pH against inactivation due to shaking and guanidine hydrochloride. Proc. Soc. Exp. Biol. Med. 146, 249–253 (1974).

Edy, V. G., Billiau, A., van Damne, J., Desomer, P.: Mass production of human interferon in diploid cells. Proc. Symp. Clinical Use of Interferon Yugoslav Acad. Sci. Arts, Zagreb, pp. 35–39 (1975).

Edy, V. G., Desmyter, J. Billiau, A., Desomer, P.: Stable and unstable forms of human fibroblast interferon. Infect. Immun. 16, 445–448 (1977).

Einhorn, S., Strander, H.: Is interferon tissue-specific? Effect of human leukocyte and fibroblast interferons on the growth of lymphoblastoid and osteosarcoma cell lines. J. Gen. Virol. 35, 573–577 (1977).

Elgio, K., Degre, M.: Polyinosinic-polycytidylic acid in two-stage skin carcinogenesis. Effect on epidermal growth parameters and interferon induction in treated mice. J. Natl. Cancer Inst. 51, 171–177 (1973).

Ellis, L. F., Kleinschmidt, W. J.: Virus-like particles in a fraction of statolon. Nature 215, 649–650 (1967).

Emödi, G., Just, M.: Interferon production by lymphocytes in human milk. Scand. J. Immunol. 3, 157–160 (1974 a).

Emödi, G., Just, M.: Impaired interferon response of children with congenital cytomegalovirus disease. Acta Paediatr. Scand. 63, 183–187 (1974 b).

Emödi, G., Just, M., Hernandez, R., Hirt, H. R.: Circulating interferon in man after administration of exogenous human leukocyte interferon. J. Nat. Cancer Inst. 54, 1045–1048 (1975 a).

Emödi, G., O'Reilly, R., Muller, A., Everson, L. K., Binswanger, U., Just, M.: Effect of human exogenous leukocyte interferon in cytomegalovirus infections. J. Infect. Dis. 133, A 199–A 204 (1976).

Emödi, G., Rufli, T., Just, M., Hernandez, R.: Human interferon therapy for herpes zoster in adults. Scand. J. Infect. Dis. 7, 1–5 (1975 b).

Enzmann, P. J.: Induction of an interferon-like substance in persistently infected Aedes albopictus cells. Arch. Ges. Virusforsch. 41, 382–389 (1973).

Eppstein, D. B., Samuel, C. E.: Mechanism of interferon action. Partial purification and characterization of a low-molecular weight interferon-mediator of translation with nucleolytic activity. Biochem. Biophys. Res. Commun. 79, 145–153 (1977).

Epstein, L. B.: Mitogen and antigen stimulated interferon: the role of human T and B lymphocytes and macrophages, in: Effects of Interferon on Cells, Viruses and the Immune System (Geraldes, A., ed.), pp. 169–182. New York: Academic Press (1975).

Epstein, L. B.: Assay of human immune interferon from lymphocyte-macrophage cultures by a virus plaque-reduction method, in: Manual of Clinical Immunology (Rose, N. R., Friedman, H., eds.), p. 120. Washington: Amer. Soc. Microbiol. Publications (1976 a).

Epstein, L. B.: Ability of macrophages to augment in vitro mitogen-stimulated and antigen stimulated production of interferon and other mediators of cellular immunity, in: Immunobiology of the Macrophage (Nelson, D. S., ed.), pp. 202–234. New York: Academic Press (1976 b).

Epstein, L. B.: Effects of interferon on the immune response in vitro and in vivo, in: Interferons and their Actions (Stewart II, W. E., ed.), pp. 91–132. Cleveland, Ohio: CRC Press, Inc. (1977).

Epstein, L. B., Ammann, A. J.: Evaluation of T lymphocyte effector function immunodeficiency diseases: Abnormality in mitogen-stimulated interferon in patients with selective IGA deficiency. J. Immunol. 112, 617–626 (1974).

Epstein, L. B., Bourne, H. R.: Interferon production by mitogen stimulated lymphocytes: Cyclic AMP mediated inhibition by cholera toxin, in: Mitogens in Immunobiology (Oppenheim, J. J., Rossenstreich, D. L., eds.), pp. 453–476. New York: Academic Press (1976).

Epstein, L. B., Cline, M. J.: Chronic lymphocytic leukemia. Studies on mitogen-stimulated lymphocyte interferon as a new technique for assessing T lymphocyte effector function. Clin. Exp. Immunol. 16, 553–563 (1974).

Epstein, L. B., Cline, M. J., Merigan, T. C.: Macrophage-lymphocyte interaction in the PHA-stimulated production of interferon in vitro. Proc. 5th Ann. Leukocyte Culture Conf. (Harris, J. E., ed.), p. 501. New York: Academic Press (1970).

Epstein, L. B., Cline, H. J., Merigan, T. C.: Interaction of human macrophages and lymphocytes in the phytohemagglutinin-stimulated production of interferon. J. Clin. Invest. 50, 744–753 (1971 a).

Epstein, L. B., Cline, M. J., Merigan, T. C.: PPD-stimulated interferon: in vitro macrophage-lymphocyte interaction in the production of a mediator of cellular immunity. Cell. Immunol. 2, 602–613 (1971 b).

Epstein, L. B., Cline, M. J., Merigan, T. C.: The in vitro interaction of immune macrophages and lymphocytes in the antigen (PPD)-induced production of interferon. Proceedings of the Sixth Leucocyte Culture Conference, p. 265 (1972).

Epstein, L. B., Epstein, Ch. J.: Localization of the gene AVG for the antiviral expression of immune and classical interferon to the distal portion of the long arm of chromosome 21. J. Infect. Disease 133, A 56–A 53 (1976).

Epstein, L. B., Kreth, H. W., Herzenberg, L. A.: The separation of human T and B lymphocytes: studies on mitogen-stimulated interferon, in: Lymphocytes Recognition and Effector Mechanisms (Lindahl–Kiessling, K., Osoba, D., eds.), p. 169. Academic Press (1974a).

Epstein, L. B., Kreth, H. W., Herzenberg, L. A.: Fluorescence-activated sorting of human T and B lymphocytes. II. Identification of the cell type responsible for interferon production and cell proliferation in response to mitogens. Cell. Immunol. **12**, 407–421 (1974b).

Epstein, L. B., Salmon, S. E.: The production of interferon by malignant plasma cells from patients with multiple myeloma. J. Immunol. **112**, 1131–1138 (1974).

Epstein, L. B., Stevens, D. A., Merigan, T. C.: Selective increase in lymphocyte interferon response to vaccinia antigen after revaccination. Proc. Nat. Acad. Sci. U. S. A. **69**, 2632–2636 (1972).

Ermolieva, Z. V., Furer, N. M.: Experimental and clinical studies on interferon and interferon inducers. Proc. Microbiol. Res. Group Hung, Acad. Sci. **2**, 49 (1968).

Ershov, F. I., Sokolova, T. M., Kadrova, A. A.: Superinduction of interferon and a study of its messenger RNA. Antibiotiki **22**, 247–252 (1977).

Ershov, F. I., Sokolova, T. M., Takulakhova, E. B., Novokhatsky, A. S., Verkhadskaya, A. A.: Isolation and characterization of mRNA for antiviral protein. Problems of Virology **4**, 441–447 (1977).

Ershov, F. I., Tazulakhova, E. B.: Proofs of the necessity of antiviral protein synthesis in the action of interferon. Vopr. Virusol. **3**, 273–275 (1976).

Ershov, F. I., Tazulakhova, E. B., Zhbanov, V. M.: Messenger RNA for antiviral protein. Dokl. Akad. Nauk. USSR 231–233, 1001 (1976).

Esteban, M., Metz, D. H.: Inhibition of early vaccinia virus protein synthesis in interferon-treated chicken embryo fibroblasts. J. Gen. Virol. **20**, 111–115 (1973).

Falcoff, E., Falcoff, R., Catinot, L., Vomecourt, A., Sanceau, J.: Synthesis of interferon in human lymphocytes stimulated *in vitro* by antilymphocytic serum. Rev. Eur. Etud. Clin. Biol. **17**, 20–26 (1972a).

Falcoff, E., Falcoff, R., Eyquem, A., Sanceau, J., Catinot, L., Vomecourt, A.: Induction d'interféron humain par le sérum antilymphocytaire. C. R. Acad. Sc. (Paris) **271 D**, 545–549 (1970).

Falcoff, E., Falcoff, R., Fournier, F., Chany, C.: Production en masse, purification partielle et caractérisation d'un interféron destiné à des essais thérapeutiques humains. Ann. Inst. Pasteur **111**, 562–584 (1966).

Falcoff, E., Falcoff, R., Lebleu, B., Revel, M.: Interferon treatment inhibits Mengo RNA and haemoglobin mRNA translation in cell-free extracts of L cells. Nature New Biol. **240**, 145–147 (1972b).

Falcoff, E., Falcoff, R., Lebleu, B., Revel, M.: Correlation between the antiviral effect of interferon treatment and the inhibition of *in vitro* mRNA translation in noninfected L cells. J. Virology **12**, 421–424 (1973).

Falcoff, E., Fauconnier, B.: *In vitro* production of an interferon-like inhibitor of viral multiplication by a poikilothermic animal cell: the tortoise *(Testuda greca)*. Proc. Soc. Exp. Biol. Med. **118**, 609–612 (1965).

Falcoff, E., Fournier, F., Chany, C.: Étude comparative des poids moléculaires de deux interférons humains produits *in vitro*. Ann. Inst. Pasteur (Paris) **111**, 241–244 (1966).

Falcoff, E., Havell, E. A., Lewis, J. A., Lande, M. A., Falcoff, R., Sabatini, D. D., Vilček, J.: Intracellular location of newly synthesized interferon in human FS-4 cells. Virology **75**, 384–393 (1976).

Falcoff, R.: Some properties of virus and immune-induced human lymphocyte interferons. J. Gen. Virol. **16**, 251–253 (1972).

Falcoff, R., Falcoff, E., Catinot, L.: Interferon induction by and infectivity of ultraviolet-irradiated double- and multistranded viral RNAs. Biochim. Biophys. Acta **217**, 192–195 (1970).

Falcoff, R., Lebleu, B., Sanceau, J., Weissenbach, J., Dirheimer, G., Ebel, J. P., Falcoff, E.: The inhibition of translation of synthetic polyribonucleotides and Mengo RNA translations in extracts from interferon-treated L cells and its reversion by yeast tRNAs. Biochem. Biophys. Res. Commun. **68**, 1323–1328 (1976).

Falcoff, R., Oriol, R., Iscaki, S.: Lymphocyte stimulation and interferon induction by TS anti-human leukocyte globulins and their uni- and divalet fragments. Eur. J. Immunol. **2**, 476–478 (1972).

Falcoff, R., Scheps, R., Sanceau, J., Catinot, L., Falcoff, E.: Protein synthesis in interferon-treated cells. Biochemie **57**, 1109–1111 (1975).

Fantes, K. M.: Purification, concentration and physico-chemical properties of interferons, in: Interferons (Finter, N. B., ed.), p. 119. Amsterdam: North Holland Publishing Co. (1966).

Fantes, K.: Purification and properties of human interferon. Ann. N. Y. Acad. Sci. **173**, 118–125 (1966).

Fantes, K. H.: Purification and physico-chemical properties of interferons, in: Interferons and Interferon Inducers (Finter, N., ed.), p.171–200. Amsterdam: North Holland Publishing Co. (1973).

Fantes, K. H.: Human leukocyte interferon: Properties and purification. *In Vitro* Monogr. **3**, 48–53 (1974).

Fantes, K. H., Furminger, I. G. S.: Biochemistry – Polyacrylamide gel electrophoresis of highly purified chick interferon. Nature **216**, 71–72 (1967).

Fantes, K., O'Neill, C. F., Mason, P. J.: Purification of chick interferon. Biochem. J. **91**, 20–24 (1964).

Farber, P. A., Glasgow, L. A.: Effect of *Corynebacterium acnes* on interferon production in mice. Infect. Immun. **6**, 272–276 (1972).

Fauconnier, B.: Parenté antigénique des interférons, induits par des agents viraux ou bactérieux et par le statolon chez la souris. C. R. Acad. Sc. (Paris) D **264**, 1814–1817 (1967a).

Fauconnier, B.: Antigenic identity of interferons induced by different viruses in the same cell system. Nature **214**, 591–592 (1967b).

Fauconnier, B.: Viral auto-inhibition studied by the effect of antiinterferon serum on plaque formation. Arch. gesamte Virusforsch. **31**, 266–272 (1970).

Fauconnier, B.: Effect of anti-interferon serum on experimental viral pathogenicity *in vivo*. Path. Biol. **19**, 575–578 (1971).

Fauconnier, B., Wroblowski, H.: Interferon and antiviral activity induced *in vitro* by a plant mycoplasma species Ø Gl. Ann. Microbiol. **125 A**, 469–472 (1974).

Feingold, D. S., Keleti, G., Youngner, J. S.: Antiviral activity of *Brucella abortus* preparations: Separation of active components. Infect. Immun. **13**, 763–768 (1976).

Fenje, P., Postic, B.: Protection of rabbits against experimental rabies by poly I·poly C. Nature **226**, 171–172 (1970).

Fenner, F.: Immune mechanisms in viral infections, in: Viral and Rickettsial Infections of Man (Horsfall, F. L., jr., Tamm, I, eds.), p. 356. Philadelphia: J. B. Lippincott Co. (1965).

Fernandes, M. Y., Wiktor, T. J., Koprowski, H.: Endosymbiotic relationship between animal viruses and host cells. J. Exp. Med. **120**, 1099–1116 (1964).

Ferris, P., Padnos, M., Molomut, N.: Tumor inhibition in mice by M-P virus-induced interferon. Fed. Proc. **30**, 341 (1971).

Fiala, M.: Susceptibility to, and production of interferon by rhinovirus 1. Proc. Soc. Exp. Biol. Med. **140**, 1185–1189 (1972).

Field, A. K., Lampson, G. P., Tytell, A. A., Hilleman, M. R.: Demonstration of double-stranded ribonucleic acid in concentrates of RNA viruses. Proc. Soc. Exp. Biol. Med. **141**, 440–444 (1972c).

Field, A. K., Lampson, G. P., Tytell, A. A., Nemes, M. M., Hilleman, M. R.: Inducers of interferon and host resistance. IV. Double-stranded replicative RNA (MS 2-RF-RNA) from E. coli MS 2 coliphage. Proc. Nat. Acad. Sci. U. S. A. **58**, 2102–2107 (1967b).

Field, A. K., Tytell, A. A., Lampson, G. P., Hilleman, M. R.: Inducers of interferon and host resistance. II. Multistranded synthetic polynucleotide complexes, Proc. Natl. Acad. Sci. **58**, 1004–1009 (1967a).

Field, A. K., Tytell, A. A., Lampson, G. P., Hilleman, M. R.: Inducers of interferon and host resistance. V. *In vitro* studies. Proc. Nat. Acad. Sci. U. S. A. **61**, 340–344 (1968).

Field, A. K., Tytell, A. A., Lampson, G. P., Hilleman, M. R.: Cellular control of interferon production and release after treatment with poly I : C inducer. Proc. Soc. Exp. Biol. Med. **140**, 710–714 (1972a).

Field, A. K., Tytell, A. A., Lampson, G. P., Nemes, M. M., Hilleman, M. R.: Double-stranded polynucleotides as interferon inducers. J. Gen. Physiol. **56**, 905–909 (1970).

Field, A. K., Tytell, A. A., Piperno, E., Lampson, G. P., Nemes, M. M., Hilleman, M. R.: Poly I·C, an inducer of interferon and interference against virus infections. Medicine **51**, 169–174 (1972 b).

Field, A. K., Young, C. W., Krakoff, I. M., Tytell, A. A., Lampson, G. P., Nemes, M. M., Hilleman, M. R.: Induction of interferon in human subjects by poly I:C. Proc. Soc. Exp. Biol. Med. **136**, 1180–1186 (1971).

Findlay, G. M., Mac Callum, F. O.: An interference phenomenon in relation to yellow fever and other viruses. J. Path.. Bact. **44**, 405–424 (1937).

Finkelstein, M. S., Bausek, G. M., Merigan, T. C.: Interferon inducers *in vitro*: Difference in sensitivity to inhibitors of RNA and protein synthesis. Science **161**, 465–468 (1968).

Finter, N. B.: Interferon production and sensitivity of Semliki Forest virus variants. J. Hyg. **62**, 337–342 (1964 a).

Finter, N. B.: A rich source of mouse interferon. Nature **204**, 1114–1115 (1964 b).

Finter, N. B.: Protection of mice by interferon against systemic virus infections. Brit. Med. J. **2**, 981–985 (1964 c).

Finter, N. B.: A comparison of the amounts of mouse interferon obtained from different sources. Nature **206**, 597–599 (1965).

Finter, N. B.: Interferon as an antiviral agent *in vivo*: Qualitative and temporal aspects of the protection of mice against Semliki Forest virus. British J. Exp. Pathol. **47**, 361–371 (1966 a).

Finter, N. B.: Interferon assays and standards, in: Interferons (Finger, N. B., ed.), p. 87. Amsterdam: North Holland Publ. Co. (1966 b).

Finter, N. B.: Quantitative hemadsorption, a new assay technique. J. Immunol. **98**, 88–93 (1967 a).

Finter, N. B.: Interferon in mice: protection against small doses of virus. J. Gen. Virol. **1**, 395–397 (1967 b).

Finter, N. B.: Interferon Assay: sensitivity and other aspects, in: The Interferons (Rita, G., ed.), pp. 203–212. New York: Academic Press (1968).

Finter, N. B.: Dye uptake methods of assessing viral cytopathogenicity and their application to interferon assays. J. Gen. Virol. **5**, 419–425 (1969).

Finter, N. B.: Exogenous interferon in animals and its clinical implications. Arch. Intern. Med. **126**, 147–157 (1970 a).

Finter, N. B.: Will interferon be clinically useful? Ann. N. Y. Acad. Sci. **173**, 619–622 (1970 b).

Finter, N. B.: The assay and standardization of interferon and interferon inducers, in: Interferons and Interferon Inducers (Finter, N. B., ed.), pp. 135–170. Amsterdam: North Holland Publ. Co. (1973 a).

Finter, N. B.: Interferons and inducers *in vivo*. I. Antiviral effects in experimental animals, in: Interferons and Interferon Inducers (Finter, N. B., ed.), pp. 295–362. Amsterdam: North Holland Publ. Co (1973 b).

Finter, N. B., Christofinis, G., Whitaker, A., Johnston, M. D.: Comparisons between interferons induced with Sendai virus in primary leucocytes and lymphoblastoid cells. Personal communication (1976).

Fischbach, J., Glasgow, L. A.: Effect of *Corynebacterium acnes* on interferon production in mouse peritoneal exudate cells. Infect. Immun. **11**, 80–84 (1975).

Fisher, J. C., Cooperband, S. R., Mannick, J. A.: The effect of polyinosinic-polycytidylic acid on the immune response of mice to antigenically distinct tumors. Cancer Res. **32**, 889–894 (1972).

Fitzgerald, G. R.: The effect of interferon on focus formation and yield of murine sarcoma virus *in vitro*. Proc. Soc. Exp. Biol. Med. **130**, 960–964 (1969).

Fleischmann, W. R., Simon, E. H.: Mechanism of interferon induction by NDV: A monolayer and single cell study. J. Gen. Virol. **25**, 337–341 (1974).

Fleming, W. A., McNeill, T. A., Killen, M.: The effects of an inhibiting factor (interferon) on the *in vitro* growth of granulocyte-macrophage colonies. Immunology **23**, 429–437 (1972).

Flick, J. A., Pincus, W. B.: Inhibition of the lesions of primary vaccinia and of delayed hypersensitivity through immunological tolerance in rabbits. J. Exp. Med. **117**, 633–640 (1963).

Fontaine–Brouty–Boyé, D., Gresser, I., Maciera–Coelho, A., Rosenfeld, C., Thomas, M. T.: Inhibition *in vitro* de la multiplication des cellules leucémiques murines L1210 par des préparations d'interféron. C. R. Acad. Sci. D **269**, 406–410 (1969).

Force, E. E., Stewart, R. C.: Relationship of interferon-like inhibitor production to Rous sarcoma virus growth and tumor formation in chicks. J. Immunol. **97**, 126–130 (1966).

Force, E. E., Stewart, R. C., Haff, R. F.: Development of interferon in rabbit dermis after infection with Herpes Simplex virus. Virology **25**, 322–325 (1965).

Fornosi, F., Talas, M., Weiszfeller, G.: Effect of tilorone hydrochloride on the experimental rabies of mice. Acta Microbiol. Acad. Sci. Hung. **18**, 327–931 (1971).

Fournier, F., Chany, C., Sarragne, M.: Origin and possible mode of action of a tissue antagonist of interferon. Nature New Biol. **235**, 47–48 (1972).

Fournier, F., Falcoff, E., Chany, C.: Demonstration, mass production and characterization of a heavy molecular weight human interferon. J. Immunol. **99**, 1036–1041 (1967).

Fournier, F., Rousset, S., Chany, C.: Un facteur tissulaire antagoniste de l'action de l'interféron. C. R. Acad. Sc. (Paris) **D 266**, 2306–2308 (1968).

Fournier, F., Rousset, S., Chany, C.: Investigations on a tissue antagonist of interferon. Proc. Soc. Exp. Biol. Med. **132**, 943–950 (1969).

Fournier, F., Sarragne, M., Rouffet, A., Leaute, J. B., Chany, C.: Mechanism of action of tissue factors inhibiting the antiviral state established by interferon. C. R. Acad. Sci. **D 278**, 1915–1918 (1974).

Frankfort, H. M., Havell, E. A., Croce, C. M. and Vilcek, J.: The synthesis and action of mouse and human interferons in mouse-human hybrid cells. Virology **89**, 45–50 (1978).

Frayssinet, C., Gresser, I., Tovey, M., Lindahl, P.: Inhibitory effect of potent interferon preparations on the regeneration of mouse liver after partial hepatectomy Nature **245**, 146–147 (1973).

Freed, E. R., Duma, R. J., Escobar, M. R.: Vaccinia necrosm and its relationship to impaired immunologic responsiveness. Am. J. Med. **52**, 411–414 (1972).

Freeman, A. L., Al–Bussam, N., O'Malley, J. A., Stutzman, L., Bjornsson, S., Carter, W. A.: Pharmacologic effects of poly I·C in man. J. Med. Virol. **1**, 79–94 (1977).

Freshman, M. M., Merigan, T. C., Remington, J. S., Brownlee, I. E.: *In vitro* and *in vivo* antiviral action of an interferon-like substance induced by *Toxoplasma gondii*. Proc. Soc. Exp. Biol. Med. **123**, 862–866 (1966).

Friedman, R. M.: Role of interferon in viral interference. Nature **201**, 848–849 (1964).

Friedman, R. M.: Effect of interferon treatment on interferon production. J. Immunol. **96**, 872–877 (1966 a).

Friedman, R. M.: Interferon production and protein synthesis in chick cells. J. Bacteriol. **91**, 1224–1229 (1966 b).

Friedman, R. M.: Interferon binding: the first step in establishment of antiviral activity. Science **156**, 1760–1761 (1967).

Friedman, R. M.: Inhibition of arbovirus protein synthesis by interferon. J. Virol. **2**, 1081–1088 (1968).

Friedman, R. M.: Antiviral activity of interferon. Bact. Rev. **41**, 543–567 (1977).

Friedman, R. M., Baron, S.: The role of antibody in recovery from infection with vaccinia virus. J. Immunol. **87**, 379–382 (1961).

Friedman, R. M., Baron, S., Buckler, C. E., Steinmuller, R. I.: The role of antibody, delayed hypersensitivity and interferon production in recovery of guinea pigs from primary infection with vaccinia virus. J. Ex. Med. **116**, 347–355 (1962).

Friedman, R. M., Chang, E. H.: Interferon action: possible mechanisms of antiviral activity, in: Interferons and their Actions (Stewart II, W. E., ed.), pp. 145–152. Cleveland, Ohio: CRC Press, Inc. (1977).

Friedman, R. M., Chang, E. H., Ramseur, J. M., Myers, M. W.: Interferon-directed inhibition of chronic murine leukemia virus production in cell cultures: lack of effecton intracellular viral markers. J. Virol. **16**, 569–574 (1975).

Friedman, R. M., Cooper, H. L.: Stimulation of interferon production in human lymphocytes by mitogens. Proc. Soc. Exp. Biol. Med. **125**, 901–905 (1967).

Friedman, R. M., Costa, J. R.: Fate of interferon-treated cells. Infect. Immun. **13**, 487–497 (1976).

Friedman, R. M., Costa, J. C., Ramseur, J. M., Meyers, M. W., Jay, F. T., Chang, E. M.: Persistence of the viral genome in interferon-treated cells infected with oncogenic or nononcogenic viruses. J. Infect. Dis. **133** suppl., A 43–A 47 (1976).

Friedman, R. M., Fantes, K. H., Levy, H. B., Carter, W. B.: Interferon action on parental Semliki Forest virus ribonucleic acid. J. Virol. 1, 1168–1173 (1967).

Friedman, R. M., Jay, F. T., Chang, E. H., Myers, M. W., Ramseur, J. M., Mims, S. J., Triche, T. J., Wong, P. K. Y.: Interferon-directed inhibition of chronic murine leukemia virus production in cell cultures, in: Prog. Cancer Res. Ther. 2 (Chirigos, M. A., ed.), p. 347. New York: Raven Press (1977).

Friedman, R. M., Kohn, L. D.: Cholera toxin inhibits interferon action. Biochem. Biophys. Res. Commun. 70, 1078–1081 (1976).

Friedman, R. M., Metz, D. H., Esteban, R. M., Tovell, D. R., Ball, L. A., Kerr, I. M.: Mechanism of interferon action: inhibition of viral messenger RNA translation in L-cell extracts. J. Virol. 10, 1184–1198 (1972).

Friedman, R. M., Pastan, T.: Interferon and cyclic-3'5'-adenosine monophosphate: Potentiation of antiviral activity. Biochem. Biophys. Res. Comm. 36, 735–739 (1969).

Friedman, R. M., Rabson, A. S.: Possible role of interferon in determining the oncogenic effect of polyoma virus variants. J. Exp. Med. 119, 71–81 (1964).

Friedman, R. M., Ramseur, J. M.: Inhibition of murine leukemia virus production in chronically infected AKR cells: a novel effect of interferon. Proc. Natl. Acad. Sci. U.S.A. 71, 3542–3544 (1974).

Friedman, R. M., Sonnabend, J. A.: Inhibition of interferon action by p-fluorophenylalanine. Nature, 203, 366–367 (1964).

Friedman, R. M., Sonnabend, J. A.: Inhibition of interferon action by puromycin. J. Immunol. 95, 696–703 (1965 a).

Friedman, R. M., Sonnabend, J. A.: Inhibition by interferon of production of double-stranded Semliki Forest virus ribonucleic acid. Nature 206, 532–535 (1965 b).

Friedman, R. M., Sonnabend, J. A.: Mechanism of interferon action. Arch. Intern. Med. 126, 51–63 (1970).

Friedman, R. M., Sreevalsan, T.: Membrane binding of input arbovirus ribonucleic acid: effect of interferon or cycloheximide. J. Virology 6, 169–175 (1970).

Friedman–Kien, A. E., Vilček, J.: Induction of interference and interferon synthesis by non-replicating molluscum contagiosum virus. J. Immunol. 99, 1092–1098 (1967).

Frothingham, T. E.: Further observations on cell cultures infected concurrently with mumps and Sindbis viruses. J. Immunol. 94, 521–524 (1965).

Fruitstone, M. J., Michaels, B. S., Rudolf, D. A. C., Siegel, M. M.: Role of the spleen in interferon production in mice. Proc. Soc. Exp. Biol. Med. 122, 1008–1011 (1966).

Fruitstone, M. J., Waddell, G. H., Siegel, M. M.: An interferon produced in response to infection by Herpes simplex virus. Proc. Soc. Exp. Biol. Med. 117, 804–807 (1964).

Fuchsberger, N., Hajnicka, V., Borecky, L.: Antiviral and cell-growth inhibitory activities of highly-purified L cell interferon. An analysis of quantitative disproportions. Acta Virol. 19, 59–61 (1975).

Fuchsberger, N., Styk, B., Borecky, L., Hajnicka, V.: Some biological activities of rabbit anti-interferon serum. Acta Virol. 20, 107–108 (1976).

Fuchsberger, N., Vetrak, J., Lackovic, V., Borecky, L., Doskocil, j.: Evaluation of the Czechoslovak dsRNA preparation as inducer of interferon in model experiments. Acta Virol. 16, 466–476 (1972).

Fujibayashi, T., Hooks, J. J., Notkins, A. L.: Production of interferon by immune lymphocytes exposed to Herpes simplex virus-antibody complexes. J. Immunol. 115, 1191–1193 (1975).

Fulton, R. W., Rosenquist, B. D.: In vitro interferon production by bovine tissues: effects of hydrocortisone. Amer. J. Vet. Res. 37, 1493–1496 (1976 a).

Fulton, R. W., Rosenquist, B. D.: In vitro interferon production by bovine tissues: induction by infectious bovine rhinotracheitis virus. Amer. J. Vet. Res. 37, 1497–1502 (1976 b).

Furer, N. M., Pokidova, N. V., Weissberg, G. E., Nemirovskaya, B. M., Kuznetsov, V. P., Zhukovskaya, N. A., Ermolieva, Z. V.: Experimental studies of polysaccharide interferon inducers. Proc. Microbiol. Res. Group Hung. Acad. Sci. 2, 55 (1968).

Furmanski, P., Juno, S., Hall, L., Rich, M. A.: The role of interferon in the spontaneous regression of Friend virus induced leukemia. Proc. Soc. Exp. Biol. Med. 150, 11–13 (1975).

Fuse, A., Kuwata, I.: Effects of interferon on the human clonal cell line, RSa. J. Gen. Virol. 33, 17–22 (1976).

Fuse, A., Kuwata, T.: Inhibition of DNA synthesis of synchronized RSa cells by human leukocyte interferon. J. Natl. Cancer Inst. 58, 891–896 (1977).

Gaffney, E. V., Picciano, P. T., Grant, C. A.: Inhibition of growth and transformation of human cells by interferon. J. Natl. Cancer. Inst. 50 (4), 871–878 (1973).

Gainer, J. H.: Effects of arsenicals on interferon formation and action. Am. J. Vet. Res. 33, 2579–2586 (1972).

Gainer, J. H.: Effects on interferon of heavy metal excess and zinc deficiency. Amer. J. Vet. Res. 38, 863–867 (1977).

Galabov, A. S.: Interferonogenesis and phylogenesis. Bull. Inst. Pasteur 71, 233–247 (1973).

Galabov, A. S., Galabov, S. M.: Induction of interferon in mice by detoxicated-O-antigens of *Salmonella typhi* and *Serratia marcescens*. Zentralbl. Bakteriol. Orig. A. 219, 500–505 (1972).

Galabov, A. S., Galabov, S. M.: Interferon induction by detoxicated bacterial endotoxins. Acta Virol. 17, 493–500 (1973).

Galabov, A., Petrunova, S., Savov, Z.: Molecular weight of virus-induced tortoise interferon in cell cultures. Experientia 29, 900–901 (1973).

Galabov, A., Savov, Z., Vassileva, V.: Interferon production in arbovirus-infected cell cultures of tortoise *(Testudo grasca)* kidney. Acta Virol. 17, 1–10 (1973).

Galabov, A. S., Velichkova, E. H.: Interferon production in tortoise peritoneal cells. J. Gen. Virol. 28, 259–264 (1975).

Galasso, G. J.: Interferon: Its expectation for the future. *In Vitro* Monograph 3, Production and use of interferon for the treatment and prevention of human virus infection, p. 66 (1974).

Galasso, G. J., Dunnick, J. K.: Interferon, an antiviral drug for use in man. Tex. Rep. Biol. Med. 35, 178–485 (1977).

Galin, M. A., Chowchuveck, E., Kronenberg, B.: Therapeutic use of inducers of interferon on herpes simplex keratitis in humans. Ann. Ophthalmol. 8, 72–76 (1976).

Gallagher, J. G., Khoobyarian, N.: Adenovirus susceptibility to interferon: sensitivity of types 2, 7 and 12 to human interferon. Proc. Soc. Exp. Biol. Med. 130, 137–142 (1969).

Gallagher, J. G., Khoobyarian, N.: Sensitivity of adenovirus types 1, 3, 4, 5, 8, 11 and 18 to human interferon. Proc. Soc. Exp. Biol. Med. 136, 920–924 (1971).

Gallagher, J. G., Khoobyarian, N.: Adenovirus susceptibility to human interferon during one-step replication. Infect. Immun. 5, 905–908 (1972).

Galliot, B., Moreau, M. C., Renard, N., Chany, C.: Interferon antagonists induced by Newcastle disease virus (NDV). Proc. Soc. Exp. Biol. Med. 142 (1), 266–270 (1973).

Galster, R. L., Lengyel, P.: Formation and characteristics of reovirus subviral particles in interferon-treated mouse L-cells. Nucl. Acid. 3, 581–583 (1976).

Gandhi, S. S., Burke, D. C.: Interferon production by myxoviruses in chick embryo cells. J. Gen. Virol. 6, 95–104 (1970).

Gandhi, S. S., Burke, D. C., Scholtissek, C.: Virus RNA synthesis by ultraviolet-irradiated Newcastle disease virus and interferon production. J. Gen. Virol. 9, 97–99 (1970).

Gandhi, S. S., Stewart, R. B.: Interferon production in cell cultures derived from various chick embryo tissues. Can. J. Microbiol. 14, 1305–1308 (1968).

Ganti, T., Mecs, I., Kotai, A.: Potentiation of poly IC-induced viral resistance by polycation modified polypeptides. Arch. Virol. 51, 227–234 (1976).

Gatmaitan, B. C., Stanley, E. D., Jackson, G. G.: The limited effect of nasal interferon induced by rhinovirus and a topical chemical inducer on the course of infection. J. Infect. Dis. 127 (4), 401–407 (1973).

Gauntt, C. J.: Effect of interferon on synthesis of ssRNA in reovirus type-3-infected L cell cultures. Biochem. Biophys. Res. Commun. 47, 1228–1236 (1972).

Gauntt, C. J.: Induction of interferon in L cells by reoviruses. Infect. Immun. 7, 711–717 (1973).

Gazdar, A. F.: Enhancement of tumor growth rate by interferon inducers. J. Nat. Cancer Institut. 49, 1435–1440 (1972).

Gazdar, A. F., Ikawa, Y.: Synthetic RNA and DNA polynucleotides: *in vivo* and *in vitro* enhancement of oncogenesis by a murine sarcoma virus. Proc. Soc. Exp. Biol. Med. 140, 1166–1169 (1972).

Gazdar, A. F., Sims, M., Spahn, G. J., Baron, S.: Interferon mediates enhancement of tumor growth and virus-induced sarcomas in mice. Nature New Biol. 245 (142), 77–78 (1973).

Gazdar, A. F., Steinberg, A. D., Spahn, G. F., Baron, S.: Interferon inducers: enhancement of viral oncogenesis in mice and rats. Proc. Soc. Exp. Biol. Med. 139 (4), 1132–1137 (1972a).

Gazdar, A. F., Weinstein, A. Y., Sims, M. L., Steinberg, A. D.: Enhancement and suppression of murine sarcoma virus induced tumors by polyriboinosinic-polyribocytidylic acid. Proc. Soc. Exp. Biol. Med. **139**, 279–282 (1972b).

Geber, W. F., Lefkowitz, S. S., Hung, C. Y.: Effect of morphine, hydromorphone, methadone, mescaline, trypan blue, vitamin A, sodium salicylate, and caffeine on the serum interferon level in response to viral infection. Arch. Internat. Pharmaco. Ther. **214**, 322–323 (1975).

Geber, W. F., Lefkowitz, S. S., Hung, C. Y.: Role of spleen in the interferon-lowering action of morphine. General Pharmacology **7**, 255–258 (1976a).

Geber, W. F., Lefkowitz, S. S., Hung, C. Y.: Action of naloxone on the interferon-lowering activity of morphine in the mouse. Pharmacology **14**, 322–325 (1976b).

Geber, W. F., Lefkowitz, S. S., Hung, C. Y.: Duration of interferon inhibition following single and multiple injections of morphine. J. Toxicol. Environ. Hlth. **2**, 577–579 (1977).

Gelboin, H. V., Levy, H. B.: Polyinosinic-polycytidylic acid inhibits chemically induced tumorigenesis in mouse skin. Science **167**, 205–207 (1970).

Georgadze, I. I., Mentkevich, L. M., Orlova, T. G., Kognovitskaya, A. I., Solovyvov, V. D.: Hyporeactivity to interferon induction: specificity of the phenomenon and production of mRNA for interferon. Acta. Virol. **18**, 376–382 (1974).

German, A., Quero, A. M., Poindron, P.: Production d'anticorps neutralisant l'activité de interféron de poulet. Relation antigénique entre une substance extraite de liquide allantoique d'oeuf embryonne sain et l'interféron de poulet semi-purifié. C. R. Acad. Sc. (Paris) **D 271**, 1224–1226 (1970).

German, A., Quero, A. M., Poindron, P.: Immunogenic properties of chick interferon; its antigenic relations with a substance extracted from uninfected egg allantoic fluid. Ann. Inst. Pasteur (Paris) **121**, 207–221 (1971).

Ghendon, Yu. Z.: On the ability of certain viruses to block the effect of interferon. Acta. Virol. **9**, 186–187 (1965).

Ghendon, Yu., Z., Balandin, I. G., Babushkina: On the mechanism of the ability of certain viruses to block the action of interferon. Acta Virol. **10**, 268–270 (1966).

Ghosh, S. N., Gifford, G. E.: Effect of interferon on the dynamics of H^3-thymidine incorporation and thymidine kinase induction in chick fibroblast cultures infected with vaccinia virus. Virology **27**, 186–192 (1965).

Gibson, J. P., Megel, H., Camyre, K. P., Michael, J. G.: Effect of tilorone hydrochloride on the lymphoid and interferon response of athymic mice. Proc. Soc. Exp. Biol. Med. **151**, 264–268 (1976).

Gifford, G. E.: Effect of environmental changes upon antiviral action of interferon. Proc. Soc. Exp. Biol. Med. **114**, 644–649 (1963a).

Gifford, G. E.: Variation of interferon yield with multiplicity of infection. Nature **200**, 91–92 (1963b).

Gifford, G. E.: Studies on the specificity of interferon. J. Gen. Microbiol. **33**, 437–443 (1963c).

Gifford, G. E.: Relative insensitivity of spleen cells to interferon. J. Immunol. **113**, 1947–1953 (1974).

Gifford, G. E., Heller, E.: Effect of actinomycin D on interferon production by "active" and "inactive" Chikungunya virus in chick cells. Nature **200**, 50–51 (1963).

Gifford, G. E., Mussett, M. Y., Heller, E.: Comparative studies on the production and assay of interferon. J. Gen. Microbiol. **34**, 475–481 (1964).

Gifford, G. E., Toy, S. T.: Assay of interferon: general comments. Symp. Ser. Immunobiol. Stand. (Karger, Basel) **14**, 80–88 (1970).

Gifford, G. E., Toy, S. T., Lindenmann, J.: Studies on vaccinia virus plaque formation and its inhibition by interferon. II. Dynamics of plaque formation by vaccinia virus in the presence of interferon. Virology **19**, 294–301 (1963).

Gilden, D. H., Cole, G. A., Monjan, A. A., Nathanson, N.: Immunopathogenesis of acute general nervous system disease produced by lymphocytic choriomeningitis virus. I. cyclophosphamide-mediated induction of the virus-carrier state in adult mice. J. Exp. Med. **135**, 860–871 (1972).

Giron, D. J.: Role of interferon in the propagation of MM virus in L cells. Appl. Microbiol. **18**, 584–588 (1969).

Giron, D. J., Allen, P. T., Pindak, F. F., Schmidt, J. P.: Interferon-inducing characteristics of MM virus. Applied Microbiol. **21**, 387–393 (1971).

Giron, D. J., Allen, P. T., Pindak, F. F., Schmidt, J. P.: Further studies on the influence of steroids on viral infection in mice. Infect. Immun. **8**, 151–155 (1973 a).

Giron, D. J., Schmidt, J. P., Ball, R. Y., Pindak, F. F.: Effect of interferon inducers and interferon on bacterial infections. Antimicrob. Agents. Chemother. **1** (1), 80–81 (1972).

Giron, D. J., Schmidt, J. P., Pindak, F. F.: Effect of progesterone and testosterone on interferon production and on the viral infection-enhancing activity of estrone and hydrocortisone. Infect. Immun. **4** (5), 537–540 (1971).

Giron, D. J., Schmidt, J. P., Pindak, F. F.: Tilorone hydrochloride: lack of correlation between interferon induction and viral protection. Antimicrob. Agents. Chemother. **1**, 78–79 (1972).

Giron, D. J., Schmidt, J. P., Pindak, F. F., Connell, J. E.: Interferon tolerance and antiviral protection in mice given single or multiple injections of endotoxin or poly I·C. Acta Virol. **17**, 209–214 (1973 b).

Gisler, R. M., Lindahl, P., Gresser, I.: Effects of interferon on antibody synthesis *in vitro*. J. Immunol. **113** (2), 438–444 (1974).

Glasgow, L. A.: Leukocytes and interferon in the host response to viral infections. J. Exp. Med. **121**, 1001–1018 (1965).

Glasgow, L. A.: Leukocytes and interferon in the host response to viral infections. II. Enhanced interferon response of leukocytes from immune animals. J. Bacteriol. **91**, 2185–2191 (1966).

Glasgow, L. A.: Transfer of interferon-producing macrophages: new approach to viral chemotherapy. Science **170**, 854–856 (1970).

Glasgow, L. A.: Immunosuppression, interferon, and viral infections. Fed. Proc. **30**, 1846–1851 (1971).

Glasgow, L. A.: Cytomegalovirus interference *in vitro*. Infect. Immun. **9**, 702–707 (1974).

Glasgow, L. A., Bullock, W. E.: Impairment of interferon production in mice infected with *Mycobacterium lepraemurim*. Proc. Soc. Exp. Biol. Med. **139** (2), 492–496 (1972).

Glasgow, L. A., Friedman, S. B.: Interferon and host resistance to Rauscher virus-induced leukemia. J. Virol. **3**, 99–107 (1969).

Glasgow, L. A., Habel, K.: Interferon production by mouse leukocytes *in vitro* and *in vivo*. J. Exp. Med. **117**, 149–160 (1962 a).

Glasgow, L. A., Habel, K.: The role of interferon in vaccinia virus infection of mouse embryo tissue culture. J. Exp. Med. **115**, 503–511 (1962 b).

Glasgow, L. A., Habel, K.: Role of polyoma virus and interferon in a Herpes simplex virus infection *in vitro*. Virology **19**, 328–339 (1963).

Glasgow, L. A., Hanshaw, J. B., Merigan, T. C., Petralli, J. K.: Interferon and cytomegalovirus *in vivo* and *in vitro*. Proc. Soc. Exp. Biol. Med. **125**, 843–849 (1967).

Glasgow, L. A., Murrer, A. T., Lombardi, P. S.: Eperythrozoon coccoides. II. Effect on interferon production and role of humoral antibody in host resistance. Infect. Immun. **9**, 266–272 (1974).

Glasgow, L. A., Odugbemi, T., Dwyer, P., Ritterson, A. L.: Eperythrozoon coccoides. I. Effect on the interferon response in mice. Infect. Immun. **4**, 425–430 (1971).

Glaz, E. T.: Study on the effect of statolon on methylcholanthrene oncogenesis in mice. Tumori **58**, 185–186 (1972).

Glaz, E. T., Szolgay, E., Stöger, I., Talas, M.: Antiviral activity and induction of interferon-like substance by quinacrine and acranil. Antimicrob. Agents. Chemoth. **3**, 537–539 (1973).

Glaz, E. T., Talas, M.: Continual serum interferon induced by prolonged drinking of tilorone solution. Acta Virol. **17**, 168–169 (1973).

Glaz, E. T., Talas, M.: Comparison of the activity of small molecular interferon inducers: tilorone and acridine drugs. Arch. Virol. **48**, 375–377 (1975).

Gledhill, A. W.: Influence of endotoxin upon the pathogenesis of viral infections, in: Bacterial Endotoxins (Landy, M., Braun, W., eds.), p. 410. New Jersey: Rutgers (1964).

Gledhill, A. W.: The effect of bacterial endotoxin on resistance of mice to ectromelia. Brit. J. Exp. Pathol. **40**, 195–205 (1959).

Gober, L. L., Friedman–Kien, A. E., Havell, E. A., Vilček, J.: Suppression of the intracellular growth of *Shigella flexneri* in cell cultures by interferon preparations and polyinosinic-polycytidylic acid. Infect. Immun. **5** (3), 370–376 (1972).

Goguel, A. F., Nuvciel, C.: Guinea pig lymphotoxin. II. Study of its mechanism of action. Its differentiation from migration inhibitory factor and interferon. Ann. Immunol. **125 C**, 789–793 (1974).

Goldsby, R. A.: The implications of the temperature-independent binding and the temperature-dependent action of interferon. Experientia **23**, 1073–1074 (1967).

Golgher, R. R., Paucker, K.: Blocking of interferon production by chromatographically purified L-cell interferon. Proc. Soc. Exp. Biol. Med. **142** (1), 167–174 (1973).

Goore, M. Y., Dickson, J. H., Lipkin, S., Dicuollo, C. J.: The production of human leukocyte interferon in a serum-free medium. Proc. Soc. Exp. Biol. Med. **142**, 46–49 (1973).

Goorha, R. M., Gifford, G. E.: Interferon induction by heat-inactivated Semliki Forest virus. Proc. Soc. Exp. Biol. Med. **134**, 1142–1147 (1970a).

Goorha, R. M., Gifford, G. E.: An explanation for increased interferon production at low multiplicities of infection. Proc. Soc. Exp. Biol. Med. **135**, 91–93 (1970b).

Gordon, I., Chenault, S. S., Stevenson, D., Acton, J. D.: Effect of interferon on polymerization of single-stranded and double-stranded mengovirus ribonucleic acid. J. Bacteriol. **91**, 1230–1238 (1966).

Gottlieb–Stematsky, T., Rotem, Z., Karby, S.: Production and susceptibility to interferon of polyoma virus variants of high and low oncogenic properties. J. Nat. Cancer Instit. **41**, 99–103 (1966).

Gould, E. A., Ratcliff, N. A., Basarab, O., Smith, H.: Studies of the basis of localization of influenza virus in ferret organ cultures. Br. J. Exp. Pathol. **53**, 31–44 (1972).

Graessmann, A., Graessmann, M., Hoffmann, H., Niebel, J., Brandiver, G., Mueuer, N.: Inhibition by interferon of SV40 tumor antigen formation in cells injected with SV40 cRNA transcribed *in vitro*. FEBS Letters **39**, 249–251 (1974).

Graff, S., Kassel, R., Kastner, D.: Interferon. Trans. N. Y. Acad. Sci. **32**, 545–556 (1971).

Gravell, M., Cromeans, T. L.: Inhibition of early viral RNA synthesis in interferon-treated cells infected with frog polyhedral cytoplasmic deoxyribovirus. Virology **50**, 916–919 (1972).

Gravell, M., Malsberger, R. G.: A permanent cell line from the fathead minnow (*Pimephalis promelas*). Ann. N. Y. Acad. Sci. **126**, 555–565 (1965).

Graziadei, W. D. III, Weideli, M., Lengyel, P,: Endonuclease of high specific activity in a purified mouse interferon preparation. Biochem. Biophys. Res. Commun. **54**, 40–46 (1973).

Green, J. A.: Inhibition of *Shigella flexneri* by lysates of cells treated with interferon-containing preparations. Infect. Immun. **7**, 1006–1008 (1973).

Green, J. A., Cooperband, S. R., Kibrick, S.: Immune-specific induction of interferon production in cultures of human blood lymphocytes. Science **164**, 1415–1417 (1969).

Green, J. A., Cooperband, S. R., Kleinman, L. F., Kobrick, S.: Immune stimulation of interferon in human leukocyte cultures by non-viral antigens. Ann. N. Y. Acad. Sci. **173**, 736–740 (1970).

Green, M. D., Mowshowitz, S. L.: Enhanced cytopathic effect of influenza virus in interferon-treated cells. Personal communication (1978).

Greenberg, H. B., Pollard, R. B., Lutwick, L. I., Gregory, P. B., Robinson, W. S., Merigan, T. C.: Human leukocyte interferon and hepatitis B virus infection. The New. Engl. J. Med. **295**, 517–520 (1976).

Greenberg, P. L., Mosny, S. A.: Cytotoxic effects of interferon *in vitro* on granulocytic progenitor cells. Cancer Res. **37**, 1794–1799 (1977).

Greene, J. J., Dieffenbach, C. W., Tso, P. O. P.: Inactivation of interferon mRNA in the shutoff of human interferon synthesis. Nature **271**, 81–83 (1978).

Gresser, I.: Induction by Sendai virus of non-transmissible cytopathic changes associated with rapid and marked production of interferon. Proc. Soc. Exp. Biol. Med. **108**, 303–307 (1961a).

Gresser, I.: Production of interferon by suspensions of human leukocytes. Proc. Soc. Exp. Biol. Med. **108**, 799–803 (1961b).

Gresser, I.: Metamorphosis of human amnion cells induced by preparations of interferon. Proc. Natl. Acad. Sci. **47**, 1817–1822 (1961c).

Gresser, I.: Antitumor effects of interferon. Adv. Cancer. Res. **16**, 97–140 (1972).

Gresser, I.: Interferon therapy: obvious and not so obvious applications. Acta Med. Scand. **576**, 49–54 (1975).

Gresser, I.: On the varied biologic effect of interferon. Cellular Immunol. **34**, 406–415 (1977a).

Gresser, I.: Antitumor effects of interferon, in: Cancer – A Comprehensive Treatise (Chemotherapy, Vol. 5), pp. 525–571. New York: Plenum Publ. Corp. (1977b).

Gresser, I., Bandu, M. T., Brouty–Boye, D.: Interferon and cell division. IX. Interferon-resistant L1210 cells: characteristics and origin. J. Natl. Cancer. Inst. **52**, 553–559 (1974).

Gresser, I., Bandu, M. T., Brouty–Boye, D., Tovey, M.: Pronounced antiviral activity of human interferon on bovine and porcine cells. Nature **251**, 543–545 (1974).

Gresser, I., Bandu, M. T., Tovey, M., Bodo, G., Paucker, K., Stewart II, W. E.: Interferon and cell division VII. Inhibitory effect of highly purified interferon preparations on the multiplication of Leukemia L1210 cells. Proc. Soc. Exp. Biol. Med. **142**, 7–10 (1973).

Gresser, I., Berman, L., DeThe, G., Brouty–Boye, D., Coppey, Y., Falcoff, E.: Interferon and murine leukemia. V. Effect of interferon preparations on the evolution of Rauscher disease in mice. J. Nat. Cancer. Inst. **41**, 505–509 (1968a).

Gresser, I., Bourali, C.: Exogenous interferon and inducers of interferon in the treatment of Balb/c mice inoculated with RC 19 tumor cells. Nature **223**, 844–846 (1969).

Gresser, I., Bourali, C.: Antitumor effects of interferon preparations in mice. J. Nat. Cancer Instit. **45**, 365–375 (1970a).

Gresser, I., Bourali, C.: Development of newborn mice during prolonged treatment with interferon. Europ. J. Cancer **6**, 553–556 (1970b).

Gresser, I., Bourali–Maury, C.: Inhibition by interferon preparations of a solid malignant tumor and pulmonary metastasis in mice. Nature New Biol. **236**, 78–79 (1972).

Gresser, I., Bourali, C., Chouroulinkov, I., Fontaine–Brouty–Boye, D., Thomas, M. T.: Treatment of neoplasia in mice with interferon preparations. Ann. N. Y. Acad. Sci. **173**, 694–699 (1970a).

Gresser, I., Bourali, C., Levy, J. P.: Increased survival in mice inoculated with tumor cells and treated with interferon preparations. Proc. Natl. Acad. Sci. **63**, 51–56 (1969a).

Gresser, I., Bourali, C., Thomas, M. T., Falcoff, E.: Effect of repeated inoculation of interferon preparations on infection of mice with encephalomyocarditis virus. Proc. Soc. Exp. Biol. Med. **127**, 491–496 (1968b).

Gresser, I., Brouty–Boye, D., Thomas, M. T., Macieira–Coelho, A.: Interferon and cell division. I. Inhibition of the multiplication of mouse leukemia L1210 cells *in vitro* by interferon preparations. Proc. Natl. Acad. Sci. **66**, 1052–1058 (1970b).

Gresser, I., Brouty–Boye, D., Thomas, M. T., Macieira–Coelho, A.: Interferon and cell division. II. Influence of various experimental conditions on the inhibition of L1210 cell multiplication *in vitro* by interferon preparations. J. Nat. Cancer Instit. **45**, 1145–1153 (1970c).

Gresser, I., Chany, C., Enders, J. F.: Persistent polioviral infection of intact human amniotic membrane without apparent cytopathic effect. J. Bacteriol. **89**, 470–475 (1965).

Gresser, I., Coppey, J., Bourali, C.: Action inhibitrice de l'interferon brut sur la leucemie lymphoide des souris AKR. C. R. Acad. Sc. (Paris) **267**, 1900–1902 (1968).

Gresser, I., Coppey, J., Bourali, C.: Interferon and murine leukemia. VI. Effect of interferon preparations on the lymphoid leukemia of AKR mice. J. Natl. Cancer Institut. **43**, 1083–1089 (1969b).

Gresser, I., Coppey, J., Brouty–Boye, D., F., Falcoff, R.: Interferon and murine leukemia. III. Efficacy of interferon preparations administered after inoculation of Friend virus. Nature **215**, 174–175 (1967a).

Gresser, I., Coppey, J., Falcoff, E., Fontaine, D.: Action inhibitrice de l'interféron brut sur le dévelopement de la leucémie de Friend chez le souris. C. R. Acad. Sci. (Paris) D **263**, 586–589 (1966).

Gresser, I., Coppey, Y., Falcoff, E., Fontaine, D.: Interferon and murine leukemia. I. Inhibitory effect of interferon preparations on development of Friend leukemia in mice. Proc. Soc. Exp. Biol. Med. **124**, 84–91 (1967b).

Gresser, I., Dull, H. B.: A virus inhibitor in pharyngeal washings from patients with influenza. Proc. Soc. Exp. Biol. Med. **115**, 192–196 (1964).

Gresser, I., Enders, J. F.: Alteration of cellular resistance to Sindbis virus in mixed cultures of human cells attributable to interferon. Virology **16**, 428–435 (1962).

Gresser, I., Falcoff, R., Brouty–Boye, D. F., Zaydela, F., Coppey, Y., Falcoff, E.: Interferon and murine leukemia. IV. Further studies on the efficacy of interferon preparations administered after inoculation of Friend virus. Proc. Soc. Exp. Biol. Med. **126**, 791–797 (1967c).

Gresser, I., Fontaine, D., Coppey, Y., Falcoff, R., Falcoff, E.: Interferon and murine leukemia. II. Factors related to the inhibitory effect of interferon preparations on development of Friend leukemia in mice. Proc. Soc. Exp. Biol. Med. **124**, 91–94 (1967d).

23*

Gresser, I., Fontaine–Brouty–Boye, D., Bourali, C., Thomas, M. T.: A comparison of the efficacy of endogenous, exogenous and combined endogenous-exogenous interferon in the treatment of mice infected with encephalomyocarditis virus. Proc. Soc. Exp. Biol. Med. 130, 236–241 (1969c).

Gresser, I., Lang, D. J.: Relationship between viruses and leukocytes. Prog. Med. Virol. 8, 62–130 (1966).

Gresser, I., Maury, C., Bandu, M. T., Tovey, M., and Maunoury, M. T.: Role of endogenous interferon in the antitumor effect of poly I·C and statolon as demonstrated by the use of anti-mouse interferon serum. J. Natl. Cancer Inst. 21, 72–77 (1978).

Gresser, I., Maury, C., Brouty–Boye, D.: On the mechanism of the antitumor effect of interferon in mice. Nature 239, 167–168 (1972).

Gresser, I., Maury, C., Tovey, M.: Interferon and murine leukemia. VII. Therapeutic effect of interferon preparations after diagnosis of lymphoma in AKR mice. Int. J. Cancer 17, 647–653 (1976).

Gresser, I., Maury, Tovey, M. G.: Efficacy of combined interferon cyclophosphamide therapy after diagnosis of lymphoma in AKR mice. Europ. J. Cancer 14, 97–102 (1978).

Gresser, I., Maury, C., Tovey, M., Morel-Maroger, L., Pontillon, F.: Progressive glomerulonephritis in mice treated with interferon preparations at birth. Nature 263, 420–422 (1976a).

Gresser, I., Naficy, K.: Recovery of an interferon-like substance from cerebrospinal fluid. Proc. Soc. Exp. Biol. Med. 117, 285–289 (1964).

Gresser, I., Thomas, M. T., Brouty–Boye, D.: Effect of interferon treatment of L1210 cells in vitro on tumour and colony formation. Nature 231, 20–21 (1971).

Gresser, I., Thomas, M. T., Brouty–Boye, E. D., Macieira–Coelmo, A.: Interferon and cell division. V. Titration of the anticellular action of interferon preparations. Proc. Soc. Exp. Biol. Med. 137, 1258–1261 (1971).

Gresser, I., Tovey, M. G., Bandu, M. T., Maury, C., Brouty–Boye, D.: Role of interferon in the pathogenesis of virus disease in mice as demonstrated by the use of anti-interferon serum. I. Rapid evolution of EMC virus infection. J. Exp. Med. 144, 1305–1315 (1976b).

Gresser, I., Tovey, M. G., Maury, C.: Efficacy of exogenous treatment with interferon after onset of multiplication of vesicular stomatitis virus in the brains of mice. J. Gen. Virol. 27, 395–403 (1975).

Gresser, I., Tovey, M. G., Maury, C., Bandu, M. T.: Role of interferon in the pathogenesis of virus diseases in mice as demonstrated by the use of anti-interferon serum. II. Studies with herpes simplex, Moloney sarcoma, vesicular stomatitis, Newcastle disease and influenza viruses. J. Exp. Med. 144, 1316–1327 (1976c).

Gresser, I., Tovey, M. G., Maury, C., Chouroulinkov, I.: Lethality of interferon preparations for newborn mice. Nature 258, 76–78 (1975).

Grodnitskaya, N. N., Dreizen, R. S.: Production and action of interferon in experimental respiratory syncytial infection. Vopros. Virosol. 3, 305–307 (1975).

Grossberg, S. E.: The interferons and their inducers: Molecular and therapeutic considerations. N. Engl. J. Med. 287, 13–19, 79–85, 122–128 (1972).

Grossberg, S. E., Burleson, G., Morahan, P., Jameson, P.: A bacterial protein inducing antiviral resistance and high titers of interferon. Progr. Immunobiol. Stand. 5, 274–278 (1972).

Grossberg, S. E., Holland, J. J.: Interferon and viral RNA. Effect on virus-susceptible and insusceptible cells. J. Immunol. 88, 708–714 (1962).

Grossberg, S. E., Morahan, P. S.: Repression of interferon action: induced dedifferentiation of embryonic cells. Science 171, 77–79 (1971).

Grossberg, S. E., Scherer, W.: Inapparent viral infection of cells in vitro. II. An interferon produced in chicken embryonic cell cultures inoculated with Japanese encephalitis virus. Amer. J. Pathol. 45, 519–531 (1964).

Grossberg, S. E., Smith, A. J., Sedmak, J. J.: Control of the interferon mechanism in hamster-monkey heterokaryons. In: Effects of Interferon on Cells, Viruses and the Immune System (Geraldes, A., eds.), pp. 33–53. New York: Academic Press (1975).

Gruenewald, R., Levine, S.: Effect of tilorone on susceptibility of mice to primary and secondary infection with Listeria monocytogenes. Infect. Immun. 13, 1613–1618 (1976).

Guerra, R., Frezzotti, R., Bonanni, R., Dianzani, F., Rita, G.: A preliminary study on treatment of human herpes simplex keratitis with an interferon inducer. Ann. N. Y. Acad. Sci. 173, 823–826 (1970).

Guggenheim, M. A., Baron, S.: Clinical studies of an interferon inducer, poly I·poly C, in children. J. Infect. Dis. **136**, 50–58 (1977).

Guggenheim, M. A., Friedman, R. M., Rabson, A. S.: Interferon: production by chick erythrocytes activated by cell fusion. Science **159**, 542–543 (1968).

Gupta, S. L., Graziadei, W. D. III, Weideli, M., Sopori, M. L., Lengyel, P.: Selektive inhibition of viral protein accumulation in interferon-treated cells; nondiscriminate inhibition of the translation of added viral and cellular messenger RNAs in their extracts. Virology **57**, 49–63 (1974).

Gupta, S. L., Sopori, M. L., Lengyel, P.: Inhibition of protein synthesis directed by added viral and cellular messenger RNAs in extracts of interferon-treated Ehrlich ascites tumor cells. Location and dominance of the inhibitor(s). Biochem. Biophys. Res. Commun. **54**, 777–783 (1973).

Gupta, S. L., Sopori, M. L., Lengyel, P.: Release of the inhibition of messenger RNA translation in extracts of interferon-treated Ehrlich ascites tumor cells by added transfer RNA. Biochem. Biophys. Res. Commun. **57** (6), 763–770 (1974).

Gutman, N. R., Sorokin, A. M.: The effect of splenectomy and antilymphocytic serum upon interferon and antibody production. Vopros. Virusol. **1**, 73–74 (1973).

Haahr, S.: The effects of antilymphocyte serum on viraemia and serum interferon of mice infected with West Nile virus. Acta Pathol. Microbiol. (Scand.) **77**, 167–171 (1969).

Haahr, S.: The influence of poly I:C on the course of infection in mice inoculated with West Nile virus. Arch. Gesamte Virusforsch. **35**, 1–9 (1971).

Haahr, S., Rasmussen, L., Merigan, T. C.: Lymphocyte transformation and interferon production in human mononuclear cell microcultures for assay of cellular immunity to herpes simplex virus. Infect. Immun. **14**, 47–51 (1976).

Haahr, S., Teisner, B.: The influence of different temperatures on mortality, virus multiplication, and interferon production in adult mice infected with coxsachie B 1 virus. Arch. Ges. Virusforsch. **42**, 273–277 (1973).

Haase, A. T., Johnson, J. S., Kasel, J. A., Margolis, S., Levy, H. B.: Induction of interferon in lymphoblastoid cell lines. Proc. Soc. Exp. Biol. Med. **133**, 1076–1083 (1970).

Haber, J., Rosenau, W., Goldberg, M.: Separate factors in phytohaemagglutinin induced lymphotoxin, interferon and nucleic acid synthesis. Nature New Biol. **238**, 60–63 (1972).

Habif, D. V., Lipton, R., Cantell, K.: Interferon crosses blood-brain barrier in monkeys. Proc. Soc. Exp. Biol. Med. **149**, 287–293 (1975).

Hadhazy, G., Fekete, B., Szabo, G., Szabo, B.: Interferon production in human leukemic leukocytes. Acta Microbiol. Acad. Sci. Hung. **23**, 15–18 (1976).

Hadhazy, G., Gergely, L., Toth, F. D., Szegedi, G.: Comparative study on the interferon production by the leucocytes of healthy and leukaemic subjects. Acta Microbiol Acad. Sci. Hung. **24**, 391–395 (1967).

Hahnemann, F. V., Reinicke, V.: In ovo production of interferon induced by influenza virus of varying incompleteness. Act. Path. et Microbiol. Scand. **63**, 241–248 (1965).

Hahon, N.: Depression of viral interferon induction in cell monolayers by coal dust. Br. J. Ind. Med. **31** (3), 201–208 (1974).

Hahon, N., Kozikowska, E. H.: Induction of interferon by *oxiella burneti* in cell cultures. J. Gen. Virol. **3**, 125–128 (1968).

Hajnicka, V., Fuchsberger, N., Borecky, L.: Affinity chromatography of mouse interferon: a modified purification procedure utilizing specifically purified antibodies. Acta Virol. **20**, 326–327 (1976).

Hale, J. H., Doraisingham, M., Kangaratnam, K., Leong, K. W., Monteiro, E. S.: Large-scale use of Sabin type 2 attenuated poliovirus vaccine in Singapore during a type I poliomeylitis epidemic. Br. Med. J. **1**, 1541–1544 (1959).

Hallum, J. V., Thacore, H. R., Youngner, J. S.: Factors affecting the sensitivity of different viruses to interferon. J. Virol. **6**, 156–162 (1970).

Hallum, J. V., Youngner, J. S.: Quantitative aspects of inhibition of virus replication by interferon in chick embryo cell cultures. J. Bacteriol. **92**, 1047–1050 (1966).

Hallum, J. V., Youngner, J. S., Arnold, N. J.: Effect of pH on the protective action of interferon in L cells. J. Virol. **2**, 772–780 (1968).

Hallum, J. V., Youngner, J. S., Stinebring, W. R.: Interferon activity associated with high molecular weight proteins in the circulation of mice injected with endotoxin or bacteria. Virology **27**, 429–431 (1965).

Hanna, L., Merigan, T. C., Jawetz, E.: Inhibition of TRIC agents by virus-induced interferon. Proc. Soc. Exp. Biol. Med. **122**, 417–421 (1966).

Hanna, L., Merigan, T. C., Jawetz, E.: Effect of interferon on TRIC agents and induction of interferon by TRIC agents. Am. J. Ophthal. **63**, 1115–1119 (1967).

Harmon, M. W., Greenberg, S. B., Couch, R. R.: Effect of human nasal secretions on the antiviral activity of human fibroblast and leukocyte interferon. Proc. Soc. Exp. Biol. Med. **152**, 598–602 (1976).

Harmon, M. W., Greenberg, S. B., Johnson, P. E., Couch, R. B.: Human nasal epithelial cell culture system: Evaluation of response to human interferons. Infect. Immun. **16**, 480–483 (1977).

Harmon, M. W., Janis, B.: Therapy of murine rabies after exposure: efficacy of polynosinic-polyribocytidylic acid alone and in combination with three rabies vaccines. J. Infect. Dis. **132**, 241–247 (1975).

Harmon, M. W., Janis, B., Levy, M.: Post-exposure prophylaxis of murine rabies with polynosinic–polycytidylic acid and chlorite-oxidized amylose. Antimicrob. Agents Chemoth. **6**, 507–511 (1974).

Harper, M., Pitha, P.: Effect of Concanavalin A on interferon induction by poly IC. Biochem. Biophys. Res. Comm. **53**, 1220–1223 (1973).

Harris, R. E., Coleman, P. H., Morahan, P. S.: Erythrocyte association and interferon production by minute virus of mice. Proc. Soc. Exp. Biol. Med. **145**, 1288–1292 (1974).

Hattwich, M. A. W., Weiss, T. T., Stechschulte, C. J., Baer, G. M., Gregg, M. B.: Recovery from rabies, a case report. Ann. Intern. Med. **76**, 931–938 (1972).

Havell, E. A.: Cellular regulation mechanisms controlling synthesis of interferons, in: Interferons and their Actions. (Stewart II, W. E., ed.), pp. 37–48. Cleveland, Ohio: CRC Press, Inc. (1977).

Havell, E. A., Berman, B., Ogburn, C. A., Berg, K., Paucker, K., Vilček, J.: Two antigenically distinct species of human interferon. Proc. Nat. Acad. Sci. U. S. A. **72**, 2185–2190 (1975a).

Havell, E. A., Berman, B., Vilček, J.: Antigenic and biological differences between human leukocytic and fibroblast interferons. Proc. Symp. Clin. Use of Interferon. Yugoslav Acad. Sci. Arts, Zagreb, pp. 49–62 (1975).

Havell, E. A., Holtermann, O. A., Starr, T. J.: The influence of the indigenous bacterial flora upon the interferon response of mice. J. Gen. Virol. **9**, 93–95 (1970).

Havell, E. A., Vilček, J.: Production of high titered interferon in cultures of human diploid cells. Antimicrob. Agents Chemother. **2**, 476–484 (1972).

Havell, E. A., Vilček, J.: Mass production and some characteristics of human interferon from diploid cells. *In Vitro* Monogr. **3**, 47–53 (1974).

Havell, E. A., Vilček, J.: Inhibition of interferon secretion by vinblastine. J. Cell Biol. **64**, 716–721 (1975).

Havell, E. A., Vilček, J., Falcoff, E., Berman, B.: Suppression of human interferon production by inhibitors of glycosylation. Virology **63**, 475–482 (1975b).

Havell, E. A., Yamazaki, S., Vilček, J.: Altered molecular species of human interferon produced in the presence of inhibitors of glycosylation. J. Biol. Chem. **252**, 4425–4433 (1977).

Havell, E. A., Yip, Y. K., Vilček, J.: Characteristics of human lymphoblastoid (Namalva) interferon. J. Gen. Virol. **38**, 51–60 (1978a).

Havell, E. A., Yip, Y. K., Vilček, J.: Correlation of physicochemical and antigenic properties of human interferon subspecies. Arch. Virol. **55**, 121–129 (1977b).

Havredaki, M., McNeill, T. A.: The effect of interferon inducers on colony stimulating factor production in L cell cultures. J. Gen. Virol. **27**, 107–110 (1975).

Heine, J. W., Adler, W. H.: The quantitative production of interferon by mitogen stimulated mouse lymphocytes as a function of age and its effect on the lymphocytes proliferative response. J. Immunol. **118**, 1366–1374 (1977).

Heineberg, H., Gold, E., Robbins, F. C.: Differences in interferon content in tissues of mice of various ages infected with coxsackie B virus. Proc. Soc. Exp. Biol. Med. **115**, 947–952 (1964).

Heller, E.: Enhancement of Chikungunya virus replication and inhibition of interferon production by actinomycin D. Virology 21, 652–656 (1963).

Hellman, A., Martin, D. H., Wopschall, L. J.: The influence of X-irradiation on survival and interferon levels in viral infected mice. Proc. Soc. Exp. Biol. Med. 128, 455–460 (1968).

Hellmann, W., Kohlhage, H.: Role of spleen in production of virus-induced interferon in rabbits. Arch. Ges. Virusforsch. 39, 396–400 (1972).

Hellmann, W., Kohlhage, H.: Effects of splenectomy on production of virus induced interferon in rabbits. Nature New Biol. 241, 239–240 (1973 a).

Hellmann, W., Kohlhage, H.: Cellular origin of rabbit serum interferon induced by Newcastle disease virus. Arch. Ges. Virusforsch. 40, 334–340 (1973 b).

Henderson, J. R., Taylor, R. M.: Studies on mechanisms of arthropod-borne virus interference in tissue culture. Virology 13, 477–484 (1961).

Henle, G., Henle, W.: Differences in response of hamster tumor cells induced by polyoma virus to interfering virus and interferon. J. Natl. Cancer Inst. 31, 143–153 (1963).

Henle, G., Henle, W.: Evidence for a persistent viral infection in a cell line derived from Burkitt's lymphoma. J. Bacteriol. 89, 252–260 (1965).

Henle, W., Henle, G.: Interference of inactive virus with the propagation of virus of influenza. Science 98, 87–89 (1943).

Henle, W., Henle, G., Deinhardt, F., Bergs, V. V.: Studies on persistent infections of tissue cultures. IV. Evidence for the production of an interferon in MCN cells by myxoviruses. J. Exp. Med. 110, 525–541 (1959).

Henslová, E., Libiková, M.: Optimal conditions for interferon formation in chick embryo cell cultures infected with tick-borne encephalitis virus. Acta Virol. 10, 475–479 (1966).

Henson, D., Smith, R. D.: Interferon production in vitro by cells infected with the murine salivary gland virus. Proc. Soc. Exp. Biol. Med. 117, 517–521 (1964).

Henson, D., Smith, R. D., Gehrke, J.: Non-fatal mouse cytomegalovirus hepatitis; combined morphologic, virologic and immunologic observations. Amer. J. Pathol. 49, 871–880 (1966).

Heremans, H., Stewart II, W. E., Billiau, A., Desomer, P.: Toxicity of poly (rI)·poly (rC) for interferon-treated cells. An ultrastructural evaluation. J. Gen. Virol. 30, 131–136 (1976).

Herman, R.: The effects of interferon and its inducers on experimental protozoan parasitic infections. Trans. N. Y. Acad. Sci. 34, 176–180 (1972).

Herman, R., Baron, S.: Effects of interferon inducers on the intracellular growth of the protozoan parasite Leishmania donovani. Nature 226, 168–170 (1970).

Herman, R., Shiroishi, T., Buckler, C. E.: Viral interference with exoerythrocytic forms of malaria (Plasmodium gallinaceum) in ovo. J. Infect. Dis. 128, 148–153 (1973).

Hermodsson, S.: Inhibition of interferon by an infection with parainfluenza virus type 3 (PIV-3). Virology 20, 333–343 (1963).

Hermodsson, S.: Action of parainfluenza virus type 3 on synthesis of interferon and multiplication of heterologous virus. Acta Pathol. Microbiol. Scand. 62, 224–238 (1964).

Heron, I., Berg, K., Cantell, K.: Regulation effect of interferon on T-cells in vitro. J. Immunol. 117, 1370–1377 (1976).

Higashihara, M.: Heat and acid labile virus inhibiting factor or interferon induced by Rift Valley fever virus in mice. Jap. J. Microbiol. 15, 482–484 (1971).

Hilfenhaus, J.: What does one reference unit of human fibroblast interferon mean? Symp. on Prep. Stand. and Clin. Use of Interferon, Zagreb, Yugoslavia ((1977).

Hilfenhaus, J., Damm, H., Johannsen, R.: Sensitivities of various human lymphoblastoid cells to the antiviral and anticellular activity of human leukocyte interferon. Arch. Virol. 54, 271–277 (1977).

Hilfenhaus, J., Damm, H., Karges, H. E., Manthey, K. F.: Growth inhibition of human lymphoblastoid Daudi cells in vitro by interferon preparations. Arch. Virol. 51, 87–97 (1976).

Hilfenhaus, J., Karges, H. E.: Growth inhibition of human lymphoblastoid cells by interferon preparations, obtained from human leukocytes. Z. Naturforsch. C. 29, 618–622 (1974).

Hilfenhaus, J., Karges, H. E., Weinmann, E., Barth, R.: Effect of administered human leukocyte interferon on experimental rabies in monkeys. Infect. Immun. 11, 1156–1162 (1975).

Hilfenhaus, J., Thierfelder, H., Barth, R.: Sensitivity of various primate cells and animal viruses to the antiviral activity of human leukocyte interferon. Arch. Virol. 48, 203–208 (1975).

Hilfenhaus, J., Weinmann, E., Majer, M., Barth, R., Jaeger, J.: Post-exposure administration of human interferon to rabies infected monkeys. J. Infect. Dis. 135, 846–851 (1977).

Hill, D. A., Baron, S., Chanock, R. M.: Sensitivity of common respiratory viruses to an interferon inducer in human cells. Lancet ii, 187–188 (1969).

Hill, D. A., Baron, S., Levy, H. B., Bellianti, J., Buckler, C. E., Cannellos, G., Carbone, P., Canock, R. M. Devita, V., Guggenheim, M. A., Homan, E., Kapikian, A. Z., Kirschstein, R. L., Mills, J., Perkins, J. C., Vankirk, J. E., Worthington, M.: Clinical studies of induction of interferon by polyinosinic–polycytidylic acid, in: Perspectives in Virology 7 (Pollard, M., ed.), p. 198. New York: Academic Press (1971).

Hill, D. A., Baron, S., Perkins, J. C., Worthington, M., Vankirk, J. E., Mills, J., Kapikian, A. Z., Chanock, R. H.: Evaluation of an interferon inducer in viral respiratory disease. JAMA 219, 1179–1184 (1972).

Hill, D. A., Walsh, J. H., Purcell, R. M.: Failure to demonstrate circulating interferon during incubation period and acute stage of transfusion associated hepatitis. Proc. Soc. Exp. Biol. Med. 136, 853–856 (1971).

Hiller, G., Winkler, I., Vienhauser, G., Jungwirth, C., Bodo, G., Dube, S., Ostertag, W.: Failure of globin mRNA to stimulate globin synthesis in cell-free extracts of interferon-treated globin-synthesizing mouse erythro-leukemic cells. Virology 69, 360–368 (1976).

Hilleman, M. R.: Prospects for the use of double-stranded ribonucleic acid (poly I:C) inducers in man. J. Infect. Dis. 121, 196–211 (1970).

Hirsch, M. S., Black, P. H., Proffitt, M. R.: Interferon effects on immunologically activated murine leukemia viruses. Monograph. Natl. Cancer. Inst. 24, 115–119 (1973 a).

Hirsch, M. S., Black, P. H., Proffitt, M. R.: Interferon effects on immunologically activated MLV, in: Modulation of Host Immune Resistance in the Prevention or Treatment of Induced Neoplasia (Chirigos, M. A., ed.), pp. 251–255. Washington, D.C.: G.P.O. Fogarty International Center Proc. # 28 (1977).

Hirsch, M. S., Black, P. H., Wood, M. L., Monaco, A. P.: Immunosuppression, interferon inducers and leukemia in mice. Proc. Soc. Exp. Biol. Med. 134, 309–312 (1970).

Hirsch, M. S., Black, P. H., Wood, M. L., Monaco, A. P.: Effects of pyran copolymer on oncogenic virus infections in immunosuppressed hosts. J. Immunol. 108, 1312–1318 (1972).

Hirsch, M. S., Ellis, D. A., Black, P. H., Monaco, A. P., Wood, M. L.: Immunosuppressive effects of an interferon preparation in vivo. Transplantation 17 (2), 234–236 (1974).

Hirsch, M. S., Ellis, D. A., Proffitt, M. R., Black, P. H.: Effects of interferon on leukemia virus activation in graft versus host disease. Nature New Biol. 244 (134), 102–103 (1973 b).

Hirsch, M. S., Murphy, F. A.: Effects of anti-thymocyte serum on 17-D yellow fever infection in adult mice. Nature 216, 179–181 (1967).

Hirsch, M. S., Murphy, F. A.: Effects of antilymphoid sera on viral infections. Lancet ii, 37–39 (1968).

Hirsch, M. S., Nahmias, A. J., Murphy, F. A., Kramer, J. H.: Effect of antilymphocytic serum on interferon induction by virus and nonviral inducers. J. Exp. Med. 128, 121–129 (1968).

Hitchcock, G., Isaacs, A.: Protection of mice against the lethal action of an encephalitis virus. British Med. J. ii, 1268–1270 (1960).

Hitchcock, G., Porterfield, J. S.: Production of interferon in brains of mice infected with an arthropod-borne virus. Virology 13, 363–365 (1961).

Ho, M.: Inhibition of the infectivity of poliovirus ribonucleic acid by an interferon. Proc. Soc. Exp. Biol. Med. 107, 639–644 (1961).

Ho, M.: Interferons. New Eng. J. Med. 266, 1258–1265 (1962).

Ho, M.: Interferons. New Eng. J. Med. 266, 1313–1318 (1962).

Ho, M.: Interferons. New Eng. J. Med. 266, 1367–1371 (1962).

Ho, M.: Interferon-like viral inhibitor in rabbits after intravenous administration of endotoxin. Science 146, 1472–1474 (1964 a).

Ho, M.: Identification and induction of interferons. Bact. Rev. 28, 367–381 (1964 b).

Ho, M.: The induction of interferons and related problems. Jap. J. Exp. Med. 37, 169–182 (1967).

Ho, M.: Animal viruses and interferon formation, in: Interferons and Interferon Inducers (Finter, N. B., ed.), pp. 29–44. Amsterdam: North-Holland Publ. Co. (1973).

Ho, M., Armstrong, J. A.: Interferon. Ann. Rev. Microbiol. 29, 131–158 (1975).

Ho, M., Breinig, M. K.: Conditions for the production of interferon appearing in chick cell cultures infected with Sindbis virus. J. Immunol. 89, 177–185 (1962).

Ho, M., Breinig, M. K.: Metabolic determinants of interferon formation. Virology 25, 331–339 (1965).

Ho, M., Breinig, M. K., Postic, B., Armstrong, J. A.: The effect of preinjections on the stimulation of interferon by a complexed polynucleotide, endotoxin, and virus. Ann. N. Y. Acad. Sci. **173**, 680–688 (1970).

Ho, M., Enders, J. F.: An inhibitor of viral activity appearing in infected cell cultures. Proc. Nat. Acad. Sci. U. S. A. **45**, 385–389 (1959a).

Ho, M., Enders, J. F.: Further studies on an inhibitor of viral activity appearing in infected cell cultures and its role in chronic viral infection. Virology **9**, 446–477 (1959b).

Ho, M., Ke, Y. H.: The mechanism of stimulation of interferon production by a complexed polyribonucleotide. Virology **40**, 693–702 (1970).

Ho, M., Ke, Y. H., Armstrong, J. A.: Mechanism of interferon induction by endotoxin. J. Infect. Dis. **128**, suppl. S 220–S 228 (1973).

Ho, M., Köhler, K.: Studies on human adenoviruses as inducers of interferon in chick cells. Archiv. für die gesamte Virusforschung **22**, 69–78 (1967).

Ho, M., Kono, Y.: Effect of actinomycin D on virus and endotoxin-induced interferon-like inhibitors in rabbits. Proc. Natl. Acad. Sci. **53**, 220–224 (1965).

Ho, M., Kono, Y., Breinig, M. K.: Tolerance to the induction of interferons by endotoxin and virus: role of a humoral factor. Proc. Soc. Exp. Biol. Med. **119**, 1227–1232 (1965).

Ho, M., Nash, C., Morgan, C. W., Armstrong, J. A., Carroll, R. G., Postic, B.: Interferon administered in the cerebrospinal space and its effect on rabies in rabbits. Infect. Immun. **9**, 268–293 (1974).

Ho, M., Postic, B.: Renal excretion of interferon. Nature **214**, 1230–1232 (1967).

Ho, M., Postic, B., Ke, Y. H.: The systemic induction of 1 F, in: Ciba Foundation Symp. on IF (Wolstenholme, G. E. W., O'Connor, M., eds.), pp. 19–35. London: J. &. A. Churchill Ltd. (1967).

Ho, M., Tan, Y. H., Armstrong, J. A.: Accentuation of production of human interferon by metabolic inhibitors. Proc. Soc. Exp. Biol. Med. **139**, 259–262 (1972).

Hoffmann, H., Kunz, C.: The protective effect of the interferon inducers tilorone hydrochloride and poly I:C on experimental tickborne encephalitis in mice. Arch. Ges. Virusforsch. **37**, 262–266 (1972).

Hoffmann, M. K., Oettgen, H. F., Old, L. J., Chin, A. F., Hammerling, U.: Endotoxin induced serum factor controlling differentiation of bone-marrow derived lymphocytes. Proc. Nat. Acad. Sci. **74**, 1200–1204 (1976).

Hoffman, W. W., Korst, J. J. Niblack, J. F., Cronin, T. H.: N,N-dioctadecyl-N', N'-Bis (2-hydroxyethyl)propanediamine: antiviral activity and interferon stimulation in mice. Antimicrobial Agents Chemothr. **3**, 498–504 (1973).

Holmes, A. W., Gilson, J., Deinhardt, F.: Inibition of interferon production by 5-iodo-2-deoxyuridine. Virology **24**, 229–231 (1964).

Holtermann, O. A., Havell, E. A.: Reduced interferon response in mice congenitally infected with lymphocytic choriomeningitis virus. J. Gen. Virol. **9**, 101–103 (1970).

Hong, C. C., Sevoian, M.: Interferon production and host resistance to type II avian (Marek's) leukosis virus. Appl. Microbiol. **22**, 818–820 (1971).

Hooks, J. J., Burns, W., Hayashi, K., Geis, S., Notkins, A. L.: Viral spread in the presence of neutralizing antibody: Mechanisms of persistence in foamy virus infection. Infect. Immun. **14**, 1172–1179 (1976).

Hopps, H. E., Kohno, S., Kohno, M., Smadel, J. E.: Production of interferon in tissue cultures infected with *Rickettsia tsutsugamushi*. Bact. Proc. **64**, 115 (1964).

Horak, I., Jungwirth, C., Bodo, G.: Poxvirus specific cytopathic effect in interferon-treated L cells. Virology **45**, 456–462 (1971).

Horoszewicz, J. S., Leong, S. S., Ito, M., Berardino, L. D., Carter, W. A.: Aging *in vitro* and large scale interferon production by 15 new strains of human diploid fibroblasts. Infect. Immun. **19**, 720–726 (1978).

Hoskins, M.: A protective action of neurotropic against viscerotropic yellow fever virus in Macacus rhesus. Amer. J. Trop. Med. Hyg. **15**, 675–680 (1935).

Hovanessian, A. G., Brown, R. E., Kerr, I.: Synthesis of low molecular weight inhibitor of protein synthesis with enzyme from interferon-treated cells. Nature **268**, 537–539 (1977).

Hovanessian, A. G., Kerr, I. M.: Synthesis of an oligonucleotide inhibitor of protein synthesis in rabbit reticulocytes lysates analogous to that formed in extracts from interferon-treated cells. Eur. J. Biochem. **84**, 149–160 (1978).

Hsiung, G. D.: Production of an inhibitory substance by myxovirus auto-inhibition of plaque formation. Proc. Soc. Exp. Biol. Med. **108**, 357–360 (1962).

Hsiung, G. D., Van de Water, T.: Production of interferon in embryonated eggs and in cell cultures infected with simian virus 5. Proc. Soc. Exp. Biol. Med. **123**, 840–844 (1966).

Huang, A. S.: Viral pathogenesis and molecular biology. Bact. Rev. **41**, 811–821 (1977).

Huang, A. S., Baltimore, D.: Defective viral particles and viral disease processes. Nature **226**, 325–330 (1970).

Huang, A. S., Wagner, R. R.: Defective T particles of vesicular stomatitis virus. II. Biologic role in homologous interference. Virology **30**, 173–181 (1966).

Huang, J. W., Davey, M. W., Hejna, C. J., von Muenchhausen, W., Sulkowski, E., Carter, W. A.: Selective binding of human interferon to albumin immobilized on agarose. J. Biol. Chem. **249**, 4665–4667 (1974).

Huang, J. W., Hejna, C. I., Sulkowski, E., Carter, W. D., Silver, G. H., Munayyer, H., Came, P.: The human interferon-albumin interaction: The influence of albumin conformation. Virology **65**, 268–273 (1975).

Huang, K. Y., Donahoe, R. M., Gordon, F. B., Dressler, H. R.: Enhancement of phagocytosis by interferon-containing preparations. Infect. Immun. **4**, 581–588 (1971).

Huang, K. Y., Gordon, F. D.: Production of interferon in mice: Effect of altered gaseous environments. App. Microbiol. **16**, 1551–1555 (1968).

Huang, K. Y., Landay, M. E.: Enhancement of the lethal effects of endotoxins by interferon inducers. J. Bacteriol. **100**, 1110–1111 (1969).

Huang, K. Y., Schultz, W. W., Gordon, F. B.: Interferon induced by Plasmodium berghei. Science **162**, 123–125 (1968).

Huet, C., Gresser, I., Bandu, M. T., Lindahl, P.: Increased binding of Concanavalin A to interferon-treated murine leukemia L_{1210} cells. Proc. Soc. Exp. Biol. Med. **147**, 52–57 (1974).

Huismans, H.: Bluetongue virus-induced interferon synthesis. Onderstepoort J. Vet. Pres. **36**, 181–185 (1969).

Hung, C. Y., Lefkowitz, S. S., Geber, W. F.: Interferon inhibition by narcotic analgesics. Proc. Soc. Exp. Biol. Med. **142** (1), 106–111 (1973).

Huppert, J., Hillova, J., Gresland, L.: Viral RNA synthesis in chicken cells infected with ultraviolet irradiated Newcastle disease virus. Nature **223**, 1015–1017 (1969).

Hutchinson, D. W., Johnston, M. D., Eaton, M. A.: Necessity for the 2'-hydroxyl group for the antiviral activity of synthetic polynucleotides. J. Gen. Virol. **23**, 331–333 (1974).

Hutchinson, D. W., Merigan, T. C.: The lack of antiviral effect of poly I-poly C when attached to insoluble supports. J. Gen. Virol. **27**, 403–410 (1975).

Ibrahim, A. L., Zee, Y. C., Osebold, J. W.: The effects of ozone on the respiratory epithelium and alveolar macrophages of mice. I. interferon production. Proc. Soc. Exp. Biol. Med. **152**, 483–488 (1976).

Ida, S., Hooks, J. J., Siraganian, R. P., Notkins, A. L.: Enhancement of IgE-mediated histamine release from human basophils by viruses: role of interferon. J. Exp. Med. **145**, 892–899 (1977).

Ikic, D., Brnobic, A., Jurkovic-Vukelic, V., Smerdel, S., Jusic, D., Soos, E.: Therapeutic effect of human leukocyte interferon incorporated into ointment and cream on condylomata acuminata. Proc. Symp. Clin. Use of Interferons. Yugoslav. Acad. Sci. Arts, pp. 235–238 (1975a).

Ikic, D., Orescanin, N., Krusic, J., Cestar, Z., Alac, Z., Soos, E., Jusic, D., Smerdel, S.: Preliminary study of the effect of human leukocytic interferon on condylomata acuminata in women. Proc. Symp. Clin. Use of Interferons. Yugoslav Acad. Sci., pp. 223–225 (1975b).

Ikic, D., Smerdel, S., Rajninger–Miholic, M., Soos, E., Justic, D.: Treatment of labial and genital herpes with human leukocytic interferon. Proc. Symp. Clin. Use of Interferon Yugoslav Acad. Sci. Arts, pp. 195–202 (1975c).

Ikic, D., Smerdel, S., Soos, E., Jusic, D.: The use of interferon in herpes simplex infections and condylomata acuminatum. Radova Imunol. Zovada–Zagreb. **27**, 69–75 (1974).

Illinger, D., Coupin, G., Richards, M., Poindron, P.: Rat interferon inhibits steroid-inducible glycerol 3-phosphate dehydrogenase synthesis in a rat glial cell line. FEBS Letters **64**, 391–394 (1976).

Imanishi, J.: Inhibition of macrophage migration by virus-induced interferon preparations. Jap. J. Microbiol. **19**, 337–342 (1975).

Imanishi, J., Oishi, K., Kishida, T., Negoro, Y., Izuka, M.: Effects of interferon preparations on rabbit corneal xenograft. Arch. Virol. **53**, 157–161 (1977).

Imanishi, J., Yokota, Y., Kishida, T., Mukainaka, T., Matsuo, A.: Phagocytosis-enhancing effect of human leukocyte interferon preparation on human peripheral monocytes *in vitro*. Acta Virol. **19**, 52–55 (1975).

Inglot, A., Chudzio, T.: A bioassay employing polyethylene glycol for measuring neutralization of interferon by specific antibodies. J. Immunol. Methods, **13**, 63–69 (1976).

Inglot, A. D., Chudzio, T.: Enhancement of leukemogenesis in mice after prolonged administration of anti-interferon or normal rabbit globulin. Arch. Virol. **55**, 67–76 (1977).

Inglot, A. D., Radzikowski, C., Szkudlarek, J.: Influence of rabbit anti-mouse lymphocyte serum on interferon production in mice; different effects dependent upon the character of the inducer. Archiv. Immunol. et Therap. Experim. **18**, 409–417 (1970).

Isaacs, A.: Interferon: the prospects. Practitioner **183**, 601–605 (1959a).

Isaacs, A.: Virus interference, in: Virus Growth and Variation, 9th Symp. Soc. Gen. Microbiol., p. 256. Cambridge Univ. Press (1959b).

Isaacs, A.: Action of interferon on the growth of sublethally irradiated virus. Virology **9**, 56–69 (1959c).

Isaacs, A.: Interferon. Scientific American **204**, 51–57 (1961).

Isaacs, A.: Production and action of interferon. Cold Spring Harbor Symp. Quant. Biol. **27**, 343–349 (1962).

Isaacs, A.: Interferon and virus infection. Recent Prog. Microbiol. **8**, 420–426 (1963a).

Isaacs, A.: Foreign nucleic acids. Scientific American **209**, 46–55 (1963b).

Isaacs, A., Baron, S.: Antiviral action of interferon in embryonic cells. The Lancet ii, 946–947 (1960).

Isaacs, A., Burke, D. C.: Mode of action of interferon. Nature **182**, 1073–1074 (1958).

Isaacs, A., Burke, D. C.: Viral interference and interferon. Brit. Med. Bull. **15**, 185–188 (1959).

Isaacs, A., Burke, D. C., Fadeeva, L.: Effect of interferon on the growth of viruses on the chick chorion. Brit. J. Exp. Pathol. **39**, 447–451 (1958).

Isaacs, A., Cox, R. A., Rotem. Z.: Foreign nucleic acids as the stimulants to make interferon. Lancet ii, 7299, 113–116 (1963).

Isaacs, A., Hitchcock, G.: Role of interferon in recovery from virus infections. Lancet ii, 69–71 (1960).

Isaacs, A., Klemperer, H. G., Hitchcock, G.: Studies on the mechanism of action of interferon. Virology **13**, 191–199 (1961).

Isaacs, A., Lindenmann, J.: Virus interference. I. The interferon. Proc. Royal Soc. B **147**, 258–267 (1957).

Isaacs, A., Lindenmann, J., Valentine, R. C.: Virus interference II. Some properties of interferon. Proc. Royal Soc. B **147**, 268–273 (1937).

Isaacs, A., Porterfield, J. S., Baron, S.: The influence of oxygenation on virus growth. II. Effect on the antiviral action of interferon. Virology **14**, 450–455 (1961).

Isaacs, A., Rotem, Z., Fantes, K. H.: An inhibitor of the production of interferon (blocker). Virology **29**, 248–254 (1966).

Isaacs, A., Westwood, M. A.: Duration of protective action of interferon against infection with West Nile virus. Nature **184**, 1232–1233 (1959a).

Isaacs, A., Westwood, M. A.: Inhibition by interferon of the growth of vaccinia virus in the rabbit skin. Lancet ii, 324–325 (1959b).

Ito, F., Kobayashi, S.: Enhancing effect of interferon pretreatment on interferon production. Jap. J. Microbiol. **18** (3), 223–228 (1974).

Ito, Y., Kimura, Y., Nagata, I., Kunii, A.: Production of interferon-like substance by mouse spleen cells through contact with BHK cells persistently infected with HVJ. Virology **60**, 73–84 (1974).

Ito, Y., Kunii, A., Mori, N., Nagata, I.: Effects of splenectomy on production of endotoxin-type interferon in mice. Virology **44** (3), 638–641 (1971).

Ito, Y., Montagnier, L.: Heterogeneity of the sensitivity of vesicular stomatitis virus to interferons. Infect. Immun. **18**, 13–27 (1977).

Ito, Y., Nagata, I., Kunii, A.: Mechanism of endotoxin-type interferon production in mice. Virology **52** (2), 439–446 (1973a).

Ito, Y., Nagata, I., Kunii, A.: Effect of omentumectomy on production of endotoxin-type interferon in mice. Virology **56**, 362–368 (1973b).

Ito, Y., Nisiyama, Y., Nagata, K., Kunii, A.: Interferon induction in mice by BHK cells persistently infected with HVJ. J. Gen. Virol. **27**, 93–98 (1975).

Ito, Y., Nisiyama, Y., Shimokata, K., Kimuka, Y., Nagata, I., Kunii, A.: Interferon producing capacity of germ-free mice. Infect. Immun. **13**, 332–340 (1976a).

Ito, Y., Nishiyama, Y., Shimokata, K., Kimura, Y., Nagata, I., Kunii, A.: The effects of cytochalasin and colchicine on interferon production. J. Gen. Virol. **33**, 1–9 (1976b).

Ito, Y., Suzuki, J., Kobayashi, S.: Requirement of newly synthesized protein for the priming activity of interferon. Jap. J. Microbiol. **19**, 87–95 (1975).

Jahiel, R. I., Taylor, D., Rainford, N., Hirschberg, S. E., Kroman, R.: Inducers of interferon inhibit the mitotic response of liver cells to partial hepatectomy. Proc. Nat. Acad. Sci. U. S. A. **68**, 740–742 (1971).

Jahiel, R. I., Vilček, J., Nussenzweig, R. S.: Exogenous interferon protects mice against *Plasmodium Berghei* malaria. Nature **277**, 1350–1351 (1970).

Jahrling, P. B.: Interference between virulent and vaccine strains of Venezuelan encephalitis virus in mixed infections of hamsters. J. Gen. Virol. **28**, 1–8 (1975).

Jahrling, P. B., Navarro, E., Scherer, W. F.: Interferon induction and sensitivity as correlates to virulence of Venezuelan encephalitis viruses for hamsters. Arch. Virol. **51**, 23–28 (1976).

Jameson, P.: Induction of the interferon protein *in vivo*: viral inducers. Texas. Rep. Biol. Med. **35**, 84–90 (1977).

Jameson, P., Dixon, M. A., Grossberg, S. E.: A sensitive interferon assay for many species of cells: EMC virus hemagglutinin yield-reduction. Proc. Soc. Exp. Biol. Med. **155**, 173–178 (1977).

Jameson, P., Grossberg, S. E.: Production of interferon in human cell cultures by a new potent viral inducer. Proc. Symp. on Prod. of Human Interferon and Invest. of its Clin. Use. W. Alton Jones Cell Science Center, Lake Placid, N. Y. (1977).

Jameson, P., Schoenherr, C. K., Grossberg, S. E.: Bluetongue virus induction of interferon and resistance to viral infection. Interferon Workshop, Lake Placid, New York (1977).

Janis, B., Habel, K.: Rabies in rabbits and mice: protective effect of polyriboinosinic – polyribocytidylic acid. J. Infect. Dis. **125**, 345–353 (1972).

Jankowski, W. J., Davey, M. W., O'Malley, J., Sulkowski, E., Carter, W. A.: Molecular structure of human fibroblast and leukocyte interferons: probe by lectin and hydrophobic chromatography. J. Virol. **16**, 1124–1130 (1975).

Jankowski, W. J., von Muenchhausen, W., Sulkowski, E., Carter, W. A.: The binding of human interferons to immobilized cibachron blue F 3 GA: the nature of molecular interaction. Biochem. **15**, 5182–5187 (1976).

Jao, R. L., Wheelock, E. F., Jackson, G.G.: Interferon study in volunteers infected with Asian influenza. J. Clin. Invest. **44**, 1062–1071 (1965).

Jariwalla, R., Grossberg, S. E., Sedmak, J. J.: The influence of physicochemical factors on the thermal inactivation of murine interferon. Arch. Virol. **49**, 261–268 (1975).

Jariwalla, R. J., Grossberg, S. E., Sedmak, J. J.: Effect of chaotropic salts and protein denaturants on the thermal stability of mouse fibroblast interferon. J. Gen. Virol. **35**, 45–52 (1977).

Jarvis, A. P., Colby, C.: Regulation of the murine interferon system: isolation and characterization of a mutant 3 T 6 cell engaged in the semiconstitutive synthesis of interferon. Cell **14**, 355–364 (1978).

Jeng, D. K. H.: Hydrophobicity of neuraminidase-treated rabbit interferon. Proc. Soc. Exp. Biol. Med. **154**, 534–536 (1977).

Jenkin, H. M., Lu, Y. K.: Induction of interferon by the bour strain of *trachoma* in Hela 229 cells. Am. J. Ophthalmology **63**, 1110–1115 (1967).

Jensen, M. M.: Transitory impairment of interferon production in stressed mice. J. Infect. Dis. **118**, 230–234 (1968a).

Jensen, M. M.: Transitory impairment of interferon production in seratonin treated mice. Proc. Soc. Exp. Biol. Med. **128**, 174–178 (1968b).

Jensen, M. M.: The influence of vasoactive amines on interferon production in mice. Proc. Soc. Exp. Biol. Med. **130**, 34–37 (1969).

Jensen, M. M.: Possible mechanisms of impaired interferon production in stressed mice. Proc. Soc. Exp. Biol. Med. **142**, 820–823 (1973).

Johnson, H. M., Baron, S.: Interferon as the mediator of the suppressive effects of some interferon inducers in the *in vitro* immune response. IRCS J. Med. Sci. **4**, 187 (1976 a).

Johnson, H. M., Baron, S.: The nature of the suppressive effect of interferon and interferon inducers on the *in vitro* immune response. Cell Immunol. **25**, 106–109 (1976 b).

Johnson, H. M., Baron S.: Regulatory role of interferons in the immune response. IRCS J. Med. Sci. **4**, 50 (1976 c).

Johnson, H. M., Baron, S.: Evaluation of effects of interferon and interferon inducers on the immune response. Pharmacol. Therap. **1**, 349–368 (1977).

Johnson, H. M., Blalock, J. E., Baron, S.: Separation of mitogen-induced suppressor and helper cell activities during inhibition of interferon production by cyclic AMP. Cell. Immunol. **33**, 170–179 (1977).

Johnson, H. M., Bukovic, J. A., Baron, S.: Interferon inhibition of the primary *in vitro* antibody response to a thymus-independent antigen. Cellular Immunol. **20**, 104–108 (1975).

Johnson, H. M., Bukovic, J. A., Smith, B. G.: Inhibitory effect of synthetic polyribonucleotides on the primary *in vitro* immune response. Proc. Soc. Exp. Biol. Med. **149**, 599–605 (1975).

Johnson, H. M., Smith, B. G, Baron, S.: Inhibition of the primary *in vitro* antibody response of mouse spleen cells by interferon preparations. IRCS Med. Sci. **2**, 1616 (1974).

Johnson, H. M., Smith, B. G., Baron, S.: Inhibition of the primary *in vitro* antibody response by interferon preparations. J. Immunol. **114**, 403–409 (1975).

Johnson, H. M., Stanton, G. J., Baron, S.: Relative ability of mitogens to stimulate production of interferon by lymphoid cells and to induce suppression of the *in vitro* immune response. Proc. Soc. Exp. Biol. Med. **154**, 138–143 (1977).

Johnson, M. L., DuBuy, H. G.: Effect of a potent interferon inducer on acute and chronic lactic dehydrogenase virus viremia. Infect. Immun. **11**, 113–119 (1975).

Johnson, R. T., Mims, C. A.: Pathogenesis for viral infections of the nervous system. N. Eng. J. Med. **278**, 23–30 (1968).

Johnson, T. C., Lerner, M. P., Lancz, G. J.: Inhibition of protein synthesis in noninfected L cells by partially purified interferon preparations. J. Cell Biol. **36**, 617–624 (1968).

Johnson, T. C., McLaren, L. C.: Plaque development and induction of interferon synthesis by RMC poliovirus. J. Bacteriol. **90**, 565–570 (1965).

Johnston, M. T., Stollar, B. D., Torrence, P. F., Witkop, B.: Structural features of double-stranded polyribonucleotides required for immunological specificity and interferon induction. Proc. Nat. Acad. Sci. U. S. A. **72**, 4564–4568 (1975).

Johnston, M. T., Atherton, K. T., Hutchinson, D. W., Burke, D. C.: The binding of poly I – poly C to human fibroblasts and the induction of interferon. Biochim. Biophys. Acta **435**, 69–73 (1976).

Joklik, W. K.: The mechanism of action of interferon. Ann. N. Y. Acad. Sci. **284**, 711–717 (1977).

Joklik, W. K., Merigan, T. C.: Concerning the mechanism of action of interferon. Proc. Nat. Acad. Sci. **56**, 558–565 (1966).

Joncas, J., Boucher, J., Boudreault, A., Granger–Julien, M.: Effect of hydrocortisone on cell viability, Epstein-Barr virus genome expression, and interferon synthesis in human lymphoblastoid cell lines. Cancer Res. **33**, 2142–2148 (1973).

Jones, B. R., Coster, D. J., Fallon, M. G., Cantell, K.: Clinical trials of tropical interferon therapy of ulcerative viral keratitis. J. Infect. Dis. **133**, A 169–A 174 (1976).

Jones, B. R., Galbraith, J. E. Y., Al-Hussaini, M. K.: Vaccinial keratitis treated with interferon. Lancet. **7235**, 875–879 (1962).

Jordan, G. W.: Quantitative aspects of interferon-induced plaque reduction: kinetics of interferon action. Virology **48**, 425–432 (1972 a).

Jordan, G. W.: Basis for the probit analysis of an interferon plaque reduction assay. J. Gen. Virol. **14** (1), 49–61 (1972 b).

Jordan, G. W.: Effect of interferon on the growth of GD VII virus. Archiv Ges. Virusforsch. **39**, 284–288 (1972 c).

Jordan, G. W.: Interferon sensitivity of Venezuelan equine encephalomyelitis virus. Infect. Immun. **7**, 911–917 (1973).

Jordan, G. W., Fried, R. P., Merigan, T. C.: Administration of human leukocyte interferon in herpes zoster. I. safety, circulating antiviral activity, and host responses to infection. J. Infect. Dis. **130**, 56–62 (1974).

Jordan, G. W., Merigan, T. C.: Cell-mediated immunity to varicella-zoster virus: *in vitro* lymphocyte responses. J. Infect. Dis. **130**, 495–499 (1974).

Jullien, P., DeMaeyer, E.: Interferon synthesis in X-irradiated animals I. Depression of circulating interferons in C3H mice after whole-body irradiation. Int. J. Rad. Biol. **11**, 567–576 (1966).

Jullien, P., DeMaeyer–Guignard, J., DeMaeyer, E.: Interferon synthesis in X-irradiated animals. V. Origin of mouse serum interferon induced by polynosinic-polycytidylic acid and encephalomyelitis virus. Infect. Immunol. **10**, 1023–1028 (1974).

Jungeblut, C. W., Kodza, H.: Interference between lymphocytic choriomeningitis virus and the leukemia-transmitting agent of leukemia L 2 C in guinea pigs. Archiv Ges. Virusforsch. **12**, 552–555 (1962).

Jungwirth, C., Horak, I., Bodo, G., Lindner, J., Shultze, B.: The synthesis of poxvirus-specific RNA in interferon treated cells. Virology **48**, 59–70 (1972a).

Jungwirth, C., Hiller, G., Pohl, D., Bodo, G.: Smallpox virus specific early function in interferon treated cells: transcription and processing of smallpox virus specific early mRNA. Hope Seylers Z. Physiol. Chem. **353**, 1531–1534 (1972b).

Jungwirth, C., Kroath, H., Bodo, G.: Effect of interferon on poxvirus replication. Tex. Rep. Biol. Med. **35**, 247–259 (1977).

Kaleta, E. F., Bankowski, R. A.: Production of interferon by the CAL-1 and turkey herpesvirus. Amer. J. Vet. Res. **33**, 567–571 (1972a).

Kaleta, E. F., Bankowski, R. A.: Production of circulating and cell-bound interferon in chickens by type 1 and 2 plaque-producing agents of the CAL-1 strain of Marek's disease herpesvirus and herpesvirus of turkeys. Amer. J. Vet. Res. **33**, 573–577 (1972b).

Kandefer–Szerszeń, M.: Typhoid-paratyphoid (TAB) vaccine as interferon inducer in mice. Acta Microbiol. Polonica A. **5**, 156–158 (1973).

Kandefer–Szerszeń, M., Kawecki, Z.: Water extracts of fungi as interference inducers. Acta Microbiol. Polonica A. **5**, 163–166 (1973).

Kaplan, M. M., Cohen, D., Koprowski, H., Dean, D., Ferrigan, L.: Studies on the local treatment of wounds for the prevention of rabies. Bull. W. H. O. **26**, 765–775 (1962).

Karakuyumchan, M. K., Bektemirova, M. S.: Production and effect of interferon in experimental infection with fixed rabies virus. Vopros. Virusol. **13**, 596–599 (1968).

Kariniemi, A–L.: Effect of human leucocyte interferon on DNA systhesis in human psoriatic skin cultured in diffusion chambers. Acta Path. Microbiol. Scand. A **85**, 270–274 (1977).

Karmazyn, M., Horrobin, D. F., Manku, M. S., Karmali, R. A., Morgan, R. A., Ally, A. I., Cunnane, S. C.: Interferon fever. Lancet i, 307 (1977).

Kassel, R. L.: Carcinolytic effects of interferon. Clinic. Obstet. & Gynecology **13**, 910–927 (1970).

Kassel, R. L., Old, L. J., Carswell, E. A., Fiore, N. C., Hardy, W. D.: Serum-mediated leukemia cell destruction in AKR mice. J. Exp. Med. **138**, 925–929 (1973).

Kassel, R. L., Old, L. J., Day, N. K., Hardy, W. D.: Plasma-mediated leukemia cell destruction: concentration and purification of the antileukemia factor. Proc. Soc. Exp. Biol. Med. **155**, 230–233 (1977).

Kassel, R. L., Pascal, R. R., Vas, A.: Interferon-mediated oncolysis in spontaneous murine leukemia. J. Natl. Cancer Inst. **48**, 1155–1159 (1972).

Kato, N., Eggers, H. J.: Depressors of interferon synthesis: inhibition of interferon synthesis by chick allantoic mucopolysaccharide, capsular polysaccharide of *Klebsiella pneumoniae* and heparin. J. Gen. Virol. **5**, 369–374 (1969a).

Kato, N., Eggers, H. J.: A factor capable of enhancing interferon synthesis. Virology **37**, 545–555 (1969b).

Kato, N., Eggers, H. J., Ohta, F., Kobayashi, T.: Depressors of interferon synthesis: further studies on the production, action and properties of the so-called enhancer. J. Gen. Virol. **5**, 195–203 (1969).

Kato, N., Nakashima, I., Ohta, F.: Interferon production in mice by the capsular polysaccharide of *Klebsiella pneumoniae*. Infect. Immun. **12**, 1–9 (1975).

Kato, N., Ohta, F.: Effect of enhancer on the replication of Newcastle disease virus in chorioallantoic membranes. Archiv Ges. Virusforsch. **18**, 116–118 (1966).

Kato, N., Ohta, F., Okada, A.: Counteraction between interferon and enhancer. Virology **28**, 785–788 (1966).

Kato, N., Okada, A., Ohta, F.: Production of a viral growth enhancing factor (Enhancer) in eggs infected with influenza virus (PR 8). Arch. Ges. Virusforsch. **17**, 631–640 (1965a).

Kato, N., Okada, A., Ohta, F.: A factor capable of enhancing virus replication appearing parainfluenza type 1 (HVJ)-infected allantoic fluid. Virology **26**, 630–637 (1965b).

Katz, L. J., Lee, S. H. S., Rozee, K. R.: Interferon-mediated increased lysis of L-cells by vesicular stomatitis virus. Can. J. Microbiol. **20**, 1077–1083 (1974).

Katz, M., Koprowski, H.: Failure to demonstrate a relationship between scrapie and production of interferon in mice. Nature **219**, 639–640 (1968).

Katz, M., Oyanagi, S., Koprowski, H.: Subacute sclerosing panencephalitis: structures resembling myxovirus nucleocapsids in cell cultured from brains. Nature (London) **222**, 888–889 (1969).

Kaufman, H. E., Centifanto, Y. M., Ellison, E. D., Brown, D. C.: Tilorone hydrochloride: human toxicity and interferon stimulation. Proc. Soc. Exp. Biol. Med. **137**, 357–360 (1971).

Kaufman, H. E., Ellison, E. D., Waltman, S. R.: Double-stranded RNA, an interferon inducer in herpes simplex keratitis. Amer. J. Opthalmol. **68**, 486–490 (1969).

Kaufman, H. E., Mayer, R. F., Laibson, P. R., Waltman, S. R., Nesburn, A. B., Shuster, J. J.: Human leucocyte interferon for the prevention of recurrences of herpetic keratitis. J. Infect. Dis. **133**, A 165–A 169 (1976).

Kauppinen, H.-L., Myllyla, G., Cantell, K.: Large-scale production and properties of human leukocyte interferon used in clinical trials. Proceeding of meeting on Interferon, Lake Placid, New York (1977).

Kawade, Y.: Purification and characterization of mouse L cell interferon. I. Preliminary studies. Jap. J. Microbiol. **17** (2), 129–140 (1973).

Kazár, J.: Interferon-like inhibitor in mouse sera induced by rickettsiae. Acta Virol. **10**, 277 (1966).

Kazár, J.: Multiplication of *Coxiella Burneti* in virus-infected and interferon-treated cell cultures. Acta Virol. **13**, 346–348 (1969).

Kazár, J., Gillmore, J. D., Gordon, F. B.: Effect of interferon and interferon inducers on infections with a nonviral intracellular microorganism, *Chlamydia Trachomatis*. Infect. Immunol. **3**, 825–832 (1971).

Kazár, J., Krautwurst, P. A., Gordon, F. B.: Effect of interferon and interferon inducers on infections with a nonviral intracellular microorganism *Rickettsia akari*. Infect. Immun. **3**, 819–823 (1971).

Ke, Y. H., Armstrong, J. A., Breinig, M. K., Ople, L., Postic, B., Ho, M.: The assay and standardization of rabbit interferon. Symp. Ser. Immunobiol. Stand. (Karger, Basel) **14**, 131–136 (1970).

Ke, Y. H., Ho, M.: Characterization of virus and endotoxin-induced interferons obtained from the serum and urine of rabbits. J. Virol. **1**, 883–890 (1967).

Ke, Y. H., Ho, M.: Studies on the physico-chemical inactivation of rabbit interferons. Proc. Soc. Exp. Biol. Med. **129**, 433–438 (1968).

Ke, Y. H., Ho, M.: Patterns of cycloheximide and puromycin effect on interferon production stimulated by virus or polyribonucleotide in different tissues. Proc. Soc. Exp. Biol. Med. **136**, 365–368 (1971).

Ke, Y. H., Ho, M., Merigan, T. C.: Heterogeneity of rabbit serum interferons. Nature **211**, 541–542 (1966).

Ke, Y. H., Singer, S. H., Postic, B., Ho, M.: Effect of puromycin on virus and endotoxin-induced interferon-like inhibitors in rabbits. Proc. Soc. Exp. Biol. Med. **121**, 181–183 (1967).

Keleti, G., Feingold, D. S. Younger, J. S.: Interferon induction in mice by lipopolysaccharide from *Brucella abortus*. Infect. Immun. **10**, 282–283 (1974).

Keleti, G., Feingold, D. S., Youngner, J. S.: Antitumor activity of a *Brucella abortus* preparation. Infect. Immun. **15**, 846–849 (1977).

Kelly, R. K., Loh, P. C.: Some properties of an established fish cell line from *Xiphophorus helleri* (red swordtail). *In Vitro* **9**, 73–80 (1973).

Kelly, T. A., Levy, H. B.: Lack of uptake of intact polyriboinsinic polyribocytidylic acid by cells. Proc. Soc. Exp. Biol. Med. 114, 534–539 (1973).

Kende, M., Glynn, J. P.: Modification of the response of autochthonous Moloney sarcoma virus-induced tumors to poly-IC by DEAE-dx. Chemotherapy 16, 281–284 (1971).

Kern, E. R., Glasgow, L. A., Overall, J. C., jr.: Antiviral activity of an extract of *Brucella abortus;* induction of interferon and immunopotentiation of host resistance. Proc. Soc. Exp. Biol. Med. 152, 372–379 (1976).

Kern, E. R., Overall, J. C., Glasgow, L. A.: Herpesvirus hominis infection in newborn mice: treatment with interferon inducer poly I. C. Antimicrobial Agents Chemother. 7, 793–798 (1975).

Kern, E. R., Hamilton, J. R., Overall, J. C., Jr., Glasgow, L. A.: Antiviral activity of BL-3849 A, a low-molecular-weight oral interferon inducer. Antimicrobial Agents Chemother. 10, 691–694 (1976).

Kerr, I. M.: Protein synthesis in cell-free systems: an effect of interferon. J. Virol. 7, 448–459 (1971).

Kerr, I. M., Brown, R. E.: ppA 2' p 5' A 2' p 5' A: an inhibitor of protein synthesis synthesized with an enzyme fraction from interferon-treated cells. Proc. Nat. Acad. Sci. 75, 256–260 (1978).

Kerr, I. M., Brown, R. E., Ball, L. A.: Increased sensitivity of cell-free protein synthesis to double-stranded RNA after interferon treatment. Nature 250 (461), 57–59 (1974).

Kerr, I. M., Brown, R. E., Clemens, M. J., Gilbert, C. S.: Interferon mediated inhibition of cell-free protein synthesis in response to double-stranded RNA. Eur. J. Biochem. 69, 551–557 (1976).

Kerr, I. M., Brown, R. E., Hovanessian, A. G.: Nature of inhibitor of cell-free protein synthesis formed in response to interferon and double stranded RNA. Nature 268, 540–542 (1977).

Kerr, I. M., Friedman, R. M., Brown, R. E., Ball, L. A., Brown, J. C.: Inhibition of protein synthesis in cell-free systems from interferon-treated infected cells: further characterization and effect of formylmethionyl tRNAf. J. Virol. 13, 9–21 (1974).

Kerr, I. M., Friedman, R. M., Esteban, R. M., Brown, R. E., Ball, L. A., Metz, D. A., Risby, D., Tovell, D. R., Sonnabend, J. A.: The control of protein synthesis in interferon-treated cells. Adv. Biosci. 11, 109–126 (1973).

Kerr, I. M., Sonnabend, J. A. Martin, E. M.: Protein-synthetic activity of ribosomes from interferon-treated cells. J. Virol. 5, 132–139 (1970).

Khaitovich, A. G., Lvovsky, E. A.: The dynamics of production and some properties of interferon-like inhibitors formed under the influence of AET and Cystaphos *in vivo* and in cell cultures. Vopr. Virusol. 2, 183–186 (1975).

Khesin, Y. A. E., Voronina, F. V., Amchenkova, A. M.: Morphological and histochemical studies on cultures of mouse peritoneal leucocytes during interferon formation. Acta Virol. 14, 445–452 (1970).

Khesin, Y. A. E., Voronina, F. V., Marchenko, V. I., Rusanova, N. A. Balandin, I. G.: Morphological, cytochemical and biochemical changes in peritoneal macrophages (normal, activated and tolerant) in the process of interferon formation. Vopr. Virusol. 18, 302–308 (1973).

Kilbourne, E. D., Smart, K. M., Pokorny, B. A.: Inhibition by cortisone of the synthesis and action of interferon. Nature 190, 650–651 (1961).

Kilham, L., Buckler, C. E., Ferm, V. H., Baron, S.: Production of interferon during rat virus infection. Proc. Soc. Exp. Biol. Med. 129, 274–276 (1968).

Killander, D., Lindahl, P., Lundin, L., Leary, P., Gresser, I.: Relationship between the enhanced expression of histocompatibility antigens on interferon-treated L1210 cells and their position in the cell cycle. Eur. J. Immunol. 6, 56–59 (1976).

Kimball, P. C., Duesberg, P. H.: Virus interference by cellular double-stranded ribonucleic acid. J. Virol. 7, 697–706 (1971).

Kingham, J. G., Ganguly, N. K., Shari, Z. D., Mendelson, R., Cartwright, T., Scott, G. M., Richards, B. M. Wright, R.: Treatment of HBsAgpositive chronic active hepatitis with human fibroblast interferon. Interferon Workshop, Zagreb, Yugoslavia (1977).

Kinkelin, P., Leberre, M.: Hematopoietic infectious necrosis of salmonidae: production of circulating interferon after experimental infection of the rainbow trout. C. R. Acad. Sci. D 279, 445–448 (1974).

Kinkelin, P., Dorson, M.: Interferon production in rainbow trout *(Salmo gairdneri)* experimentally infected with egtved virus. J. Gen. Virol. **19**, 125–127 (1973).

Kirchner, H., Hirt, H. M., Becker, H., Munk, K.: Production of an antiviral factor by murine spleen cells after treatment with *Corynebacterium parvum*. Cell Immunol. **31**, 172–180 (1977).

Kishida, T.: Can interferon be clinically useful? Asian Med. J. **18**, 161–177 (1975).

Kishida, T., Morikawa, K., Ito, M., Yokota, Y.: Influence of interferon on the inhibition by macrophages of the *in vitro* multiplication of murine malignant cells (FM3A). C. R. Soc. Biol. (Paris) **167**, 1503–1505 (1973).

Kishida, T., Toda, S., Toida, T., Hattori, T.: Effect of interferon on malignant mouse cells. C. R. Soc. Biol. (Paris) **165**, 1489–1492 (1971).

Kleinschmidt, W. J.: *In vitro* and *in vivo* studies with statolon against influenza virus. Ann. N. Y. Acad. Sci. **173**, 547–550 (1970).

Kleinschmidt, W. J.: Biochemistry of interferon and its inducers. Ann. Rev. Biochem. **41**, 517–542 (1972).

Kleinschmidt, W. J., Boeck, L. D., Van Frank, R. M., Murphy, E. B., Hull, R. N.: Interferon production by PH16 *Pseudomonas phaseolica* phage and its double-stranded RNA. Proc. Soc. Exp. Biol. Med. **144**, 304–307 (1973).

Kleinschmidt, W. J., Cline, J. C., Murphy, E. B.: Interferon production induced by statolon. Prac. Natl. Acad. Sci. U. S. A. **52**, 741–744 (1964).

Kleinschmidt, W. J., Douthart, R. J., Murphy, E. B.: Interferon production by T4 coliphage. Nature **228**, 27–30 (1970).

Kleinschmidt, W. J., Ellis, L. F. (1967) Statolon as an inducer of interferon, in: Interferon (Wolstenholme, G. E. W., O'Connor, M., eds.), pp. 39–46. London: J. A. Churchill (1967).

Kleinschmidt, W. J., Ellis, L. F., Van Frank, R. M., Murphy, E. B.: Interferon stimulation by a double-stranded RNA of a mycophage in statolon preparations. Nature **220**, 167–168 (1968).

Kleinschmidt, W. J., Murphy, E. B.: Investigations on interferon induced by statolon. Virology **27**, 484–489 (1965).

Kleinschmidt, W. J., Murphy, E. B.: Interferon induction with statolon in the intact animal. Bact. Rev. **31**, 132–137 (1967).

Kleinschmidt, W. J., Streightoff, F.: Inhibition of influenza virus and interferon response intranasally with statolon. Infect. Immun. **4**, 738–741 (1871).

Kleinschmidt, W. J., Van Etten, J. L., Vidaver, A. K.: Influence of molecular weights of phage PHI-6 double-stranded RNA on interferon induction. Infect. Immun. **10**, 284–285 (1973).

Klesel, N., Wolf, W., Miller, G., Jungwirth, C., Bodo, G.: Synthesis of poly (A) sequences in poxvirus-infected cells treated with interferon or poly (rI)-poly (rC). Virology **57**, 570–573 (1974).

Klimpel, G. R., Day, K. D., Lucas, D. O.: Differential production of interferon and lymphotoxin by human tonsil lymphocytes. Cellular Immunol. **20**, 187–189 (1975).

Klimpel, G. R., Dean, J. H., Day, K. D., Chen, P. B., Lucas, D. O.: Lymphotoxin and interferon production by rosette-separated human peripheral blood leukocytes. Cell. Immunol. **32**, 293–297 (1977).

Knight, E., Jr.: Interferon: effect on the saturation density to which mouse cells will grow *in vitro*. J. Cell. Biol. **56**, 846–849 (1973).

Knight, E., Jr.: Interferon-sepharose: induction of the antiviral state. Biochem. Biophys. Res. Commun. **56**, 860–864 (1974a).

Knight, E., Jr.: Interferon-sepharose: priming of L cells for induction of interferon by MM virus. J. Gen. Virol. **25**, 143–145 (1974b).

Knight, E., Jr.: Heterogeneity of purified mouse interferons. J. Biol. Chem. **250**, 4139–4144 (1975).

Knight, E., Jr.: Interferon purification and initial characterization from human diploid cells. Proc. Natl. Acad. Sci., U. S. A. **73**, 520–523 (1976a).

Knight, E., Jr.: Antiviral and cell growth inhibitory activities reside in the same glycoprotein of human fibroblast interferon. Nature **262**, 302–303 (1976b).

Knight, E., Jr.: A multisurface glass roller bottle for growth of animal cells in culture. Appl. Environ. Microbiol. **33**, 666–670 (1977a).

Knight, E., Jr.: Workshop on purification and production of interferons. NIH, March (1977b).

Knight, E., Jr., Korant, B. D.: A cell surface alteration in mouse L cells induced by interferon. Biochem. Biophys. Res. Commun. 74, 707–713 (1977).

Kobayashi, S., Yasui, O., Masuzumi, M.: Studies on early-appearing interferon *in vitro*. I. Production of endotoxin-induced interferon by mouse spleen cells cultured *in vitro*. Proc. Soc. Exp. Biol. Med. 131, 487–490 (1969).

Koblet, H., Kohler, U., Wyler, R.: Interferon assay and kinetics. Pathol. Microbiol. (Basel) 38, 48–49 (1972).

Kobza, K., Emodi, G., Just, M., Hilti, E., Leuenberger, A., Binswanger, U., Thiel, G., Brunner, F. P.: Treatment of herpes infection with human exogenous interferon. Lancet, 1, 1343–1344 (1975).

Kohase, M., Vilček, J.: Regulation of human interferon production stimulated with poly I·poly C: Correlation between shutoff and hyporesponsiveness to reinduction. Virology 76, 47–54 (1977).

Kohn, L. D., Friedman, R. M., Holmes, J. M., Lee, G.: Use of thyrotropin and cholera toxin to probe the mechanism by which interferon initiates its antiviral activity. Proc. Natl. Acad. Sci. U. S. A., 73, 3695–3699 (1976).

Kohno, S., Buckler, C. E., Levy, H. B., Baron, S.: Elution of cell-bound interferon as a cause of development of antiviral activity subsequent to washing of interferon-treated cell culture. IRCS Med. Sci. 3, 57 (1975a).

Kohno, S., Buckler, C. E., Levy, H. B., Baron, S.: Studies on the role of cell-bound interferon in the induction of antiviral activity, in: Effects of Interferon on Cells, Viruses and the Immune System (Geraldes, A., ed.), pp. 123–133. New York: Academic Press (1975b).

Kohno, S., Kohase, M., Sakata, H., Shimizo, Y.: Inhibition of interferon synthesis in phospholipase C treated primary chick embryo cells. Virology 44, 227–238 (1971).

Kohno, S., Kohase, M., Sakata, H., Shimizo, Y., Hikita, M., Shishido, A.: Production of interferon in primary chick embryonic cells infected with *Rickettsia mooseri*. J. Immunol. 105, 1553–1558 (1970).

Kohno, S., Kohase, M., Suganuma, M.: Inhibition of interferon production by chloroquine diphosphate. Jap. J. Med. Sci. Biol. 21, 239–244 (1968).

Kojima, Y., Homma, J. Y., Abe, C.: Property to induce interferon of *Pseudomonoas aeruginosa* endotoxin and its components. Jap. J. Exp. Med. 41, 493–496 (1971).

Kojima, Y., Yoshida, F.: Enhanced production of interferon by temperature shift-down from 37 C to 25 C in rabbit cell cultures stimulated with Newcastle Disease virus. Jap. J. Microbiol. 18, 217–222 (1974).

Kojima, Y., Yoshida, F., Nakase, Y.: Interferon production by *Bordetella pertussis* components in rabbits and in rabbit cell cultures. Jap. J. Microbiol. 17, 160–161 (1973).

Kolot, F. B., Baron, S., Yeagers, H., Schwartz, S. L.: Comparative production of interferon by explanted lymphoreticular tissue and alveolar macrophages from rabbits and humans. Infect. Immun. 13, 63–69 (1976).

Kono, Y.: Interferon-like inhibitor produced in bovine leukocyte cultures after inoculation with endotoxin. Archiv für die gesamte Virusforsch. 21, 276–281 (1967).

Kono, Y., Ho, M.: The role of the reticuloendothelial system in interferon formation in the rabbit. Virology 25, 162–166 (1965).

Korsantiya, B. M., Smorodintsev, A. A.: Transplacental transmission of endogenous interferon in pregnant mice inoculated with influenza or Newcastle Disease viruses. Nature 232, 560–561 (1971).

Korsantiya, B. M., Smorodintsev, A. A., Gvozdilova, D. A.: Some aspects of the interferon-cell interaction. Vopr. Virusol. 9, 1304–1309 (1967).

Kozikowska, E. H., Hahon, N.: Quantitative assay of interferon by the immunofluorescent cell-counting technique. J. Gen. Virol. 4, 441–443 (1969).

Kozikowska, E. H., Hahon, N.: Interferon induction by psittacosis agent in guinea pig leukocyte cultures. Infect. Immun. 2, 731–734 (1970).

Kravchenko, A. T., Voronin, E. S., Kosmiada, N.: Effects of anti-rabies vaccine and fixed rabies virus on the development of tumor caused by Rous sarcoma virus. Acta Virol. 11, 145 (1967).

Kreibich, G., Süss, R., Kinzel, V., Hecker, E.: On the biochemical mechanism of tumorigenesis in mouse skin. III. Decrease in tumor yields by poly I/C administered during initiation of skin by an intragastric dose of 7,12 dimethylbenz[a]anthrancene. Z. Krebsforsch. **74**, 383–386 (1970).

Kreider, J. W., Benjamin, S. A.: Tumor immunity and the mechanism of polynosinic-polycytidylic acid inhibition of tumor growth. J. Natl. Cancer Inst. **49**, 1303–1306 (1972).

Kronenberg, L. H., Friedmann, T.: Relative quantitative assay of the biological activity of interferon messenger RNA. J. Gen., Virol. **27**, 225–232 (1975).

Krueger, R. F., Mayer, G. D.: Tilorone hydrochloride: an orally active antiviral agent. Science **169**, 1213–1214 (1970).

Krueger, R. F., Mayer, G. D., Yoshimura, S., Ludwig, K. A.: *In vivo* evaluations of tilorone hydrochloride against Semliki Forest virus. Antimicrob. Agents Chemotherap. **4**, 486–490 (1971).

Kuehne, R. W., Panier, W. L., Stephen, E. C.: Evaluation of various analogues of tilorone HCl against VEE virus in mice. Antimicrob. Agts. Chemother. **11**, 92–97 (1977).

Kumar, R., Worthington, M., Tilles, J. G., Abelmann, W. H.: Effect of the interferon stimulator polynosinic-polycytidylic acid on experimental *Trypanosoma cruzi* infection. Proc. Soc. Exp. Biol. Med. **137**, 884–888 (1971).

Kunz, C., Hofmann, H.: The influence of the interferon-inducing compound poly I:C on the experimental infection with tick-borne encephalitis (TBE) virus. Zentroblatt für Bacteriologic, Parasitenkunde Infektionskrankheiten und Hygiene, Abt. 1 Referet. **211**, 270–273 (1969).

Kuwata, T., Fuse, A., Morinaga, N.: Effects of interferon on cell and virus growth in transformed human cell lines. J. Gen. Virol. **33**, 7–11 (1976).

Kuwata, T., Fuse, A., Morinaga, N.: Effects of cycloheximide and puromycin on the antiviral and anticellular activities of human interferon. J. Gen. Virol. **37**, 195–198 (1977).

Kuwata, T., Oda, T., Sekiya, S., Morinaga, N.: Characteristics of a human cell line successively transformed by Rous sarcoma virus and Simian virus 40. J. Nat. Cancer Inst. **56**, 919–926 (1976).

Kuznetsov, O. K., Diadikova, A. M., Gvozdilova, D. A., Smorodintsev, A. A.: Interferon and avian leukosis-sarcoma viruses. Vopr. Virusol. **17**, 35–40 (1972).

Lab, M., Koehren, F.: Potentiation of the antiviral action of interferon by cycloheximide. Ann. Inst. Pasteur (Paris) **122**, 567–573 (1972).

Lab, M., Koehren, F.: Maintenance and recovery of the interferon-induced antiviral state. Proc. Soc. Exp. Biol. Med. **153**, 112–118 (1976).

Lab, M. R., Tinland, N., Kirn, A.: Influence de le température sur le développement du virus Sindbis et le production d'interféron en cultures cellulaires. Can. J. Microbiol. **14**, 1211–1226 (1968).

Lackovic, V., Borecky, L.: Interferon-like and antibody substances in mouse peritoneal cells stimulated by myxoviruses *in vivo*. Acta Virol. **9**, 382–399 (1965).

Lackovic, V., Borecky, L.: Peritoneal leukocytes-central role in interferon production. IRCS **2**, 1080–1088 (1974).

Lackovic, V., Borecky, L.: Increased resistance of an interferonresistant cell subline to the toxic effect of double-stranded RNA. Acta Virol. **20**, 347–362 (1976).

Lackovic, V., Borecky, L., Sikl, D., Masler, L., Bauer, S.: The temperature requirement for interferon production by Newcastle disease virus or microbial agents *in vitro*. Acta Virol. **11**, 500–505 (1967).

Lagwinska, E., Stewart, C. C., Adles, C., Schlesinger, S.: Replication of lactic dehydrogenase virus and Sindbis virus in mouse peritoneal macrophages. Induction of interferon and phenotypic mixing. Virology **65**, 204–210 (1975).

Lai, M. H., Joklik, W. K.: The induction of interferon by temperature-sensitive mutants of reovirus, UV-irradiated and subviral reovirus particles. Virology **51**, 191–212 (1973).

Lai, P. K., Alpers, M. P., Mackay–Scollay, E. M.: Epstein–Barr herpesvirus infection: inhibition by immunologically induced mediators with interferon-like properties. Int. J. Cancer **20**, 21–29 (1977).

Lampson, G. P., Field, A. K., Tytell, AH A., Nemes, M. M., Hilleman, M. R.: Relationship of molecular size of rIn:rCn (poly I:C) to induction of interferon and host resistance. Proc. Soc. Exp. Biol. Med. **135**, 911–916 (1970).

Lampson, G. P., Tytell, A. A., Field, A. K., Nemes, M. M., Hilleman, M. R.: Inducers of interferon and host resistance. I. Double-stranded RNA from extracts of *Penicillium funiculosum.* Proc. Nat. Acad. Sci. USA, **58**, 782–789 (1967).

Lampson, G. P., Tytell, A. A., Nemes, M. M., Hilleman, M. R.: Purification and characterization of chick embryo interferon. Proc. Soc. Exp. Biol. Med. **112**, 468–481 (1963).

Lancz, G. J., Johnson, T. C.: Temporal relationship between virus and interferon biosynthesis in L cells infected with Newcastle disease virus. Proc. Soc. Exp. Biol. Med. **132**, 266–269 (1969).

Langston, D. P., Sobin, L. H.: The detection of a virus-interfering substance in the Shope papilloma and the VX 7 and VX 2 carcinoma. J. Exp. Med. **126**, 887–895 (1967).

Larke, R. P.: Interferon production in Powassan virus infections in chickens. Proc. Soc. Exp. Biol. Med. **119**, 1234–1238 (1965).

Larke, R. P. B.: Interferon in the cerebrospinal fluid of children with central nervous system disorders. Can. Med. Assoc. J. **96**, 21–32 (1967).

Larson, V. M., Clark, W. R., Dagle, G. E., Hilleman, M. R.: Influence of synthetic double-stranded ribonucleic acid, poly I:C on Friend leukemia in mice. Proc. Soc. Exp. Biol. Med. **132**, 602–607 (1969).

Larson, V. M., Clark, W. R., Hilleman, M. R.: Influence of synthetic (poly-I. C) and viral double-standard ribonucleic acids on adenovirus 12 oncogenesis in hamsters. Proc. Soc. Exp. Biol. Med. **131**, 1002–1008 (1969).

Larson, V. M., Panteleakis, P. N., Hilleman, M. R.: Influence of synthetic double-stranded ribonucleic acid (poly IC) on SV 40 viral oncogenesis and transplant tumor in hamsters. Proc. Soc. Exp. Biol. Med. **133**, 14–20 (1970).

Larsson, A., Forsgren, M., Hard, S., Strander, H., Cantell, K.: Administration of interferon to an infant with congenital rubella syndrome involving persistent viremia and cutaneous vasculitis. Acta Pediat. Scand. **65**, 105–119 (1976).

Laufs, R., Steinke, H., Jacobs, C., Hilfenhaus, J., Karges, H.: Influence of interferon on the replication of oncogenic herpesvirus in tissue cultures and in nonhuman primates. Med. Microbiol. Immunol. **160**, 235–247 (1974).

Lebleu, B., Sen, G. C., Shaila, S., Cabrer, B., Lengyel, P.: Interferon, double-stranded RNA and protein phosphorylation. Proc. Natl. Acad. Sci. U. S. A. **73**, 3107–3111 (1976).

Lebon, P., Moreau, M. C., Cohen, L., Chany, C.: Different effect of Ouabain on interferon production and action. Proc. Soc. Exp. Biol. Med. **149**, 108–112 (1975).

Lee, S. H. S., O'Saughnessy, M. V., Rozee, K. R., Kind, L. S.: Interferon-induced growth depression in diploid and heteroploid human cells. Proc. Soc. Exp. Biol. Med. **139**, 1438–1440 (1972).

Lee, S. H. S., Ozere, R. L.: Additional studies of interferon production by human leukemic leucocytes *in vitro.* Cancer Res. **29**, 645–659 (1965).

Lee, S. H. S., Ozere, R. L., Van Rooyen, C. E.: Interferon production by human leucocytes *in vitro.* Reduced levels in lymphatic leukemia. Proc. Soc. Exp. Biol. Med. **122**, 32–39 (1966).

Lee, S. H. S., Rozee, K. R.: Enhanced responsiveness of L929 cells treated with interferon to arginine starvation. Exp. Cell Res. **93**, 143–158 (1975).

Lee, S. H. S., Van Rooyen, C. E., Ozere, R. L.: Additional studies of interferon production by human leucocytes *in vitro.* Cancer Res. **29**, 645–664 (1969).

Lefkowitz, E., Baron, S.: Mechanism of late therapy of viral infections with interferon. IRCS **2**, 1518–1522 (1974).

Lefkowitz, E., Worthington, M., Confiffe, M. A., Baron, S.: Comparative effectiveness of six antiviral agents in herpes simplex TYPE I infection of mice. Proc. Soc. Exp. Biol. Med. **152**, 337–352 (1976).

Lefkowitz, S. S.: Drugs of abuse: effects on immunity. Adv. Exp. Med. Biol. **73**, 457–462 (1976).

Lefkowitz, S. S., Hung, C. Y., Geber, W. F.: The effect of psychotomimetic drugs on interferon production. Res. Commun. Chem. Pathol. Pharmacol. **5**, 885–888 (1973).

Lengyel, P., Sen, G. C., Desrosiers, R., Ratner, L., Shaila, S., Brown, G. E., Lebleu, B., Kawakita, M., Cabrer, B., Taira, H., Slattery, E.: Double-stranded RNA and the mechanisms of interferon action. Personal communication (1978).

Lennette, E. H., Koprowski, H.: Interference between viruses in tissue culture. J. Exp. Med. **83**, 195–219 (1946).

Leonard, B. J., Eccleston, E., Jones, D.: Toxicity of interferon inducers of the double-stranded RNA type. Nature **224**, 1023–1024 (1969).

Lerner, A. M., Bailey, E. J.: Synergy of a 9-Beta-D-Arabinofuranosyladenine and human interferon against herpes simplex virus type 1. J. Infect. Dis. **130**, 549–552 (1974).

Lerner, A. M., Bailey, E. J.: Differential sensitivity of herpes simplex Types I and 2 to human interferon: antiviral effects of interferon plus 9-β-B-arabino-furanosyladenine. J. Infect. Dis. **134**, 400–410 (1976).

Leunen, J., Desmyter, J., Desomer, P.: Effects of oxyamylose and polyacrylic acid on foot-and-mouth disease and hog cholera virus infections. Applied Microbiol. **21**, 203–208 (1971).

Levine, D. W., Wong, J. S., Wang, D. I. C., Thilly, W. G.: Microcarrier cell culture: new methods for research scale application. Somatic Cell Genet. **3**, 149–155 (1977).

Levine, S.: Some characteristics of an interferon derived from embryonated eggs infected with Newcastle disease virus. Virology **17** (4), 593–595 (1962).

Levine, S.: Persistence of active interferon in cells washed after treatment with interferon. Proc. Soc. Exp. Biol. Med. **121**, 1041–1045 (1966).

Levine, S., Magee, W. E., Hamilton, R. D., Miller, O. V.: Effect of interferon on early enzyme and viral DNA synthesis in vaccine virus infection. Virology **32**, 33–39 (1967).

Levy, H. B., Asofsky, R., Riley, F., Garapin, A., Cantor, H., Adamson, R.: The mechanism of the antitumor action of poly I:poly C. Ann. N. Y. Acad. Sci. **173**, 640–659 (1970).

Levy, H. B., Axelrod, D., Baron, S.: Messenger RNA for interferon production. Proc. Soc. Exp. Biol. Med. **118**, 384–385 (1965).

Levy, H. B., Baer, G., Baron, S., Buckler, C. E., Gibbs, C. J., Iadarola, M. J., London, W. T., Rice, J.: A modified polyriboinosinic–polyribocytidylic acid complex that induces interferon in primates. J. Infect. Dis. **132**, 434–452 (1975).

Levy, H. B., Baer, G., Baron, S., Gibbs, C. J., Iadarola, M., London, W., Rice, J. M.: Induction of interferon in non-human primates by a nuclease-resistant polyriboinosinic-polyribocytidylic acid complex. IRCS **2**, 1643–1658 (1974).

Levy, H. B., Buckler, C. E., Baron, S.: Effect of interferon on early interferon production. Science **152**, 1274–1276 (1966).

Levy, H. B., Carter, W. A.: Molecular basis of the action of interferon. J. Mol. Biol. **31**, 561–576 (1968).

Levy, H. B., Duenwald, J., Buckler, C. E.: Chlorite-oxidized amylose as an adjuvant for interferon production. Infect. Immun. **7** (3), 457–460 (1973).

Levy, H. B., Law, L. W., Rabson, A. S.: Inhibition of tumor growth by polyinosinic–polycytidylic acid. Proc. Natl. Acad. Sci. U. S. A. **62**, 357–359 (1969).

Levy, H. B., London, W., Fuccillo, D. A., Baron, S., Rice, J.: Prophylactic control of simian hemorrhagic fever in monkeys by an interferon inducer, polyriboinosinic–polyribocytidylic acid-poly-L-lysine. J. Infect. Dis. **133**, A 256 (1976).

Levy, H. B., Merigan, T. C.: Interferon and uninfected cells. Proc. Soc. Exp. Biol. Med. **121**, 53–55 (1966).

Levy, H. B., Riley, F. L.: Effect of interferon treatment on cellular messenger RNA. Proc. Natl. Acad. Sci. U. S. A. **70** (12), 3815–3819 (1973).

Levy, H. B., Snellbaker, L. F., Baron, S.: Studies on the mechanism of action of interferon. Virology **21**, 48–59 (1963).

Levy, H. B., Wheeler, J.: Interferon induction by input virion. Arch. Gesamte Virusforsch. **41**, 150–153 (1973).

Levy, L., Merigan, T. C.: Inhibition of multiplication of *Mycobacterium leprae* by poly I-poly C. Antimicrob. Agts. Chemother. **11**, 122–134 (1977).

Levy, M. H., Wheelock, E. F.: Impaired macrophage function in Friend virus leukemia: restoration by statolon. I. Immunol. **114**, 962–970 (1975).

Levy–Koenig, R. E., Golgher, R. R., Paucker, K.: Immunology of interferons. II. Heterospecific activities of human interferons and their neutralization by antibody. J. Immunol. **104**, 791–797 (1970a).

Levy–Koenig, R. E., Mundy, M. J., Paucker, K.: Immunology of interferons I. Immune response to protective and nonprotective interferons. J. Immunol. **104**, 785–790 (1970b).

Lewis, J. A., Falcoff, E., Falcoff, R.: The molecular mechanism of interferon action. Pathol. Biol. **25**, 9–13 (1977).

Libikova, H.: Lowered susceptibility to exogenous interferon during the first stages of virus infection of cells. Acta Virol. **9**, 279–281 (1965).

Libikova, H.: Interferon in young and aged chick embryo cell cultures infected with herpes simplex and pseudorabies viruses. Acta Virol. **17**, 464–471 (1973).

Libikova, H.: Viral infection and interferon in cell cultures aged *in vitro*. Adv. Exp. Med. Biol. **53**, 469–479 (1975).

Lidin, B., Adams, A.: Spontaneous interferon production and Epstein-Barr virus antigen expression in two human lymphoid cell lines and their somatic cell hybrids. Intervirology **5**, 205–218 (1975).

Lieberman, D., Voloch, Z., Aviv, H., Nudel, V., Revel, M.: Effect of interferon on hemoglobin synthesis and leukemia virus production in Friend cells. Molec. Biol. Res. **1**, 447–454 (1974).

Lieberman, M., Merigan, T. C., Kaplan, H. S.: Inhibition of radiogenic lymphoma development in mice by interferon. Proc. Soc. Exp. Biol. Med. **138**, 575–578 (1971).

Lin, L. S., Stewart II, W. E.: Two dimensional gel electrophoresis of human leukocyte interferon. Abstr. Ann. Meeting Amer. Soc. Biol. Chem. (1978).

Lin, L. S., Wiranowska–Stewart, M., Chudzio, T., Stewart II, W. E.: Characterization of the size and charge heterogeneities of human leukocyte interferon populations. Arch. Virol. **56**, 269–272 (1977).

Lin, L. S., Wiranowska–Stewart, M., Chudzio, T., Stewart II, W. E.: Characterization of the heterogeneous molecules of human interferons: Differences in the cross-species antiviral activities of various molecular populations in human leukocyte interferons. J. Gen. Virol. **39**, 125–130 (1978).

Lin, L. S., Wiranowska–Stewart, M., Stewart II, W. E.: Purification of human leukocyte interferon to apparent homogeneity: Criteria for purity. Abs. Ann. Meeting of Amer. Soc. Microbiol. (1978).

Lindahl, P.: Influence of interferon on normal cell functions. Thesis: Institut de Recherches Scientifiques sur le Cancer, Villejuif, France. Department of Virology, Karolinska Institutet, Stockholm (1974).

Lindahl, P., Gresser, I., Leary, P., Tovey, M.: Enhanced expression of histocompatibility antigens of lymphoid cells in mice treated with interferon. J. Infect. Disease **133**, A 66–A 72 (1976 a).

Lindahl, P., Gresser, I., Leary, P., Tovey, M.: Interferon treatment of mice-enhanced expression of histocompatibility antigens on lymphoid cells. Proc. Nat. Acad. Sci. U. S. A. **73**, 1284–1299 (1976 b).

Lindahl, P., Leary, P., Gresser, I.: Enhancement by interferon of the specific cytotoxicity of sensitized lymphocytes. Proc. Natl. Acad. Sci. U. S. A. **69**, 721–725 (1972).

Lindahl, P., Leary, P., Gresser, I.: Enhancement by interferon of the expression of surface antigens on murine leukemia L1210 cells. Proc. Natl. Acad. Sci. U. S. A., **70**, 2785–2788 (1973).

Lindahl, P., Leary, P., Gresser, I.: Enhancement of the expression of histocompatibility antigens of mouse lymphoid cells by interferon *in vitro*. Europ. J. Immunol. **4**, 779–794 (1974).

Lindahl–Magnusson, P., Leary, P., Gresser, I.: Interferon and cell division. VI. Inhibitory effect of interferon on the multiplication of mouse embryo and mouse kidney cells in primary cultures. Proc. Soc. Exp. Biol. Med. **138**, 1044–1050 (1971).

Lindahl–Magnusson, P., Leary, P., Gresser, I.: Interferon inhibits DNA synthesis induced in mouse lymphocyte suspensions by phytohaemagglutinin or by allogenic cells. Nature New Biol. **237**, 120–121 (1972).

Lindenmann, J.: Neuere aspekte der virus-interferenz. Ergeb. Microbiol. Immunitaetsforsch. **33**, 369–373 (1960).

Lindenmann, J., Burke, D., Isaacs, A.: Studies on the production, mode of action and properties of interferon. Brit. J. Exp. Path. **38**, 551–562 (1957).

Lindenmann, J., Gifford, G. E.: Studies on vaccinia virus plaque formation and its inhibition by interferon. III. A simplified plaque inhibition assay of interferon. Virology **19** (3), 302–309 (1963 a).

Lindenmann, J., Gifford, G. E.: Studies on vaccinia virus plaque formation and its inhibition by interferon. I. Dynamics of plaque formation by vaccinia virus. Virology **19**, 283–293 (1963 b).

Lindh, H. F., Lindsay, H. L., Mayberry, B. R., Forbes.: Polyinosinic-cytidylic acid complex (poly I:C) and viral infections in mice. Proc. Soc. Exp. Biol. Med. **132**, 83–87 (1969).

Lindner–Frimmel, S. J.: Enhanced production of human interferon by UV-irradiated cells. J. Gen. Virol. **25**, 147–150 (1974).

Lindsay, H. L., Trown, P. W., Brandt, J., Forbes, M.: Pyrogenicity of Poly I: Poly C in rabbits. Nature (London) **223**, 717 (1969).

Link, F., Blaskovic, D., Raus, J.: Effect of an exogenous interferon on experimental influenza virus infection and interferon production in white mice. Nature **197**, 821 (1963).

Link, F., Blaskovic, D., Raus, J.: Virus multiplication and interferon formation in lungs' from mice infected with A₂ influenza virus. Acta Virol. **9**, 380–390 (1965).

Link, F., Blaskovic, D., Raus, J., Albrecht, P.: Investigations into the adaptation of a neurovaccinia virus to mouse lungs. Acta Virol. **9**, 323–342 (1965).

Link, F., Szanto, J., Blaskovic, D., Raus, J., Dobrocka, E., Pristasova, S.: Interaction of heart glycosides and viruses. Acta Virol. **10**, 455–472 (1966).

Lobodzinska, M., Biernacka, I., Skurska, Z.: Rat interferon. I. Biological properties of interferons in rat serum. Arch. Immunol. Ther. Exp. (Warsz.) **21**, 461–469 (1973 a).

Lobodzinska, M., Biernacka, I., Skurska, Z.: Rat interferons. III. Antiviral activity and effect of priming on interferon production in homologous and heterologous cell lines. Arch. Immunol. Ther. Exp. (Warsz.) **23**, 225–231 (1975).

Lobodzinska, M., Sypula, A., Zielinska, J., Szpila–Stankiewicz, K., Kidankiewicz, T., Skurska, Z.: Characterization of NDV strains used as interferon inductors in mouse embryonic cell cultures. Arch. Immunol. Ther. Exp. (Warsz.) **21**, 209–218 (1973 b).

Lockart, R. Z., jr.: Production of an interferon by L cells infected with WEE virus. J. Bact. **85**, 556–566 (1963).

Lockart, R. Z., jr.: The necessity for cellular RNA and protein synthesis for viral inhibition from interferon. Biochem. Biophys. Res. Commun. **15**, 513–518 (1964).

Lockart, R. Z., jr.: Variations in the abilities of several lines of L cells to produce and to be affected by interferon. J. Bacterial **89**, 117–122 (1965).

Lockart, R. Z., jr.: Biological properties of interferons: criteria for acceptance of a viral inhibition as an interferon, in: Interferons (Finter, N. B., ed.), p. 1. Amsterdam: North Holland Publ. Co. (1966).

Lockart, R. Z., jr.: Analysis of additional interference occurring after the removal of interferon. J. Virol. **1**, 1158–1163 (1967).

Lockart, R. Z., jr.: Viral interferons in aged cultures of chick embryo cells, in: Medical and Applied Virology (Saunders, M., Lennette, E. H., eds.), pp. 45–55. St. Louis, Mo.: W. H. Green (1968).

Lockart, R. Z., jr.: Criteria for acceptance of a viral inhibitor as an interferon and a general description of the biological properties of known interferons, in: Interferons and Interferon Inducers (Finter, N. B., ed.), pp. 11–27. Amsterdam: North Holland Publ. Co. (1973).

Lockart, R. Z., jr., Bayliss, N. L., Toy, S. T., Yin, F. H.: Viral events necessary for the induction of interferon in chick embryo cells. J. Virol. **2**, 962–965 (1968).

Lockart, R. Z., jr., Horn, B.: Interaction of interferon with L cells. J. Bact. **85**, 996–1002 (1963).

Lockart, R. Z., jr., Sreevalsan, T.: A comparison of methods for interferon assay. Virology **17** (1), 207–208 (1962).

Lockart, R. Z., jr., Streevalsan, T., Horn, B.: Inhibition of viral RNA synthesis by interferon. Virology **18** (3), 493–494 (1962).

Lodmell, D. L., Ewalt, L. C., Notkins, A. L.: Inhibition of vaccinia virus replication in skin of tuberculin-sensitized animals challenged with PPD. J. Immunol. **117**, 1757 (1976).

Lodmell, D. L., Notkins, A. L.: Cellular immunity to herpes simplex virus mediated by interferon. J. Exp. Med. **140**, 764–778 (1974).

Lomniczi, B.: Factors influencing the interferon production of Aujeszky's disease (pseudorabies) virus. Arch. Ges. Virusforsch. **44**, 150–152 (1974 a).

Lomniczi, B.: Biological properties of Aujeszky's disease (pseudorabies) virus strains with special regard to interferon production and sensitivity. Arch. Ges. Virusforsch. **44**, 205–214 (1974 b).

Lomniczi, B., Burke, D. C.: Interferon production by temperature-sensitive mutants of Semliki Forest virus. J. Gen. Virol. **8**, 55–68 (1970).

Lonai, P., Steinman, L.: Physiological regulation of antigen binding to T cells: Role of a soluble macrophage factor and of interferon. Proc. Nat. Acad. Sci. **74**, 5662–5666 (1977).

Long, W. F., Burke, D. C.: Interferon production by double-stranded RNA: a comparison of induction by reovirus to that by a synthetic double-stranded polynucleotide. J. Gen. Virol. 12, 1–11 (1971).

Luby, J. P., Sanders, C. V., Sulkin, S. E.: Interferon assays and quantitative virus determinations in a fatal infection in man with westernequine encephalomyelitis virus. Am. J. Trop. Med., Hyg. 20, 765–769 (1971).

Luby, J. P., Stewart II, W. E., Sulkin, S. E., Sanford, J. P.: Interferon in human infections with St. Louis encephalitis virus. Ann. Int. Med. 71, 703–710 (1969).

Lukas, B., Hruskova, J.: A virus inhibitor circulating in the blood of chickens induced by Francisella tularensis and Listeria monocytogenes. Folio Microbiol. 12, 157–160 (1967).

Lukas, B., Hruskova, J.: In vivo induction of an interferon-like inhibitor by kanamycin. Acta Virol. 12, 263–266 (1968).

Lvovsky, E., Levy, H. B.: Interferon assay of high sensitivity. Proc. Soc. Exp. Biol. Med. 153, 511–514 (1976).

Lvovsky, E., Levy, H. B., Doherty, D. G., Baron, S.: Interferon induction by radioprotective mercaptoalkylamines and derived th ophosphates. Infect. Immun. 15, 191–211 (1977).

Lwoff, A.: Death and transfiguration of a problem. Bact. Rev. 33, 390–420 (1969).

Lysov, V. V., Aksenon, O. A., Rudenko, V. I., Moshkin, S. A., Yurlova, T. I., Smorodintsev, A. A., Selivanon, A. A.: Interference activity and sensitivity to interferon of original and cold strains of adenovirus types 1 and 2. Acta Virol. 15, 387–392 (1971).

Maciera–Coelho, A., Brouty–Boye, D., Thomas, M. T., Gresser, I.: Interferon and cell division III. Effect of interferon on the division cycle of L1210 cells in vitro. J. Cell. Biol. 48, 415–419 (1971).

Maehara, N., Ho, M.: Cellular origin of interferon induced by bacterial lipopolysaccharide. Infect. Immun. 15, 78–85 (1977).

Maehara, N., Ho, M., Armstrong, J. A.: Differences in mouse interferons according to cell source and mode of induction. Infect. Immun. 17, 572–579 (1977).

Maehara, N., Nagano, Y.: Heat-labile virus-inhibiting factor or interferon induced by virus. Jap. J. Microbiol. 14, 257–260 (1970).

Maehara, N., Nagano, Y.: Formation of virus-inhibiting factor or interferon in splenectomized mice. Jap. J. Microbiol. 16, 469–474 (1972).

Maenner, H., Brandner, G.: Interferon action may not be effected by induction of a cellular ribonuclease. Nature 260, 637–645 (1976).

Maeno, K., Yoshii, S., Nagata, I., Matsumoto, T.: Growth of Newcastle disease virus in HVJ carrier culture of HeLa cells. Virology 29, 255–269 (1966).

Magee, W. E., Griffith, M. J.: The liver as a site for interferon production in response to poly I:poly C. Life Sciences 11 (part II), 1081–1087 (1972).

Magee, W. E., Levine, S., Miller, O. V., Hamilton, R. D.: Inhibition by interferon of the uncoating of vaccinia virus. Virology 35, 505–512 (1968).

Magee, W. E., Talcott, M. J., Strau, S. X., Vriend, C. Y.: A comparison of negatively and positively charged lysosomes containing entrapped pIC for interferon induction in mice. B. B. A. 451, 610–621 (1976).

Mahdy, M. S., Ho, M.: Potentiating effect of fractions of Eastern equine encephalomyelitis virus or interferon production. Proc. Soc. Exp. Biol. Med. 116, 174–187 (1964).

Majer, M., Weinman, N., Hilfenhaus, J.: The role of interferon in the prevention and treatment of rabies. Symp. on Prep. Stand. and Clin. Use of Interferon, Zagreb, Yugoslavia (1977).

Malucci, L.: Mouse hepatitis virus and interferon production in normal and regenerating liver. Arch. Ges. Virusforsch. 15, 91–97 (1964).

Manders, E. K., Tilles, J. G., Huang, A. S.: Interferon-mediated inhibition of virion-directed transcription. Virology 49, 573–581 (1972).

Marchenko, V. I., Povolotsky, A. L., Krivokhatskaya, L. D.: Interferon-producing capacity of human tonsil cells and properties of interferon produced by these cells. Acta Virol. 20, 114–127 (1976a).

Marchenko, V. I., Pokidysheva, L. N., Zubanova, N. A., Voronina, E. V.: The causes of decrease in resistance to Krebs-2 ascitic carcinoma in mice in the state of hyporesponsiveness (tolerance) to virus interferon inducer. Vopr. Virusol. 2, 176–189 (1976b).

Marcus, P. I., Carver, D. H.: Hemadsorption-negative plaque test: new assay for rubella revealing a unique interference. Science **149**, 983–986 (1965).

Marcus, P. I., Carver, D. H.: Intrinsic interference: a new type of viral interference. J. Virol. **1**, 334–343 (1967).

Marcus, P. I., Engelhardt, D. L., Hunt, J. M., Sekellick, M. J.: Interferon action: inhibition of vesicular stomatitis virus RNA synthesis induced by virion-bound polymerase. Science **174**, 593–598 (1971).

Marcus, P. I., Salb, J. M.: Molecular basis of interferon action: inhibition of viral RNA translation. Virology **30**, 502–516 (1966).

Marcus, P. I., Salb, J. M.: On the translation inhibitory protein of interferon action, in: The Interferons (Rita, G., ed.), p. 111. New York: Academic Press (1968).

Marcus, P. I., Sekellick, M. J.: Cell killing by viruses. III. The interferon system and inhibition of cell killing by vesicular stomatitis virus. Virology **69**, 378–393 (1976).

Marcus, P. I., Sekellick, M. J.: Defective interfering particles with covalently linked (±) RNA induce interferon. Nature **226**, 815–818 (1977).

Marcus, P. I., Terry, T. M., Levine, S.: Interferon action. II. Membrane-bound alkaline ribonuclease activity in chick embryo cells manifesting interferon-mediated interference. Proc. Nat. Acad. Sci. U. S. A., **72**, 182–186 (1975).

Margolis, S. A., Oie, M., Levy, H. B.: The effect of interferon, interferon inducers or interferon-induced virus resistance on subsequent interferon production. J. Gen. Virol. **15** (2), 119–128 (1972).

Markovits, P., Coppey, J.: Induction of interferon in cells of chicken infected with a DNA virus. C. R. Acad. Sci. (Paris) **D 273**, 1076–1079 (1971).

Marshall, L. W., Pitha, P. M., Carter, W. A.: Inactivation of interferon: the effect of protonation. Virology **48** (2), 607–611 (1972).

Martelly, I., Bailey, D. W., DeMaeyer-Guignard, J.: Poids moléculaires de l'interféron sérique induit par le virus de la maladie de Newcastle dans des lignes de souris hautes et basses productrices. Ann. Inst. Pasteur **123**, 835–848 (1972).

Martelly, I., Jullien, P.: Effect of repeated injections of polyriboinosinic–polyribocytidilic acid on mouse hematopoietic stem cells. J. Nat. Cancer Institut. **53**, 1021–1028 (1974).

Martin, E. M., Sonnabend, J. A.: Ribonucleic acid polymerase synthesis of double-stranded arbovirus ribonucleic acid. J. Virol. **1**, 97–109 (1967).

Matarese, G. P., Rossi. G. B.: Effect of interferon on growth and division cycle of Friend erythroleukemic murine cells *in vitro*. J. Cell Biol. **75**, 334–354 (1977).

Mathe, G.: Active immunotherapy. Adv. Cancer Res. **14**, 1–17 (1971).

Mathe, G., Amiel, L., Schwarzenberg, L., Schneider, M., Hayat, M., DeVassal, F., Jasmin, C., Rosenfeld, C., Sakouhi, M., Choay, J.: Remission induction with poly IC in patients with acute lymphoblastic leukaemia. Europ. J. of Clin. and Biol. Res. **15**, 671–684 (1970).

Matisova, E., Butorova, E., Lackovic, V., Borecky, L.: Some properties of interferon released by mouse peritoneal leukocytes stimulated with endotoxin, mannan and Newcastle disease virus *in vitro*. Acta Virol. **14**, 1–7 (1970).

Matsuda, S., Kida, M., Shirafuji, H., Yoneda, M., Yadi, H.: Induction of interferon and host resistance *in vivo* by double-stranded complexes of copoly-ribonucleotide of inosinic acid and guanylic with polyribocytidylic acid. Arch. Ges. Virusforsch. **34**, 105–118 (1971).

Matsuno, T., Shirasawa, N., Kohno, S.: Interferon suppresses glutamine synthetase induction in chick embryonic neural retina. Biochem. Biophys. Res. Commun. **70**, 310–320 (1976).

Matsuo, A., Hayashi, S., Kishida, T.: Production and purification of human leukocyte interferon. Jap. J. Microbiol. **18**, 21–27 (1974).

Matsuzawa, T., Kawade, Y.: Cell growth inhibitory activity of electrophoretic fractions of L-cell interferon preparation. Acta. Virol. **18**, 383–390 (1974).

May, D. C., Stanton, G. J.: The effect of cell age on the production and assay of interferon by Sindbis virus and WEE in chick embryo cells. Tex. Rep. Biol. Med. **32**, 875–876 (1974).

Mayer, G. D., Krueger R. F.: Tilorone hydrochloride: mode of action. Science **169**, 1214–1215 (1970).

Mayer, V.: Interaction of mammalian cells with tick-borne encephalitis virus. Acta Virol. **6**, 317–326 (1962).

Mayer, V., Dobrocka, E.: Reproduction of tick-borne encephalitis virus and inhibition of formation and action of interferon in the presence of deuterium oxide. Acta Virol. **12**, 247–256 (1968).

Mayer, V., Sokol, F., Vilček, J.: Effect of interferon on the infection with Eastern equine encephalomyelitis (EEE) virus and its ribonucleic acid (RNA). Acta Virol. **5**, 264–278 (1961).

Mayer, V., Sokol, F., Vilček, J.: Infection of interferon-treated cells with Eastern equine encephalomyelitis virus and its ribonucleic acid. Virology **16** (4), 359–362 (1962).

Mayer, V., Stancek, D., Doskocil, J.: Distribution of doublestranded f 2 phage RNA in mouse tissue after intraperitoneal administration. Acta Virol. **20**, 169–174 (1976).

Mayhew, E., Papahadjopoulos, D., O'Malley, J. A., Carter, W. A., Vail, W. J.: Cellular uptake and protection against virus infection by poly IC entrapped within phospholipid vesicles. Mol. Pharmacol. **13**, 488–495 (1977).

Mayr, U., Bermayer, H. P., Weidinger, G., Jungwirth, C., Gross, H. J., Bodo, G.: Release of interferon-induced translation inhibition by tRNA in cell-free extracts from mouse erythroleukemia cells. Eur. J. Biochem. **72**, 541–552 (1977).

Mazzur, S. R., Ellsworth, B., Paucker, K.: Studies on the effect of interferon on the formation of antibody in mouse spleen cells. I. survival of spleen cells in culture and preservation of cellular function. J. Immunol. **98**, 683–688 (1967).

Mazzur, S. R., Paucker, K.: Studies on the effect of interferon on the formation of antibody in mouse spleen cells. II. The effect of interferon on antibody plaque formation and antibody production by transferred spleen cells. J. Immunol. **98**, 689–696 (1967).

McCullough, B.: Interferon response in cats. J. Infect. Dis. **125**, 174–179 (1972).

McGill, J. I., Collins, P., Cantell, K., Jones, B. R., Finter, N. B.: Optimal schedules for use of interferon in the corneas of rabbits with herpes simplex keratitis. J. Infect. Diseas. **133**, A 13–A 19 (1976).

McIntyre, O. R., Rai, K., Glidewell, O., Holland, J. F.: Poly IC as adjunct to remission maintenance therapy in acute myelogenous leukemia, in: Immunotherapy of Cancer: Present status of Trials in Man (Terry, W. D., Windhorst, D., eds.). New York: Raven Press (1977).

McKimm, J., Rapp, F.: Variation in ability of measles virus plaque progeny to induce interferon. Proc. Natl. Acad. Sci. U. S. A. **74**, 3056–3061 (1977 a).

McKimm, J., Rapp, F.: Inability of measles virus temperature sensitive mutants to induce interferon. Virology **76**, 409–421 (1977 b).

McLaren, C.: Influence of cell age on production and assay of mouse interferon in L-cells. Archiv. für die gesamte Virusforsch. **32**, 13–18 (1970).

McManus, N. H.: Microtiter assay for interferon: microspectrophotometric quantitation of cytopathic effect. App. Envir. Microbiol. **31**, 35–47 (1976).

McNeil, T. A.: Release of bone marrow colony stimulating activity during immunological reactions *in vitro*. Nature New Biol. **244**, 175–178 (1973).

McNeil, T. A., Fleming, W. A.: The relationship between serum interferon and an inhibitor of mouse haemopoietic colonies *in vitro*. Immunology **21**, 761–766 (1971).

McNeill, T. A., Fleming, W. A., McCance, D. J.: Interferon and haemopoietic colony inhibitor responses to poly I·poly C in rabbits and hamsters. Immunology **22**, 711–721 (1972).

McNeill, T. A., Gresser, I.: Inhibition of haemopoietic colony growth by interferon preparations from different sources. Nature New Biol. **244**, 173–174 (1973).

McVicar, J. W., Richmond, J. Y., Campbell, C. H., Hamilton, L. D.: Observation of cattle, goats and pigs after administration of synthetic interferon inducers and subsequent exposure to foot and mouth disease virus. Can. J. Comp. Med. **37**, 362–374 (1973).

McWilliams, M., Finkelstein, M. S., Allen, P. T., Giron, D. J.: Assay of chick interferons by the inhibition of viral ribonucleic acid synthesis. Applied. Microbiol. **21**, 959–961 (1971).

Meager, A., Burke, D. C.: Production of interferon by ultraviolet radiation inactivated NDV. Nature **235**, 280–282 (1972).

Mecs, I.: Inhibition of interferon action and production by adenine. Acta. Virol. **8**, 475–488 (1964).

Mecs, I., Sonnabend, J. A., Martin, E. M., Fantes, K. H.: The effect of interferon on the synthesis of RNA in chick cells infected with Semliki Forest virus. J. Gen. Virol. **1**, 25–40 (1967).

Mecs, I., Ganti, T., Kotai, A.: Enhancement of interferon induction in mice by polycationic modified polypeptides. Acta. Virol. **20**, 164–173 (1976).

Mecs, I., Kasler, M., Lozosa, A., Kovacs, G.: Metabolic effect of interferon preparations and some interferon inducers: Activation of adenylate cyclase system. Acta. Microbiol. Acad. Sci., Hung. **21**, 265–268 (1974).

Mecs, I., Rosztoczy, I.: Physical and biological properties of DEAE-dextran-polyriboinosinic:polyribocytidylic acid complex. Acta. Virol. **15**, 280–285 (1971).

Meindl, P., Bodo, G., Huppy, H.: Synthetic low-molecular weight interferon inducers: derivatives of diaminofluoren-9-one, diamino-benzophenone and diaminobiphenyls. Arzneimittel-Forschung **26**, 312–318 (1976).

Meldolesi, M. F., Friedman, R. M., Kohn, L. D.: An interferon-induced increase in cyclic AMP levels precedes the establishment of the antiviral state. Biochem. Biophys. Res. Commun. **79**, 239–246 (1977).

Mendelson, J., Glasgow, L.: The *in vitro* and *in vivo* effects of cortisol on interferon production and action. J. Immunol. **96**, 345–362 (1966).

Mendelson, J., Kapusta, R., Dick, J.: Maternal and fetal interferon production in the rat. American J. of Obstetrics and Gynecology **107**, 902–907 (1970).

Menezes, J.: Interferon production by Sendai virus-treated hamster and monkey cells. Experientia **28**, 1477–1479 (1972).

Menezes, J., Patel, P., Dussault, H., Joncas, J., Leibold, W.: Effect of interferon on lymphocyte transformation and nuclear antigen production by Epstein-Barr virus. Nature **260**, 430–432 (1976).

Mentkevich, L. M., Orlova, T. G., Shcheglovitova, O. N.: Interferon production and infection caused by influenza virus in radiation chimeras. Acta. Virol. **17**, 435–438 (1973).

Mentkevich, L. M., Orlova, T. G., Shcheglovitova, O. N., Solovyov, V. D.: Interferon production and infection caused by vesicular stomatitis virus in radiation chimeras. Acta. Virol. **17**, 157–162 (1973).

Mentkevich, L. M., Shcheglovitova, O. N.: Influence of radiation and subsequent bone marrow transplantation on the production of serum and cellular interferon in CBA mice. Vopr. Virusol. **3**, 776–779 (1974).

Mentkevich, L. M., Shcheglovitova, O. N., Amchenkova, A. M.: Species specificity of interferon-indicator of chimerism of the hematopoietic tissues of radiation chimeras. Radiobiologiia **14**, 293–294 (1974).

Mentkevich, L. M., Shcheglovitova, O. N., Orlova, T. G.: Production of interferon induced by viruses and poly I:poly C in radiation chimeras. Acta Virol. **18**, 261–263 (1974).

Mentkevich, L. M., Zhdanova, L. V.: Effect of heparin on reproduction of, and interferon production and interference by, Newcastle disease virus in chick embryo cell cultures. Acta Virol. **15**, 233–236 (1971).

Merigan, T. C.: Purified interferons: physical properties and species specificity. Science **145**, 811–813 (1964).

Merigan, T. C.: Induction of circulating interferon by synthetic anionic polymers of known composition. Nature **214**, 416–418 (1967 a).

Merigan, T. C.: Various molecular species of interferon induced by viral and non-viral agents. Bact. Rev. **31**, 138–144 (1967 b).

Merigan, T. C.: Interferon's promise in clinical medicine: fact or fancy? Am. J. Medicine **43**, 817–821 (1967 c).

Merigan, T. C.: Interferon stimulated by double-stranded RNA. Nature **228**, 219–222 (1970).

Merigan, T. C.: Non-viral substances inducing interferon, in: Interferons and Interferon Inducers (Finter, N. B., ed.), pp. 45–77. Amsterdam: North-Holland Publ. Co. (1973).

Merigan, T. C., Chester, T. J., Paucker, K., in: Effects of Interferon on Cells, Viruses and the Immune System (Geraldes, A., ed.), pp. 347–388. London: Academic Press (1975).

Merigan, T. C., Finkelstein, M. S.: Interferon-stimulating and *in vivo* antiviral effects of various synthetic anionic polymers. Virology **35**, 363–374 (1968).

Merigan, T. C., Hanna, L.: Characteristic of interferon induced *in vitro* and *in vivo* by a TRIC agent. Proc. Soc. Exp. Biol. Med. **122**, 421–424 (1966).

Merigan, T. C., Jordan, G. W., Fried, R. P.: Clinical utilization of exogenous human interferon. Perspectives in Virology **9** (Pollard, M., ed.), p. 249. Academic Press (1975).

Merigan, T. C., Kleinschmidt, W. J.: Different molecular species of mouse interferon induced by statolon. Nature **208**, 667–669 (1965).

Merigan, T. C., Kleinschmidt, W., J.: A second molecular species of mouse interferon in statolon-injected mice. Nature **212**, 1383–1384 (1966).

Merigan, T. C., Oldstone, M. B. A., Walsh, R. M.: Interferon production during lymphocytic choriomeningitis virus infection of nude and normal mice. Nature **268**, 67–68 (1977).

Merigan, T. C., Pollard, R. B., Robinson, W. S., Gregory, P., Greenberg, H., Smith, J., Neal, A., Rand, K., Arvin, A., Breeden, J.: Clinical experiences with human interferon application in man. Fifth Aharon Katzir–Katchalsky Conference, Rehovot, Israel (1977).

Merigan, T. C., Reed, S. E., Hall, T. S., Tyrrell, D. A. J. (1973a). Inhibition of respiratory virus infection by locally applied interferon. Lancet **1** (803), 563–567 (1973).

Merigan, T. C., Regelson, W.: Interferon induction in man by a synthetic polyanion of defined composition. N. Eng. J. Med. **227**, 1283–1285 (1967).

Merigan, T. C., Rottman, F.: Influence of increasing 2'-O-methylation on the interferon stimulating capacity of poly (rI)-poly (rC). Virology **60**, 297–301 (1974).

Merigan, T. C., Stevens, D. A., Rasmussen, L., Epstein, L. B.: Interferon: an immune-specific or non-specific host defense? in: Reexamination of non-specific factors influencing host resistance (Braun, W., Ungar, J., eds.), p. 430. Basel: Karger (1973b).

Merigan, T. C., Waddell, D., Grossman, M., Ritchie, Y. H., Mo, G.: Modified skin lesions during concurrent varicella and measles infections. J. Amer. Med. Assn. **240**, 333–347 (1968).

Merigan, T. C., Winget, C. A., Dixon, C. B.: Purification and characterization of vertebrate interferons. J. Mol. Biol. **13**, 679–691 (1965).

Metz, D.: Interferon and interferon inducers. Advances in Drug Research, Vol. **10** (Simmonds, Alma B., ed.), pp. 101–124. Academic Press (1975a).

Metz, D. H.: The mechanism of action of interferon. Cell **6**, 429–457 (1975b).

Metz, D. H., Esteban, M.: Interferon inhibits viral protein synthesis in L-cells infected with vaccinia virus. Nature **238**, 385–388 (1972).

Metz, D. H., Esteban, M., Danielescu, G.: The effect of interferon on the formation of virus polyribosomes in L-cells infected with vaccinia virus. J. Gen. Virol. **27**, 197–213 (1975).

Metz, D. H., Levin, M. Y., Oxman, M. N.: Mechanism of interferon action: Further evidence for transcription as the primary site of action in simian virus 40 infection. J. Gen. Virol. **32**, 227–241 (1976).

Metz, D. H., Oxman, M. N., Levin, M. J.: Interferon inhibits the *in vitro* accumulation of virus specific RNA in nuclei isolated from SV40 in fected cells. Biochem. Biophys. Res. Commun. **75**, 172–188 (1977).

Michaels, R. H., Weinberger, M. M., Ho, M.: Circulating interferon-like viral inhibitor in patients with meningitis due to *Haemophilus influenzae*. New. Engl. J. Med. **272**, 1148–1162 (1965).

Mills, J., Kirk, J. E. V., Wright, P. F., Chanock, R. M.: Experimental respiratory syncytial virus infection of adults. J. Immunol. **107**, 123–136 (1971).

Milstone, L. M., Waksman, B. H.: Release of virus inhibitors from tuberculin-sensitized peritoneal cells stimulated by antigen. J. Immunol. **105**, 1068–1079 (1970).

Miner, A. N., Koehler, J.: Pyran: mode of action *in vivo*. Bacteriol. Proc., p. 150 (1969).

Miner, N., Ray, W. J., jr., Simon, E. M.: Effect of interferon on the production and action of viral RNA polymerase. Biochem. Biophys. Res. Comm. **24**, 264–268 (1966).

Minnefor, A. B., Halsted, C. C., Seto, D. S., Glade, P. R., Moore, G. E., Carver, D. H.: Production of interferon by long-term suspension cultures of leukocytes derived from patients with viral and non-viral diseases. J. Infect. Dis. **121**, 442–451 (1970).

Mobraaten, L. E., DeMaeyer, E., DeMaeyer–Guignard, J.: Prolongation of allograft survival in mice by inducers of interferon. Transplantation **16**, 415–431 (1973).

Moehring, J. M., Forsyth, B. R.: The role of the interferon-system in respiratory syncytial virus infections. Proc. Soc. Exp. Biol. Med. **138**, 1009–1014 (1971).

Moehring, J. M., Stinebring, W. R.: Examination of species specificity of avian interferons. Nature **226**, 360–361 (1970).

Moehring, J. M., Stinebring, W. R.: Prolonged application of interferon and "aging" of human diploid fibroblast. Proc. Soc. Exp. Biol. Med. **137**, 191–193 (1971).

Moehring, J. M., Stinebring, W. R., Merchant, D. J.: Survey of interferon production and sensitivity of human cell lines. Appl. Microbiol. **22**, 102–105 (1971).

Moehring, T. J., Moehring, J. M., Stinebring, W. R.: Response of interferon treated cells to diphtheria toxin. Infect. Immun. **4**, 747–752 (1971).

Mogensen, K. E., Cantell, K.: Stability of human leukocyte interferon towards heat. Acta. Pathol. Microbiol. Scand. **B 81**, 382–383 (1973).

Mogensen, K. E., Cantell, K.: Loss of specific antigenicity on carboxymethylation of mercaptoethanol-reduced interferon of human leukocyte origin. Intervirology 2, 52–55 (1973–1974).

Mogensen, K. E., Cantell, K.: Human leukocyte interferon: a role for disulphide bonds. J. Gen. Virol. 22, 95–103 (1974).

Mogensen, K. E., Cantell, K.: Production and preparation of human leukocyte interferon. Pharmacology and Therapeutics 1, 369–383 (1977).

Mogensen, K. E., Pyhala, L.: Cantell, K.: Raising antibodies to human leukocyte interferon. Acta Pathol. Microbiol. Scand. 83, 443–458 (1975).

Mogensen, K. E., Pyhala, L., Torma, E., Cantell, K.: No evidence for carbohydrate moiety affecting the clearance of circulating human leukocyte interferon in rabbits. Acta Pathol. Microbiol. Scand. B 82, 305–310 (1974).

Mohr, S. J., Brown, D. G., Coffey, D. S.: Size requirement of polyinosinic acid for DNA synthesis, viral resistance, and increased survival of leukaemic mice. Nature New Biol. 240, 250–251 (1972).

Molomut, N., Padnos, M.: Inhibition by transplantable and spontaneous murine tumors by the M-P virus. Nature (Lond.) 208, 948–950 (1965).

Monath, T. P., Borden, E. C.: Effects of thorotrast on humoral antibody, viral multiplication and interferon during infection with St. Louis encephalitis virus. J. Infect. Dis. 123, 297–300 (1971).

Montagnier, L., Collandre, M., DeMaeyer–Guignard, J., DeMaeyer, E.: Two forms of mouse interferon messenger RNA. Biochem. Biophys. Res. Commun. 59, 1031–1038 (1974).

Morahan, P. S., Glasgow, L. A., Crane, J. L., Kern, E. R.: Comparison of antiviral and antitumor activity of activity of activated macrophages. Cellul. Immunol. 28, 404–415 (1977a).

Morahan, P. S., Kaplan, A. M.: Macrophage activation and antitumor activity of biologic and synthetic agents. Int. J. Cancer 17, 82–89 (1976).

Morahan, P. S., Munson, J. A., Baird, L. G., Kaplan, A. M., Regelson, W.: Antitumor action of pyran copolymer and tilorone against Lewis lung carcinoma and B-16 melanoma. Cancer Res. 34, 506–511 (1974).

Morahan, P. S., Munson, A. E., Regelson, W., Commerford, S. L., Hamilton, L. D.: Antiviral activity and side effects of polyriboinosinic-cytidylic acid complex as affected by molecular size. Proc. Nat. Acad. Sci. U. S. A. 69, 842–847 (1972).

Morahan, P. S., Schuller, G. B., Snodgrass, M. Y., Kaplan, A. M.: Padoxical effects of immunopotentiators in antitumor and antitumor virus treatment. J. Infect. Dis. 133 A, 249–255 (1977b).

Mordhorst, C. M. Reinicke, V., Schonne, E.: In ovo inhibition by concentrated chick interferon of the growth of tric agents. Am. J. Ophthalmology 63, 1107–1109 (1968).

Morgan, M. J.: The production and action of interferon in Chinese hamster cells. J. Gen. Virol. 33, 351–367 (1976a).

Morgan, M. J.: The production of Chinese hamster interferon. Acta Virol. 20, 446–462 (1976b).

Morgan, M. J., Colby, C., jr., Hulse, J. L. N.: Isolation and characterization of virus-resistant mouse embryo fibroblast. J. Gen. Virol. 20, 377–388 (1973).

Morgan, M. J., Faik, P.: The expression of the interferon system in clones of Chinese hamster/human hybrid cells. Brit. J. Cancer 36, 254 (1977).

Mozes, L. W., Havell, E. A., Gradoville, M. L., Vilček, J.: Increased interferon production in human cells irradiated with ultraviolet light. Infect. Immun. 10, 1189–1191 (1974).

Mozes, L. W., Vilček, J.: Interferon induction in rabbit cells irradiated with U. V. light. J. Virology 13, 646–651 (1974).

Mozes, L. W., Vilček, J.: Distinguishing characteristics of interferon induction with poly I·poly C and Newcastle disease virus in human cells. Virology 65, 100–110 (1975).

Mucsi, I., Pusztai, R., Beladi, I., Bakay, M.: Production of high titres of interferon in chicken leukocyte cultures inoculated with human adenovirus type 12. Acta Virol. 14, 453–458 (1970).

Murphy, B. R., Baron, S., Chalhub, E. G., Uhlendorf, C. P., Chanock, R. M.: Temperature-sensitive mutants of influenza virus. IV. Induction of interferon in nasopharynx by wild-type and a temperature-sensitive virus. J. Infect. Dis. 128, 488–493 (1973).

Murphy, B. R., Glasgow, L. A.: Factors modifying host resistance to viral infection. III. Effecto of whole body X-irradiation on experimental encephalomyocardis infection in mice. J. Exp. Med. 127, 1035–1042 (1966).

Murphy, B. R., Glasgow, L. A.: Factors modifying host resistance to viral infection. I. Effect of immunosuppressive drugs on experimental infection of mice with encephalomyocarditis virus. Antimicrob. Agents Chemother. **7**, 661–674 (1967).

Murphy, B. R., Richman, D. D., Chalhub, E. G., Uhlendorf, C. P., Baron, S., Chanock, R. M.: Failure of attenuated temperature-sensitive influenza A virus (H 3 NZ) virus to induce heterologous interference in human to Parainfluenza Type 1 virus. Infect. Immun. **12**, 62–74 (1975).

Murray, A. M., Morahan, P. S.: Studies of interferon production in *Aedes albopictus* mosquito cells. Proc. Soc. Exp. Biol. Med. **142**, 11–15 (1973).

Myers, M. W., Friedman, R. M.: Potentiation of human interferon production by superinduction. J. Natl. Cancer Inst. **47** (4), 757–764 (1971).

Nagano, Y.: Studies on virus inhibiting factor. Jap. J. Exp. Med. **37**, 183–187 (1967).

Nagano, Y.: Virus-Inhibiting Factor, pp. 1–260. Tokyo: University of Tokyo Press (1975).

Nagano, Y., Kojima, Y.: Pouvoir immunisant de virus vaccinal inactive par des rayo ultraviolets. C. R. Soc. Biol. (Paris) **148**, 1700–1702 (1954).

Nagano, Y., Kojima, Y.: Inhibition de l'infection vaccinale par le virus homologue. C. R. Seances Soc. Biol. Filiales **152**, 1627–1630 (1958).

Nagano, Y., Mizunoe, K., Maehara, N., Kumazawa, Y.: Induction of virus-inhibiting factor or interferon by cell fractions of *Mycobacterium tuberculosis*. Jap. J. Microbiol. **15** (6), 542–544 (1971).

Nagata, I., Kunii, Ono, S.: Effects of thymectomy and splenectomy on *in vivo* interferon induction with Sindbis virus or E. coli endotoxin, in rats (cited in Ito *et al.*, 1971) (1971).

Nathanson, N., Cole, G. A.: Immunosuppression and experimental virus infection of the nervous system. Adv. Virus. Res. **16**, 397–402 (1970).

Nathanson, N., Davis, M., Thind, I. S., Price, W. H.: Histological studies of the monkey neuro-virulence of group B arboviruses II. Selection of indicator centers. Am. J. Epidemiol. **84**, 524–530 (1966).

Nathanson, N., Stolley, P. D., Boolukas, P. J.: Effect of immunosuppression on arboviral infection. J. Comp. Pathol. **79**, 109–115 (1969).

Nebert, D. W., Friedman, R. M.: Stimulation of aryl hydrocarbon hydroxylase induction in cell cultures by interferon. J. Virol. **11**, 193–197 (1973).

Nemes, M. M., Hilleman, M. R.: Effect of Westphal lipid A on viral activities in mice and hamsters. Proc. Soc. Exp. Biol. Med. **110**, 500–510 (1962).

Nemes, M. M., Tytell, A. A., Lampson, G. P., Field, A. K., Hilleman, M. R.: Inducers of interferon and host resistance. VI. Antiviral efficacy of poly I:C in animal models. Proc. Soc. Exp. Biol. Med. **132**, 776–783 (1969a).

Nemes, M. M., Tytell, A. A., Lampson, G. P., Field, A. K., Hilleman, M. R.: Inducers of interferon and host resistance. VII. Antiviral efficacy of double-stranded RNA of natural origin. Proc. Soc. Exp. Biol. Med. **132**, 784–789 (1969b).

Neumann–Haefelin, D., Shrestha, B., Manthey, K. F.: Effective antiviral prophylaxis and therapy by systemic application of human interferon in immunosuppressed monkeys. J. Infect. Dis. **133**, A 211–A 215 (1976).

Neumann–Haefelin, D., Sundmacher, R., Sauter, B., Karges, H. E., Manthey, K. F.: Effect of human leukocyte interferon on vaccinia- and herpes virus-infected cell cultures and monkey corneas. Infect. Immun. **12**, 148–154 (1975).

Neumann–Haefelin, D., Sundmacher, R., Skoda, R., Cantell, K.: Comparative evaluation of human leukocyte and fibroblast interferon in the prevention of herpes simplex virus keratitis in a monkey model. Infect. Immun. **17**, 468–470 (1977).

Neva, F. A., Weller, T. H.: Rubella interferon and factors influencing the indirect neutralization test for rubella antibody. J. Immunol. **93**, 466–472 (1964).

Ng, M. H., Berman, B., Vilček, J.: Membrane-bound intracellular interferon in rabbit kidney cell cultures. Virology **49**, 322–325 (1972).

Ng, M. H., Vilček, J.: Interferons: physicochemical properties and control of cellular synthesis. Advances in protein chemistry **26**, 173–201 (1972).

Ng, M. H., Vilček, J.: Temperature-sensitive interferon production in rabbit kidney cell cultures treated with toyocamycin. Biochem. Biophys. Acta **294**, 284–291 (1973).

Ngan, J., Lee, S. H. S., Kind, L. S.: Suppressive effect of interferon on ability of mouse spleen cells synthesizing IgE to sensitize rat skin for heterologous adoptive cutaneous anaphylaxis. J. Immunol. **117**, 1063–1075 (1976).

Niblack, J. F., McCreary, M. B.: Relationship of biological activities of poly I-poly C to homopolymer molecular weights. Nature New Biol. **233**, 52–53 (1971).

Niblack, J. E., McCreary, M., Stone, N. L.: Interferon induction by polyacrylic acid: dependence on molecular weight, in: Colloque No. 6, Institut National de la Sante et de Recherche Medicale, p. 219 (1970).

Nichols, F. R., Tershak, D. R.: Effect of 5-fluorouracil and 6-azauridine on interferon action. J. Virol. **1**, 450–462 (1967).

Nichols, F. R., Weed, S. D., Underwood, G. E.: Stimulation of murine interferon by a substituted pyrimidine. Antimicrob. Agents Chemother. **9**, 433–446 (1976).

Nissen, C., Speck, B., Emodi, G., Iscove, N. N.: Toxicity of human leukocyte interferon preparations in human bone-marrow cultures. Lancet **1**, 203–204 (1977).

Nordlund, J. J., Wolff, S. M., Levy, H. B.: Inhibition of biologic activity of poly I:poly C by human plasma. Proc. Soc. Exp. Biol. Med. **133**, 439–444 (1970).

Northrop, R. L., Deinhardt, F.: Production of interferon-like substances by human bone marrow tissues *in vitro*. J. Nat. Cancer Inst. **39**, 685–689 (1967).

Nozaki, J., Atanasiu, P.: Evaluation of interferon induced by rabies vaccines. Ann. Microbiol. (Paris) **126** (3), 381–388 (1975).

Nuwer, M. R., Declercq, E., Merigan, T. C.: Interferon clearance rate decreased after repeated injections. J. Gen. Virol. **12**, 191–194 (1972).

O'Farrell, P. H.: High resolution two-dimensional electrophoresis of proteins. J. Biol. Chem. **250**, 4007–4021 (1975).

Ogburn, C. A., Berg, K., Paucker, K.: Purification of mouse interferon by affinity chromatography on anti-interferon globulin-sepharose. J. Immunol. **111**, 1206–1218 (1973).

Oh, J. O.: An interferon-like viral inhibitor in body fluids of endotoxin-injected rabbits. Proc. Soc. Exp. Biol. Med. **123**, 493–496 (1966).

Oh, J. O.: Enhancement of virus multiplication and interferon production by cortisone in ocular Herpesvirus infection. J. Immunol. **104**, 1359–1363 (1970).

Oh, J. O.: Sensitivity of types 1 and 2 herpesvirus Hominis to an interferon inducer poly I : C. Infect. Immun. **3**, 847–848 (1971).

Oh, J. O., Gill, E. J.: Role of interferon-like viral inhibitor in endotoxin-induced corneal resistance to newcastle disease virus. J. Bacteriol. **91**, 251–256 (1966).

Oh, J. O., Yoneda, C.: Induction of ocular resistance to vaccinia virus by typhoid vaccine: role of interferon. J. Immunol. **102**, 145–159 (1969).

Ohno, S., Nozima, T.: Inhibitory effect of interferon on the induction of thymidine kinase in vaccinia virus-infected chick embryo fibroblasts. Acta. Virol. **8**, 479–483 (1964).

Ohwaki, M., Kawade, Y.: Inhibition of multiplication of mouse cells in culture by interferon preparations. Acta. Virol. **16**, 477–486 (1972).

Oie, H. K., Buckler, C. E., Uhlendorf, C. P., Hill, D. A., Baron, S.: Improved assays for a variety of interferons. Proc. Soc. Exp. Biol. Med. **140**, 1178–1181 (1972a).

Oie, H. K., Easton, J. M., Ablashi, D. V., Baron, S.: Murine cytomegalovirus: induction of and sensitivity to interferon *in vitro*. Infect. Immun. **12**, 1012–1035 (1975).

Oie, H. K., Gazdar, A. F., Buckler, C. E., Baron, S.: High interferon producing line of transformed murine cells. J. Gen. Virol. **17**, 107–109 (1972 b).

Oie, H. K., Loh, P. C.: Reovirus type 2: production of and sensitivity to interferon in human amnion cells. Proc. Soc. Exp. Biol. Med. **127**, 1210–1219 (1968).

Oie, H. K., Loh, P. C.: Reovirus type 2: induction of viral resistance and interferon production in Fathead Minnow cells. Proc. Soc. Exp. Biol. Med. **136**, 369–373 (1971).

Oie, H. K., Loh, P. C., Ratnayake, R. T.: Studies on Reovirus Type 2 viral interference with uv-inactivated virus. Archiv für die gesamte Virusforschung **42**, 170–179 (1973).

Old, L. J., Benacerraf, B., Stockert, E.: Increased resistance to Mengo virus following infection with bacillus, in: Colloq. Inter. Centre. Nat. Rech. Sci. **115**, 319–326 (1963).

Olsen, G. A., Kern, E. R., Glasgow, L. A., Overall, J. C., jr.: Effect of treatment with exogenous interferon Poly I·Poly C, or poly I-poly C – poly-lysine complex on EMC virus infections in mice. Antimicrob. Agents Chemother. **10**, 668–679 (1976).

O'Malley, J. A., Al-Bussam, N., Beutner, K., Wallace, H. J., Gailani, S., Henderson, E. S., Carter, W. A.: Cytomegalovirus infection with acute myeloctyc leukemia: antiviral (interferon and antibody) responses. New York State J. Med. **75**, 738 (1975a).

O'Malley, J. A., Ho, Y. K., Chakrabarti, P., Diberardino, L., Chandra, P., Orinda, D. A. O., Byrd, D. M., Bardos, T. J., Carter, W. A.: Antiviral activity of partially thiolated polynucleotides. Molec. Pharm. **11**, 61–69 (1975b).

O'Malley, J. A., Jankowski, W., Davey, M. W., Horoszewicz, J., Sulkowski, E., Carter, W. A.: Probes of structural differences in human fibroblast and leukocyte interferons. Abstr. Ann. Meet. Amer. Soc. Microbiol., p. 338 (1975c).

O'Reilly, R. J., Chibbaro, A., Anger, E., Lopez, C.: Cell-mediated immune responses in patients with recurrent herpes simplex infections. II. Infection-associated deficiency of lymphokine production in patients with recurrent herpes. J. Immunol. **118**, 1095–1102 (1977).

O'Reilly, R. J., Everson, L. K., Emodi, G., Hansen, J., Smithwick, E. M., Grimes, E., Pahwa, S., Pahwa, R., Schwartz, S., Armstrong, D., Siegal, F. P., Gupta, S., DuPont, B., Good, R. A.: Effect of exogenous interferon in cytomegalovirus infection complicating bone marrow transplantation. Clin. Immunol. Immunopath. **6**, 51–58 (1976).

Orlova, T. G., Georgadze, I. I., Kognovitskaya, A. I.: Formation of interferon with chicken species-specificity in bacterial cells. Acta Virol. **20**, 167 (1976).

Orlova, T. G., Georgadze I. I., Kognovitskaya, A. I., Soloviev, V. D.: Formation of messenger RNA for interferon in cells treated with various viruses and poly I-poly C. Vopr. Virusol. (4), 431–435 (1974a).

Orlova, T. G., Georgadze, I. I., Kognovitskaya, A. I., Solovyov, V. D.: Interferon-inducing and interferon-translating functions of RNA isolated from Newcastle disease virus-infected cells. Acta. Virol. **18**, 210–216 (1974b).

Orlova, T. G., Kognovitskaya, A. I., Georgadze, I. I., Solovyov, V. D.: The dynamics of production and the sensitivity to cycloheximide and actinomycin D of interferon-inducing and interferon messenger RNA. Acta Virol. **20**, 9 (1976).

Orlova, T. G., Kognovitskaya, A. I., Georgadze, I. I., Soloviev, V. D.: Translation by bacterial cells of messenger RNA for interferon of animal origin. Acta Virol. **21**, 353 (1977).

Osborn, Y. E., Medearis, D. N., jr.: Studies of relationship between mouse cytomegalovirus and interferon. Proc. Soc. Exp. Biol. Med. **121**, 819–824 (1966).

O'Shaughnessy, M. V., Easterbrook, K. B., Lee, S. H. S., Katz, L. J., Rozee, K. R.: Interferon inhibition of autogenously induced virions (C particles) in synchronized L929 cell cultures. J. Nat. Cancer Inst. **53**, 1687–1696 (1974).

O'Shaugnessy, M. V., Lee, S. H., Rozee, K. R.: Interferon inhibition of DNA synthesis and cell division. Can. J. Microbiol. **18**, 145–151 (1972).

Osterhoff, J., Jager, M., Jungwirth, C., Bodo, G.: Inhibition of Poxvirus specific functions induced in chick-embryo fibroblasts by treatment with homologous interferon. Eur. J. Biochem. **69**, 535–543 (1976).

Overall, J. C., Glasgow, L. A.: Fetal response to viral infection: interferon production in sheep. Science **167**, 1139–1140 (1970).

Oxman, M. N., Baron, S., Black, P. H., Takemoto, K. K., Habel, K., Rowe, W. P.: The effect of interferon on SV40 T antigen production in SV40 transformed cells. Virology **32**, 122–127 (1967).

Oxman, M. N., Black, P. H.: Inhibition of SV40 T antigen formation by interferon. Proc. Natl. Acad. Sci. **55**, 1133–1140 (1966).

Oxman, M. N., Levin, M. J.: Interferon and transcription of early virus-specific RNA in cells infected with Simian virus 40. Proc. Natl. Acad. Sci. **68**, 299–302 (1971).

Oxman, M. N., Levin, M. J., Lewis, A. M.: Control of Simian virus 40 gene expression in adenovirus-simian virus 40 hybrid viruses. Synthesis of hybrid adenovirus 2-Simian virus 40 RNA molecules in cells infected with a nondetective adenovirus 2-Simian virus 40 hybrid virus. J. Virology **13**, 322–330 (1974).

Oxman, M. N., Rowe, W. P., Black, P. H.: Studies of adenovirus-SV40 hybrid viruses. VI. Differential effects of interferon on SV40 and adenovirus T antigen formation in cells infected with SV40 virus, adenovirus and adenovirus SV40 hybrid viruses. Proc. Nat. Acad. Sci. U. S. A. **57**, 941–948 (1967).

Oxman, M. N., Takemoto, K. K.: Comparative sensitivity of SV40 and polyoma virus, in: Colloque No. 6, institut National de la Sante et de la Recherche Medicale, p. 429 (1970).

Pacheco, D., Faloff, R., Catinot, L., Floch, F., Werner, G. H., Falcoff, E.: Inhibitory effect of interferon on DNA and RNA synthesis in murine spleen cells stimulated by lectins. Ann. Immunol. **127**, 163–172 (1976).

Padnos, M., Shimonaski, G., Came, P. E.: Interferon in mice acutely infected with M-P virus. J. Gen. Virol. **13**, 163–165 (1971).

Pallin, O., Lundmark, K., Brege, K. G.: Interferon in severe herpes simplex of cornea. Lancet **ii**, 1187–1188 (1976).

Pantelouris, E. M., Pringle, C. R.: Interferon production in athymic nude mice. J. Gen. Virol. **32**, 149–157 (1976).

Panusarn, C. M., Stanley, E. D., Dirda, B. S., Rubenis, B. S., Jackson, G. G.: Prevention of illness from rhinovirus infection by a topical interferon inducer. New England Journal of Medicine **291**, 57–61 (1974).

Park, J. H., Baron, S.: Herpetic keratoconjunctivitis: therapy with synthetic double-stranded RNA. Science **162**, 811–813 (1968).

Park, J. H., Galin, M., Billiau, A., Baron, S.: Prophylaxis of herpetic keratoconjunctivitis with interferon inducers. Arch. Ophthalmol. **81**, 840–849 (1969).

Parkman, P. D., Buescher, E. L., Arlenstein, M. S.: Recovery of rubella virus from army recruits. Proc. Soc. Exp. Biol. Med. **111**, 225–230 (1962).

Parkman, P. D., Buescher, E. L., Arlenstein, M. S., McCown, J. M., Mundon, F. K., Druzo, A. D.: J. Immun, **93**, 595–607 (1964).

Pathak, P. N., Tompkins, W. A.: Interferon production by macrophages from adult and newborn rabbits bearing fibroma virus-induced tumors. Infect. Immun. **9**, 669–673 (1974).

Paucker, K.: Interference and cell division. Viruses, Nucleic Acids, and Cancer, pp. 430–446 (1963).

Paucker, K.: The serologic specificity of interferon. J. Immunol. **94**, 371–378 (1965).

Paucker, K., Berman, B. J., Golgher, R. R., Stancek, D.: Purification, characterization, and attempts at isotopic labeling of mouse interferon. J. Virol. **5**, 145–152 (1970).

Paucker, K., Boxaca, M.: Cellular resistance to induction of interferon. Bacteriol. Rev. **31**, 145–184 (1967).

Paucker, K., Cantell, K.: Neutralization of interferon by specific antibody. Virology **18**, 145–147 (1962).

Paucker, K., Cantell, K.: Quantitative studies on viral interference in suspended L-cells. V. Persistence of protection in growing cultures. Virology **21**, 22–29 (1963).

Paucker, K., Cantell, K., Henle, W.: Quantitative studies on viral interference in suspended L-cells. III. Effect of interfering viruses and interferon on the growth rate of cells. Virology **17**, 324–334 (1962).

Paucker, K., Dalton, B. J., Ogburn, C. A., Torma, E.: Multiple active sites on human interferons. Proc. Natl. Acad. Sci. U. S. A. **72**, 4587–4592 (1975).

Paucker, K., Dalton, B. J., Torma, E. T., Ogburn, C. A.: Biological properties of human leukocyte interferon components. J. Gen. Virol. **35**, 341–351 (1977).

Paucker, K., Golgher, R.: Effect of purified murine interferon on noninfected L-cell. Colloques de l'institut National de la sante et de la Recherche Medicale, **No. 6**, L'interferon, p. 119–123 (1969).

Paucker, K., Golgher, R.: Effect of purified murine interferon on noninfected L-cells. Coll. Inst. Nat. Sante. Rech. Med. **6**, 119 (1970).

Paucker, K., Henle, W.: Interference between inactivated and active influenza viruses in the chick embryo. Virology **6**, 198–214 (1958).

Paucker, K., Stancek, D.: Characterization of interferon-associated proteins. J. Gen. Virol. **15**, 129–138 (1972).

Pauloin, A., Chany-Fournier, F., Epstein, L., Chany, C.: Degradation par la Phytohémagglutinine de l'état antiviral induit par l'interféron. C. R. Acad. Sci. D **284**, 119–1126 (1977).

Pearson, J. W., Turner, W., Ebert, P. S., Chirigos, M. A.: Effectiveness of therapy with a multistranded synthetic polynucleotide complex against a murine sarcoma virus. Appl. Microbiol. **18**, 474–483 (1969).

Peries, J., Canivet, M., Bernard, C., Boiron, M.: Perte de la sensibilité cellulaire à l'action d'un interféron exogène après infection par les virus du complexe leucémies-sarcomes de la souris. C. R. Acad. Sci. (Paris) D **226**, 1439–1441 (1968).

Pestka, S., McInnes, J., Havell, E. A., Vilček, J.: Cell-free synthesis of human interferon. Proc. Nat. Acad. Sci. U. S. A. **72**, 3898–3906 (1975).

Pestka, S., McInnes, J., Weiss, D., Havell, E. A., Vilček, J.: *De novo* cell-free synthesis of human interferon. Ann. N. Y. Acad. Sci. **284**, 697–720 (1977).

Petralli, J. K., Merigan, T. C., Wilbur, J. R.: Circulating interferon after measles vaccination. New. Engl. J. Med. **273**, 198–201 (1965 a).

Petralli, J. K., Merigan, T. C., Wilbur, J. R.: Action of endogenous interferon against vaccinia infection in children. The Lancet ii, 401–405 (1965 b).

Pidot, A. L.: Dye uptake assay: An efficient and sensitive method for human interferon titration. Appl. Microbiol. **22** (4), 671–677 (1971).

Pidot, A. L., Maurer, L. H., McIntyre, O. R.: Leukocyte interferon production, RNA synthesis, and PHA response in patients with infectious mononucleosis. Blood **42**, 175–185 (1973).

Pincus, W. B., Flick, J. A.: Inhibition of the primary vaccinal lesion and of delayed hypersensitivity by an antimononuclear cell serum. J. Infect. Dis. **113**, 15–23 (1963).

Pindak, F. F., Schmidt, J. P.: Treatment of Mengovirus infection in mice with statolon. Appl. Microbiol. **15**, 1240–1243 (1967).

Pindak, F. F., Schmidt, J. P., Giron, D. Y., Allen, P. T.: Interferon levels and resistance to viral infection associated with selected interferon inducers. Proc. Soc. Exp. Biol. Med. **138**, 317–321 (1971).

Pinto, C. A., Haff, R. F., Valenta, J. R., Pagano, J. F., Dicuollo, C. J., Ferlauto, R. J.: Human interferon. II. Biological activity, in: Symp. Series Immunobiol. Standard (Karger, Basel) **14**, 105 (1970).

Pitha, J., Pitha, P. M.: Antiviral resistance by the polynosinic acidpoly (l-vinylcytosine) complex. Science **172**, 1146–1148 (1971).

Pitha, P. M.: Interferon action revisited. Nature **269**, 374 (1977).

Pitha, P. M., Carter, W. A.: The DEAE-dextran-poly I·C complex: physical properties and interferon induction. Virology **45**, 777–781 (1971 a).

Pitha, P. M., Carter, W. A.: Antiviral activity produced by the polycytidylic acid-hexainosinate system. Nature New Biol. **234**, 105–106 (1971 b).

Pitha, P. M., Harper, M. D., Pitha, J.: Dependence of interferon induction on cell membrane integrity. Virology **59**, 40–50 (1974).

Pitha, P. M., Hutchinson, D. W.: The mechanism of interferon induction by synthetic polyribonucleotide, in: Interferons and Their Actions (Stewart II, W. E. ed.), pp. 13–36. Cleveland, Ohio: CRC Press, Inc. (1977).

Pitha, P. M., Marshall, L. W., Carter, W. A.: Interferon induction: rate of cellular attachment of poly I·C. J. Gen. Virol. **15**, 89–92 (1972).

Pitha, P. M., Marshall, L. W., Carter, W. A.: Interferon: the dissociation of rIn-rCn-induced proteins by protonation. J. Gen. Virol. **21**, 169–171 (1973).

Pitha, P. M., Pitha, J.: Interferon induction site: Poly IC on solid substrate carriers. J. Gen. Virol. **21**, 31–37 (1973).

Pitha, P. M., Pitha, J.: Interferon induction by single-stranded polynucleotides modified with polybases. J. Gen. Virol. **21**, 385–390 (1974).

Pitha, P. M., Rowe, W. P., Oxman, M. N.: Effect of interferon on exogenous, endogenous, and chronic murine leukemia virus infection. Virology **70**, 321–337 (1976).

Pitha, P. M., Staal, S. P., Bolognesi, D. P., Denny, T. P., Rowe, W. P.: Effect of interferon on murine leukemia virus infection. II. Synthesis of viral components in exogenous infection. Virology **79**, 1–16 (1977).

Pitha, P. M., Vengris, V. E., Reynolds, F. H.: The role of cell membrane in the antiviral effect of interferon, in: Cell Surface Receptors (Nicholson, J., *et al.*, eds.), pp. 427–434. New York: Alan R. Liss, Inc. (1976 a).

Pitha, P. M., Vengris, V. E., Reynolds, F. H.: The role of cell membrane in the antiviral effect of interferon. J. Supramol. Structure **4**, 467–473 (1976 b).

Polezhaev, F. I., Makariev, G. S., Aleksandrova, G. I.: Interferon-inducing ability in human leukocyte cultures of influenza viruses of different virulence. Acta. Virol. **18**, 362–374 (1974).

Pollikoff, R. P., Cannavale, P., Dixon, P., DiPuppo, A.: Effect of complexed synthetic RNA analogues on herpes simplex virus infection in rabbit cornea. Amer. J. Ophthalmol. **69**, 650–664 (1970).

Pollikoff, R., Donikian, M. A., Liu, O. C.: Multiplication of influenza virus in interferon treated mice lungs. Bacteriol. Proc., p. 158 (1961).

Pollikoff, R., Donikian, M. A., Padron, A., Liu, O. C.: Tissue specificity of interferon prepared in various tissue cultures. Proc. Soc. Exp. Biol. Med. 110, 232–234 (1962).

Polikoff, R., Jankauskas, P., DiPuppo, A., Nazario, R.: Studies on the effect of bacterial endotoxin on primary herpetic keratitis. Invest. Ophthalmol. 7, 397–406 (1968).

Pollikoff, R., Lieberman, M., Lem. N. E.: Role of interferon and partial immunity in influenza virus infection of mouse lung. Proc. Soc. Exp. Biol. Med. 119, 790–793 (1965).

Porterfield, J. S.: A simple plaque inhibition test for antiviral agents: Application to assay of interferon. The Lancet 7098, 326–327 (1959).

Porterfield, J. S.: Interference and interferon, in: Techniques in Experimental Virology (Harris, R., ed.), p. 313. London: Academic Press (1964).

Portnoy, J., Merigan, T. C.: The effect of interferon and interferon inducers on avian influenza. J. Infect. Dis. 124, 545–552 (1971).

Porwit–Bobr, Z., Ptak, W.: Studies on cellular resistance factors in polyoma virus infection. Arch. Immun. Ther. Exp. 14, 753–760 (1966).

Postic, B., DeAngelis, C., Breinig, M. K., Ho, M.: Effect of temperature on the induction of interferon by endotoxin and virus. J. Bact. 91, 1277–1281 (1966).

Postic, B., DeAngelis, C., Breinig, M. K., Ho, M.: Effects of cortisol and adrenalectomy on induction of interferon by endotoxin. Proc. Soc. Exp. Biol. Med. 125, 89–92 (1967).

Postic, B., Dowling, J. N.: Susceptibility of clinical isolates of cytomegalovirus to human interferon. Antimicrob. Agents. Chemother. 11, 656–660 (1977).

Postic, B., Fenje, P.: Effect of administered interferon on rabies in rabbits. Appl. Microbiol. 22, 428–431 (1971a).

Postic, B., Fenje, P.: Prophylaxis of rabies in rabbits by poly I·C, in: Rabies (Nagano, Y., Davenport, F., eds.), pp. 217–223. Univ. Park Press, 1971 (1971b).

Postic, B., Sather, G. E.: Effect of poly I:C in mice injected with Japanese encephalitis virus. Ann. N. Y. Acad. Sci. 173, 606–610 (1970).

Potmesil, M., Goldfeder, A.: Inhibitory effect of polyinosinic-polycytidylic acid on the growth of transplantable mouse mammary carcinoma. Proc. Soc. Exp. Biol. Med. 139, 1392 (1972).

Pudov, V. I.: The effect of interferon on Brown-Pearce carcinoma metastasis. Vopr. Onkol. 17, 74–77 (1971).

Purcell, R. H., London, W. T., McAuliffe, V. J., Palmer, A. E., Kaplan, P. M., Gerin, J. L., Wagner, J., Popper, H., Lvovsky, E., Wong, D. C., Levy, H. B.: Modification of chronic hepatitis-B virus infection in chimpanzees by administration of an interferon inducer. Lancet, Oct. 9, 757–758 (1976).

Pusztai, R., Beladi, I., Bakay, M., Mucsi, I.: Effect of ultraviolet irradiation and heating on the interferon-inducing capacity of human adenoviruses. J. Gen. Virol. 4, 169–176 (1969).

Pusztai, R., Belladi, I., Lengyel, A., Naszi, Tarodi, B.: Effect of trypsin and antipenton serum on the interferon inducing ability of human adenovirus. Acta Microbiol. Acad. Sci. Hung. 21, 269–272 (1974).

Pusztai, R., Berencsi, K., Beladi, I., Szabo, E.: Relationship between interferon production and transformation of chick cells infected with human adenovirus type 12, in: Interferon and Interferon Inducers (Foldes, I., Talas, M., eds.), pp. 100–108. Budapest: Res. Group. Hung. Acad. Sci. (1976).

Pyhala, L., Cantell, K.: Clearance of human interferon in rabbits induced to make rabbit interferon. Proc. Soc. Exp. Biol. Med. 146, 394–397 (1974).

Rabin, H., Adamson, R. H., Neubauer, R. H., Neubauer, R. H., Cicmanec, J. L., Wallen, W. C.: Pilot studies with human interferon in herpesvirus saimiri-induced lymphoma in owl monkeys. Cancer Res. 36, 715–721 (1976).

Rabinovitch, M., Manejias, R. E., Russo, M., Abbey, E. F.: Increased spreading of macrophages from mice treated with interferon inducers. Cell Immun. 29, 86–93 (1977).

Rabson, A. S., Tyrrell, S. A., Levy, H.: Inhibition of human cytomegalovirus in vitro by double-stranded polyribocytidylic-inosinic acid (Poly rI:rC). Proc. Soc. Exp. Biol. Med. 131, 495 (1969).

Radke, K. L., Colby, C., Kates, J. R., Krider, H. M., Prescott, D. M.: Establishment and maintenance of the interferon-induced antiviral state: studies in enucleated cells. J. Virol. **13**, 623–645 (1974).

Raj, N. B. K., Pitha, P. M.: Relationship between interferon production and interferon messenger RNA synthesis in human fibroblasts. Proc. Natl. Acad. Sci. **74**, 1483–1487 (1977).

Ramoni, C., Rossi, G. B., Matarese, G. P., Dolei, A.: Production of Friend leukaemia antigens in chronically-infected cells treated with interferon. J. Gen. Virol. **37**, 285–296 (1977).

Ramseur, J. M., Friedman, R. M.: Interferon inhibits induction of endogenous murine leukemia virus production. Virology **73**, 553–566 (1976).

Ramuz, M. M., Bousquet, C., Sassine, J., Roux, J.: Induction of the synthesis of interferon in the mouse by spheroplasts and R mutants of Brucella. C. R. Acad. Sci. (Paris) **D 278**, 1135–1137 (1974).

Rana, M. W., Pinkerton, H., Rankin, A.: Effect of rifamycin and tilorone derivatives on Friend virus leukemia in mice. Proc. Soc. Exp. Biol. Med. **150**, 32–38 (1975).

Rasmussen, L., Farley, L. B.: Inhibition of herpesvirus hominis by human interferon. Infect. Immun. **12**, 104–117 (1975).

Rasmussen, L., Holmes, A. R., Hofmeister, B., Merigan, T. C.: Multiplicity-dependent replication of varicella-zoster in interferon-treated cells. J. Gen. Virol. **35**, 361–376 (1977).

Rasmussen, L. E., Jordan, G. W., Stevens, D. A., Merigan, T. C.: Lymphocyte interferon production and transformation after herpes simplex infections in humans. J. Immun. **112**, 728–736 (1974).

Rassiga–Pidot, A. L., O'Keefe, G. III, McManus, N., McIntyre, O. R.: Human leukocyte interferon: the variation in normals and correlation with PHA transformation. Proc. Soc. Exp. Biol. Med. **140**, 1263–1269 (1972).

Rassiga–Pidot, A. L., McIntyre, O. R.: *In vitro* leukocyte interferon production in patients with Hodgkin's disease. Cancer Res. **34**, 2995–3002 (1974).

Rathova, V., Kociskova, D., Borecky, L.: Interrelations between serum interferon and complement levels. Acta Virol. **18**, 143–150 (1974).

Rathova, V., Kociskova, D., Borecky, L.: Interferon-hyporesponsiveness in mice in connection with dose interval and site of administration of NDV-reflection in serum complement levels. Acta. Virol. **19**, 158–164 (1975).

Ratner, L., Sen., G. C., Brown, G. E., Lebleu, B., Kawakita, M., Cabrer, B., Slattery, E., Lengyel, P.: Interferon, dsRNA and RNA degradation-characteristics of an endonuclease activity. Europ. J. Biochem. **79**, 565–577 (1977).

Ray, C. G.: The ontogeny of interferon production by human leukocytes. J. Pediatrics **76**, 94–98 (1970).

Ray, C. G., Gravelle, C. R., Chin, T. D. Y.: Circulating interferon in infants with acute respiratory illness. J. Pediat. **71**, 27–30 (1967).

Regelson, W.: Prevention and treatment of Friend leukemia virus (FLV) infection by interferon-inducing synthetic polyanions. Advan. Exp. Med. Biol. **1**, 315–321 (1967).

Regelson, W.: The antitumor activity of polyanions, in: Advances in Chemotherapy, **3** (Goldin, A., Hawking, F., Schnitzer, R. J., eds.), pp. 303–320. New York: Academic Press (1968).

Regelson, W.: Host modulation of resistance to infection and neoplasia. Ann. Rep. Medicinal Chem. **8**, 160–174 (1973).

Regelson, W., Foltyn, O.: Prevention and treatment of Friend leukemia virus (FLV) infection by polyanions and phytohemagglutinin. Proc. Amer. Assoc. Cancer Res. **7**, 58–64 (1966).

Reinicke, V.: The influence of hydrocortisone on production of influenza virus and interferon *in ovo*. Acta. Path. Microbiol. Scand. **60**, 528–539 (1964).

Reinicke, V.: The influence of steroid hormones and growth hormones on the production of influenza virus and interferon in tissue culture. Acta. Path. Microbiol. Scand. **64**, 339–346 (1965a).

Reinicke, V.: Increase of size of Sindbis virus plaques due to the effect of steroid hormones. Acta Path. Microbiol. Scand. **65**, 554–558 (1965b).

Reinicke, V., Mordhorst, C. H., Schonne, E.: In ovo inhibition of the growth of TRIC agents by purified species-specific interferon. Acta, Path. Microbiol. Scand. **69**, 478–482 (1967).

Remington, J. S., Merigan, T. C.: Interferon: Protection of cells infected with an intracellular protozoan *(Toxoplasma gondii)*. Science **161**, 804–806 (1968).

Remington, J. S., Merigan, T. C.: Resistance to virus challenge in mice infected with protozoa or bacteria. Proc. Soc. Exp. Biol. Med. **131**, 1184–1187 (1969).

Remington, J. S., Merigan, T. C.: Synthetic polyanions protect mice against intracellular bacteria infection. Nature **226**, 361–363 (1970).

Repik, P., Flamand, A., Bishop, D. H.: Effect of interferon upon the primary and secondary transcription of vesicular stomatitis and influenza viruses. J. Virol. **14**, 1169–1178 (1974).

Revel, M.: Interferon-induced translation regulation. Tex. Rep. Biol. Med. **35**, 212–220 (1977).

Revel, M., Bash, D., Ruddle, F. H.: Antibodies to a cell-surface component coded by human chromosome 21 inhibit action of interferon. Nature **260**, 139 (1976).

Revel, M., Gilboa, E., Kimchi, A., Schmidt, A., Shulman, L., Yakobson, E., Zilberstein, A.: Interferon-induced translational regulation. 11th FEBS Meeting, Copenhagen.

Reyes, M. P., Lerner, A. M.: Interferon and neutralizing antibody in sera of exercised mice with coxsackievirus B-3 myocarditis. Proc. Soc. Exp. Biol. Med. **151**, 333–339 (1976).

Reynolds, F. H., jr., Pitha, P. M.: The induction of interferon and its messenger RNA in human fibroblasts. Biochem. Biophys. Res. Commun. **59** (3), 1023–1030 (1974).

Reynolds, F. H., jr., Pitha, P. M.: Molecular weight study of human fibroblast interferon. Biochem. Biophys. Res. Comm. **65**, 107–114 (1975).

Reynolds, F. H., jr., Premkumar, E., Pitha, P. M.: Interferon activity produced by translation of human interferon messenger RNA in cell-free ribosomal systems and in *Xenopus* oocytes. Proc. Nat. Acad. Sci. U. S. A. **72**, 4881–4887 (1975).

Rheins, M. S., Barker, A. D., Wilson, M. E.: Therapeutic effects of a series of non-viral interferon inducers on a viral-induced leukemia. Can. J. Microbiol. **17**, 1259–1265 (1971).

Rhim, J. S., Greenawalt, C., Huebner, R. J.: Synthetic double-stranded RNA: inhibitory effect on murine leukaemia and sarcoma viruses in cell cultures. Nature **222**, 1166–1168 (1969).

Rhim, J. S., Heubner, R. J.: Inhibitory effect of statolon on virus-induced sarcoma of mice. Antimicrob. Ag. Chemother. **7**, 177–180 (1969).

Rhim, J. S., Heubner, R. J.: Comparison of the antitumor effect of interferon and interferon inducers. Proc. Soc. Exp. Biol. Med. **136**, 524–529 (1971).

Rice, J. M., Turner, W., Chirigos, M. A., Rice, N. R.: Enhancement by poly I:C-induced interferon production in mice. Applied Microbiol. **19**, 867–869 (1970).

Rice, J. M., Turner, W., Chirigos, M. A., Spahn, G.: Dose responsiveness and variation among inbred strains of mice in production of interferon after treatment with poly IC complexes. Appl. Microbiol. **22**, 300–306 (1971).

Richman, D. D., Murphy, B. R., Baron, S., Uhlendorf, C.: Three strains of influenza A virus (H 3 N 2): Interferon sensitivity *in vitro* and interferon production in volunteers. J. Clin. Microb. **3**, 223–232 (1976).

Richmond, J. Y.: An interferon-like inhibitor of foot and mouth disease virus induced by phytohemogglutinin in swine leukocyte cultures. Arch. Ges. Virusforsch. **27**, 282–284 (1969).

Richmond, J. Y.: DEAE-dextran requirement for poly I-C-induced interferon effective against foot-and-mouth disease virus *in vitro*. Arch. Ges. Virusforsch. **33**, 242–250 (1971).

Richmond, J. Y., Hamilton, L. D.: Foot-and-mouth disease virus inhibition induced in mice by synthetic double-stranded RNA. Proc. Natl. Acad. Sci. U. S. A. **64**, 81–87 (1969).

Riley, B. P., Gifford, G. E.: Studies on tissue specificity of interferon. J. Gen. Microbiol. **46**, 293–297 (1967).

Riley, B. P., Toy, S. T., Gifford, G. E.: Relative effects of interferon on virus plaque formation. Proc. Soc. Exp. Biol. Med. **122**, 1142–1144 (1966).

Riley, F. L., Levy, H. B.: Studies on the mechanism of interferon action: characterization of polysome-associated cellular RNAs modified by interferon. Virology **76**, 459–463 (1977).

Rinaldo, C. R., jr.: Mycoplasma in biological systems: induction of interferon. Hlth. Lab. Sci. **13**, 137–142 (1976).

Rinaldo, C. R., jr., Cole, B. C., Overall, J. C., Glasgow, L. A.: Induction of interferon in mice by mycoplasmas. Infec. Immun. **10**, 1296–1302 (1974 a).

Rinaldo, C. R., jr., Cole, B. C., Overall, J. C., jr., Ward, J. R., Glasgow, L. A.: Induction of interferon in ovine leukocytes by species of mycoplasma and acholeoplasma. Proc. Soc. Exp. Biol. Med. **146**, 613–618 (1974 b).

Rinaldo, C. R., jr., Isackson, D. W., Overall, J. C., jr., Glasgow, L. A., Brown, T. T., Bistner, S. I., Gillespie, J. H., Scott, F. W.: Fetal and adult bovine interferon production during bovine viral diarrhea virus infection. Infec. Immun. **14**, 660–671 (1976).

Rinaldo, C. R., jr., Overall, J. C., Cole, B. C., Glasgow, L. A.: Mycoplasma-associated induction of interferon in ovine leukocytes. Infec. Immun. **8**, 796–808 (1973).

Rinaldo, C. R. jr., Overall, J. C., Glasgow, L. A.: Viral replication and interferon production in fetal and adult ovine leukocytes and spleen cells. Infec. Immun. **12**, 1070–1082 (1975).

Rivière, Y., Bandu, M. T.: Induction of interferon by lymphocytic choriomeningitis virus in mice. Ann. Microbiol. A **128**, 323–334 (1977).

Rivière, Y., Gresser, J., Guillon, J. C., Tovey, M. G.: Inhibition by anti-interferon serum of lymphocytic choriomeningitis virus disease in suckling mice. Proc. Nat. Acad. Sci. U. S. A. **74**, 2135–2139 (1977).

Roberts, W. K., Clemens, M. J., Kerr, I.: Interferon-induced inhibition of protein synthesis in L-cell extracts: an ATP-dependent step in the activation of an inhibitor by double-stranded RNA. Proc. Natl. Acad. Sci. U. S. A. **70**, 3136–3140 (1976).

Roberts, W. K., Hovanessian, A., Brown, R. F., Clemens, M. J., Kerr, I. M.: Interferon-mediated protein kinase and low molecular-weight inhibitor of protein synthesis. Nature, **264**, 477–480 (1976).

Robinson, T, W. E., Cureton, R. J. R., Heath, R. B.: The effect of cyclophosphamide on Sendai virus infection of mice J. Med. Microbiol. **2**, 137–143 (1969).

Robinson, T. W. E., Heath, R. B.: Effect of cyclophosphamide on the production of interferon. Nature **217**, 178–180 (1969).

Rodgers, R., Merigan, T. C.: Interferon production by individual cells. Virology **57** (2), 464–474 (1974).

Rodgers, R., Merigan, T. C., Hardy, W. D., Old, L. J., Kassel, R.: Cat interferon inhibits feline leukemia virus infection in cell cultures, Nature New Biol. **237**, 270–271 (1972).

Rollag, H., Degre, M.: Effect of antibiotics on interferon production in mice. Acta. Path. Microbiol. Scand. B **84**, 369–372 (1976).

Rosenquist, R. D.: Polyriboinosinic-polyribocytidylic acid-induced interferons in calves. Amer. J. Vet. Res. **328**, 35–42 (1971).

Rosenquist, R. D., Loan, R. W.: Interferon production with strain SF-4 of parainfluenza-3 virus. Am. J. Veterinary Res. **28**, 619–628 (1967).

Rossen, R. D., Douglas, R. G., Cate, T. R., Couch, R. B., Butler, W. T.: The sedimentation behavior of rhinovirus neutralizing activity in nasal secretion and serum following the rhinovirus common cold. J. Immunol. **97**, 532–540 (1966).

Rossen, R. D., Kasel, J. A., Couch, R. B.: The secretory immune system: Its relation to respiratory viral infection. Prog. Med. Virol. **13**, 194–201 (1971).

Rossi, G. B., Dolei, A., Cioe, L., Benedetto, A., Matarese, G. P., Belardelli, F.: Inhibition of transcription and translation of globin messenger RNA in dimethyl sulfoxide-stimulated Friend erythroleukemia cells treated with interferon. Proc. Nat. Acad. Sci. U. S. A. **74**, 2036–2040 (1977 a).

Rossi, G. B., Dolei, A., Cioe, L., Benedetto, A., Matarese, G. P., Belardelli, F., Rita, G.: Interferon and Friend leukemia cells in culture. Tex. Rep. Biol. Med: **35**, 420–429 (1977 b).

Rossi, G. B., Marchegiani, M., Matarese, G., Gresser, I.: Inhibitory effect of interferon on multiplication of Friend leukemia cells *in vivo*. J. Nat. Cancer Inst. **54**, 993–999 (1975).

Rossi, G. B., Matarese, G. P., Grappelli, C., Belardelli, F., Benedetto, A.: Interferon inhibits dimethyl sulphoxide-induced erythoid differentiation of Friend leukemia cells. Nature **267**, 50–52 (1977 c).

Rossman, T. G., Vilček, J.: Influence of the rate of cell growth and cell density on interferon action in chick embryo cells. J. Virol. **4**, 7–18 (1969).

Rossman, T. G., Vilček, J.: Blocking of interferon action by a component of normal serum. Arch. Gesamte Virusforsch. **31**, 18–24 (1970).

Rosztoczy, I.: Interferon induced by poly IC in interferon pretreated L-cells in absence of DEAE-dextran. Acta. Virol. **15**, 431–440 (1971).

Rosztoczy, I.: Further evidences that priming is a non-antiviral function of interferon. Acta. Microbiol. Acad. Sci. Hung. **21**, 305–309 (1974).

Rosztoczy, I.: Interferon pretreatment primes interferon production by human adenovirus in chick embryo cells. Acta. Virol. **20**, 162–163 (1976 a).

Rosztoczy, I.: Study of priming effect of interferon in L-cells. I. Primed interferon response and kinetics of development of priming. Acta. Virol. **20**, 472–485 (1976 b).

Rosztoczy, I.: Study of the priming effect of interferon in L-cells. II. Metabolic requirements for the development of primed state. Acta. Virol. 21, 1–7 (1977).

Rosztoczy, I., Mecs, I.: Enhancement of interferon synthesis by polyinosinic-polycytidylic acid in L-cells pretreated with interferon. Acta. Virol. 14, 398–400 (1970).

Rotem, Z., Cox, R. A., Isaacs, A.: Inhibition of virus multiplication by foreign nucleic acid. Nature 197, 564–566 (1963).

Rouse, B. T., Babiuk, L. A.: The role of neutrophils in antiviral defense – in vitro studies on the mechanism of antiviral inhibition. J. Immunol. 118, 1957–1961 (1977).

Rousset, S.: Refractory state of cells to interferon induction. J. Gen. Virol. 22 (1), 9–20 (1974).

Rousset, S., Fournier, F., Chany, C.: Recherche d'une corrélation entre l'état réfractaire à la synthèse de l'interféron et l'état de résistance antivirale. C. R. Acad. Sc. (Paris) D 271, 267–269 (1970).

Rozee, K. R., Katz, L. J., McFarlane: Interferon stimulation of methylase activity in L-cells. Can. J. Microbiol. 15, 969–974 (1969).

Rozee, K. R., Lee, S. H. S., in: Interferons and their Actions (Stewart II, W. E., ed.), pp. 133–144. Cleveland, Ohio: CRC Press, Inc. (1977).

Rozee, K. R., Lee, S. H., Ngan, J.: Effect of priming on interferon inhibition of Con A induced spleen cell blastogenesis. Nature New Biol. 245 (140), 16–18 (1973).

Ruiz–Gomez, J., Isaacs, A.: Optimal temperature for growth and sensivity to interferon among different viruses. Virology 19, 1–7 (1963 a).

Ruiz–Gomez, J., Isaacs, A.: Interferon production by different viruses. Virology 19, 8–12 (1963 b).

Ruiz–Gomez, J., Sosa–Martinez, J.: Virus multiplication and interferon production at different temperatures in adult mice infected with Coxackie B₁ virus. Archiv für die gesamte Virusforsch. 17, 295–299 (1965).

Russell, P. K., Bellanti, J. A., Buescher, E. L., McCowin, J. M.: Challenge virus resistance and interferon produced in BS-C-1 cells by dengue virus. Proc. Soc. Exp. Biol. Med. 122, 557–561 (1966).

Rytel, M. W.: Interferon response during Coxsackie B-3 infection in mice. I. The effect of cortisone. J. Infect. Dis. 120, 379–386 (1969).

Rytel, M. W.: Antagonism of interferon action by mouse tissue extracts and serum. Arch. Virol. 48, 103–110 (1975).

Rytel, M. W., Ferstenfeld, J. E., Rose, H. D., Balay, J., Pierce, W. E., Lynch, K. L.: Efficacy of a mixed bacterial vaccine in prophylaxis of acute respiratory infections: possible role of interferon. Am. J. Epidemiol. 99, 347–359 (1974).

Rytel, M. W., Hooks, J. J.: Induction of immune interferon by murine cytomegalovirus. Proc. Soc. Exp. Biol. Med. 155, 611–618 (1977).

Rytel, M. W., Jones, T. C.: Induction of interferon in mice infected with Toxoplasma gondii. Proc. Soc. Exp. Biol. Med. 123, 859–862 (1966).

Rytel, M. W., Kilbourne, E. D.: The influence of cortisone on experimental viral infection. VIII. Suppression by cortisone of interferon formation in mice injected with Newcastle disease virus. J. Exp. Med. 123, 767–776 (1966).

Rytel, M. W., Kilbourne, E. D.: Differing susceptibility of adolescent and adult mice to non-lethal infection with Coxsackievirus B 3. Proc. Soc. Exp. Biol. Med. 137, 443–448 (1971).

Rytel, M. W., Marsden, P. D.: Induction of an interferon-like inhibitor by Trypanosoma cruzi in mice. Amer. J. Trop. Med. Hyg. 19, 929–932 (1970).

Rytel, M. W., Rose, H. D., Stewart, R. D.: Absence of circulating interferon in patients with malaria and with American Trypanosomiasis. Proc. Soc. Exp. Biol. Med. 144, 122–123 (1973).

Rytel, M. W., Shope, R. E., Kilbourne, E. D.: An antiviral substance for Penicillium funiculosum. V. Induction of interferon by Helenine. J. Exp. Med. 123, 577–588 (1966).

Saito, N., Kohno, S.: Priming by mouse interferon. Proc. Fifth Aharon-Katzir Katchalsky Conf., Rehobeth, Israel 2–6 May (1977).

Saito, N., Ktame, F., Kikuchi, M., Ishida, N.: Studies on a new antiviral antibiotic, 9-methyl-streptimidone. I. Physicochemical and biological properties. J. Antibiot. 27, 206–214 (1974).

Saito, N., Suzuki, F., Sasaki, K., Ishida, N.: Antiviral and interferon-inducing activity of a new glutarimide antibiotic, 9-methylstreptimidone. Antimicriob. Agents Chemother. **10**, 14–27 (1976).

Salerno, R. A., Whitmire, C. E., Garcia, I. M., Heubner, R. J.: Chemical carcinogenesis in mice inhibited by interferon. Nature New Biol. **239**, 31–32 (1972).

Salvin, S. B., Nishio, J., Shonnard, T.: Two new inhibitory activities in blood of mice with delayed hypersensitivity, after challenge with specific antigen. Infect. Immun. **9**, 631–635 (1974).

Salvin, S. B., Ribi, E., Granger, D. L., Youngner, J. S.: Migration inhibitory factor and type II interferon in the circulation of mice sensitized with mycobacterial components. J. Immunol. **114**, 354–362 (1975a).

Salvin, S. B., Youngner, J. S., Lederer, W. H.: Migration inhibitory factors and interferon in the circulation of mice with delayed hypersensitivity. Infec. Immun. **7**, 68–79 (1973).

Salvin, S. B., Youngner, J. S., Nishio, J., Neta, R.: Tumor suppression by a lymphokine released into the circulation of mice with delayed hypersensitivity. J. Natl. Cancer Inst. **55**, 1233–1235 (1975b).

Salzberg, S., Bakhanashvili, M., Aboud, M.: Effect of interferon on mouse cells chronically infected with murine leukemia virus. J. Gen. Virol. **40**, 121–130 (1978).

Sammons, M. L., Stephen, E. L., Levy, H. B., Baron, S., Hilmas, D. E.: Interferon induction in cynomolgus and rhesus monkey after repeated doses of a modified poly I·poly C complex. Antimicrob. Agts. Chemother. **11**, 80–91 (1977).

Samuel, C. E.: Mechanism of interferon action. Studies on the mechanism of interferon-mediated inhibition of reovirus messenger RNA translation in cell free protein synthesis systems from mouse ascites tumor cells. Virology **75**, 166–173 (1976).

Samuel, C. E., Farris, D. A.: Mechanism of interferon action: species specificity of interferon and of the interferon-mediated inhibitor of translation from mouse, monkey and human cells. Virology **77**, 556–565 (1977).

Samuel, C. E., Joklik, W. K.: A protein synthesizing system from interferon-treated cells that discriminates between cellular and viral messenger RNAs. Virology **58** (2), 476–491 (1974).

Sanders, C. V., Luby, J. P., Stanford, J. P., Hull, A. R.: Suppression of interferon response in lymphocytes from patients with uremia. J. Lab. Clin. Med. **77**, 768–776 (1971).

Sano, E., Matsui, Y., Kobayashi, S.: Production of mouse interferon with high titers in a large-scale suspension culture system. Japn. J. Microbiol. **18**, 165–172 (1974).

Sarma, P. S., Neubauer, R. H., Rabstein, L.: Inhibitory effect of interferon on murine sarcoma virus infection *in vitro*. Proc. Soc. Exp. Biol. Med. **137**, 469–472 (1971).

Sarma, P. S., Shiu, G., Baron, S., Huebner, R. J.: Inhibitory effect of interferon in murine sarcoma and leukaemia virus infection *in vitro*. Nature **223**, 845–846 (1969).

Sather, G. E., Hammon, M. W.: ATC interference test for Dengue viruses. Fed. Proc. **22**, 557 (1963).

Sauter, C., Gifford, G. E.: Interferon-like inhibitor and lysosomal enzyme induced in mice injected with endotoxin. Nature **212**, 626–628 (1966).

Sawicki, L.: Influence of age of mice on the recovery from experimental Sendai virus infection. Nature **192**, 1258–1259 (1961).

Schachter, N., Galin, M., Weissenbacher, M., Baron, S., Billiau, A.: Comparison of antiviral action of interferon, interferon inducers and IDU against Herpes Simplex and other viruses. Ann. Ophthal. **2**, 795–798 (1970).

Schafer, T. W., Lockart, R. Z., jr.: Interferon required for viral resistance induced by poly I: poly C. Nature **226**, 449–450 (1970).

Schafer, T. W., Lieberman, M., Cohen, M., Came, P. E.: Interferon administered orally: protection of neonatal mice from lethal virus challenge. Science, **176**, 1326–1327 (1972).

Schell, K.: Studies on the innate resistance of mice to injection with mouse pox. I. Resistance and antibody production. Aust. J. Exp. Biol. Med. Sci. **38**, 271–280 (1960).

Schellekens, H., Hoffmeyer, J. H. P. M., Van Griensven, L. J. L. D.: The influence of emetine on the induction of interferon by poly I-poly C in Swiss mice. J. Gen. Virol. **26**, 197–212 (1975).

Schiller, A. J. G., Ribovich, R., Feingold, D. S., Youngner, J. S.: Interferon production in mice by components of Salmonella minnesota R 595 Lipid A. Infect. Immun. **14**, 586–599 (1976).

Schlesinger, R. W.: Interference between animal viruses. The Viruses, Vol. III, pp. 157–194. Academic Press (1959).

Schleupner, C. J., Postic, B., Armstrong, J. A., Atchison, R. W., Ho, M.: Two variables of Sindbis virus which differ in interferon induction and serum clearance. J. Infect. Dis. 120, 348–354 (1969).

Schmidt, J. P., Pindak, F. F.: Duration of prophylactic effect of statolon against mengovirus in mice. Appl. Microbiol. 16, 468–476 (1968).

Schmunis, G., Weissenbacher, M., Chowchuvech, E., Sawicki, L., Galin, M. A., Baron, S.: Growth of toxoplasma gondii in various tissue cultured treated with In-Cn or interferon. Proc. Soc. Exp. Biol. Med. 143 (4), 1153–1157 (1973).

Schonne, E.: Properties of rat-tumor interferon. Biochim. Biophys. Acta. 115, 429–439 (1966).

Schonne, E., Billiau, A., Desomer: The properties of interferon IV. Isoelectric focusing of rabbit interferon (NDV-RK 13), in: Symp. Series Immunbiol. 14, p. 61. Basel: Karger (1970).

Schuller, G. B., Morahan, P. S., Snodgrass, M.: Inhibition and enhancement of Friend leukemia virus by pyran copolymer. Cancer. Res. 35, 1915–1919 (1975).

Schulman, J. L., Kilbourne, E. D.: Induction of viral interference in mice by aerosols of inactivated influenza virus. Proc. Soc. Exp. Biol. Med. 113, 431–435 (1963).

Schultz, R. M., Papamatheakis, J. D., Chirigos, M. A.: Interferon: the ultimate inducer of macrophage activation by polyanions. Science 197, 674–675 (1977).

Schultz, W. W., Huang, K., Gordon, F. B.: Role of interferon in experimental mouse malaria. Nature 220, 709–711 (1968).

Schumacher, H. P., Albrecht, P., Taurasa, N. M.: The effect of altered immune reactivity on experimental measles encephalitis in rats. Arch. Gesamte Virusforsch. 37, 218–223 (1972).

Schwartz, A. A., Villani–Price, D.: Interferon assay anomaly. Interferon Workshop, Lake Placid, New York (1977).

Scientific Committee on Interferon: Effect of interferon on vaccination in volunteers. The Lancet, 28 April, pp. 873–875 (1962).

Scientific Committee on Interferon: Experiments with interferon in man. Lancet i, 505–510 (1965).

Scientific Committee on Interferon: Progress towards trials of human interferon in man. Ann. N. Y. Acad. Sci. 173, 770–774 (1970).

Scott, G. M., Butler, J. K., Cartwright, T., Richards, B. M., Kingham, G., Wright, R., Tyrrell, D. A. J., Slavin, G.: Concerning skin hypersensitivity to interferon. Lancet 8034, 402 (1977 a).

Scott, G. M., Cartwright, T., LeDu, G., Dicker, D.: Effect of human fibroblast interferon on vaccination in volunteers. Symp. Prep. Stand. and Clin. Use of Interferon, Zagreb, Yugoslavia (1977 b).

Scott, G. M., Cartwright, T., Tyrrell, D. A. J., Butler, J. K., Porteous, M., Stevens, R. M.: Preliminary experience with fibroblast interferon against vaccinia virus in human and monkey skin. Symp. Prep. Stand. and Clinical Use of Interferon, Zagreb, Yugoslavia (1977 c).

Sedmak, J. J., Grossberg, S. E.: Interferon bioassay: Reduction in yield of myxovirus neuraminidases. J. Gen. Virol. 21, 1–7 (1973).

Sedmak, J. J., Grossberg, S. E., Jameson, P.: The neuraminidase yield-reduction bioassay of human and other interferons. Proc. Soc. Exp. Biol. Med. 149, 433–438 (1975).

Sehgal, P. B.: Thesis, Rockefeller University (1977).

Sehgal, P. B., Dobberstein, B., Tamm, I.: Interferon messenger RNA content of human fibroblasts during induction, shutoff and superinduction of interferon production. Proc. Natl. Acad. Sci. U. S. A. 74, 3409–3413 (1977).

Sehgal, P. B., Tamm, I.: Evaluation of messenger RNA competition in shutoff of human interferon production. Proc. Natl. Acad. Sci. U. S. A. 73, 1621–1627 (1976).

Sehgal, P. B., Tamm, I., Vilček, J.: Human interferon production superinduction by S, 6-dichloro-1β-D-ribofuranosylbenzimidazole. Science 190, 282–285 (1975 a).

Sehgal, P. B., Tamm, I., Vilček, J.: Enhancement of human interferon production by neutral red and chloroquine: analysis of inhibition of protein degradation and macromolecular synthesis. J. Exp. Med. 142, 1283–1290 (1975 b).

Sehgal, P. B., Tamm, I., Vilček, J.: On the mechanism of enhancement of human interferon production of actinomycin D and cycloheximide. Virology 70, 256–265 (1976 a).

Sehgal, P. B., Tamm, Vilček, J.: Regulation of human interferon production. I. Superinduction by 5,6-Dichloro-1-β-D-ribofuranosylbenzimidazole. Virology 70, 532–544 (1976 b).

Sehgal, P. B., Tamm, I., Vilček, J.: Regulation of human interferon production. II. Inhibition of interferon messenger RNA synthesis by 5,6-dichloro-1-β-D-ribofuranozylbenzimidazole. Virology 70, 542–559 (1976c).

Sela, I., Grossberg, S. E., Sedmak, J. J., Mehler, A. H.: Discharge of aminoacyl-viral RNA by a factor from interferon-treated cells. Science 194, 193–195 (1976).

Selivanov, A. A., Lysov, W., Rudenko, L. G., Kovaleva, T., Yurlova, T., Arsenov, O., Smorodintsev, A., Boldasov, V. K.: A study into the biology of intratype variants of adenoviruses 1, 2, 3, 4, and 7. Vopr. Virusol. 5, 46–48 (1970).

Sellers, R. F., Fitzpatrick, M.: An assay of interferon produced in Rhesus monkey and calf kidney tissue cultures using bovine enterovirus M6 as challenge. Brit. J. Exp. Path. 43, 674–683 (1962).

Sen, G. C., Gupta, S. L., Brown, G. E., Lebleu, B., Rebello, M. A., Lengyel, P.: Interferon treatment of Ehrlich ascites tumor cells: Effects on exogenous mRNA translation and tRNA inactivation in the cell extract. J. Virol. 17, 191–203 (1976a).

Sen, G. C., Lebleu, B., Brown, G. E., Kawakita, M., Slattery, E., Lengyel, P.: Interferon, double-stranded RNA and mRNA degradation. Nature 264, 370–377 (1976b).

Sen, G. C., Lebleu, B., Brown, G. E., Rebello, M. A., Furvichi, M. Y., Morgan, M., Shatkin, A., Lengyel, P.: Inhibition of reovirus messenger RNA methylation in extracts of interferon-treated Ehrlich ascites tumor cells. Biochem. Biophys. Res. Commun. 65, 427–439 (1975).

Sen, G. C., Shaila, S., Lebleu, B., Browne, G. E., Desrosiers, R. E., Lengyel, P.: Impairment of reovirus mRNA methylation in extracts of interferon-treated Ehrlich ascites tumor cells: Further characteristics of the phenomenon. J. Virol. 21, 69–76 (1977).

Shaila, S., Lebleu, B., Brown, G. E., Sen, G. C., Lengyel, P.: Characteristics of extracts from interferon-treated HeLa cells: presence of a protein kinase and endoribonuclease activated by dsRNA and of an inhibitor of mRNA methylation. J. Gen. Virol. 37, 535–546 (1977).

Shapiro, S. Z., Strand, M., Billiau, A.: Synthesis and cleavage processing of oncornavirus proteins during interferon inhibition of virus particle release. Infect. Immun. 16, 742–752 (1977).

Sharpe, T. J., Birch, P. J., Planterose, D. W.: Resistance to virus infection during the hyporeactive state of interferon induction. J. Gen. Virol. 12 (3), 331–333 (1971).

Sheaff, E. T., Meager, A., Burke, D. C.: Factors involved in the production of interferon by inactivated Newcastle disease virus. J. Gen. Virol. 17, 163–177 (1972).

Sheaff, E. T., Stewart, R. B.: Interaction of interferon with cells: induction of antiviral activity. Can. J. Microbiol. 15, 941–954 (1969).

Sheaff, E. T., Stewart, R. B.: Interaction of interferon with cells: characteristics of the induction of interferon uptake in relation to interferon antiviral activity. Can. J. Microbiol. 16, 1087–1093 (1970a).

Sheaff, E. T., Stewart, R. B.: Interaction of interferon with cells: the relationship of cell-associated interferon and antiviral activity. Can. J. Microbiol. 16, 1303–1310 (1970b).

Sheaff, E. T., Stewart, R. B.: Interaction of interferon with cells: the synthesis of an interferon-induced protein. Can. J. Microbiol. 16, 1311–1318 (1970c).

Shiokawa, T., Yaoi, I.: Correlation of double-stranded polynucleotide size and interferon production. Arch. ges. Virusforsch. 38, 109–113 (1972).

Shirodkar, N. V.: The blocking effect of West Nile virus on production of sarcoma by Rous virus. J. Immunol. 95, 1121–1132 (1965).

Siegel, B. V.: Enhanced interferon response to murine leukemia virus by ascorbic acid. Infect. Immun. 10, 409–410 (1974).

Siegel, B. V., Brown, M., Morton, Y.: Interferon induction in New Zealand black mice by murine leukemia virus. J. Immunol. 111, 644–651 (1973).

Siegert, R., Shu, H. L., Kohlhage, H.: Correlation between fever and interferon titer in rabbits after induction with myxoviruses. Life Sci. 6, 615–620 (1967).

Siewers, C. M. F., John, C. E., Medearis, D. N.: Sensitivity of human cell strains to interferon. Proc. Soc. Exp. Biol. Med. 133, 1178–1183 (1970).

Siminoff, P.: In vivo and in vitro stimulation of mouse spleen leukocytes by BL-20803, a low molecular weight interferon inducer. Infect. Immun. 12, 1051–1063 (1975).

Siminoff, P.: Target cells for interferon induction by BL-20803. J. Infect. Disease 133, A 37 (1976).

Siminoff, P., Bernard, A. M., Hursky, V. S., Price, K. E.: BL-20803, a new, low-molecular-weight interferon inducer. Antimicrob. Agents Chemotherap. **3**, 742–751 (1973).

Siminoff, P., Crenshaw, R. R.: Stimulation of interferon production in mice and spleen leukocytes by analogues of BL-20803. Antimicrob. Agents Chemother. **11**, 571–577 (1977).

Simon, E. H., Kung, S., Koh, T. T., Brandman, P.: Interferon-sensitive mutants of mengovirus. I. Isolation and biological characterization. Virology **69**, 727–739 (1976).

Singer, S. H., Barile, M. F., Kirschstein, R. L.: Enhanced virus yields and decreased interferon production in mycoplasma-infected hamster cells. Proc. Soc. Exp. Biol. Med. **131**, 1129–1140 (1969).

Singer, S. H., Ford, M., Noguchi, P., Kirschstein, R. L., Baron, S.: Successful induction of locally produced (lung) interferon during the hyporesponsive state. Proc. Soc. Exp. Biol. Med. **143**, 915–918 (1973).

Sinkovic, J. G., Howe, C. D.: Growth characteristics, virus yield and interferon assay of leukemic mouse spleen tissue cultures. J. Infect. Dis. **114**, 359–372 (1964).

Sipe, J. D., DeMaeyer–Guignard, J., Fauconnier, B., DeMaeyer, E.: Purification of mouse interferon by affinity chromatography on a solid-phase immunoadsorbent. Proc. Natl. Acad. Sci. U. S. A. **70**, 1037–1040 (1973).

Skehel, J. J., Burke, D. C.: Interferon production by Semliki forest virus inactivated with hydroxylamine. J. Gen. Virol. **3**, 35–47 (1968a).

Skehel, J. J., Burke, D. C.: A temperature-sensitive event in interferon production. J. Gen. Virol. **3**, 191–209 (1968b).

Skreko, F., Zajac, T., Bahnsen, H. P., Haff, R. F., Cantell, K.: The kinetics of human interferon clearance in gibbons. Proc. Soc. Exp. Biol. Med. **142**, 946–947 (1973).

Skurkovich, S. V., Aleksandrovskaia, I. M.: Effect of interferon on immunological reactivity. Prob. Gematol. Pereliv. Krovi **18**, 43–50 (1973).

Skurkovich, S. V., Eremkina, E. I.: The probable role of interferon in allergy. Annals of Allergy **35**, 377–383 (1975).

Skurkovich, S. V., Eremkina, E. I., Klinova, E. G.: Preparation of anti-interferon serum in animals immunized with heterologous interferon. Vopr. Virusol. **2**, 241–243 (1974).

Skurkovich, S. V., Kalinina, I. A., Eremkina, E. I., Bulycheva, T. I.: Increased sensitivity of leukemia cells incubated in interferon to the action of immune serum. Biull Eksp. Biol. Med. **12**, 1459–1461 (1976a).

Skurkovich, S. V., Kalinina, I. A., Eremkina, E. I., Bulycheva, T. I.: Enhancement of the immune response following immunization with L1210 cells preliminarilly incubated with interferon. Biull. Eksp. Biol. Med. **81**, 706–707 (1976b).

Skurkovich, S. V., Kisljak, N. S., Bulicheva, T. I., Makhonova, L. A., Majakova, S. A., Skorikova, A. S., Erjemkina, E. I.: Active immunization of children suffering from acute leukemia remission with "living" mixed leukoblast vaccine and means of enhancement of antileukemic immunity. Ann. N. Y. Acad. Sci. **277**, 384–395 (1976c).

Skurkovich, S. V., Klinova, E. G., Aleksandrovskaia, I. M., Levina, N. V., Arkhipova, N. A.: Stimulation of transplantation immunity and the plasmacyte reaction in mice by interferon. Biull. Eksp. Biol. Med. **75**, 66–69 (1973a).

Skurkovich, S. V., Klinova, E. G., Aleksandrovskaia, I. M., Levina, N. V., Arkhipova, N. A., Bulicheva, T. I.: Stimulation of transplanation, immunity and plasma cell reaction by interferon in mice. Immunology **25**, 317–322 (1973b).

Skurkovich, S. V., Klinova, E. G., Eremkina, E. I.: Stimulation of humoral immunity to surface antigens of leukemic cells. Bull. Exp. Biol. Med. **81**, 429 (1976).

Slamon, D. J.: Protective effect of the double-stranded polyribonucleotide, polyinosinic–polycytidylic acid, against rat erythroblastosis induced by murine erythroblastosis virus. J. Natl. Cancer Inst. **51**, 851–867 (1973).

Slamon, D. J.: Hemolytic anemia induced by murine erythroblastosis virus – possible mechanisms of hemolysis and effects of an interferon inducer. J. Nat. Cancer Inst. **55**, 329–339 (1975).

Slate, D. L., Shulman, L., Lawrence, J. B., Revel, M., Ruddle, F. H.: Presence of human chromosome 21 alone is sufficient for hybrid cell sensitivity to human interferon. J. Virol. **25**, 319–325 (1978).

Slavina, E. G., Leneva, M. V., Svet–Moldavsky, G. J.: Sensitivity of target cells to the cytotoxic effects of lymphocytes induced by interferon. Folia Biol. (Praha) **20**, 231–237 (1974).

Slavina, E. G., Svet–Moldavsky, G. J.: Introduction by interferon of sensitivity of target cells to the cytotoxic action of lymphocytes. Vopr. Virusol. **18**, 366–368 (1973).

Smart, K. M., Kilbourne, E. D.: The influence of cortisone on experimental viral infection VI. Inhibition by hydrocortisone of interferon synthesis in the chick embryo. J. Exp. Med. **123**, 299–307 (1966).

Smetana, O., Eylan, E., Weinberg, M.: Inhibition of herpes simplex virus strains isolated from herpetic keratitis by poly I·C. Antimicrob. Agents Chemother. **11**, 797–811 (1977).

Smirnova, T. D., Kagan, G.: Effect of Mycoplasma-viral infection of a primary culture of chick embryo cells on interferon production induced by langet virus. Zh. Mikrobiol. Epidemiol. Immunobiol. **48**, 54–58 (1971).

Smith, K. A., Fredrickson, T. N., Mobraaten, L. E., DeMaeyer, E.: The interaction of erythropoietin with fetal liver cells. II. Inhibition of the erythropoietin effect by interferon. Exp. Hematol. **14**, 164–168 (1976).

Smith, T. J., Lubinecki, A. S., Armstrong, J. A., Russ, S. B.: Interferon induced by endotoxin and Newcastle disease virus in rabbit macrophage and kidney cell cultures. Proc. Soc. Exp. Biol. Med. **142**, 481–486 (1973).

Smith, T. J., Wagner, R. R.: Rabbit macrophage interferons. I. Conditions for biosynthesis by virus-infected and uninfected cells. J. Exp. Med. **125**, 559–577 (1967 a).

Smith, T. J., Wagner, R. R.: Rabbit macrophage interferons. II. Some physicochemical properties and estimations of molecular weights. J. Exp. Med. **125**, 579–593 (1967 b).

Smorodintsev, A. A.: The production and effect of interferon in organ cultures of calf trachea. Brit. J. Exp. Path. **49**, 511–515 (1968).

Smorodintsev, A. A., Beare, A. S., Bynoe, M. L., Head, B., Tyrrell, D. A. J.: The formation of interferon during acute respiratory virus infection of volunteers. Archiv ges. Virusforsch. **33**, 9–16 (1971 a).

Smorodintsev, A. A., Gvozdilova, D. A., Aksenov, O. A., Makarjev, G. S., Korsantya, B. M., Gaber, V. K., Gorodnev, A. G., Zlydnikov, D. M., Osidak, L. V., Shvetsova, E. G., Romanov, Y. A., Karpats, N. M.: Enhancement of nonspecific resistance to influenza due to induction of endogenous interferon. Proc. Symp. of Live Influenza Vaccine. Yugoslav Acad. Sci. and Arts, Zagreb (1971 b).

Smorodintsev, A. A., Gvozdilova, D. A., Romanov, Y. A., Makajev, G. S., Rudenko, V. I., Aksenov, O. A., Zlydnikov, D. M.: Induction of endogenous interferon by use of standard live vaccines for prevention of respiratory viral infections. Ann. N. Y. Acad. Sci. **173**, 811–822 (1970).

Smorodintsev, A. A., Rudenko, V. I., Moshkin, S. A., Gvozdilova, D. A., Aksenov, D. A.: Interferon and resistance to the toxic effects of influenza virus *in vivo*. J. Gen. Virol. **5**, 459–462 (1969).

Snodgrass, M. J., Morahan, P. S., Kaplan, A. M.: Histopathology of the host response to Lewis lung carcinoma: modulation by pyran. J. Natl. Cancer Inst. **55**, 455–467 (1975).

Snyderman, R., Wohlenberg, C., Notkins, A. L.: Inflammation and viral infection: Chemostatic activity resulting from the interaction of antiviral antibody and complement with cells infected with Herpes Simplex virus. J. Infect. Dis. **126**, 207–221 (1972).

Soave, O. A.: Influence of statolon-induced interferon on rabies virus infection in mice. Am. J. Vet. Res. **29**, 1507–1508 (1968).

Soehner, R. L., Gambardella, M. M., Hou, E. F.: Oral induction of interferon by a low-molecular-weight compound. Proc. Soc. Exp. Biol. Med. **145**, 1114–1119 (1974).

Sokawa, Y., Watanabe, Y., Kawade, Y.: Suppressive effect of interferon on the transition from a quiescent to a growing state in 3 T 3 cells. Nature **268**, 236–238 (1977).

Sokhey, J., Soloviev, A. I., Vasilieva, V. I.: Induction of interferon in mice and cell cultures by *Mycoplasma pneumoniae*. Acta Virol. **21**, 485–490 (1977).

Solomon, G. F., Merigan, T. C., Levine, S.: Variation in adrenal cortical hormones within physiologic ranges, stress and interferon production in mice. Proc. Soc. Exp. Biol. Med. **126**, 74–79 (1967).

Soloviev, V. D.: Some results and prospects in the study of endogenous and exogenous interferon, in: The Interferons (Rita, G., ed.), p. 233. New York: Academic Press (1967).

Soloviev, V. D.: The results of controlled observation on the prophylaxis of influenza with interferon. Bull. World Health Organ. **41**, 683–690 (1969).

Soloviev, V. D., Balandin, I. G., Marchenko, V. I., Dyllisalieva, R. G., Koltsov, W. D., Arevsh-atyan, N. N., Rusanova, N. A.: The phenomenon of tolerance (hyporesponsiveness) in interferon induction. Voprosy Virusol. 2, 156–159 (1974).

Soloviev, V. D., Malinovskaya, V. V., Khesin, Ya. E., Pokidysheva, L. N., Marchenko, V. I.: Acid phosphatase activity and the capacity for interferon production by cells of peritoneal exudate of mice of different ages. Voprosy Virusol. 3, 533–537 (1972 a).

Soloviev, V. D., Mentkevich, L. M.: The effect of colchicine on viral interference and interferon formation. Acta Virol. 9, 308–312 (1965).

Soloviev, V. D., Mentkevich, L. M., Orlova, T. G., Georgadze, I., Amchenkova, A. M., Zhdanova, L. V.: Serum and bone marrow interferons in radiation chimeras. Acta Virol. 16, 382–387 (1972 b).

Sonnabend, J. A.: An effect of interferon on uninfected chick embryo fibroblasts. Nature 203, 496–498 (1964).

Sonnabend, J. A., Friedman, R. M.: Mechanism of interferon action, in: Interferons and Interferon Inducers (Finter, N. B., ed.), pp. 201–238. Amsterdam: North-Holland, Publ. Co. (1973).

Sonnabend, J. A., Martin, E. M., Meces, E., Fantes, K. H.: The effect of interferon on the synthesis of an RNA polymerase isolated from chick cells infected with Semliki Forest virus. J. Gen. Virol. 1, 41–48 (1967).

Sonnenfeld, G., Mandel, A. D., Merigan, T. C.: The immunosuppressive effect of Type II mouse interferon preparations on antibody production. Cell Immunol. 34, 193–206 (1977).

Soos, E., Ikic, D., Jusic, D., Smerdel, S., Petricevic, I., Kunsten, D., Soldo, I.: Treatment of local complications provoked by vaccinia virus with leukocytic interferon. Proc. Symp. on Combined Vaccines, Yugoslav Acad. Sci. and Arts, Zagreb, pp. 179–182 (1972).

Southam, C. M.: Present status of oncolytic virus studies. Trans. N. Y. Acad. Sci. 83, 551–572 (1960).

Southam, C. M., Moore, A. E.: Clinical studies of viruses as antineoplastic agents with particular reference to Egypt 101 virus. Cancer 5, 1025–1030 (1952).

Speel, L. F., Osborn, J. E., Walker, D. L.: An immuno-cytopathogenic interaction between sensitized leukocytes and epithelial cells carrying a persisent noncytocidal myxovirus infection. J. Immunol. 101, 409–418 (1968).

Spina, C. A., Chang, R. S., Mishra, L., Golden, H. D.: Interferon production by human cells in vitro. Appl. Microbiol. 24, 735–741 (1972).

Sreevalsan, T.: Variable response of human cells to polynosinic-polycytidylic acid. Antimicrob. Agents Chemotherap. 3, 642–651 (1973).

Sreevalsan, T., Lockart, R. Z., jr.: A comparison of methods for interferon assay. Virology 17, 207–208 (1962).

Stampfer, M., Baltimore, D., Huang, A. S.: Ribonucleic acid synthesis of vesicular stomatitis virus. I. Species of RNA formed in Chinese hamster ovary cells infected with plaque-forming and defective particles. J. Virol. 4, 154–162 (1969).

Stancek, D.: The role of interferon in tick-borne encephalitis virus-induced L-cells. III. The effects of temperature on the production of virus and interferon by L-cells during acute and persistent infection. Acta Virol. 9, 298–307 (1965).

Stancek, D., Gressnerova, M., Paucker, K.: Isoelectric components of mouse, human and rabbit interferons. Virology 41, 740–750 (1970).

Stancek, D., Matisova, E.: Potentiation of the antiviral activity of interferon by histones. Acta Virol. 12, 309–321 (1968).

Stancek, D., Paucker, K.: Preparative electrophoresis of isotopically labeled L-cell interferons. Appl. Microbiol. 21, 1067–1071 (1971).

Stancek, D., Vilček, J.: The role of interferon in tick-borne encephalitis virus infected L-cells. I. Acute infection. Acta Virol. 9, 1–8 (1965).

Stanley, E. D., Jackson, G. G., Dirda, V. A., Rubenis, M.: Effect of topical interferon inducer on rhinovirus infections in volunteers. J. Infect. Dis. 133, A 121 (1976).

Stanton, G. J., May, D. C.: A more precise and sensitive hemagglutination reduction assay for interferon. Proc. Soc. Exp. Biol. Med. 143, 1048–1052 (1973).

Steeves, D. P., Barker, L. F., Brown, E. R., Hopps, H. E., Meyer, H. M., jr.: Lymphoblastoid cell cultures from patients with infectious hepatitis. Bacteriol. Proc., p. 151 (1969).

Stephen, E. L., Hilmas, D. E., Mangiafico, J. A., Levy, H. B.: Swine influenza virus vaccine potentiation in rhesus monkeys of antibody responses in a nuclease resistant derivative of poly I·poly C. Science 197, 1289–1291 (1977a).

Stephen, E. L., Sammons, M. L., Pannier, W. L., Baron, S., Spertzel, R. O., Levy, H. B.: Effect of a nuclease-resistant derivative of poly I·C on yellow fever in rhesus monkeys. J. Infect. Dis. 136, 122–126 (1977b).

Stevens, D. A., Easton, J. M., Levine, P. H., Waggoner, D. E., Manaker, R. A., Schidlovsky, G.: Antilymphocyte serum and lymphoid cell-virus carrier culture: cell kinetics morphology, EB virus replication, interferon. Cell. Immunol. 3, 629–643 (1972).

Stevens, D. A., Merigan, T. C.: Interferon, antibody and other host factors in herpes zoster. J. Clin. Invest. 51, 1170–1178 (1967).

Stewart, R. B., Gandhi, S. S.: Variation in sensitivity of an interferon assay system. Can. J. Microbiol. 13, 1421–1425 (1967).

Stewart, R. B., Sheaff, E. T.: Effect of interferon on Sindbis virus growth in chick-embryo cell cultures. Can. J. Microbiol. 15, 605–610 (1971).

Stewart, R. B., Sheaff, E. T.: Interaction of interferon with cells: the relationship between interferon uptake and activity. Can. J. Microbiol. 18, 725–730 (1972).

Stewart II, W. E.: Mechanisms of persistence of Japanese encephalitis virus in bats and bat cell cultures. Thesis, University of Texas (1969).

Stewart II, W. E.: The Natural Recovery Process from Acute Viral Infection, in: Selective Inhibitors of Viral Functions (Carter, W. C., ed.), pp. 1–26. Cleveland, Ohio: CRC Press, Inc. (1973).

Stewart II, W. E.: Distinct molecular species of interferons. Virology 61, 80–86 (1974).

Stewart II, W. E.: Uptake of interferon: the fate of cell-bound interferon during induction of antiviral and non-antiviral activities, in: Effects of Interferon on Cells, Viruses and the Immune System (Geraldes, A., ed.), pp. 75–98. New York: Academic Press (1975a).

Stewart II, W. E.: Antiviral and non-antiviral activities of distinct molecular populations of interferons. Symp. Antivirals with Clinical Potential, Stanford, Calif. (1975b).

Stewart II, W. E.: Purification and characterization of interferons. In: Interferons and Their Actions (Stewart II, W. E., ed.), pp. 49–72. Cleveland, Ohio: CRC Press, Inc. (1977).

Stewart II, W. E., Allen, R., Sulkin, S. E.: Persistent infection in bats and bat cell cultures with Japanese encephalis virus. Bacteriological Proceed., V 283 (1969).

Stewart II, W. E., Chudzio, T., Lin, L. S., Wiranowska–Stewart, M.: Interferoids: In vitro and in vivo production of modified interferons. Proc. Nat. Acad. Sci. U. S. A. 75, 4814–4818 (1978).

Stewart II, W. E., DeClercq, E.: Non-antiviral effects of interferons (1973). Medikon 6, 279 (1973).

Stewart II, W. E., DeClercq, E.: Relationship of cytotoxicity and interferoninducing activity of polyriboinosinic acid. Polyribocytidylic acid to the molecular weights of the homopolymers. J. Gen. Virol. 23, 83–89 (1974).

Stewart II, W. E., DeClercq, E., Billiau, A., Desmyter, J., DeSomer, P.: Increased susceptibility of cells treated with interferon to the toxicity of polyriboinosinic–polyribocytidylic acid. Proc. Natl. Acad. Sci. U. S. A. 69, 1851–1854 (1972).

Stewart II, W. E., DeClercq, E., DeSomer, P.: Cellular alteration by interferon; a virus-free system for assaying interferon. J. Virol. 10, 896–901 (1972a).

Stewart II, W. E., DeClercq, E., DeSomer, P.: Recovery of cell-bound interferon. J. Virol. 10, 707–712 (1972b).

Stewart II, W. E., DeClercq, E., DeSomer, P.: Specificity of interferon-induced enhancement of toxicity for double-stranded ribonucleic acids. J. Gen. Virol. 18, 237–246 (1973).

Stewart II, W. E., DeClercq, E., DeSomer, P.: Stabilization of interferons by defensive reversible denaturation. Nature 249, 460–474 (1974).

Stewart II, W. E., DeClercq, E., DeSomer, P., Berg, K., Ogburn, C. A., Paucker, K.: Antiviral and non-antiviral activity of highly-purified interferon. Nature New Biol. 246, 141–143 (1973).

Stewart II, W. E., Desmyter, J.: Molecular heterogeneity of human leukocyte interferon: two populations differing in molecular weights, requirements for renaturation and cross-species antiviral activity. Virology 67, 68–78 (1975).

Stewart II, W. E., DeSomer, P., DeClercq, E.: Renaturation of inactivated interferons: requirement for reduction of a major component; lack of requirement for reduction of a minor component. J. Gen. Virol. 24, 567–570 (1974a).

Stewart II, W. E., DeSomer, P., DeClercq, E.: Protective effect of anionic detergents on interferons: reversible denaturation. Biochim. Biophys. Acta 359, 364–368 (1974b).

Stewart II, W. E., DeSomer, P., DeClercq, E.: Renaturation of inactivated interferons by "defensive reversible denaturation". Prep. Biochem. 4, 383–389 (1974c).

Stewart II, W. E., DeSomer, P., Edy, V. G., Paucker, K., Berg, K., Ogburn, C. A.: Distinct molecular species of human interferons: requirements for stabilization and reactivation of human leukocyte and fibroblast interferons. J. Gen. Virol. 26, 327–333 (1975a).

Stewart II, W. E., Gosser, L. B., Lockart, R. Z., jr.: Priming: a non-antiviral function of interferon. J. Virol. 7, 792–801 (1971a).

Stewart II, W. E., Gosser, L. B., Lockart, R. Z., jr.: Distinguishing characteristics of the interferon responses of primary and continuous mouse cell cultures. J. Gen. Virol. 13, 35–50 (1971b).

Stewart II, W. E., Gosser, L. B., Lockart, R. Z., jr.: The effect of priming with interferon on interferon production by two lines of L-cells. J. Gen. Virol. 15, 85–87 (1972).

Stewart II, W. E., Gresser, I., Tovey, M. G., Bandu, M. T., LeGoff, S.: Identification of the cell-multiplication-inhibitory factors in interferon preparations as interferons. Nature 262, 300–303 (1976).

Stewart II, W. E., Lin, L. S. and Wiranowska-Stewart, M.: Antiviral and other activities of pure interferons and interferoids. Proceedings of the IVth Int. Cong. Virology, Den Haag, Netherlands (1978).

Stewart II, W. E., Lin, L. S., Wiranowska–Stewart, M., Cantell, K.: Elimination of size and charge heterogeneities of human leukocyte interferons by chemical cleavage. Proc. Natl. Acad. Sci. U. S. A. 74, 4200–4204 (1977).

Stewart II, W. E., Lockart, R. Z., jr.: Relative antiviral resistance induced in homologous and heterologous cells by cross-reacting interferons. J. Virol. 6, 795–799 (1970).

Stewart II, W. E., Lutskus, J. M., Sulkin, S. E.: Chromosomal stability of bat cells in culture. Caryologia 23, 163–172 (1970).

Stewart II, W. E., Scott, W. D., Sulkin, S. E.: Relative sensitivities of viruses to different species of interferon. J. Virol. 4, 147–153 (1969).

Stewart II, W. E., Sulkin, S. E.: Interferon production in hamsters experimentally infected with rabies virus. Proc. Soc. Exp. Biol. Med. 123, 650–653 (1966).

Stewart II, W. E., Sulkin, E.: Evaluating the role of interferon in rabies infection. Bacteriological Proceedings V 23 (1968).

Stewart II, W. E., Wiranowska, M., Kobus, M., Szmigielski, S., Korbecki, M.: Increased sensitivites of interferon-treated cells to the toxicities of double-stranded RNAs and lectins. Abstr. Ann. Meeting, Amer. Soc. Microbiol. (1975b).

Stewart II, W. E., Wiranowska, M., Kobus, M., Korbecki, M., Luczak, M., Szmigielski, S.: Synergistic antitumor activity of interferon and poly rI·poly rC against murine sarcoma. Symp. Antivirals with Clinical Potential, Stanford, Calif. (1975c).

Stim, T. B.: Interference of coccal virus with Friend leukemia virus-induced splenomegaly in DBA/2 J mice. Proc. Soc. Exp. Biol. Med. 134, 413–418 (1970).

Stinebring, W. R., Absher, P. M.: Production of interferon following an immune response. Ann. N. Y. Acad. Sci. 173, 714–725 (1970).

Stinebring, W. R., Youngner, J. S.: Patterns of interferon appearance in mice injected with bacteria and bacterial endotoxin. Nature 204, 712–715 (1964).

Stobo, J., Green, I., Jackson, L., Baron, S.: Identification of a subpopulation of mouse lymphoid cells required for interferon production after stimulation with mitogens. J. Immunol. 112, 1589–1593 (1974).

Stoker, D., Kiernat, J., Gauntt, C.: Interferon induction by rhinoviruses and effect of interferon on rhinovirus yields in human cell lines. Proc. Soc. Exp. Biol. Med. 143, 23–27 (1973).

Stokes, J., jr., Reilly, C. M., Buynak, E. B., Hilleman, M. R.: Immunologic studies of measles. Am. J. Hyg. 74, 293–300 (1961).

Strander, H.: Interferons: Anti-neoplastic drugs? Blut 35, 277–288 (1977a).

Strander, H.: Antitumor effects of interferon and its possible use as an antineoplastic agent in man. Texas Rep. Biol. Med. 35, 429–435 (1977b).

Strander, H.: Administration of exogenous leucocyte interferon into patients with neoplastic diseases. Fifth Aharon Katzir–Katchalsky Conference, Rehovot, Israel (1977c).

Strander, H., Cantell, K.: Production of interferon by human leukocytes in vitro. Ann. Med. Exp. Biol. Fenn. 44, 265–273 (1966).

Strander, H., Cantell, K.: Studies on antiviral and antitumor effects of human leukocyte interferon in vitro and in vivo. In Vitro Monograph 3, 49–56 (1974).

Strander, H., Cantell, K., Carlstrom, G., Jakobsson, P. A.: Clinical and laboratory investigations on man; systemic administration of potent interferon to man. J. Natl. Cancer Inst. 51, 733–739 (1973).

Strander, H., Cantell, K., Carlstrom, G., Ingimarsson, S., Jakobsson, P., Nilsonne, U.: Acute infections in interferon-treated patients with osteosarcoma: a preliminary report of a comparative study. J. Infect. Dis. 133, A 245–248 (1976).

Strander, H., Cantell, K., Ingimarsson, S., Jakobsson, P. A., Nilsonne, U., Soderberg, G.: Interferon treatment of osteogenic sarcoma: a clinical trial. Fogarty Intern. Center Proc. 28, 377–380 (1977).

Strander, H., Cantell, K., Jakobsson, P. A., Nilsonne, U., Soderberg, G.: Exogenous interferon therapy of osteogenic sarcoma. Acta Orthop. Scand. 45, 958–967 (1974).

Strander, H., Cantell, K., Leisti, J., Nikkila, E.: Interferon response of lymphocytes in disorders with decreased resistance to infections. Clin. Exp. Immunol. 6, 263 (1970).

Strander, H., Einhorn, S.: Effect of human leukocyte interferon on the growth of human osteosarcoma cells in tissue culture. Internatl. J. Cancer 19, 468–471 (1977).

Strander, H., Mogensen, K. E., Cantell, K.: Production of human lymphoblastoid interferon. J. Clin. Microbiol. 1, 116–124 (1975).

Strandstrom, H., Sandelin, K., Oker–Blum, M.: Inhibitory effect of Coxsackie virus, influenza virus, and interferon on Rous sarcoma virus. Virology 16, 384–391 (1962).

Straub, O. C., Ahl, R.: Local induction of interferon in cattle after intranasal infection with foot-and-mouth disease virus. Zentr. Vet. B 23, 470–476 (1976).

Straub, S. X., Garry, R. F., Magee, W. E.: Interferon induction by poly I·poly C enclosed in phospholipid particles. Infect. Immun. 10, 783–792 (1974).

Stringfellow, D. A.: Hyporeactivity to interferon induction: characterization of a hyporeactive factor in the serum of encephalomyocarditis virus-infected mice. Infect. Immun. 11, 294 (1975).

Stringfellow, D. A.: Murine leukemia: depressed response to interferon induction correlated with a serum hyporeactive factor. Infect. Immun. 13, 392–404 (1976).

Stringfellow, D. A.: Comparative interferon inducing and antiviral properties of 2-amino-5-bromo-6-methyl-4-pyrimidinol (U-25, 166), tilorone HCl and poly I·C. Antimicrob. Agts. Chemother. 11, 984–996 (1977a).

Stringfellow, D. A.: Production of the interferon protein: hyporesponsiveness. Tex. Rep. Biol. Med. 35, 126–131 (1977b).

Stringfellow, D. A., Glasgow, L. A.: Hyporeactivity of interferon: potential limitation to therapeutic use of interferon-inducing agents. Infect. Immun. 6, 743–751 (1972a).

Stringfellow, D. A., Glasgow, L. A.: Tilorone hydrochloride: an oral interferon-inducing agent. Antimicrob. Agents Chemotherap. 2, 73–85 (1972b).

Stringfellow, D. A., Glasgow, L. A.: Hyporeactivity due to infection: recognition of a tranferable hyporeactive factor in the serum of Encephalomyocarditis virus-infected mice. Infect. Immun. 10, 1337–1342 (1974).

Stringfellow, D. A., Gorman, R., Li, L. H., Mathews, J., Vanderberg, H. C.: Hyporeactivity to interferon induction: characteristics of suppressed cells. Personal communication (1977a).

Stringfellow, D. A., Kern, E. R., Kelsey, D. K., Glasgow, L. A.: Suppressed response to interferon induction in mice infected with EMC, SFV, A 2 influenza, herpes hominis type 2 or murine cytomegaloviruses. J. Infect. 135, 540–551 (1977b).

Stringfellow, D. A., Overall, J. C., jr., Glasgow, L. A.: Interferon inducers in therapy of infection with encephalomyocarditis virus in mice. I. Effect of single doses of polyriboinosinic-polyribocytidylic acid and tilorone hydrochloride on viral pathogenesis. J. Infect. Dis. 130, 470–482 (1974a).

Stringfellow, D. A., Overall, J. C., jr., Glasgow, L. A.: Interferon inducers in therapy of infection with encephalomyocarditis virus in mice. II. Effect of multiple doses of polyriboinosinic-polyribocytidylic acid on viral pathogenesis. J. Infect. Dis. 130, 481–493 (1974b).

Stringfellow, D. A., Weed, S. D.: Feline interferon response to 2-amino-5-bromo-6-methyl-4-pyrimidinol (U-25, 166). Amer. J. Vet. Res. **38** 1963–1968 (1977).

Styk, B., Borecky, L., Vetrak, J., Fuchsberger, N., Lackovic, V., Hajnick, A. V.: Contribution to the problem of purity of interferon preparations. Acta Virol. **17**, 163–166 (1973).

Subrahmanyan, T. P.: A study of the possible basis of age-dependent resistance of mice to pox-virus diseases. Aust. J. Exp. Biol. Med. Sci. **46**, 251–260 (1968).

Subrahmanyan, T. P., Mims, C. A.: Fate of intravenously administered interferon and the distribution of interferon during virus infections in mice. Brit. J. Exp. Pathol. **47**, 168–171 (1966).

Sueltenfuss, E. A., Pollard, M.: Cytochemical assay of interferon produced by duck hepatitis virus. Science **139**, 595–596 (1963).

Sugar, J., Kaufman, H. E., Varnell, E. D.: Effect of exogenous interferon on herpetic keratitis in rabbits and monkeys. Investigative Ophthalmology **12**, 378–386 (1973).

Sugiyama, M., Yamamoto, K., Kinoshita, Y., Kimura, S., Shibata, T., Watanabe, M.: Blast formation and interferon production of human tonsil lymphocytes with cellular immunoresponses, Jap. J. Tonsil. **13**, 104–112 (1974).

Sugiyama, M., Yamamoto, K., Kinoshita, Y., Kimura, S., Watanabe, M.: Interferon producing ability of the lymphocyte isolated from the tonsil. J. Otolaryngol. Jap. **75**, 1066–1067 (1972).

Suh, M., Bodo, G., Wolf, W., Viehhauser, G., Jungwirth, C.: Interferon effect on cellular functions: enhancement of virus induced inhibition of host cell protein synthesis in interferon-treated cells. Z. Naturforsch. **29 C**, 623–629 (1974).

Sulkowski, E., Davey, M. W., Carter, W. A.: Interaction of human interferons with immobilized hydrophobic amino acids and dipeptides. J. Biol. Chem. **251**, 5381–5390 (1976).

Sundmacher, R., Neumann–Haefelin, D., Cantell, K.: Interferon treatment of dendritic keratitis. Lancet **26**, 1406–1407 (1976a).

Sundmacher, R., Neumann–Haefelin, D., Cantell, K.: Successful treatment of dendritic keratitis with human leukocyte interferon. Albrecht v. Graefes Arch. Klin. Exp. Ophthal. **201**, 39–45 (1976b).

Sundmacher, R., Neumann–Haefelin, D., Manthey, K. F., Muller, O.: Interferon in treatment of dendritic keratitis in humans: a preliminary report. J. Infect. Dis. **133**, A 160–A 165 (1976c).

Sundmacher, R., Neumann–Haefelin, D., Shrestha, B.: The effect of human leukocyte interferon on experimental viral keratitis in monkeys. Alb. v. Graefes Arch. Klin. Exp. Ophthal. **195**, 263–270 (1975).

Suntharasamai, P., Rytel, M. W.: Interferon response and interferon action in Eperythrozoon coccoides infection of mice. Proc. Soc. Exp. Biol. Med. **142**, 811–816 (1973).

Sutton, R. N. P., Tyrrell, D. A. J.: Some observations on interferon prepared in tissue cultures. Brit. J. Exp. Pathol. **42**, 99–104 (1961).

Suzuki, F., Ishida, N., Suzuki, M., Sato, T., Suzuki, S.: Effect of the interferon inducer, Dextran Phosphate on influenza virus infection in mice. Proc. Soc. Exp. Biol. Med. **149**, 1069–1074 (1975).

Suzuki, F., Koide, T., Tsunoda, A., Ishida, N.: Mushroom extract as an interferon inducer. I. Biological and physicochemical properties of spore extracts of *Lentinus edodes*. Mushroom Sci. **9**, 509–520 (1974).

Suzuki, F., Saito, N., Ishida, N.: Effect of an interferon inducer, 9-methylstreptimidone, on influenza virus infection in mice. Ann. N. Y. Acad. Sci. **284**, 667–672 (1977).

Suzuki, F., Suganuma, T., Ishida, N.: Interferon induction by an antitumor antibiotic, lymphomycin. J. Antibiot. (Tokyo) **27**, 376–378 (1974).

Suzuki, J., Akaboshi, T., Kobayash, S.: A rapid and simple method for assaying interferon. Japan J. Microbiol. **18**, 449–456 (1974).

Suzuki, S., Suzuki, M., Imaya, M.: Interferon-inducing activity of acidic polysaccharides. I. Induction of rabbit serum interferon by *Hansenula Phosphomanans*. Jap. J. Microbiol. **15**, 485–492 (1971).

Suzuki, S., Suzuki, M., Imaya, M., Chaki, F.: Interferon-inducing activity of acid polysaccharides. II. Induction of rabbit serum interferon by chemically phosphorylated polysaccharides. Jap. J. Microbiol. **16**, 1–5 (1972).

Svet-Moldavsky, G. J., Chernyakhovskaya, I. Yu.: Interferon and the interaction of allogeneic normal and immune lymphocytes with L-cells. Nature 215, 1299–1300 (1967).

Svet-Moldavsky, G. J., Nemirovskaya, B. M., Osipova, T. V.: Interferonogenicity and antigen recognition. Nature 247, 205–206 (1974).

Svet–Moldavsky, G. J., Nemirovskaya, B. M., Osipova, T. V., Slavina, E. G., Zinzar, S. N., Karmanova, N. V., Morozova, L. F.: Interferonogenicity of antigens and early cytotoxicity of lymphocytes. Folia Biol. (Praha) 20, 225–230 (1974).

Swetly, P.: Induction of interferon and erythropoietic differentiation in cells transformed by Friend virus. J. Virol. 17, 27–35 (1976).

Swetly, P., Ostertag, W.: Friend virus release and induction of haemoglobin synthesis in erythroleukemic cells respond differently to interferon. Nature 251, 642–644 (1974).

Sydiskis, R. J., Schultz, I.: Interferon and antibody production in mice with Herpes simplex skin infections. J. Infect. Dis. 116, 455–460 (1966).

Szalaty, H., Golubska, B.: The in vitro effect of cyclophosphamide on col. MM virus replication and interferon production. Acta Microbiol. Pol. A 5, 176–180 (1973).

Szalaty, H., Lobodzinska, M., Albin, M.: The influence of immunization on production of interferon in vivo and in vitro. Arch. Immunol. Ther. Exp. 25, 719–724 (1977).

Szolgay, E., Talas, M.: Interferon synthesis in mouse peritoneal cells damaged by X-irradiation. Intervirology 7, 338–345 (1976–1977).

Taborsky, S. I., Stancek, D.: Can a part of an inducer become incorporated into interferon? Med. Microbiol. Immunol. 160, 53–57 (1974).

Takano, K., Jensen, K. E., Warren, J.: Induced resistance to intranasal viral infections by nucleic acid prophylaxis. Bacteriol. Proc., p. 138 (1963).

Takehara, M.: Studies on interferon induction and antiviral activity by certain arboviruses. Kobe J. Med. Sci. 21, 23–32 (1975 a).

Takehara, M.: Interferon inducing capacity and antiviral action of double-stranded RNA from Rice dwarf virus in vitro. Kobe. J. Med. Sci. 21, 33–36 (1975 b).

Takehara, M., Suzuki, N.: Interferon induction by rice dwarf virus RNA. Antiviral activity in vitro and its stability. Arch. Ges. Virusforsch. 40, 291–299 (1973).

Takeyama, H., Nishiwaki, H., Yamada, K., Ito, Y., Nagata, I.: Experimental studies on antitumor effects of interferon (cited in Gresser, 1977 b) (1975).

Talas, M.: Interferon stimulation and other phenotypic properties of two variants of polyoma virus. Acta Microbiol. Acad. Sci. Hung. 16, 319–332 (1969).

Talas, M., Konstantinova, I., Fuks, B. B., Stoger, I., Szolgay, E.: Interferon, nucleic acid and protein synthesis in mouse spleen cells after acute-irradiation. J. Gen. Virol. 18, 393–397 (1973).

Talas, M., Stoger, I.: Hormone petreatment and interferon production in mice. Acta Virol. 16, 211–216 (1972).

Talas, M., Szolgay, E., Rozsa, K.: Further study of spontaneous interferon produced by hamster peritoneal cells. Arch. Ges. Virusforsch. 38, 149–158 (1972).

Talas, M., Szolgay, E., Varteresz, V., Koczk, As G.: Influence of acute and fractional X-irradiation on induction of interferon in vivo. Arch. gesamte Virusforsch. 38, 143–148 (1972).

Talas, M., Weiszfeiler, G., Batkai, L.: Hamster interferons induced by polyoma virus. Acta Virol. 12, 378–380 (1968).

Talash, M. Ya., Savchenko, N. Ya., Sheyeen, V. I., Fedorenko, B. S., Ryzhov, N. I., Konstantinova, I. V.: Influence of interferon inductors on the progress of radiation disease in mice irradiated with high energy protons. Vopr. Virusol. 3, 237–241 (1974).

Tamm, I., Sehgal, P. B.: A comparative study of the effects of certain halogenated benzimidazole ribosides on RNA synthesis, cell proliferation, and interferon production J. Exp. Med. 145, 344–351 (1977).

Tan, Y. H.: Chromosome-21-dosage effect on inducibility of anti-viral gene(s). Nature 253, 280–282 (1975).

Tan, Y. H.: Chromosome 21 and the cell growth inhibitory effect of human interferon preparations. Nature 260, 141–142 (1976).

Tan, Y. H.: Genetics of the human interferon system, in: Interferons and Their Actions (Stewart II, W. E., ed.), pp. 73–90. Cleveland, Ohio: CRC Press, Inc. (1977).

Tan, Y. H., Armstrong, J. A., Ho, M.: Accentuation of interferon production by metabolic inhibitors and its dependence on protein synthesis. Virology **41**, 503–509 (1971 a).

Tan, Y. H., Armstrong, J. A., Ho, M.: Intracellular interferon: kinetics of formation and release. Virology **45** (3), 837–840 (1971 b).

Tan, Y. H., Armstrong, J. A., Ke, Y. M., Ho., M.: Regulation of cellular interferon production: enhancement by antimetabolites. Proc. Natl. Acad. Sci. **67**, 464–471 (1970).

Tan, Y. H., Berthold, W.: A mechanism for the induction and regulation of human interferon genetic expression. J. Gen. Virol. **34**, 401–412 (1977).

Tan, Y. H., Chou, E. L., Lundh, N.: Regulation of chromosome 21-directed antiviral gene(s) as a consequence of age. Nature **257**, 310–312 (1975).

Tan, Y. H., Creagan, R. P., Ruddle, F. M.: Assignment of the genes for the human interferon system to chromosomes 2 and 5. Cytogenet. Cell. Genet. **13**, 155–157 (1974 a).

Tan, Y. H., Creagan, R. P., Ruddle, F. M.: The somatic cell genetics of human interferon loci to chromosomes 2 und 5. Proc. Natl. Acad. Sci. U. S. A. **71**, 2251–2255 (1974 b).

Tan, Y. H., Greene, A. E.: Subregional localization of the genes governing the human interferon-induced antiviral state in man. J. Gen. Virol. **32**, 153–157 (1976).

Tan, Y. H., Jeng, D. K., Ho, M.: The release of interferon: an active process inhibited by p-hydroxymercuribenzoate. Virology **48**, 41–48 (1972).

Tan, Y. H., Schneider, E. L., Tischfield, J., Epstein, C. J., Ruddle, F. H.: Human chromosome 21 dosage: effect on the expression of the interferon induced antiviral state. Science **186**, 61–63 (1974).

Tan, Y. H., Tischfield, J., Ruddle, F. H.: The linkage of genes for the human interferon-induced antiviral protein and indophenol oxidase-B traits to chromosome G-21. J. Exp. Med. **137**, 317–330 (1973).

Tarodi, B., Pusztai, R., Berencsi, K.: Physico-chemical characteristics of interferons induced by human adenovirus in chick fibroblasts and leukocytes. Acta. Virol. **19**, 393–400 (1975).

Taylor, J.: Inhibition of interferon action by actinomycin. Biochem. Biophys. Res. Commun. **14**, 447–453 (1964).

Taylor, J.: Studies on the mechanism of action of interferon. I. Interferon action and RNA synthesis in chick embryo fibroblast infected with Semliki Forest virus. Virology **25**, 340–349 (1968).

Taylor, P. E., Zuckerman, A. J.: Non-production of interfering substances by serum from patients with infectious hepatitis. J. Med. Microbiol. **1**, 217–220 (1968).

Taylor-Papadimitriou, J., Kallos, J.: Induction of interferon by sepharose-bound poly (I)·poly (C). Nature New Biol. **245**, 143–158 (1973).

Taylor–Papadimitriou, J., Spandidos, D., Georgatsos, J. G.: An endonuclease activity associated with preparations of chick interferon. Biochem. Biophys. Res. Commun. **43**, 149–155 (1971).

Taylor–Papadimitriou, J., Stoker, M.: Effect of interferon on some aspects of transformation by polyoma virus. Nature New Biol. **230**, 114–117 (1971).

Tazulakhova, E. B., Novokhatsky, A. S., Yershov, F. I.: Interferon induction by, and antiviral effect of, poly I·C in experimental viral infection. Acta. Virol. **17**, 487–492 (1973).

ter Meulen, V., Katz, M., Kackell, Y. M., Barbant–Brodano, G., Koprowski, H., Lennette, E. H.: Subacute sclerosing panencephalitis: *In vitro* characterization of viruses isolated from brain cells in culture. J. Infect. Dis. **126**, 11–23 (1972).

Thacore, H. R.: Rescue of vesicular stomatitis virus from homologus and heterologous interferon-induced resistance in human cell cultures by Poxviruses. Infect. Immun. **14**, 311–314 (1976).

Thacore, H. R., Youngner, J. S.: Cells persistently infected with Newcastle disease virus. II. Ribonucleic acid and protein synthesis in cells infected with mutants isolated from persistently infected L-cells. J. Virol. **6**, 42–48 (1970).

Thacore, H. R., Youngner, J. S.: Viral RNA synthesis by NDV mutants isolated from persistently infected L-cells: effect of interferon. J. Virol. **9**, 503–509 (1972).

Thacore, H. R., Youngner, J. S.: Rescue of VSV from interferon-induced resistance by super-infection with vaccinia virus. I. Rescue in cell cultures from different species. Virology **56**, 505–511 (1973 a).

Thacore, H. R., Youngner, J. S.: Rescue of vesicular stomatitis virus from interferon-induced resistance by superinfection with vaccinia virus. II. Effect of uv-inactivated vaccinia and metabolic inhibitors. Virology **56**, 512–521 (1973 b).

Thacore, H. R., Youngner, J. S.: Different sensitivity of ribonucleic and deoxyribonucleic acid viruses to resistance induced in rabbit cells (RK-13) by polyriboinosinic-acid-polyribocytidilic acid. Infect. Immun. **7**, 685–699 (1973c).

Thacore, H. R., Youngner, J. S.: Persistence of vesicular stomatitis virus in interferon-treated cell cultures. Virology **63**, 345–357 (1975).

Thang, M. N., Bachner, L., Declercq, E., Stollar, B. D.: A continuous high molecular weight base-paired structure is not an absolute requirement for potential polynucleotide inducer of interferon. FEBS Letters **76**, 159–164 (1977).

Thang, M. N., DeMaeyer–Guignard, J., DeMaeyer, E.: Interaction of interferon with tRNA. FEBS Letters **80**, 365–370 (1977).

Thang, M. N., Thang, D. C., DeMaeyer, E., Montagnier, L.: Biosynthesis of mouse interferon by translation of its messenger RNA in a cell-free system. Proc. Natl. Acad. Sci. U. S. A. **72**, 3975–3979 (1975).

Thorbecke, G. J., Friedman–Kien, A. E., Vilček, J.: Effect of rabbit interferon on immune responses. Cell Immunol. **12** (2), 290–295 (1974).

Tilles, J. G.: Enhancement of interferon titers by poly-L-ornithine. Proc. Soc. Exp. Biol. Med. **125**, 996–999 (1967).

Tilles, J. G.: Diethylaminoethyl-dextran enhancement of interferon induction by a complexed polyribonucleotide. Proc. Soc. Exp. Biol. Med. **133**, 1334–1340 (1970).

Tilles, J. G., Braun, P.: Induction of interferon in perfused whole rat-lung cultures. Proc. Soc. Exp. Biol. Med. **144**, 460–472 (1973).

Tilles, J. G., Finland, M.: Microassay for human and chick cell interferons. Applied Microbiol. **16**, 1706–1708 (1968).

Timovsky, A. L., Aksenov, O. A., Bresler, S. E., Kogan, E. M., Smorodintsev, A. A., Tikhomirova–Sidorova, N. S.: Molecular weight characteristics of the poly (G) and poly (C) complex and their relationship with the interferon inducing activities. Vopr. Virusol. **18**, 250–255 (1973).

Tkacheva, E. I., Guozdilova, D. A., Smorodintsev, A. A.: Therapeutic effect of interferonogen in herpetic keratitis. Vestin. Oftalmol. **4**, 73–75 (1971).

Todaro, G. J., Baron, S.: The role of interferon in the inhibition of SV 40 transformation of mouse cell line 3 T 3. Proc. Nat. Acad. Sci. U. S. A. **54**, 752–757 (1965).

Todaro, G. J., Green, H.: Interferon resistance of SV 40 induced DNA synthesis. Virology **33**, 752–767 (1967).

Todd, J. D., Volenec, F. J., Paton, I. M.: Interferon in nasal secretion and sera of calves after intranasal administration of avirulent infectious bovine rhinotracheitis virus: Association of interferon in nasal secretions with early resistance to challenge with virulent virus. Infect. Immun. **5**, 699–706 (1972).

Tokumaru, T.: The effect of trauma on production of herpes interferon in guinea pigs. Arch. Ges. Virusforsch. **21**, 61–65 (1967).

Tolentino, P., Dianzani, F., Zucca, M., Giacchino, R.: Decreased interferon response by lymphocytes from children with chronic hepatitis. J. Infect. Dis. **132**, 459–463 (1975).

Tomkins, G. M., Thompson, E. B., Hayashi, S., Gelehrter, T., Granner, D., Peterkosfsky, D.: Tyrosine transaminase induction in mammalian cells in tissue culture. Cold Spring Harbor Symp. Quant. Biol. **31**, 349 (1966).

Tommila, V.: Treatment of dendritic keratitis with interferon. Acta. Ophthalmol. **65**, 478–491 (1963).

Tommila, V., Penttinen, K.: Effect of ultraviolet irradiated influenza Lee viruses on experimental herpes simplex virus infection in rabbit's eyes. Acta Ophthalmol. **40**, 520–533 (1962).

Tongaonkar, S. S., Ghosh, S. N.: Production of interferon by arboviruses in suckling mouse brains. Curr. Sci. **42** (19), 680–688 (1973).

Torlone, V., Titoli, F., Gialletti: Circulating interferon production in pigs infected hog cholera virus. Life Sci. **4**, 1707–1713 (1965).

Torma, E. T., Paucker, K.: Purification and characterization of human leukocyte interferon components. J. Biol. Chem. **251**, 4810–4820 (1976).

Torrence, P. F., Bobst, A. M., Waters, J. A., Witkop, B.: Synthesis and characterization of potential interferon inducers poly (2'-azido-2'-deoxyuridylic acid. Biochemistry **12**, 3962–3967 (1973a).

Torrence, P. F., Declercq, E.: Inducers and induction of interferons. Pharmacol. Therap. Pt. A. **2**, 1–88 (1977).

Torrence, P. F., Declercq, E., Waters, J. A., Witkop, B.: Failure of duplexes based on poly-laurusin (poly L) "Polyformycin B" to induce interferon. Biochem. Biophys. Res. Commun. **62**, 658–654 (1975).

Torrence, P. F., Waters, J. A., Buckler, C. E., Witkop, B.: Effect of pirimidine and ribose modifications on the antiviral activity of synthetic polynucleotides. Biochem. Biophys. Res. Comm. **52**, 890–896 (1973 b).

Toth, F. D., Vaczi, L., Balogh, M.: The role of tumor-specific antibody and interferon production in the pathogenesis of Rauscher leukemia. Acta Virologica **18**, 57–64 (1974).

Toth, F. D., Vaczi, L., Berencsi, C.: Effect of interferon treatment on the tumor-specific antibody response of Balb-C mice infected with Rauscher virus. Acta Microbiol. Acad. Sci. Hung. **18**, 109–112 (1971 a).

Toth, F. D., Vaczi, L., Berencsi, C.: Interferon and antibody production in inbred mice infected with Rauscher virus. Acta Microbiol. Acad. Sci. Hung. **18**, 23–27 (1971 b).

Tovell, D., Cantell, K.: Kinetics of interferon production in human leukocyte suspensions. J. Gen. Virol. **13**, 485–489 (1971).

Tovey, M. G., Bandu, M. T., Begon-Lours, J., Brouty–Boye, D., Gresser, I.: Antiviral activity of bovine interferons on primate cells. J. Gen. Virol. **36**, 341–356 (1977 a).

Tovey, M. G., Begon–Lours, J., Gresser, I.: A method for the large-scale production of potent interferon preparations. Proc. Soc. Exp. Biol. Med. **146**, 809–815 (1974).

Tovey, M. G., Begon–Lours, J., Gresser, I., Morris, A. G.: Marked enhancement of interferon production in 5-bromodeoxyuridine treated human lymphoblastoid cells. Nature **267**, 455–456 (1977 b).

Tovey, M., Brouty–Boye, D.: Characteristics of the chemostat culture of animal cells. Exp. Cell Res. **101**, 346–354 (1976).

Tovey, M., Brouty–Boye, D., Gresser, I.: Interferon and cell division. 10. Early effect of interferon on mouse leukemia cells cultivated in a chemostat. Proc. Nat. Acad. Sci. U. S. A. **72**, 2265–2270 (1975).

Toy, S. T., Weislow, O. S., Wheelock, E. F.: Suppression of established Friend virus leukemia by statolon. VII. Relative roles of interferon and the immune response in development of FV-dormant infections. Proc. Soc. Exp. Biol. Med. **143**, 726–732 (1973).

Traub, B.: Interference with Eastern equine encephalomyelitis (EEE) virus in the brains of mice immune to lymphocytic choriomeningitis. Arch. Ges. Virusforsch. **11**, 419–422 (1961).

Traub, W. H., Morgan, H. R.: Comparative studies with the zilber (Carr) strain of Rous sarcoma virus (Z-RSV). III. Suppression of viral replication and focus formation by interferon in vitro. Arch. Ges. Virusforsch. **20**, 1–10 (1967).

Treagan, L.: Anti-lymphocyte serum and suppression of interferon production. Experientia **28**, 569–575 (1972).

Trinchieri, G., Santoli, D., Knowles, B. B.: Tumor cell lines induce interferon in human lymphocytes. Nature **270**, 611–613 (1977).

Trubina, L. M., Yakovenko, Z. F., Zakharchenko, E. M., Lychokovskaya, E. V.: Two mechanisms of interferon production by leukocytes from immunized animals. Acta Virol. **19**, 116–124 (1975).

Truden, J. L., Sigel, M. M., Dietrich, L. S.: An interferon antagonist: its effect on interferon action in mengo-infected Ehrlich ascites tumor cells. Virology **33**, 95–103 (1967).

Trudgett, A.: Partial purification of lymphokinase activities by isoelectric focusing. J. Immunol. Methods. **10**, 1–6 (1976).

Ts'o, O. P., Alderfer, J. L., Levy, J., Marshall, L. W., O'Malley, J. M., Horoszewicz, J. S., Carter, W. A.: An integrated and comparative study of the antiviral effects and other biological properties of the polynosinic acid-polycytidylic acid and its mismatched analogues. Mol. Pharmacol. **12**, 299–310 (1976).

Tsukui, K.: Influenza virus-induced interferon production in mouse spleen cell culture: T cells as the main producer. Cell. Immunol. **32**, 243–250 (1977).

Tsunoda, A., Ishida, N.: A mushroom extract as an interferon inducer. Ann. N.Y. Acad. Sci. **173**, 719–726 (1970).

Turner, W., Chirigos, M. A., Scott, D.: Enhancement of Friend and Rauscher leukemia virus replication in mice by guaroa virus. Cancer Res. **28**, 1064–1068 (1968).

Tyrrell, D. A. J.: Interferon produced by cultures of calf kidney cells. Nature 184, 452–453 (1959).

Tyrrell, D. A. J.: Rhinoviruses. Virology Monograph 2, 67–85 (1968).

Tyrrell, D. A. J.: Interferon and Its Clinical Potential, pp. 1–101. London: William Heinemann Medical Books Ltd. (1976).

Tyrell, D. A. J., Reed, S. E. in: Non-specific factors influencing hast resistance (Braun, W., ed.), p. 438–442. Basel: Karger (1973).

Tytell, A. A., Lampson, G. P., Field, A. K., Hilleman, M. R.: Inducers of interferon and host resistance. III. Double-stranded RNA from reovirus type 3 virions. Proc. Natl. Acad. Sci. U. S. A. 58, 1719–1724 (1967).

Tytell, A. A., Lampson, G. P., Field, A. K., Nemes, M. M., Hilleman, M. R.: Influence of size of individual homopolynucleotides on the physical and biological properties of complex rIn:rCn. Proc. Soc. Exp. Biol. Med. 135, 917–921 (1968).

Uhlendorf, C. P., Zimmerman, E. M., Baron, S.: Heterologous activity of monkey interferons. Proc. Soc. Exp. Biol. Med. 144, 628–632 (1973).

Umino, Y., Kohno, S.: Binding and interspecies specificity of two rodent interferons. IRCS Med. Sci. 4, 138–145 (1976).

Ustacelebi, S.: Virion heat-sensitivity of adenovirus type 5 temperature-sensitive mutants and interferon induction. Acta. Virol. 20, 297–305 (1976).

Ustacelebi, S., Williams, J. F.: Induction of interferon in chick cells by polyoma virus. J. Gen. Virol. 21, 163–168 (1973).

Vaczi, L., Horvath, E., Hadhazy, G.: Studies on the conditions of interferon production by cells infected with herpes virus. Acta. Microbiol. Acad. Sci. Hung. 12, 345–351 (1965).

Vainio, T., Gwatkin, R., Koprowski, H.: Production of interferon by brains of genetically resistant and susceptible mice infected with West Nile Virus. Virology 14, 385–387 (1961).

Valle, M. J., Jordan, G. W., Haahr, S., Merigan, T. C.: Characteristics of immune interferon produced by human lymphocyte cultures compared to other human interferons. J. Immunol. 115, 230–244 (1975 a).

Valle, M. J., Bobrove, A. M., Strober, S., Merigan, T. C.: Immune specific production of interferon by human T cells in combined macrophage-lymphocyte cultures in response to herpes simplex antigen. J. Immunol. 114, 435–446 (1975 b).

Vandeputte, M., De La Fonteyne, J., Billiau, A., Desomer, P.: Influence and production of interferon in Rauscher virus infected mice. Archiv für die gesamte Virusforschung 20, 235–245 (1967).

Vandeputte, M., Datta, S. K., Billiau, A., Desomer, P.: Inhibition of polyoma-virus oncogenesis in rats by polyriboinosinic-ribocytidylic acid. Europ. J. Cancer 6, 323–327 (1970).

Van Griensven, L. J., Baudelaire, M. F., Peries, J., Emanoil-Ravicovitch, R., Boiron, M.: Studies on the biosynthesis of murine leukemia virus RNA. I. Some properties of Rauscher leukemia virus isolated from interferon treated JLSV 5 cells, in: Le petit Colloq. on Biol. and Med., Biol. of Oncogen. Viruses, Vol. 2, pp. 145–153. Amsterdam: North-Holland (1971).

Van Rossum, W., Desomer, P.: Some aspects of the interferon production in vivo. Life Sciences 5, 105–113 (1966).

Vassef, A., Beaud, G., Paucker, K., Lengyel, P.: Interferon assay based on the inhibition of double-stranded Reovirus RNA accumulation in mouse L-cells. J. Gen. Virol. 19 (1), 81–87 (1973).

Vassef, A., Spencer, C., Gelehrter, T. D., Lengyel, P.: Selectivity of interferon action: Hormonal induction of tyrosine aminotransferase in rat hepatoma cells is much less sensitive to interferon than the replication of vesicular stomatitis virus or reovirus. Biochim. Biophys. Acta. 353 (1), 115–120 (1974).

Vassileva, V., Galabov, A.: Interferon induction and action in transformed poikilothermal cells. Acta. Microbiol. 22, 323–330 (1975).

Vengris, V. E., Mare, J.: Protection of chickens against Marek's disease virus JM-V strain with statolon and exogenous interferons. Avian Dis. 17, 758–767 (1973).

Vengris, V. E., Reynolds, jr., F. H., Hollenberg, M. D., Pitha, P. M.: Interferon action: role of membrane gangliosides. Virology 72, 486–496 (1976).

Vengris, V. E., Stollar, B. D., Pitha, P. M.: Interferon externalization by producing cell before induction of antiviral state. Virology 65, 410–421 (1975).

Verlinde, J. D., Dret, A.: On the formation of a substance with the characteristics of interferon in the brains of mice infected with vaccinia. Acta Leidensia 32, 297–300 (1963).

Veskova, T. K., Nemirovskaya, B. M.: Interferon production by blood leukocytes in Hodgkin's disease. Rev. Eur. Etud. Clin. Biol. 16, 697–700 (1971).

Viehauser, G.: Simple procedure for large-scale assays for chick interferon. Appl. Environ. Microb. 33, 740–752 (1977).

Vieuchange, J.: Role d'un interféron dans le phénomène de l'interférence entre le virus vaccinal et le virus rabique fixe. C. R. Acad. Sc. (Paris) D 264, 426–428 (1967 a).

Vieuchange, J.: Interférence entre le virus vaccinal et le virus Rabique; role éventuel d'un interféron. Archiv für die gesamte Virusforschung 22, 87–96 (1967 b).

Vignaux, F., Gresser, I.: Differential effects of interferon on the expression of H-2K, H-2D, and I a antigens on mouse lymphocytes. J. Immunol. 118, 721–723 (1977).

Vilček, J.: An interferon-like substance released from tick-borne encephalitis virus-infected chick embryo fibroblast cells. Nature 187, 73–74 (1960).

Vilček, J.: Studies on an interferon from tick-borne encephalitis virus infected cells. IV. Comparison of IF with interferon from influenza virus-infected cells. Acta. Virol. 6, 144–160 (1962).

Vilček, J.: Studies on an interferon from tick-borne encephalitis virus-infected cells. V. Failure of thermally inactivated virus to induce or to influence interferon formation. Acta. Virol. 7, 107–112 (1963).

Vilček, J.: Use of interference for the assay of group B arboviruses in chick embryo cells. Acta. Virol. 8, 417–423 (1964 a).

Vilček, J.: Production of interferon by newborn and adult mice infected with Sindbis virus. Virology 22, 651–652 (1964 b).

Vilček, J.: Interferon, p. 1–141. Wien–New York: Springer (1969).

Vilček, J.: Metabolic determinants of the induction of interferon by a synthetic double-stranded polynucleotide in rabbit cells. Ann. N.Y. Acad. Sci. 173, 390–403 (1970 a).

Vilček, J.: Cellular mechanisms of interferon production. J. Gen. Physiol. 56, 76–89 (1970 b).

Vilček, J., Barmak, S. L., Havell, E. A.: Control of interferon synthesis: effect of diethylaminoethyl-dextran on induction by polyinosinic-polycytidylic acid. J. Virol. 10, 614–621 (1972).

Vilček, J., Havell, E. A.: Stabilization of interferon messenger RNA activity by treatment of cells with metabolic inhibitors and lowering of the incubation temperature. Proc. Nat. Acad. Sci. U. S. A. 70, 3909–3913 (1973).

Vilček, J., Havell, E. A., Kohase, A.: Superinduction of interferon with metabolic inhibitors: possible mechanisms and practical applications. J. Infect. Disease 133, A 22–A 29 (1976).

Vilček, J., Havell, E. A., Yamazaki, S.: Antigenic, physicochemical and biologic characterization of human interferons. Ann. N.Y. Acad. Sci. 284, 703–710 (1977).

Vilček, J., Jahiel, R. I.: Action of interferon and its inducers against nonviral infectious agents. Arch. Intern. Med. 126, 69–77 (1970).

Vilček, J., Lowy, D. R.: Interaction of interferon with chick embryo cells. Archiv für die gesamte Virusforschung 21, 254–264 (1967).

Vilček, J., Ng, M. H.: Potentiation of the action of interferon by extracts of Escherichia coli. Virology 31, 552–555 (1967).

Vilček, J., Ng, M. H.: Post-transcriptional control of interferon synthesis. J. Virol. 7, 588–594 (1971).

Vilček, J., Ng, M., Friedman-Kein, A. E., Krawciw, T.: Induction of interferon synthesis by synthetic double-stranded polynucleotides. J. Virology 2, 648–654 (1968).

Vilček, J., Rada, B.: Studies on an interferon from tick-borne encephalitis virus infected cells. III. Antiviral action of IF. Acta Virol. 6, 9–15 (1962).

Vilček, J., Rossman, T. C., Varacalli, F.: Differential effects of Actinomycin D and puromycin on the release of interferon induced by double-stranded RNA. Nature 222, 682–683 (1969).

Vilček, J., Stancek, D.: Formation and properties of interferon in the brain of tick-borne encephalitis virus-infected mice. Acta. Virol. 7, 331–345 (1963 a).

Vilček, J., Stancek, D.: Unresponsiveness to the action of interferon developed in persistently infected L cells. Life Sci. 2, 895–913 (1963 b).

Vilček, J., Tomisova, J., Sokol, F., Hana, L.: Concentration and partial purification of interferon from mouse brains. Acta. Virol. **8**, 76–88 (1964).

Vilček, J., Varacalli, F.: Sequential suppression by actinomycin D of interferon production and cellular resistence induced by poly I·C. J. Gen. Virol. **13**, 185–188 (1971).

Vilček, J., Yamazaki, S., Havell, E. A.: Interferon induction by vesicular stomatitis virus and its role in virus replication. Infect. Immun. **18**, 863–867 (1977).

Vilner, L. M., Brodskaia, L. M., Kogan, E. M., Timkovski, A. L., Miroshnichenko, R. L.: Comparatie antiviral and interferonogenic activity of different complexes of hetero- and homo-polyribonucleotides. Antibiotiki **21**, 842–846 (1976).

Vilner, L. M., Brodskaya, L. M., Kogan, E. M., Timkovsky, A. L., Tikhomirova-Sidorova, N. S., Bresler, S. E.: Investigation of the biological activity of polyribonucleotide complex poly (G)·poly (C) in relation to the structural features of the original polyribonucleotides. Vopr. Virusol. **19**, 45–50 (1974).

Virelizier, J. L., Allison, A. C., DeMaeyer, E.: Production by mixed lymphocyte cultures of a Type II interferon able to protect macrophages against virus infections. Infect. Immun. **17**, 282–296 (1977).

Virelizier, J. L., Virelizier, A. M., Allison, A. C.: Role of circulating interferon in modifications of immune responsiveness by mouse hepatitis virus (MHV-3). J. Immunol. **117**, 748–764 (1976).

Vladutiu, A. L.: Hepatitis B virus, HLA types and interferon. N. Eng. J. Med. **297**, 399–411 (1977).

Volckaert-Vervliet, G., Billiau, A.: Induction of interferon in human lymphoblastoid cells by Sendai and measles virus. J. Gen. Virol. **37**, 199–203 (1977).

Volkert, M., Larsen, J. H., Pfau, C.: Studies on immunological tolerance to LCM virus 4. The question of immunity in adoptively immunized virus carriers. Acta Pathol. Microbiol. Scand. **61**, 268–274 (1964).

Wacker, A. M., Singer, A., Svec, J., Lodemann, E.: „Einfluß der Kettenlänge von Oligonucleotiden auf die Interferon-induction". Naturwissenschaften **56**, 638–649 (1969).

Wacker, A., Lodemann, E., Diederich, J., Mohrbutter, K., Lauschke, U.: Induction of interferon in L-cells by poly I·C in presence of cationic compounds. I·poly-cations. Arch. Ges. Virusforsch. **36**, 71–79 (1972).

Waddell, D. J., Wilbur, J. R., Merigan, T. C.: Interferon production in human mumps infection. Proc. Soc. Exp. Biol. Med. **127**, 320–326 (1968).

Wadell, G.: Hazards of human leukocyte interferon therapy. N. Eng. J. Med. **296**, 1295–1311 (1977).

Wagner, A. F., Bugianesi, R. L., Shen, T. Y.: Preparation of Sepharose-bound poly (rI·rC). Biochem. Biophys. Res. Commun. **45**, 184–188 (1971).

Wagner, R. R.: Viral interference. Some considerations of basic mechanisms and their potential relationship to host resistance. Bact. Rev. **24**, 151–166 (1960).

Wagner, R. R.: Biological studies of interferon. I. Suppression of cellular infection with eastern equine encephalomyelitis virus. Virology **13**, 323–337 (1961).

Wagner, R. R.: The interferons: cellular inhibitors of viral infections. Am. Rev. Microbiol. **17**, 285–347 (1963 a).

Wagner, R. R.: Biological studies of interferon. II. Temporal relationship of virus and interferon production by cells infected with eastern equine encephalomyelitis and influenza viruses. Virology **19**, 215–224 (1963 b).

Wagner, R. R.: Inhibition of interferon biosynthesis by actinomycin D. Nature **204**, 49–50 (1964).

Wagner, R. R., Huang, A. S.: Reversible inhibition of protein synthesis by puromycin. Evidence for interferon specific mRNA. Proc. Natl. Acad. Sci. **54**, 1112–1118 (1965).

Wagner, R. R., Huang, A. S.: Inhibition of RNA and interferon synthesis in Krebs-2-cells infected with vesicular stomatitis virus. Virology **28**, 1–10 (1966).

Wagner, R. R., Levy, A. H., Snyder, R. M., Ratcliff, G. A., Hyatt, D. F.: Biological properties of two plaque variants of vesicular stomatitis virus. J. Immunol. **91**, 112–121 (1963).

Wagner, R. R., Snyder, R. M.: Viral interference induced in mice by acute or persistent infection with the virus of lymphocytic choriomeningitis. Nature **19**, 393–395 (1962).

Wagner, R. R., Snyder, R. M., Hook, E. W., Luttrell, C.: Effect of bacterial endotoxin on resistance of mice to viral encephalitides. J. Immunol. **83**, 87–98 (1959).

Wallen, W. C., Dean, J. M., Lucas, D. O.: Interferon and the cellular immune response: separation of interferon-producing cells from DNA-synthetic cells. Cell Immunol. **6**, 110–122 (1973).

Walters, S., Burke, D. C., Skehel, J. J.: Interferon production and RNA inhibitors. J. Gen. Virol. **1**, 349–362 (1967).

Waschke, K., Lackovic, V., Borecky, I.: Relation of incubation temperature to interferon production in mouse peritoneal cells infected with Newcastle disease virus. Acta. Virol. **13** (5), 387–392 (1969).

Waschke, K., Borecky, I., Lackovic, V.: Release of interferon by mouse peritoneal cells *in vitro*. The requirement of contact with endotoxin and the temperature dependence of release. Acta Virol. **13**, 393–400 (1969).

Webb, H. E., Wight, D. G. D., Platt, G. S., Smith, C. E. G.: Langat virus encephalitis in mice. I. The effect of the aministration of specific antiserum. J. Hyg. **66**, 343–360 (1968).

Weber, J. M., Stewart, R. B.: Interaction of interferon with cells: limited heterologous reactivity of chick and mouse interferons. J. Gen. Virol. **19**, 165–174 (1973).

Weber, J. M., Stewart, R. B.: Cyclic AMP potentiation of interferon antiviral activity and effect of interferon on cellular cyclic AMP levels. J. Gen. Virol. **28**, 363–372 (1975).

Weinstein, A. J., Gazdar, A. F., Sims, H. L., Levy, H. B.: Lack of correlation between interferon induction and antitumor effect of poly I·poly C. Nature New Biol. **231**, 53–55 (1971).

Weinstein, M. J., Weitz, J. A., Came, P. E.: Induction of resistance to bacterial infections of mice with poly I·poly C. Nature **226**, 170–171 (1970).

Weislow, O. S., Wheelock, E. F.: Suppression of established friend virus leukemia by statolon: potentiation of statolon's leukemosuppressive activity by chlorite-oxidized oxyamylose. Infect. Immun. **11**, 129–136 (1975).

Weissenbach, J., Dirheimer, G., Falcoff, R., Sanceau, J., Falcoff, E.: Yeast tRNA leu (anticodon U-A-G) translates all six leucine codons in extracts from interferon-treated cells. FEBS Letters **82**, 71–76 (1977).

Weissenbacher, M., Schachter, N., Galin, M. A., Baron, S.: Intraocular production of interferon. Arch. Ophthalmol. **84**, 495–509 (1970).

Werenne, J., Rousseau, G.: Studies of leukemia L1210 cells in culture: a comparison of clones differing in sensitivity to interferon. Arch. Int. Physiol. Biochim. **84**, 683–684 (1976a).

Werenne, J., Rousseau, G.: Double-stranded RNA-dependent protein phosphorylation in interferon-treated cells. Arch. Int. Physiol. Biochim. **84**, 1123–1124 (1976b).

Werner, G. H., Jasmin, C., Chermann, J. C.: Effect of ammonium S-tungsts-2-antimoniate on EMC and VSV infections in mice. J. Gen. Virol. **31**, 59–64 (1976).

Wertz, G. W., Youngner, J. S.: Interferon production and inhibition of host synthesis in cells infected with vesicular stomatitis virus. J. Virol. **6**, 476–484 (1970).

Whalen, R. G., Butlerbrowne, G. E., Gros, F.: Proteins synthesis and actin heterogeneity in calf muscle cells in culture. Proc. Natl. Acad. Sci. U. S. A. **73**, 2018–2022 (1976).

Wheelock, E. F.: Interferon in dermal crusts of human vaccinia virus vaccinations. Possible explanation of relative benignity of variolation smallpox. Proc. Soc. Exp. Biol. Med. **117**, 650–653 (1964).

Wheelock, E. F.: Interferon-like virus-inhibitor induced human leukocytes by phytohemagglutinin. Science **149**, 310–311 (1965).

Wheelock, E. F.: Virus replication and high-titered interferon production in human leukocyte cultures inoculated with Newcastle disease virus. J. Bact. **92**, 1415–1419 (1966a).

Wheelock, E. F.: The effects of non-tumor viruses on virus-induced leukemia in mice: reciprocal interference between Sendai virus and Friend leukemia virus in DBA/2 mice. Proc. Natl. Acad. Sci. U. S. A. **55**, 774–778 (1966b).

Wheelock, E. F.: Inhibitory effects of Sendai virus on Friend virus leukemia in mice. J. Nat. Cancer Inst. **38**, 771–778 (1967a).

Wheelock, E. F.: Effect of statolon on Friend virus leukemia in mice. Proc. Soc. Exp. Biol. Med. **124**, 855–858 (1967b).

Wheelock, E. F.: Applied and induced interferon in the prophylaxis and treatment of leukemia. Arch. Intern. Med. **126**, 64–67 (1970).

Wheelock, E. F., Caroline, N. L., Moore, R. D.: Suppression of established Friend virus leukemia by statolon. J. Virol. **4**, 1–10 (1969).

Wheelock, E. F., Dingle, J. H.: Observations on the repeated administration of viruses to a patient with acute leukemia. New. Engl. J. Med. **271**, 645–651 (1964).

Wheelock, E. F., Edelman, R.: Specific role of each human leukocyte type in viral infections. III. 17 D Yellow fever virus and interferon production in homogeneous leukocyte cultures treated with phytohemagglutinin. J. Immunol. **103**, 429–435 (1969).

Wheelock, E. F., Larke, R. P. B.: Efficacy of interferon in the treatment of mice with established friend virus leukemia. Proc. Soc. Exp. Biol. Med. **127**, 230–236 (1968).

Wheelock, E. F., Schenker, S., Combes, P.: Absence of circulating interferon in patients with infectious and serum hepatitis. Proc. Soc. Exp. Biol. Med. **128**, 251–257 (1968).

Wheelock, E. F., Sibley, W. A.: Circulating virus interferon and antibody after vaccination with the 17-D strain of yellow-fever virus. New Engl. J. Med. **273**, 194–198 (1965).

Wheelock, E. F., Toy, S. T., Caroline, N. L., Sibal, L. R., Fink, M. A., Beverly, P. C., Allison, A. C.: Suppression of established Friend virus leukemia by statolon. IV. Role of humoral antibody in the development of a dormant infection. J. Natl. Cancer Inst. **48**, 665–672 (1972).

Wiebe, M. E., Joklik, W. K.: The mechanism of inhibition of reovirus replication by interferon. Virology **66**, 229–234 (1975).

Wietzerbin, J., Falcoff, R., Catinot, L., Falcoff, E.: Affinity chromatographic analysis of murine interferons induced by viruses and by T and B cell stimulants. Ann. Immunol. (Inst. Pasteur) **128 C**, 699–708 (1977 a).

Wietzerbin, J., Stephanos, S., Falcoff, R., Falcoff, E.: Some properties of interferons induced by stimulants of T and B lymphocytes. Tex. Rep. Biol. Med. **35**, 205–211 (1977 b).

Wiktor, T. J., Fernandes, M. V., Koprowski, H.: Cultivation of rabies viruses in human diploid cell strain WI-38. J. Immunol. **93**, 353–360 (1964).

Wiktor, T. J., Koprowski, H., Mitchell, J. R., Merigan, T. C.: Role of interferon in prophylaxis of rabies after exposure. J. Infect. Dis. **133**, A 260–A 266 (1976).

Wiktor, T. J., Koprowski, H., Rorke, L. B.: Localized rabies interferon in mice. Proc. Soc. Exp. Biol. Med. **140**, 759–764 (1972).

Wiktor, T. J., Postic, B., Ho, M., Koprowski, H.: Role of interferon induction in the protective activity of rabies vaccines. J. Infect. Dis. **126**, 408–418 (1972).

Wildstein, A., Stevens, L. E., Applebaum, H., McCabe, R. E., Hashim, G. A., Fitzpatrick, H.: Prolonged survival of canine renal allografts by Tilorone. Transplantation **22**, 205–207 (1976).

Wildstein, A., Stevens, L. E., Hashim, G.: Skin and heart allograft prolongation in Tilorone treated rats. Transplantation **21**, 129–134 (1976).

Winchurch, R. A., Karpetsky, T. P., Levy, C. C., Cantell, K.: RNase activity in human interferon preparations. J. Virol. **21**, 1247–1259 (1977).

Wiranowska-Stewart, M., Chudzio, T., Stewart II, W. E.: Repeated superinduction of interferon in human diploid fibroblast cultures. J. Gen. Virol. **37**, 351–374 (1977).

Wiranowska-Stewart, M., Lin, L. S., Chudzio, T., Stewart II, W. E.: Contributions of carbohydrate moieties to the physical and biological properties of human leukocyte, lymphoblastoid and fibroblast interferons. Abst. Ann. Meeting Amer. Soc. Microbiol. (1978).

Wiranowska-Stewart, M., Stewart II, W. E.: The role of human chromosome 21 in sensitivity to interferons. J. Gen. Virol. **37**, 629–634 (1977).

Wong, P. K. Y., Yuen, P. H., MacLeod, R., Chang, E. H., Myers, M. W., Friedman, R. M.: The effect of interferon on de novo infection by Moloney murine leukemia virus. Cell **10**, 245–263 (1977).

Woodruff, J. F., Kilbourne, E. D.: Interferon production in neonatally thymectomized mice. Proc. Soc. Exp. Biol. Med. **126**, 542–554 (1967).

Worthington, M., Baron, S.: Late therapy with an interferon stimulator in an arbovirus encephalitis in mice. Proc. Soc. Exp. Biol. Med. **136**, 323–327 (1971 a).

Worthington, M., Baron, S.: Effectiveness of an interferon stimulator in immunosuppressed mice. Proc. Soc. Exp. Biol. Med. **136**, 349–353 (1971 b).

Worthington, M., Hasenclever, H. F.: Effect of an interferon stimulator, polyinosinic: polycytidylic acid on experimental fungus infections. Infect. Immun. **5**, 199–211 (1972).

Worthington, M., Levy, H., Rice, J.: Late therapy of an arbovirus encephalitis in mice with interferon and interferon stimulators. Proc. Soc. Exp. Biol. Med. **143**, 638–643 (1973).

Worthington, M., Rabson, A. S., Baron, S.: Mechanism of recovery from systemic vaccinia virus infection. I. The effects of cyclophosphamide. The J. Experim. Medicine **136**, 277–293 (1972).

Wright, J., Falk, L. A., Deinhardt, P.: Interferon production by simian lymphoblastoid cell lines. J. Natl. Cancer Inst. **53**, 271–275 (1974).

Wu, A. M., Schultz, A., Gallo, R. C.: Synthesis of type C virus particles from murine-cultured cells induced by iododeoxyuridine. V. Effect of interferon and its interaction with dexamethasone. J. Virol. **19**, 108–117 (1976).

Wu, A. M., Schultz, A., Reitz, M. S., Gallo, R. C.: Posttranscriptional effect of dexamethasone and interferon on the viral replication induced by iododeoxyuridine from murine cells transformed by non-producer fibroblasts. Bib. Haematol. **43**, 475–480 (1975).

Yabrov, A. A.: The enhancement of the stability of cells to the diphtheria toxin under the influence of a latent viral infection. Cytology **8**, 767–769 (1966).

Yabrov, A. A.: A nonspecific stability of cells to bacterial toxins. The idea of cell stress. Citologia (Leningrad) **9**, 692–706 (1967).

Yabrov, A. A.: Influence of interferon or the disturbance of protein synthesis. Proc. Symp. Clin. Use of Interferon, Zagreb, Yugoslavia (1975).

Yabrov, A. A.: Prevention of the disturbance of protein synthesis is a possible mechanism of interferon protective activity. Life Sciences **18**, 1397–1404 (1976).

Yabrov, A. A., Yekimova, V. A., Zaitlenok, N. A.: The effect of dibazole on interferon activity. Leningrad Nauka **14**, 62–74 (1971).

Yakobson, E., Prives, C., Hartman, J. R., Winocour, E., Revel, M.: Inhibition of viral protein synthesis in monkey cells treated with interferon late in Simian virus 40 lytic cycle. Cell **12**, 73–82 (1977).

Yakobson, E., Revel, M., Winocour, E.: Inhibition of Simian virus 40 replication by interferon treatment late in the lytic cycle. Virology **80**, 225–228 (1977).

Yamada, M., Azuma, M., Nishioka, R., Togashi, T.: Relationship between immunity and interferon production in macrophages. I. Effect of immunity on interferon production. Jap. J. Microbiol. **14**, 311–318 (1970).

Yamaguchi, T., Handa, K., Shimizu, Y., Abo, T., Kumagai, K.: Target cell for interferon production in human leukocytes stimulated by Sendai virus. J. Immunol. **118**, 1931–1946 (1977).

Yamamoto, Y., Kawade, Y.: Purification of two components of mouse L-cell interferon: electrophoretic demonstration of interferon proteins. J. Gen. Virol. **33**, 225–234 (1976).

Yamamoto, Y., Yamaguchi, N., Oda, K.: Mechanism of interferon-induced inhibition of early Simian virus 40 (SV_{40}) functions. Virology **68**, 58–69 (1975).

Yamamoto, Y., Tsukui, K., Ohwaki, M., Kawade, Y.: Electrophoretic characterization of purified mouse L-cell interferon of high specific activity. J. Gen. Virol. **23**, 23–32 (1974).

Yamazaki, S.: Effect of endogenous interferon and actinomycin D on growth of Japanese Encephalitis virus in chick embryo cells. Jap. J. Microbiol. **12**, 171–178 (1968).

Yamazaki, S., Wagner, R. R.: Purified rabbit interferon: attempts to demonstrate interferon-specific ^{3}H-protein. J. Virol. **5**, 270–273 (1970a).

Yamazaki, S., Wagner, R. R.: Action of interferon: kinetics and differential effects on viral functions. J. Virol. **6**, 421–429 (1970b).

Yaron, M., Yaron, I., Gurari-Rotman, D., Revel, M., Lindner, H. R., Zor, U.: Stimulation of prostoglandin E production in cultured human fibroblasts by poly I·C and human interferon. Nature **267**, 457 (1977).

Yaron, M., Yaron, I., Smetana, O., Eylan, E., Herzberg, M.: Hyaluronic acid produced by human synovial fibroblasts. Effect of poly I·C and interferon. Arthritis Rheum. **19**, 1315–1320 (1976).

Yershov, F. I., Tazulakhova, E. G., Novokhatsky, A. S.: The effect of combination of different inducers on the refractory state in interferon production. Acta Virol. **20**, 15–28 (1976).

Yershov, F. I., Zhdanov, V. M.: Influence of PPLO on production of interferon in virus-infected cells. Virology **27**, 451–457 (1965).

Yokota, Y., Kishida, T., Esaki, K., Kawamata, J.: Induction of interferon in congenitally athymic mice. Biken J. **18**, 183–197 (1975 a).

Yokota, Y., Kishida, T., Esaki, K., Kawamata, J.: Lower production of circulating interferon in congenitally athymic (nude) mice induced by intravenous administration of Newcastle disease virus. Biken J. **18**, 275–295 (1975 b).

Yokota, Y., Kishida, T., Esaki, K., Kawamata, J.: Antitumor effects of interferon on transplanted tumors in congenitally athymic nude mice. Biken J. **19**, 125–139 (1976).

Yoshino, K., Morishima, T.: A simple and sensitive method for assay of chick interferon. Proc. Soc. Exp. Biol. Med. **135**, 695–698 (1970).

Youn, J. K., Barski, G.: Interference between LCM and Rauscher leukemia in mice. J. Natl. Cancer Inst. **37**, 381–388 (1966).

Youn, J. K., Barski, G., Huppert, J.: Inhibition of viral leukemogenesis in mice by treatment with synthetic polynucleotides. C. R. Acad. Sci. (Paris) D **267**, 816–829 (1968).

Young, C. W.: Interferon induction in cancer with some observations on the clinical effects of poly I·C. Med. Clin. N. Amer. **55**, 721–728 (1971).

Young, C. H. S., Pringle, C. R., Follett, E. A. C.: Effect of interferon in enucleated cells. J. Virol. **15**, 428–441 (1975).

Young, P. A., Taylor, J. J., Yu, M. C., Eyerman, E.: Morphological changes in chick cerebellum induced by poly I·poly C. Nature (Lond.) **228**, 1191–1195 (1970).

Youngner, J. S.: Interferon production in mice infected with viral and nonviral stimuli, in: Medical and Applied Virology (Sanders, M., Lennette, E., eds.), p. 210. Missouri: Green (1968).

Youngner, J. S.: Influence of inhibitors of protein synthesis on interferon formation in mice. II. Comparison of effects of glutarimide antibotics and tenuazonic acid. Virology **40**, 335–343 (1970).

Youngner, J. S.: Bacterial lipopolysaccharide: oral route for interferon production in mice. Infect. Immun. **6**, 646–654 (1972).

Youngner, J. S., Feingold, D. S., Chen, J. K.: Involvement of a chemical moiety of bacterial lipopolysaccharide in production of interferon in animals. J. Infect. Dis. **128**, 227–231 (1973).

Youngner, J. S., Hallum, J. V.: Interferon production in mice by double-stranded synthetic polynucleotides: induction or release. Virology **35**, 177–185 (1968).

Youngner, J. S., Hallum, J. V.: Inhibition of induction of interferon synthesis in L-cells pretreated with interferon. Virology **37**, 473–475 (1969).

Youngner, J. S., Keleti, G., Feingold, D. S.: Antiviral activity of an etherextracted nonviable preparation of *Brucella abortus*. Infect. Immun. **10**, 1202–1220 (1974).

Youngner, J. S., Kelly, M. E.: Inhibition by exogenous interferon of replication of poliovirus ribonucleic acid in chick brain. J. Bacteriol. **90**, 443–445 (1965).

Youngner, J. S., Salvin, S. B.: Production and properties of migration inhibitory factor and interferon in the circulation of mice with delayed hypersensitivity. J. Immunol. **111** (6), 1914–1922 (1973).

Youngner, J. S., Scott, A., Hallum, J. V., Stinebring, W. R.: Interferon production by inactivated Newcastle disease virus in cell cultures in mice. J. Bacteriol. **92**, 862–868 (1966).

Youngner, J. S., Stinebring, W. R.: Interferon production in chickens infected with *Brucella abortus*. Science **144**, 1022–1023 (1964).

Youngner, J. S., Stinebring, W. R.: Interferon appearance stimulated by endotoxin, bacteria, or viruses in mice pretreated with *Escherichia coli*, endotoxin, or infected with *Mycobacterium tuberculosis*. Nature **208**, 456–458 (1965).

Youngner, J. S., Stinebring, W. R.: Comparison of interferon production in mice by bacterial endotoxin and statolon. Virology **1**, 310–316 (1966).

Youngner, J. S., Stinebring, W. R., Taube, S. G.: Influence of inhibitors of protein synthesis on interferon formation in mice. Virology **27**, 541–564 (1965).

Youngner, J. S., Taube, S. E., Stinebring, W. R.: Inhibition of viral replication by interferon with different molecular weights. Proc. Soc. Exp. Biol. Med. **123**, 795–797 (1966).

Youngner, J. S., Thacore, H. R., Kelly, M. E.: Sensitivity of ribonucleic acid and deoxyribonucleic acid viruses to different species of interferon in cell cultures. J. Virol. **10** (2), 171–178 (1972).

Youngner, J. S., Wertz, G.: Interferon production in mice by vesicular stomatitis virus. J. Virol. **2**, 1360–1361 (1968).

Zedginidze, I. S., Bakhutashvili, V. I., Korsantiya, B. M., Gogitashvili, K. V., Sabashvili, M. G.: Interferon administration during acute leukemia. Vopr. Virusol. **4,** 64–68 (1975).

Zeitlenok, N. A., Roihel, V. M., Gorbachkova, E. A.: Effects of testosterone analogues on interferon formation, induction of antiviral protein and synthesis of cell protein in tissue culture. Nature **219,** 978–980 (1968).

Zeleznick, L. D., Bhuyan, B. K.: Treatment of leukemic (L1210) mice with double-stranded polyribonucleotides. Proc. Soc. Exp. Biol. Med. **130,** 126–132 (1969).

Zemla, J., Sehramek, S.: The action of interferon under anaerobic conditions. Virology **16,** 204–205 (1962).

Zemla, J., Vilček, J.: Studies on an interferon from tick-borne encephalitis virus-infected cells (IF). II. Physical and chemical properties of IF. Acta Virol. **5,** 367–372 (1961).

Ziegler, J. E., Lavin, G. I., Horsfall, F. L.: Interference between the influenza viruses. II. Effect of virus rendered non-infective by ultraviolet radiation upon multiplication of influenza viruses in chick embryos. J. Exp. Med. **79,** 379–400 (1944).

Zilberstein, A., Dudock, B., Berissi, H., Revel, M.: Control of messenger RNA translation by minor species of leucyl-transfer RNA in extracts from interferon-treated cells. J. Molec. Biol. **108,** 43–49 (1976a).

Zilberstein, A., Federman, P., Shulman, L., Revel, M.: Specific phosphorylation *in vitro* of a protein associated with ribosomes of interferon-treated mouse L-cells. FEBS Letters **68,** 119–127 (1976b).

Zimmerman, E. M., Freeman, A. E., Price, P. J., Holbrook, Z., Uhlendorf, C. P.: A simple interferon assay as an adjunct for determining the genus of origin of cell cultures. *In Vitro* **8,** 85–90 (1972).

Zlotnick, I., Peacock, S., Grant, D. P., Batter-Hatton: The pathogenesis of Western equine encephalitis virus (W. E. E.) in adult hamsters with special reference to the long and short term effects on the C. N. S. of the attenuated clone 15 variant. Br. J. Exp. Pathol. **53,** 59–65 (1972).

Zuckerman, A. J.: Interferon therapy for hepatitis. Nature **263,** 640 (1976).

Appendix

Aboud, M., Michalski-Stern, T., Nitzan, Y., Salzberg, S. Enhancement of cellular protein synthesis sensitivity to diphtheria toxin by interferon. Infect. Immun. **28**, 11–16 (1980).

Abreu, S. L., Bancroft, F. C.: Intracellular location of human fibroblast interferon messenger RNA. Biochem. Biophys. Res. Comm. **82**, 1300–1305 (1978).

Abreu, S. L., Bancroft, F. C., Stewart II, W. E.: Interferon priming: effects on interferon messenger RNA. J. Biol. Chem. **254**, 4114–4118 (1979).

Adam, C., Thova, Y., Ronco, P., Verroust, P., Tovey, M., Morelmaroger, L.: The effect of exogenous interferon-acceleration of autoimmune and renal diseases in (NZB/W) F1 mice. Clin. Exp. Immunol. **40**, 373–382 (1980).

Adamson, R. H., Ablashi, D. V., Armstrong, G. R., Ellmore, N. W.: Effect of cytosine araebinoside, adenine arabinoside, tilorone and rifamycin SV on multiplication of herpesvirus saimiri in vitro. Antimicrob. Agents Chemother. **1**, 82–88 (1972).

Adolf, G. R., Swetly, P.: Glucocorticoid hormones inhibit DNA synthesis and enhance interferon production in a human lymphoid cell line. Nature **282**, 736–738 (1979).

Adolf, G. R., Swetly, P.: Interferon production by human lymphoblastoid cells is stimulated by inducers of Friend cell differentiation. Virology **99**, 158–166 (1979).

Agabalian, A. S., Gasparian, E. T., Galstian, A. G., Bostandzhian, M. G.: Synthesis and antiviral activity of interferon, induced by Arboviruses, in the cell cultures of chick embryo fibroblasts. Zh. Eksp. Klin. Med. **14**, 22–27 (1974).

Aguet, M.: High-affinity binding of ^{125}I-labelled mouse interferon to a specific cell surface receptor. Nature **284**, 459–461 (1980).

Ahl, R.: The effect of interferon and quanidine on the inactivation of RNA of foot-and-mouth disease virus infected cells. Hoope Seylers Z. Physiol. Chem. **354**, 1164–1165 (1973).

Ahl, R.: Inhibitors of foot-and-mouth disease virus. I. Effect of EDTA, teryeratine and interferon on the viral growth cycle. Arch. Virusforsch. **46**, 302 (1974).

Ahl, R., Straub, O. C.: Local interferon production in the respiratory and genital tract following infection with rhinotracheitis and herpes exanthema virus. Dtsch. Tierärztl. Wschr. **78**, 653–655 (1971).

Ahronheim, G. A.: Toxoplasma gondii: human interferon studies by plaque assay. Proc. Soc. Exp. Biol. Med. **161**, 522–525 (1979).

Alarcon-Segovia, P., Ruiz-Gomez, J., Fishbein, E., Bustamonte, M. E.: Interferon production by lymphocytes from patients with systemic lupus erythematosus. Arthrit. Rheum. **17**, 590–592 (1974).

Albright, D. J., Whalen, R. A., Blacklow, N. R.: Sensitivity of human foetal intestine to interferon. Nature **247**, 218–220 (1974).

Allen, L. B., Cochran, K. W.: Accleration of scrapie in mice by target organ treatment with interferon inducers. Ann. N. Y. Acad. Sci. **284**, 676 (1977).

Allen, L. B., Huffman, J. M., Sidwell, R. W.: Failure of 1-β-D-Ribofurano-syl-1, 2, 4-triazole-3-carboxamiole (Virazole, icn 1229) to stimulate interferon. Antimicrob. Agents Chemother. **3**, 534 (1973).

Allison, A. C.: Mechanisms by which activated macrophages inhibit lymphocyte responses. Immunol. Rev. **40**, 3–27 (1978).

Altstein, A. D., Dodonova, N. N., Nadtochey, G. A., Bykovski, A. F.: Interaction between SV 40 and other viruses in tissue culture: Interference and double infection. Arch. ges. Virusforsch. **28**, 7–18 (1969).

Andreev, E. V., Berns, P. T.: Interferon and postvaccinal immunity. Veterinaria **9**, 35–36 (1973).

Andrews, R. D., Dudgeon, J. A.: Preparation of interferon. Biochemical J. **78**, 564 (1961).

Andzhaparidze, O. G., Bektemirov, R. A., Burgasova, M. P.: The effect of polyIC complex with polylysine on the course of vaccinia infection in mice. Prob. Virol. **3**, 339 (1977).

Andzhaparidze, O. G., Bektemirov, T. A., Burgasova, M. P.: Methodic recommendations for evaluation of interferon-inducers of clinical importance. Vopr. Virusol. **4**, 494 (1978). (In Russian.)

Ankel, H., Krishnamurti, C., Bescancon, F., Stefanos, S., Falcoff, S.: Mouse fibroblast (type I) and immune (type II) interferons. Pronounced differences in affinity for gangliosides and in antiviral and antigrowth effects on mouse leukemia L 1210R cells. Proc. Natl. Acad. Sci. U.S.A. **77**, 2528–2532 (1980).

Anonymous: Trypansoma cruzi as inductor of interferon. Medicine **37**, 429 (1977).

Anonymous: Interferon treatment of Herpes Zoster. Lancet ii, 126: 84 (1978).

Anonymous: Can interferons cure cancer. Lancet i, 1171 (1979).

Anonymous: Interferon interferes with virus translation. Naturewissenschaften **66**, 571 (1979).

Anonymous: Interferon: *U. S.* company increases production ten-fold. Nature **284**, 115 (1980).

Anonymous: U.S.-Yugoslav interferon agreement. Nature **284**, 296 (1980).

Anonymous: Interferon via molecular biology. Lancet i (1980).

Anonymous: The interferon boom. Lancet i, 611 (1980).

Anonymous. Interferon: Weizmann's interferon entries. Nature **284**, 391 (1980).

Anonymous: Human interferon gene sequences. Nature **285**, 536 (1980).

Anonymous: What not to say about interferon. Nature **285**, 603 (1980).

Anonymous: Immune interferon in the blood may aid in diagnosing active autoimmune disease. J. Amer. Med. Assoc. **243**, 20 (1980).

Anonymous: Publicity for interferon. Lancet i, 1371 (1980).

Anonymous: New Names for interferon. Lancet ii, 159 (1980).

Anszhelov, V. O., Maichuk, I. U. F., Pozoniakov, V.: Experimental clinical study of leukocyte interferon and aminoadamantane in adenoviral conjunctivities. Oftalmol. Zh. **26**, 418–420 (1971).

Antignus, Y., Sela, I., Harpaz, I.: Further studies on the biology of an antiviral factor (AVF) from virus-infected plants and its association with the N-gene of Nicotiana species. J. Gen. Virol. **35**, 107–112 (1977).

Aoki, F. Y., Reed, S. E., Craig, J. W., Tyrrell, D. A. J., Lees, L. J.: Effect of polynucleotide interferon-inducer of fungal origin on experiment rhinovirus infections in humans. J. Infect. Dis. **137**, 82–86 (1978).

Apte, R. N., Ascher, O., Pluznik, D.: Genetic analysis of generation of serum interferon by bacterial lipopolysaccharide. J. immunol. **119**, 1898–1902 (1977).

Archer, D. L., Johnson, H. M.: Blockade of mitogen induction of the interferon lymphokine by aphenolic food additive metabolite. Exp. Biol. Med. **157**, 684 (1979).

Archer, D. L., Smith, B. G., Ulrich, J. T., Johnson, H. M.: Immune interferon induction by T-cell mitogens involves different T-cell subpopulations. Cell Immunol. **48**, 420–426 (1979).

Armen, R. C., Evermann, J. F., Truant, A. L., Laughlin, C. A., Hallum, J. V.: Temperature-sensitive mutants of measles virus produced from persistently infected mice. Arch. Virol. **53**, 121–132 (1977).

Armstrong, J. A., Freeburg, L. C., Ho, M.: Effect of interferon on synthesis of Eastern Equine Encephalitis virus RNA. Proc. Soc. Exp. Biol. Med. **137**, 13 (1972).

Arnaoudova, V.: Treatment and prevention of acute respiratory virus infections in children with leukocytic interferon. Virologie **77**, 83–88 (1976).

Arnaoudova, V., Basheva, L., Tasheva, M., Ivanova, N., Novachev, D.: Treatment and prevention of acute viral respiratory infection in children with leukocytic interferon. Archiv. Immunol. Therap. Exper. **25**, 731–736 (1977).

Arnheiter, H., Haller, O., Lindenmann, J.: Host gene influence on interferon action in adult mouse hepatocytes: specificity for influenza virus. Virology **103**, 11–20 (1980).

Arvin, A., Feldman, S., Merigan, T. C.: Human leukocyte interferon in the treatment of varicella in children with cancer: A preliminary controlled trial. Antimicrob. Agents Chemother. **13**, 605–612 (1978).

Arvin, A., Pollard, R. B., Rasmussen, L. E., Rand, K. H., Merigan, T. C.: Lymphocyte transformation and interferon production as measures of cellular immunity in lymphoma patients. IARC Sci. Publ. **24**, 745–751 (1978).

Asculai, S. S., Kuchler, R. J.: The relationship between cytotoxicity and interferon induction in L-M strain mouse fibroblast. Proc. Soc. Exp. Biol. Med. **143**, 252–225 (1973).

Ashimova, F. M.: Interferon reaction on leukocytes in pyelonephritis in children. Pediatriia **5**, 77–78 (1975).

Assaad, F., Bres, P., Cantell, K., Cartwright, T., Chany, C., Dzagurov, S. G., Galasso, G. J., Higymandie, L. J., Hilleman, M. R., Hlabic, G. N., Levy, H. B., Majer, M., Merigan, T. C., Perkins, F., DeSomer, P., Zuckerman, A. J.: Interferon and other antiviral agents with special reference to influenza. Bull. WHO **56**, 753–760 (1978).

Atanasiu, P., Tsiang, H.: Action of interferon on the replication cycle of the rabies virion. C. R. Acad. Sci. (Paris) **274**, 2108–2111 (1972).

Atanasiu, P., Yokota, Y., Gamet, A.: Evaluation of interferon production in humans after cell culture vaccination. Ann. Microbiol. **A130**, 273–276 (1976).

Atherton, K. T., Burke, D. C.: Interferon induction by viruses and polynucleotides: a differential effect of camptothecin. J. Gen. Virol. **29**, 297–299 (1975).

Atherton, K. T., Burke, D. C.: The effects of some different metabolic inhibitors of interferon superinduction. J. Gen. Virol. **41**, 229–238 (1978).

Attallah, A. M., Folks, T.: Interferon enhanced human natural killer and antibody-dependent cell-mediated cytotoxic activity. Int. Arch. Allergy Appl. Immun. **60**, 377–382 (1979).

Attallah, A. M., Hartzmann, R. J., Noguchi, P. D.: Effect of human interferon on the primed LD typing test. IRCS Med. Sci. Biochem. **7**, 524 (1979).

Attallah, A. M., Needy, C. F., Nogvchi, P. D., Elisberg, B. L.: Enhancement of carcinoembryonic antigen expression by interferon. Int. J. Cancer **24**, 49–52 (1979).

Attallah, A. M., Strong, D. M.: Differential effects of interferon on the MLC expression on human lymphocytes: Enhanced expression of HLA without effect on Ia. Int. Arch. Allergy Appl. Immun. **60**, 101–105 (1979).

Aujean, O., Sanceau, J., Falcoff, E., Falcoff, R.: Location of enhanced ribonuclease activity and of phosphoprotein kinase in interferon-treated mengovirus-infected cells. Virology **92**, 583–586.

Ault, K. A., Weiner, H. L.: Natural killing of measles-infected cells by human lymphocytes. J. Immunol. **122**, 2611–2616 (1979).

Aviv, H., Lieberman, D., Volloch, Z., Nudel, V., Revel, M.: Inhibition of the production of leukemia virus by interferon. Isr. J. Med. Sci. **11**, 1211 (1975).

Azhary, R. E., Mannering, G. J.: Effects of interferon inducing agents on hepatic hemoproteins, heme metabolism and cytochrome P-450, linked monoxygenase systems. Molec. Pharmacol. **15**, 698–707 (1979).

Azhary, R. E., Renton, K. W., Mannering, G. J.: Effect of interferon inducing agents (polyriboinosinic acid · polyribocytidylic acid and tilorone) on the heme turnover of hepatic cytochrome P-450. Molec. Pharm. **17**, 395–399 (1980).

Azuma, M., Suenaga, T., Yoshida, I., Mizuno, F.: Interferon synthesis in human diploid cells pretreated with insulin. Antimicrob. Agents Chemother. **13**, 566–570 (1978).

Babbar, O. P.: Possible role of viruses or virus-like factor(s) in malignancies of animals and microbial cells. Ind. J. Med. Res. **69**, 876–885 (1979).

Babbar, O. P., Bajpai, S. K., Chowdhury, B. L., Khan, S. K.: Occurrence of interferon-like antiviral and antitumor factor(s) in extracts of some indigenous plants. Ind. J. Exp. Biol. **17**, 451–454 (1979).

Babbar, O. P., Dhar, M. M., Kar, A. B., Mistra, S. C., Goel, T. C.: Effect of endogenous interferon on growth of malignant tumours in man. Ind. J. Exp. Biol. **9**, 504–506 (1972).

Babbar, O. P., Sharma, S.: Possible association of the antitumor activities of chick interferon with different protein fractions constituting it. Ind. J. Med. Res. **69**, 374–382 (1979).

Babin, P.: Lysozyme, interferon and cancer. Nouv. Presse Med. **2**, 1672 (1973).

Bachmann, U., Dorries, R., Strate, C., Jungwirth, C., Bodo, G.: Impairment by interferon of mitogen-induced DNA synthesis in chick lymphocytes. Exp. Cell Biol. **46**, 210–212 (1970).

Baer, G. M., Moore, S. A., Shaddock, J. H., Levy, H. B.: Effective rabies treatment in exposed monkeys-a single dose of interferon inducer and vaccine. Bull. WHO **57**, 807–814 (1979).

Baglioni, C.: Interferon-induced enzymatic activities and their role in the antiviral state. Cell 17, 255–264 (1979).

Baglioni, C., Maroney, P. A.: Human leukocyte interferon induces 2'5'-oligo(A)polymerase and protein kinase. Virology 101, 540–544 (1980).

Baglioni, C., Maroney, P. A., West, D. K.: 2'5'-oligo(A)polymerase activity and inhibition of viral RNA synthesis in interferon-treated HeLa cells. Biochemistry 18, 1765–1770 (1979).

Baglioni, C., Minks, M. A., Maroney, P. A.: Interferon action may be mediated by activation of a nuclease by pppA2'p5'A2'p5'A. Nature 273, 684–686 (1978).

Bakay, M., Tarodi, B., Pragai, B., Beladi, I.: The effect of interferon on chicken spleen lymphocytes. Arch. Immunol. Therap. Exper. 25, 669–672 (1977).

Baker, P. N., Bradshaw, T. K., Morser, J., Burke, D. C.: The effect of 5-Bromodeoxy-uridine on interferon production in human cells. J. Gen. Virol. 45, 177–184 (1979).

Bal, E., Puricelli, L., DellaPena, N. C., Delustig, E. S.: Influence of human leukocyte interferon and IgG on the replication of herpes simplex virus in nervous tissue in vitro. Acta Virol. 23, 461–467 (1979).

Baldekierojoffe, E., Puricelli, L., Delustig, E. S.: Mouse interferon action on a murine neuroblastoma in vitro. Cell. Molec. Biol. 24, 257–264 (1979).

Balezina, T. I., Korneeva, L. E., Zemskow, V., Loidina, G. L., Nikolaeva, O. V., Fainshtein, S. L., Fadeeva, L. L., Ermolieva, Z. V.: Comparison of interferon-inducing activities and antiviral effects of tobacco mosaic virus, tilorone, and sodium nucleinate. Acta Virol. 21, 338 (1977).

Balkwill, F. R.: Interferons as cell-regulatory molecules. Cancer Immunol. Immunother. 7, 7–14 (1979).

Balkwill, F. R., Taylor-Papadimitriou, J.: Interferon affects both G, and S+G2 in cells stimulated from quiescence to growth. Nature 274, 798–799 (1978).

Balkwill, F. R., Taylor-Papadimitriou, J., Fantes, K., Sebesteny, A.: Human lymphoblastoid interferon can inhibit the growth of human breast cancer xenografts in athymic (nude) mice. Europ. J. Cancer 16, 514–569 (1980).

Balkwill, F. R., Watling, D., Taylor-Papadimitriou, J.: Inhibition by lymphoblastoid interferon of growth of cell derived from human breast. Internat. J. Cancer 22, 58 (1978).

Ball, L. A.: Induction of 2'5'-oligoadenylate synthetase activity and a new protein by chick interferon. Virology 94, 282–296 (1979).

Ball, L. A., White, C. N.: Effect of interferon pretreatment on coupled transcription and translation in cell-free extracts of primary chick embryo cells. Virology 84, 496–508 (1978).

Ball, L. A., White, C. N.: Nuclease activation by double-stranded RNA and by 2'5'-oligoadenylate in extracts of interferon-treated chick cells. Virology 93, 348–356 (1979).

Banatvala, J. E., Potter, J. E., Webster, M. J.: Foetal interferon responses induced by rubella virus. Ciba Found. Symp. 10, 77–99 (1972).

Bandyopadhyay, A. K., Chang, E. H., Levy, C. C., Friedman, R. M.: Structural abnormalities in murine leukemia viruses produced by interferon-treated cells. Biochem. Biophys. Res. Commun. 87, 983–988 (1979).

Bankowski, R. A.: Interferon and its role in poultry health. Amer. J. Vet. Res. 36, 494 (1975).

Bankowski, R. A., Kaleta, E. F.: Relations in interferon production and other known properties between CAL 11914 and TCND strains of Newcastle disease virus. Avian Dis. 16, 481–491 (1972).

Bardon, A., Sierakowska, H., Shugar, D.: Human pancreatic-type RNases with activity against dsRNAs. Biochem. Biophys. Acta 438, 461–473 (1976).

Barinski, I. I., Riabova, M. W., Sinaiko, G. A., Bektemirov, T. A., Etkind, G. V.: Interferon formation in viral hepatitis and liver cirrhosis of viral etiology. Sov. Med. 37, 26–31 (1974).

Barinsky, I. F., Shubladze, A. K., Fomina, A. N., Davydova, A. A., Bychkova, E. N., et al.: Comparative investigations on the combined use of vaccines, interferon and interferon inducers in some neurovirus infections. Vopr. Virusol. 3, 262–266 (1979). (In Russian.)

Baron, S.: Host defenses during virus infection; in: Modern Trends in Medical Virology (Heath, R. B., Waterson, A. P., eds.), pp. 77–110. London: Butterworths (1967).

Baron, S.: The biological significance of the interferon system. Arch. Intern. Med. 126, 84–93 (1970).

Baron, S.: Interferon: its role in infectious disease. Continuing Education 67 (1976).

Baron, S., Buckler, C. E.: Protective effect of antibody or elevated temperature on intracerebral infection of mice with encephalomyocarditis virus. J. Immunol. **93**, 45–48 (1964).

Baron, S., DuBuy, H., Buckler, C. E., Johnson, M. L.: Relationship of interferon production to virus growth *in vivo*. Proc. Soc. Exp. Biol. Med. **117**, 338–341 (1965).

Baron, S., Galasso, G.: Antiviral Agents. Ann. Reports Med. Chem. **10**, 161 (1975).

Baron, S., Isaacs, A.: Mechanism of recovery from viral infection in the chick embryo. Nature **191**, 97–98 (1961).

Baron, S., Porterfield, J. S., Isaacs, A.: The influence of oxygenation on virus growth. I. effect on plaque formation by different viruses. Virology **14**, 449–449 (1961).

Baron, S., Worthington, M. G., Williams, J., Gaines, J. W.: Postexposure serum prophylaxis of neonatal herpes simplex virus infection of mice. Nature **261**, 505 (1976).

Barot-Ciobaru, R., Wietzerbin, J., Petit, J. F., Chedid, L., Falcoff, E., Lederer, E.: Induction of interferon synthesis in mice by fractions from *Nocardia*. Infect. Immun. **19**, 353–356 (1978).

Barot-Ciorbaru, R., Yakota, Y., Petit, J. F., Chedid, L., Atanasio, P.: Interferon induced in the hamster by subunits of Nocardia: assay of protection against rabies. Ann. Microbiol. **B130**, 263–265 (1979).

Bart, R. S., Porzio, N. R., Kopf, A. W., Vilček, J. T., Cheng, E. H., Farcet, Y.: Inhibition of growth of B16 murine malignant melanoma by exogenous interferon. Cancer Res. **40**, 614–619 (1980).

Bartfeld, H., Vilček, J.: Immunologically specific production of interferon in cultures of rabbit blood lymphocytes: association with *in vitro* tests for cell-mediated immunity. Infect. Immun. **12**, 1112 (1975).

Barton, J. K., Lippard, S. J.: Cooperative binding of a platinum metallointercalation reagent to poly A. poly U. Biochem. **18**, 2661–2668 (1979).

Baugh, C. L., Tytell, A. A., Hilleman, M. R.: In vitro safety assessment of double-stranded polynucleotides poly I·C and Mu-9. Proc. Soc. Exp. Biol. Med. **137**, 1194–1196 (1971).

Baze, W. B., Lvovsky, E., Higbee, G. A., Levy, H. B., Hilmas, D. E.: Evaluation of a nuclease resistant derivative of polyI.polyC (polyICLC) as a radioprotective agent. Radiat. Res. **77**, 276–284 (1979).

Beatrics, S. T., Wagner, R. R.: Immunogenicity in mice of ts mutants of vesicular stomatitis virus: early appearance in bronchial secretions of an interferon-like inhibitor. J. Gen. Virol. **47**, 529 (1980).

Beck, G., Ebel, J. P., Louisot, P., Gresle, J., Pradal, M. B., Colobert, L.: Inhibition of viral multiplication by chemically methylated DNA from the host cells. Nature **228**, 859–860 (1970).

Bektemirov, T. A., Burgasova, M. P., Barkova, E. P., Andzhaparidze, O. G.: The influence of poly I.poly C modification with poly-L-lysine on the interferon inducing activity in vitro and in vivo. Vopr. Virusol. **5**, 607–610 (1978). (In Russian.)

Bektemirov, T. A., Burgasova, M. D., Kuznetsov, V. P., Rozina, E. E., Andzhaparidze, O. G.: Smallpox vaccination under the interferon and its inducers protection. Vopr. Virusol. **1**, 76–78 (1980). (In Russian.)

Bektemirov, T. A., Kitsak, V. I. A.: The relationship between the induction of interferon synthesis by a heat sensitive Sindbis virus mutant and the quantity of virus specific RNA in the chicken fibroblast culture. Vopr. Virusol. **18**, 538–541 (1973). (In Russian.)

Bektemirov, T. A., Parushina, A. E.: The relationship between individual interferon production and the skin reactions of rabbits to vaccinia virus. Vopr. Virusol. **16**, 466–468 (1971). (In Russian.)

Bektemirov, T. A., Shenkman, L. S., Marennikova, S. S.: Interferon-inducing capability of vaccinia virus strains of different pathogenicity. Vopr. Virusol. **16**, 555–560 (1971). (In Russian.)

Bektemirov, T. A., Shulitsev, G. P.: Interferon its clinical significance and use. Ter. Arkh. **45**, 10–15 (1973). (In Russian.)

Bektemirova, M. S., Karakuiumchian, M. K., Polkovnikova, V. I. A.: Individual characteristics of interferon production induced by pyrogenal in outbred and inbred mice. Vopr. Virusol. **17**, 608–611 (1972). (In Russian.)

Beladi, I., Pusztai, R., Mucsi, I., Bakay, M., Bajszar, G.: Effect of human adenoviruses on the response of chickens and sheep erythrocytes. Infect. Immun. **7**, 22–28 (1973).

Berg, K., Heron, I.: The complete purification of human leukocyte interferon. Scand. J. Immunol. **11**, 489–502 (1980).

Berg, K., Heron, I., Hamilton, R.: Purification of human interferon by antibody affinity chromatography using highly absorbed anti-interferon. Scand. J. Immunol. **8**, 429–436 (1978).

Berger, S. L., Hitchcock, M. J. M., Zoon, K. C., Birkenmeier, C. S., Friedman, R. M., Chang, E. H.: Characterization of interferon messenger RNA synthesis in Namalva cells. J. Biol. Chem. **255**, 2955–2961 (1980).

Bergeret, M., Gregoire, A., Chany, C.: Protection effect of interferon on target cells of cytotoxic lymphocytes. C. R. Acad. Sci. D **290**, 203–206 (1980).

Berkovich, S., Ressel, M.: Effect of gonadectomy on susceptibility of the adult mouse to coxsackie B1 virus infection. Proc. Soc. Exp. Biol. Med. **119**, 690–694 (1965).

Berman, L., D., Chany, C. H.: Stimulatory and inhibitory effects of adenovirus and SV40 on various virus-cell systems. Archiv ges. Virusforsch. **30**, 203–216 (1970).

Berthold, W., Tan, C., Tan, Y. H.: Purification and in vitro labeling of interferon from a human fibroblastoid cell line. J. Biol. Chem. **253**, 5206–5210 (1978).

Berthold, W., Tan, C., Tan, Y. H.: Chemical modifications of tyrosyl residue(s) and action of human-fibroblast interferon. Eur. J. Biochem. **87** (1978).

Besancon, F., Ankel, H.: Decreased sensitivity of an interferon resistant subline of murine leukemia L-1210 cells to toxic effects of ricin and abrin. Biochem. Biophys. Res. Commun. **88**, 818–825 (1979).

Besancon, F., Vignal, M., Chany, C.: Sensitivity of cells in a state of antiviral resistane to interferon. C. R. Acad. Sci. (Paris) **273**, 2694–2697 (1971).

Best, J. M., Banatvala, J. E.: The effect of a human interferon preparation on vaccine-induced rubella infection. J. Biol. Stand. **31**, 107 (1975).

Billiau, A., DeSomer, P., DeMaeyer, E.: Current status and prospects for interferon. Prog. Immunobiol. Stand. **5**, 264–266 (1972).

Billiau, A., DeSomer, P., Edy, V. G., DeClercq, E., Heremans, H.: Human fibroblast interferon for clinical trials: pharmacokinetics and tolerability in experimental animals and humans. Antimicrob. Agents Chemother. **16**, 56–58 (1979).

Billiau, A., Edy, V. G., DeSomer, P.: The clinical use of fibroblast interferon, in: Antiviral Mechanisms in the Control of Neoplasia. New York: Plenum Pub. Co. (1978).

Billiau, A., Schonne, E., Eyckmans, L., DeSomer, P.: Interferon induction and resistance to virus infection in mice infected with Brucella abortus. Infect. Immun. **2**, 698–704 (1970b).

Billiau, A., VanDamme, J., VanLeuven, F., Edy, V. G., DeLey, M., Cassiman, J. J., Van Den Berghe, H., DeSomer, P.: Human fibroblast interferon for clinical trials: production, partial purification and characterization. Antimicrob. Agts. Chemother. **16**, 49–55 (1979).

Blach-Olszewska, A., Mazur, R., Skurska, Z.: The influence of route of administration of interferon on its therapeutic effect. Arch. Immunol. Ther. Exp. (Warsz.) **20**, 491–196 (1972).

Black, D. B., Eckstein, F., DeClercq, E., Merigan, T.: Studies on the toxicity and antiviral activity of various polynucleotides. Antimicrob. Agents Chemother. **3**, 198–204 (1973).

Blalock, J. E.: Cellular interactions determine the rate and degree of interferon action. Infect. Immun. **23**, 496–501 (1979).

Blalock, J. E.: A small fraction of cells communicates the maximal interferon sensitivity to a population. Proc. Soc. Exp. Biol. Med. **161**, 80–84 (1979).

Blalock, J. E., Baron, S.: Mechanisms of interferon-induced transfer of viral resistance between animal cells. J. Gen. Virol. **42**, 363–372 (1979).

Blalock, J. E., Georgiades, J., Johnson, H. M.: Immune-type interferon-induced transfer of viral resistance. J. Immunol. **122**, 1018–1021 (1979).

Blalock, J. E., Georgiades, J. A., Langford, M. P., Johnson, H. M.: Purified human immune interferon has more potent anticellular activity than fibroblast or leukocyte interferon. Cell Immunol. **49**, 390–394 (1980).

Blalock, J. E., Langford, M. P., Georgiades, J., Stanton, G. J.: Nonsensitized lymphocytes produce leukocyte interferon when cultured with foreign cells. Cellular Immunol. **43**, 197–201 (1979).

Blalock, J. E., Stanton, G. J.: Efficient transfer of interferon-induced virus resistance between human cells. J. Gen. Virol. **41**, 325–332 (1978).

Blank, K. J., Murasko, D. M.: Induction of interferon in AKR mice by murine leukemia viruses. Nature **283**, 494–495 (1980).

Blaskovic, D.: Interference phenomena against arthropod-borne viruses. Recent Progr. Microbiol. **8**, 427–442 (1963).

Blattner, R. J.: Comments on current literature: Interferon an antiviral substance. J. Pediat. **68**, 488–491 (1966).

Bloom, B. R.: Interferon effects on the immune system. Nature **284**, 593–595 (1980).

Bloom, B. R.: The unspecificity of cellular reactions. J. Immunol. **124**, 2527–2529 (1980).

Blough, H. A., Tudor, C. H.: Potentiation of interferon by vitamin A and polysaccharides. Fed. Proc. **26**, 604 (1967).

Bocharov, A. F., Lialina, M. I., Moisiadi, S. A., Shcheglovitova, O. N., Bektemirova, T. A.: Antibody- and interferon – formation in chronic relapsing aphthous stomatitis. Vopr. Virusol. **17**, 79–84 (1972). (In Russian.)

Bocharov, A. F., Moisiadi, S. A. Amchenkova, A. M., Voronina, F. V., Khesin, I. A. E.: The influence of the immunologic reactivity of rabbit leukocytes and macrophages on interferon production under the influence of herpesvirus. Vopr. Virusol. **16**, 725–731 (1971). (In Russian.)

Bodo, G.: Interferons. Cellular proteins with antiviral effect. Naturwissenschaften **58**, 425–429 (1971).

Bodo, G., Jungwirth, C.: Die Bestimmung des isoelektrischen Punktes von huhnerinterferon durch Zonenelektrophorese in Dichtegradienten. Biochem. Zeitschrift **340**, 56–59 (1964).

Boehlandt, D., Brandner, G., Burger, J.: Inhibition of DNA and RNA synthesis in SV40 infected African green monkey kidney cell cultures by interferon. Proc. 5th Internatl. Cong. Infect. Dis., Vienna (1970).

Bollin, E., Sulkowski, E.: Metal chelate chromatography of hamster interferon. Arch. Virol. **58**, 149–152 (1978).

Bollin, E., Sulkowski, E.: Physico-chemical characterization of hamster interferon. Prep. Biochem. **9**, 339–358 (1979).

Bollin, E., Vastola, K., Oleszek, D., Sulkowski, E.: The interaction of mammalian interferons with immobilized Cibacron Blue F3GA: modulation of binding strength. Prep. Biochem. **8**, 259–274 (1978).

Bonnardiere, C. L.: Association of mouse interferon with liposomes. FEBS Letters **77**, 191 (1977).

Bonnardiere, C. L.: Liposomes can potentiate in vivo antiviral effect of exogenous interferon as shown in MHV3-infected mice. Ann. Microbiol. Inst. Pasteur **A129**, 397 (1978).

Bonnardiere, C. L., Vaureix, C., De L'Haridon, R., Scherrer, R.: Weak susceptibility of rotavirus to bovine interferon in calf kidney cells. Arch. Virol. **64**, 167–170 (1980).

Borden, E. C.: Interferons – rationale for clinical trials in neoplastic disease. Ann. Intern. Med. **91**, 472–479 (1979).

Borden, E. C., McBain, J. A., Leonhardt, P. H.: Effect of amphotericin B and its methylester on the antiviral activity of polyI polyC. Antimicrob. Agts. Chemother. **16**, 203–209 (1979).

Borecky, L.: Interferon 1976. I. Interferon and regulatory systems of the organism. Bratisl. Lek Listy **66**, 629–644 (1976).

Borecky, L.: Interferon 1976. II. The significance of interferon in medicine. Bratisl. Lek Listy **66**, 645–652 (1976).

Borecky, L.: The interferon research and our possibilities. Some concluding thoughts. Arch. Immunol. Therap. Exp. **25**, 737–739 (1977).

Borecky, L.: Twenty years after discovery of interferon: the progress and the persistent problems. Acta. Biol. Med. Germ. **38**, 709–731 (1979).

Borecky, L., Lackovic, V.: Peritoneal macrophages and interferon formation. Cesk. Epidemiol. Mikrobiol. Immunol. **23**, 196 (1974).

Borecky, L., Lackovic, V., Fuchsberger, N., Hajnicka, V.: Stimulation of interferon production in macrophages. (Excerpta Medica International Congress Series No. 325.) Activation and Macrophages, Germany, October 25–26 (1973).

Borecky, L., Lackovic, V., Fuchsberger, Hajnicka, V., Zemla, J.: The mouse leukocyte interferon: its release and characterization, in: Non-specific factors influencing host resistance (Braun, W., ed.), pp. 391–411. Basel: Karger (1973).

Borecky, L., Lackovic, V., Waschke, K., Fuchsberger, N.: Initiation of interferon production in the cell. Proc. Microbiol. Res. Grp. Hung. Acad. Sci. 4 (1971).

Borzov, M. V., Kuznetsov, V. P., Lobanovski, I. G. I.: Treatment of dermatoses of viral and non-viral etiology with interferon. Vrach. Delo. 4, 149–151 (1974).

Bostandzhian, M. G., Antonova, I. N., Bostandzhian, L. G., Karagezian, L. A., Fadeeva, L. L.: Treatment of herpetic diseases of the skin with interferon and inductors of its formation. Vestn. Dermatol. Venerol. 46, 58–61 (1972). (In Russian.)

Bostandzhian, M. G., Bikbulatov, R. M., Fadeeva, L. L., Antonova, T. N., Kasparov, A. A.: Study of the effectiveness of the action of polyvinylpyrrolidone, polyvinyl alcohol and their combinations with interferon in various manifestations of herpetic infection. Vopr. Virusol. 18, 211–215 (1973). (In Russian.)

Bostandzhian, M. G., Dorofeeva, T. N., Fadeeva, L. L., Abramian, A. N., Chemshkian, K. A.: Prevention of influenza during epidemics by leukocytic interferon combined with polyvinyl-pyrrolidone and polyvinyl alcohol. Vopr. Virusol. 17, 303–305 (1972). (In Russian.)

Bostandzhian, M. G., Khachatrian, E. A., Pylaeva, E. I. A., Fadeeva, L. L.: Treatment of acute catarrhs of the upper respiratory tract and tonsilitis with interferon. Klin. Med. (Mosk.) 51, 20–22 (1973). (In Russian.)

Bourgeade, M.-F.: Effect of murine and primate interferons on mouse-monkey hybrid cells. C. R. Acad. Sci. 278, 165–158.

Bourgeade, M. F.: Effect of sodium butyrate on sensitivity to interferon of normal or murine sarcoma transformed cells. C. R. Acad. Sci. D 287, 391–394 (1978).

Bourgeade, M. F., Cerutti, I., Chany, C.: Enchancement of interferon antitumor action by sodium butyrate. Cancer Res. 39, 4720–4723 (1979).

Bourgearde, M. F., Chany, C.: Effect of sodium butyrate on the antiviral and anticellular action of interferon in normal and MSV-transformed cells. Int. J. Cancer 24, 314–318 (1979).

Bourgeade, M. F., Chany C., Merigan, T. C.: Type I and type II interferons: differential antiviral actions in transformed cells. J. Gen. Virol. 46, 449–454 (1980).

Bousquet, C., Cannat, A., Ramuz, M., Serre, A.: Adherent cell and T-lymphocyte cooperation for the in vitro production of brucella-induced interferon by murine spleen cells. Ann. Immunol. C 129, 715–720 (1978).

Bousquet, C., Ramuz, M., Cannat, A., Roux, J.: Specific inhibition of interferon synthesis in mice immunized against Brucella and Newcastle disease viruses. FEMS Microbiol. Letters 1, 133 (1977).

Bousquet, C., Senglat, C., Ramuz, M.: Localization of the interferon inductor in Brucella suiss. C. R. Acad. Sci. D 282, 513 (1976).

Bousquet-Ucla, C., Wietzerbin, J., Falcoff, E.: Studies on Brucella interferon: chromatographic behaviour and purification. Arch. Virol. 63, 57–88 (1980).

Boxaca, M., Paucker, K.: Neutralization of different murine interferons by antibody. J. Immunol. 98, 1130–1135 (1967).

Bradish, C. J., Allner, K.: The production of mouse interferon in rolling monolayers of L-cells. Symp. Ser. Immunobiol. Stand. 14, 35–38 (1970).

Brailovsky, C., Chany, C.: Un facteur produit per l'adenovirus 12 en culture cellulaire stimulant la multiplication du virus K du rat. C. R. Acad. Sci. (Paris) 260, 2634–2637 (1965).

Brandner, G., Mueller, N.: Cytosine arabinoside- and interferon-mediated control of polyoma and SV 40 genome expression. Cold Spring Harbor Symp. Quant. Biol. 39, 305 (1974).

Brandner, G., Mueller, N., Burger, J., Koch, E., Burger, A.: The effect of polyinosinic-polycytidylic acid on the transcription of the SV 40 genome in African green monkey. Acta Virol. 18, 284–292 (1974).

Braude, I. A., Declercq, E.: Purification of mouse interferon by sequential chromatography. J. Chromatography 172, 207–220 (1979a).

Braude, I. A., Declercq, E.: Mechanism of interaction of sodium dodecyl sulfate with mouse interferon. J. Biol. Chem. 245, 7758–7764 (1979b).

Braude, I. A., Edy, V. G., Declercq, E.: Mechanism of binding of mouse interferon to controlled pore glass. Biochim. Biophys. Acta 574, 15–23 (1979).

Braude, I. A., Lin, L. S., Stewart II, W. E.: Differential inactivation and separation of homologous and heterologous antiviral activity of human leukocyte interferon by a proteolytic enzyme. Biochem. Biophys. Res. Commun. **89**, 612–619 (1979).

Brezina, R. Kazar, J., Schramer, S.: Induction of interferon activity in mouse spleen by phase *Coxiella burnetti*. Acta Virol. **12**, 382–383 (1968).

Bridgen, P. J., Anfinsen, C. B., Corley, L., Bose, S., Zoon, K. C., Ruegg, U. T., Buckler, C. E.: Human lymphoblastoid interferon: large scale production and partial purification. J. Biol. Chem. **252**, 6585–6587 (1977).

Broad, W.: Industry readies for interferon market. Science **207**, 1326 (1980).

Brock, D. W., Harradine, D. L.: The effect of an interferon inducer on experimental mouse piroplasmosis (Babesia rodhaini infection). Res. Vet. Sci. **14**, 397–399 (1973).

Brodeur, B. R., Legar, E. C., Brailovsky, C. A.: Anti-interferon activity of extracts of cells transformed by SV 40 virus. Can. J. Microbiol. **19**, 7–14 (1973).

Brodeur, B. R., Merigan, T. C.: Suppressive effect of interferon on the humoral immune response to sheep red blood cells in mice. J. Immunol. **113**, 1319–1325 (1974).

Brodeur, B. R., Merigan, T. C.: Mechanism of the suppressive effect of interferon on antibody synthesis *in vivo*. J. Immunol. **114**, 1323–1330 (1975).

Brodeur, B. R., Weinstein, Y., Melnon, K. L., Merigan, T. C.: Interferon inhibition of lymphocyte mitogenesis. Ann. Immunol. (Paris) **128**, 53–56 (1977).

Brodskaya, L. M., Vilner, L. M.: Comparative antiviral and interferon-inducing activity of synthetic polyribonucleotide complexes poly I.C and poly G.C in differnt cell systems. Vopr. Virusol. **6**, 685 (1976). (In Russian.)

Brostrom, L. A.: The combined effect of interferon and methotrexate on human osteosarcoma and lymphoma cell lines. Cancer Letters **10**, 83–90 (1980).

Brostrom, L. A., Ingimarson, S., Strander, H., Soderberg, G.: Adjuvant interferon treatment and the late development of cerebral metastases in a patient with osteosarcoma. Acta Orthopaed. Scand. **51**, 589–594 (1980).

Brouty-Boye, D., Gresser, I., Baldwin, C.: Reversion of the transformed phenotype to parental phenotype by cocultivation of x-ray-transformed C3H/10T1/2 cells at low cell density. Int. J. Cancer **24**, 253–260 (1979).

Brouty-Boye, D., Gresser, I., Baldwin, C.: Decreased sensitivity to interferon associated with *in vitro* transformation of x-ray transformed C3H/10T1/2 cells. Int. J. Cancer **24**, 261–265 (1979).

Brouty-Boye, D., Zetter, B. R.: Inhibition of cell mobility by interferon. Science **208**, 516–518 (1980).

Brown, G. E., Lebleu, B., Kawakita, M., Shaila, S., Sen, G. C., Lengyel, P.: Increased endonuclease activity in an extract from mouse Ehrlich ascites tumor cells which had been treated with a partially purified interferon preparation: dependence on double-stranded RNA. Biochem. Biophys. Res. Commun. **69**, 114–116 (1976).

Brown, P., and Besancon, F.: Effect of acid pH on induction of an antiviral resistance condition by interferon. C. R. Acad Sci. **D 275**, 2275–2278 (1972).

Brown, P., Besancon, F., and Chany, C.: The effects of an acid pH upon the induction of antiviral resistance in vitro by interferon. Proc. Soc. Exp. Biol. Med. **142**, 1195–1198 (1973).

Brown, R. McK.: A quantitative study of inhibition of herpes simplex virus by interferon. Thesis, University of Texas (1966).

Brown, G. E., Simon, E. H., Chung, C.: Interferon production by individual L cells. J. Gen. Virol. **47**, 171–182 (1980).

Brunda, M. J., Berberman, R. B., Holden, H. T.: Inhibition of murine natural killer cell activity by prostaglandins. J. Immunol. **124**, 2682–2687 (1980).

Bryson, Y. J., Kronenberg, L. H.: Combined antiviral effects of interferon, adenine arabinoside, hypoxanthine arabinoside and adenine-arabinoside-5' monophosphate in human fibroblast cultures. Antimicrob. Agts. Chemother. **11**, 299–303 (1977).

Buchan, A., Burke, D. C.: Interferon production in chick-embryo cells. The effect of puromycin and p-fluorophenylalanine. Biochem. J. **98**, 530–536 (1966).

Buchvald, J., Borecky, L., Doskocil, J.: Möglichkeiten der Ausnutzung des Interferon-Induktion-Satofues in der Therapie der Virusdermatosen. Z. Hautkr. **50**, 909–911 (1975).

Buck, K. W., Chain, E. B., and Himmelweit, F.: Comparison of interferon induction in mice by purified *Penicillium chrysogenum* virus and derived double-stranded RNA. J. Gen. Virol. 12, 131–139 (1971).

Buckley, S. M., Casals, J.: Mouse interferon in ascitic fluids. Appld. Microbiol. 28, 319–321 (1974).

Buffett, R. F., Ito, M., Cairo, A. M., Carter, W. A.: Antiproliferative activity of highly purified mouse interferon: brief communication. J. Nat. Cancer Inst. 60, 243–246 (1978).

Bukata, L. A., Nosik, N. N., Fomina, A. N., Ershow, F. I.: Comparative antiviral and inter-feronogenic activity of natural and synthetic interferon-inducers in vitro and in vivo. Antibiotiki. 24, 444–448 (1979).

Burgasova, M. P., Andzhaparidze, O. G., Bektemirov, T. A., Bogomolova, N. N., Boriskin, Y. S.: Influence of poly I·poly C complex with poly-L-lysine on the experimental tick-borne encephalitis. Vopr. Virusol. 4, 438 (1977). (In Russian.)

Burke, D. C.: The purification of interferon. Biochem. J. 76, 50P (1960).

Burke, D. C.: The production of interferon by animal viruses. Proc. Roy. Soc. (London) B 177, 17–22 (1971).

Burke, D. C.: Is interferon only an antiviral agent. Sci. Progress 63, 141 (1976).

Burke, D. C., Graham, C. F., Lehman, J. M.: Appearance of interferon inducibility and sensitivity during differentiation of murine teratocarcinoma cells *in vitro*. Cell 13, 243–248 (1978).

Burke, D. C., Morser, J.: Translation of interferon messenger RNA. Nature 271, 10–11 (1978).

Burke, D. C., Ross, J.: Molecular weight of chick interferon. Nature 208, 1297–1299 (1960).

Cabrer, B., Taira, H., Broeze, R. J., Kempe, T. D., Williams, K., Slattery, E., Konigsberg, W. H., Lengyel, P.: Structural characteristics of interferons from mouse Ehrlich ascites tumor cells. J. Biol. Chem. 254, 3681–3684.

Calam, D. H.: Nomenclature of interferons. Lancet ii, 259 (1980).

Calvet, M. C., Gresser, I.: Interferon enhances the excitability of cultured neurones. Nature 278, 558–560 (1979).

Cambrelin, G.: Interferon, anaphylaxis and allergy. Acta. Otolaryngol. 73, 148–150 (1972).

Came, P. E., Moore, D. H.: Studies on interferon induction by the mouse mammary tumor virus. Proc. Soc. Exp. Biol. Med. 133, 252–254 (1970).

Campbell, J. B.: Further studies on the relative antiviral efficacies of interferon induced by poly I·C and Mengo virus. Canad. J. Microbiol. 22, 712–715 (1976).

Campbell, J. B., Buera, J. G.: A comparison of the protective effect against Mengo virus infection in mice of interferons induced by poly I·C and Mengo virus. Canad. J. Microbiol. 17, 1525–1532 (1971).

Cantell, K., Hirvonen, S.: Large-scale production of human leukocyte interferon containing 10^8 units per ml. J. Gen. Virol. 39, 541–544 (1978).

Cantell, K., Hirvonen, S., Kauppinen, H.-L., Myllyla, G.: Production of interferon in human leukocytes from normal donors with the use of Sendai virus. Methods in Enzymology (1980, in press).

Cantell, K., Hirvonen, S., Koistinen, V.: Partial purification of human leukocyte interferon on a large scale. Methods in Enzymology (1980, in press).

Cantell, K., Hirvonen, S., Mogensen, K. E., Pyhala, L.: Human leukocyte interferons: production, purification, stability and animal experiments. In: In vitro Monographs 3: The production and use of interferon for the treatment of human virus infections, pp. 35–38 (1974).

Cantell, K., Paucker, K.: Quantitative studies on viral interference in suspended L-cells IV. Production and assay of interferon. Virology 21, 11–21 (1963a).

Cantell, K., Paucker, K.: Studies on viral interference in two lines of Hela cells. Virology 19, 81–87 (1963b).

Cantell, K., Pyhala, L.: Circulating interferon in rabbits after administration of human interferon by different routes. J. Gen. Virol. 20, 97–104 (1973).

Cantell, K., Pyhala, L.: Pharmacokinetics of human leukocyte interferon. J. Infect. Dis. 133, A6–A8 (1976).

Cantell, K., Pyhala, L., Strander, H.: Circulating human interferon after intramuscular injection into animals and man. J. Gen. Virol. 25, 453–458 (1974).

Cantell, K., Skurska, Z., Paucker, K., Henle, W.: Quantitative studies on viral inferference in suspended L cells. II. Factors affecting interference by UV-irradiated NDV against VSV. Virology **17**, 312–323 (1962).

Cantell, K., Strander, H., Hadhazy, G. Y., Nevanlinna, H. R.: How much interferon can be prepared in human leukocyte suspensions. In: The Interferons (Rita, G., ed.), p. 223. New York: Academic Press (1968).

Cantell, K., Strander, H., Saxen, L., Meyer, B.: Interferon response of human leucocytes during intrauterine and post-natal life. J. Immunol. **100**, 1304–1308 (1968).

Cantell, K., Tovell, D. R.: Substitution of milk for serum in the production of human leukocyte interferon. Appl. Microbiol. **22**, 625–628 (1971).

Carroll, D., Ventura, P., Haase, A., Rinaldo, C. R., Overall, J. C., Glasgow, L. A.: Resistance of visna virus to interferon. J. Infect. Dis. **138**, 5614–5617 (1978).

Carter, W. A.: Interferon: enhanced synthesis and action in mouse and human cells under suboptimal growth conditions. Johns Hopkins Med. J. **130**, 166–173 (1972).

Carter, W. A.: Chemotherapy of human oncogenic viral infections: the possible role of interferon and reverse transcriptase inhibitors. J. Surg. Oncol. **5**, 113–136 (1973).

Carter, W. A.: By passing the "species barrier" with carbohydrate-altered interferon from leukocytes. Cancer Res. **39**, 3796–3798 (1979).

Carter, W. A.: Glycosylation, intraspecies molecular heterogeneity and trans-species activity of mammalian interferons. Life Sci. **25**, 717–728 (1979).

Carter, W. A.: Mechanisms of cross-species activity of mammalian interferons. Pharm. Ther. **7**, 245–252 (1979).

Carter, W. A., Davis, L. R., Chadha, K. C., Johnson, F. H.: Porcine leukocyte interferon and antiviral activity in human cells. Molec. Pharmacol. **15**, 685–690 (1979).

Carter, W. A., Dolen, J. G., Leong, S. S., Horoszewiez, J. S., Vladutiu, A. O., Leibowitz, A. I., Nolan, J. P.: Purified human fibroblast interferon in vivo: skin reactions and effect on bone marrow precursor cells. Cancer Lett. **7**, 243–250 (1979).

Carter, W. A., Horoszewicz, J. S.: Human interferon and its inducers: clinical program overview at Roswell Park Institute. Cancer Treatment Res. **62**, 249–250 (1978).

Carter, W. A., Horoszewicz, J. S.: Production, purification and clinical application of human fibroblast interferon. Pharmacol. Therap. **8**, 359–378 (1980).

Carter, W. A., Pitha, P. M., Brockman, W. W., Borden, E. C., Marshall, L. W.: Selective inhibition of viral functions: the antiviral action of interferon and streptovaricin. Medicine (Baltimore) **51**, 181–188 (1972).

Casals, J., Buckley, S. M., Barry, D. W.: Resistance to Arboviruses challenge in mice immediately after vaccination. Applied Microbiol. **25**, 753–756 (1973).

Cate, T. R., Kelly, J. R.: Hong-Kong influenza antigen sensitivity and decreased interferon response of peripheral lymphocytes. Antimicrob. Agents Chemother. **10**, 156–160 (1970).

Cebecaver, L., Rovensky, J., Doskocil, J., Pekarek, J., Borecky, L., Zitnan, D.: Effect of different polyribonucleotides on the induction of antibodies to DNA and RNA and serum complement levels in mice. Acta Biol. Med. Germ. **38**, 843–846 (1979).

Cembrzynska-Nowak, M.: IME – an inhibitor of interferon activity isolated from mouse embryonic tissue. II. Biological characterization. Arch. Immunol. Ther. Exp. **27**, 229–240 (1979).

Cerutti, I.: Proprietis antivirales du *C. parvum*. C. R. Acad. Sci. (Paris) **D 279**, 963 (1974).

Cerutti, I., Chany, C., Schlumberger, J.: Isoprinosine increases the antitumor action of interferon. Cancer Treat. Res. **62**, 1971–1976 (1978).

Cerutti, I., Chany, C., Schlumberger, J.: Isoprinosine increases the antitumor action of interferon. Int. J. Immunopharm. **1**, 230–236 (1979).

Cerutti, I., Chany-Fournier, F., Chany, C.: Effet potentiateur de la cyclohextmine sur l'interference virale. C. R. Acad. Sci. (Paris) **D 284**, 679 (1977).

Cesario, T. C.: Comparison of effect of body fluids on 2 species of fibroblast interferons. Curr. Ther. Res. **24**, 153 (1978).

Cesario, T. C., Slater, L. M.: Diminished antiviral effect of human interferon in the presence of therapeutic concentrations of antineoplastic agents. Infect. Immun. **27**, 842–845 (1980).

Cesario, T. C., Vaziri, N., Slater, L., Tilles, J. G.: Inactivators of fibroblast interferon found in human serum. Infect. Immun. **24**, 851–855 (1979).

Chadha, K. C., Grob, P. M.: Affinity of human leukocyte interferon for polyribonucleotides. Cell Biol. Int. Rep. 3, 663–670 (1979).

Chadha, K. C., Grob, P. M., Hamill, P. M., Sulkowski, E.: Glycosylation of human leukocyte interferon: effects of tunicamycin. Arch. Virol. 64, 109–118 (1980).

Chadha, K. C., Grob, P. M., Mikulski, A. J., Davis, L. R., Sulkowski, E.: Copper chelate affinity chromatography of human interferon. J. Gen. Virol. 43, 701–706 (1979).

Chadha, K. C., Sclair, M., Sulkowski, E., Carter, W. A.: Molecular size heterogeneity of human leukocyte interferon. Biochem. 17, 196–200 (1978).

Champney, K. J., Levine, D. P., Levy, H. B., Lerner, A. M.: Modified poly I·poly C complex: sustained interferonemia and its physiological associates in humans. Infect. Immun. 25, 831–837 (1979).

Chang, E. H., Jay, F. T., Friedman, R. M.: Physical, morphological and biochemical alterations in membrane of AKR mouse cells after interferon treatment. Proc. Nat. Acad. Sci. U.S.A. 75, 1859–1863 (1978).

Chang, T. T., Simon, E. H., Fleischmann, W. K.: The mechanism of interferon action in single cells: accumulation of intracellular virus. J. Gen. Virol. 20, 139–149 (1973).

Chany, C., Fournier, F., Rousset, S.: Interferon regulatory mechanism. Ann. New York Acad. Sci. 505–515 (1970).

Chany, C., Gresser, I., Vendrely, C., Robbe-Fossat, F.: Further studies of persistent polioviral infection of the intact aminiotic membrane, existence of a mechanical barrier to viral infection. Proc. Soc. Exp. Biol. Med. 123, 960–968 (1966).

Chany-Fournier, F., Pauloin, A., Chany, C.: Isolation, preliminary characterization, and interferon antagonistic effect of a mammalian lectin-like substance. Proc. Nat. Acad. Sci. U.S.A. 75, 2333–2337 (1978).

Chawda, R., Job, L., Horoszewicz, J. S., Carter, W. A., Arya, S. K.: Effect of bromodeoxyuridine and interferon on cellular and viral functions in human prostactic cells. Oncology 36, 35–39 (1979).

Check, W. A.: At year's end, what's new with interferon? J. Amer. Med. Assoc. 242, 2829–2830 (1979).

Check, W. A.: How they did it: the synthesis of interferon? J. Amer. Med. Assoc. 243, 721–722 (1980).

Cheeseman, S. H., Black, P. H., Rubin, R. H., Cantell, K., Hirsch, M. S.: Interferon and BK papovavirus: clinical and laboratory studies. J. Infect. Dis. 141, 157–161 (1980).

Cheeseman, S. H., Henle, W., Rubin, R. H., Tolkoffurin, N. E., Cosimi, B., Cantell, K., Winkle, S., Herrin, J. T., Black, P. H., Russell, P. S., Hirsch, M. S.: Epstein-Barr virus infection in renal transplant recipients – effects of antithymocyte globulin and interferon. Ann. Intl. Med. 93, 39–42 (1980).

Cheeseman, S. H., Rubin, R. H., Stewart, J. A., Tolkoff-Rubin, N. E., Cosimi, A. B., Cantell, K., Gilbert, J., Winkle, S., Herrin, J. T., Black, P. H., Russell, P. S., Hirsch, M. S.: Prophylactic interferon in renal transplantation: effects on cytomegalovirus and herpes simplex virus infections. N. Eng. J. Med. 300, 1345–1349 (1979).

Chernos, V. I., Libshits, B. A., Yakobson, E., Ghendon, Y. Z.: Mechanism of antiviral action of acetone on rabbitpox virus replication. J. Virol. 9, 251–258 (1972).

Chernajovsky, Y., Kinehi, A., Schmidt, A., Zilberstein, A., Revel, M.: Differential effects of two interferon-induced translational inhibitors on initiation of protein synthesis. Europ. J. Biochem. 96, 35–38 (1979).

Chertkov, K. S., Talosh, M., Mosina, Z. M., Preobrazhevski, I. I.: Radioprotective effectiveness of tilorone. Radiobiologia 19, 455–458 (1979).

Chiarini, A., Sinatra, A., Ammatuna, P.: Protective effectiveness of interferon and its stimulation in infection in vitro by thogoto-like AR126 arbrovirus. Boll. Soc. Ital. Biol. Sper. 50, 1745–1751 (1974).

Chirigos, M. A., Pearson, J. W.: Cure of murine leukemia with drug and interferon treatment. J. Natl. Cancer Inst. 51, 1367–1368 (1973).

Chisholm, M., Cartwright, T.: Interferon production in Hodgkin's disease. Clin. Exp. Immunol. 20, 419–422 (1975).

Chizhov, N. P.: Evaluation of this inhibiting action of virazole on the reproduction of vaccinia virus in tissue culture. Vopr. Virusol. 3, 259–262 (1979). (In Russian.)

Cho, Y., Tanamoto, K., Oh, Y., Homma, J. Y.: Differences of chemical structures of *Peudomonas aeruginosa* lipopolysaccharide essential for adjuncticity and antitumor and interferon-inducing activity. FEBS Lett. **105**, 120–123 (1979).

Christoffersen, J. J., Bro-Jorgensen, K.: Erythropoietic activity and interferon production in LCM virus-infected nude mice. Acta Pathol. Microbiol. Scand. **85**, 435–440 (1977).

Christophersen, I. S., Jordal, R., Osther, K., Lindenberg, J., Pedersen, P. H., Berg, K.: Interferon therapy in neoplastic disease. Acta Medica Scand. **240**, 471–476 (1978).

Chu, T. S.: Interferon and its clinical application. Chin. Med. J. **9**, 576–579 (1974).

Chudzio, T., Inglot, A. D.: Biological properties of three spontaneous mutants of Sindbis virus. Arch. Immunol. Therap. Exp. **23**, 113–118 (1975).

Chun, M., Pasanen, V., Hammerling, U., Hammerling, G. F., Hoffmann, M. K.: Tumor recrosis serum induces a serologically distinct population of NK cells. J. Exp. Med. **150**, 426–431 (1979).

Cioe, L., Dolei, A., Rossi, G. B., Belardelli, F., Affabris, E., Gambari, R., Fantoni, A.: Potential for differentiation, virus production, and tumorigenicity in murine erythroleukemic cells treated with interferon, in: In Vitro Aspects of Erythropoiesis (Murphy, M. J., ed.), pp. 159–171. New York: Springer (1978).

Cioe, L., O'Brien, T. G., Diamond, L.: Inhibition of adipose conversion of BALB/c 3T3 cells by interferon and 12-Otetradecanoylphorpol-13-acetate. Cell Biol. **4**, 255–264 (1980).

Clemens, M.: Interferons and cellular regulation. Nature **282**, 364–365 (1979).

Clynes, M. M., Duke, E. J.: Effect of poly I·C on establishment and on spontaneous and chemical transformation of Balb C mouse embryo cells in culture. Biochem. Soc. Trans. **4**, 897–899 (1976).

Coffey, J. J., Kelley, S. A., Wodinsky, I.: Effect of autoclaving on molecular weight distribution and chemotherapeutic activity of clinical samples of poly I·C (NSC-120949). Cancer Chem. Repo. **56**, 31–34 (1972).

Cohen, D., Mazzur, S., Kaplan, M. M., Koprowski, H.: Factors inhibiting the interference of WEE virus by rabies virus in chick embryo tissue cultures. Nature **198**, 270–271 (1963).

Colby, C., Stollar, B. D., Simon, M. I.: Interferon induction: DNA-RNA hybrid or double-stranded RNA? Nature New Biol. **229**, 172–174 (1971).

Cole, B. C., Lombardi, P. S., Overall, J. C., Glasgow, L. A.: Inhibition of interferon induction in mice by mycoplasmas and mycoplasmal fractions. Proc. Soc. Exp. Biol. Med. **157**, 83–86 (1978).

Collavo, D., Finco, B., Chieco-Bianchi, L.: Immune reactivity following poly I·poly C treatment in mice. Nature New Biol. **239**, 154–156 (1972).

Collins, A. R., Flanagan, T. D.: Interferon production and response to exogenous interferon in two cell lines of mouse brain origin persistently infected with Sendai virus. Arch. Virol. **53**, 313–316 (1977).

Colman, A., Morser, J.: Export of proteins from oocytes of *Xenopus laevis*. Cell **3**, 517–526 (1979).

Commoy-Chevalier, M. J., Robert-Galliot, B., Chany, C.: Effect of ammonium salts on the interferon-induced antiviral state in mouse L-cells. J. Gen. Virol. **41**, 541–548 (1978).

Cook, R. M.: Spontaneous cytotoxicity of murine cells treated with the interferon inducers BRL5907 and BRL10739. Immunology **39**, 151–158 (1980).

Cooper, J. A., Morser, J.: The toxic effect of double-stranded RNA for interferon-treated L-cells: studies on membrane transport and with cell-free-system. J. Gen. Virol. **43**, 563–570 (1979).

Cooper, J. A., Morser, J., Colby, M. S., Burke, D. C.: The toxic effect of double-stranded RNA for interferon-treated cells: evidence for a heterogeneous cellular response and the role of the cell nucleus. J. Gen. Virol. **43**, 553–562 (1979).

Coppey, J.: Repairs of interferon synthetic capacity in ultraviolet-irradiated normal and hybrid mammalian cells. Nature New Biol. **234**, 14–15 (1971).

Coppey, J.: Growth of Newcastle disease and herpes virus and interferon production in a monkey-mouse hybrid line. J. Gen. Virol. **14**, 9–14 (1972).

Cortada, D., DeLustig, E. S.: Interferon production by leukocytes from neoplastic patients. Europ. J. Cancer **10**, 189–192 (1974).

Coto, V., Galeota, C. A., Coraggio, F.: Inhibition of interferon production by a halogenated pyrimidine derivative 5-fluoro-21-deoxyuridine. Tex. Rep. on Biol. Med. **24**, 158–163 (1966).

Coupin, G., Illinger, D., Poindron, P.: Lack of association between the elevation of adenosine 3'5'-cyclic monophosphate and the potentiation of the interferon induced antiviral state by nonadrenaline in normal and tumoral rat cells. Intervirology **13**, 54–57 (1980).

Coupin, G., Illinger, D., Poindron, P., Fauconnier: Rat interferon in vivo and in vitro induction study of some biological properties. Ann. Pharm. Franc. **36**, 431–442 (1978).

Cox, D. R., Epstein, L. B., Epstein, C. J.: Genes coding for sensitivity to interferon (IFRec) and soluble superoxide dismutase (SOD-1) are linked in mouse and man and map to mouse chromosome 16. Proc. Natl. Acad. Sci. U.S.A. **77**, 2168–2172 (1980).

Craig, C. P., Gordon, S. L., Greer, R. B.: Interferon responsiveness of rabbit synovial cells and chondrocytes. Infect. Immun. **8**, 425–427 (1973).

Crane, J. L., Glasgow, L. A., Kern, E. R., Youngner, J. S.: Inhibition of murine osteogenic sarcoma by treatment with type I or type II interferon. J. Nat. Cancer Inst. **61**, 871–874 (1978).

Creasey, A. A., Bartholomew, J. C., Merigan, T. C.: Role of GoG1 arrest in the inhibition of tumor cell growth by interferon. Proc. Nat. Acad. Sci. U.S.A. **77**, 1471–1475 (1980).

Cruz, J. R., Waner, J. L., Dammin, G. J.: Effect of exogenous interferon on neonatal infection with murine cytomegalovirus. IARC Sci. Publ. **24**, 1067–1071 (1978).

Culliton, B. J., Waterfall, W. K.: War on cancer- interferon. Brt. Med. J. **2**, 195 (1979).

Cummins, J. M., Rosenquist, B. D.: Leukocyte changes and interferon production in calves injected with hydrocortisone and infected with infectious bovine rhinotracheitis virus. Amer. J. Vet. Res. **40**, 238–240 (1979).

Cummins, J. M., Rosenquist, B. D.: Protection of calves against rhinovirus infection by nasal secretion of interferon-induced by infectious bovine rhinotracheitis virus. Amer. J. Vet. Res. **41**, 161–165 (1980).

Cundliffe, B., Morser, J.: The effect of inhibitors of glycosylation on interferon production in human lymphoblastoid cells. J. Gen. Virol. **43**, 457–462 (1979).

Cunliffe, H. R., Richmond, J. Y., Campbell, C. H.: Interferon inducers and foot- and- mouth disease vaccines: influence of two synthetic polynucleotides on antibody response and immunity in guinea pigs. Can. J. Comp. Med. **41**, 117–121 (1977).

Dahl, H.: Human interferon and cell growth inhibition. III. Separation of activities by treatment with sodium dodecyl sulphate. Biochem. Biophys. Res. Comm. **82**, 6–10 (1978).

Dahl, H.: Human interferon and cell growth V. Effect of ouabain on interferon activities. Biochem. Biophys. Res. Comm. **92**, 586–590 (1980).

Dahl, H., Degre, M.: Preventive effect of a nonviral interferon inducer, a bacterial vaccine, on experimental influenza in mice. Acta. Pathol. Microbiol. Scand. **80B**, 467–474 (1972 b).

Dalton, B. J., Ogburn, C. A., Paucker, K.: Production of antibodies to human interferons in mice. Infect. Immun. **19**, 570–574 (1978).

Dalton, B. J., Paucker, K.: Antigenic properties of human lymphoblastoid interferons. Infect. Immun. **23**, 244–248 (1979).

Danielescu, G., Anton, D., Athanasiu, P., Aderca, L.: Transformation by adenovirus type 12 of rat embryo fibroblasts cultivated in the presence of interferon. Rev. Roum. Virol. **11**, 133–140 (1974).

David-West, T. S., Cooke, P. M., Stevenson, J. W.: The mode of action of an antiviral substance from Penicilium cyaneofulvum. Canad. J. Microbiol. **14**, 197–204 (1968).

Davies, A.: The partial purification of calf interferon. Biochem. J. **90**, 29p (1964).

Dawson, C. R.: How does the external eye resist infection? Invest. Ophthalmol. **15**, 971–974 (1976).

DeClercq, E.: Increased resistance of trisomic-21 cells to virus replication: role of interferon. Virology **86**, 276 (1978).

DeClercq, E.: Degradation of poly I·poly C by human plasma. Europ. J. Biochem. **93**, 165–172 (1979).

DeClercq, E., DeSomer, P.: Antiviral activity of polyribocytidylic acid in cells primed with polyriboinosinic acid. Science **173**, 260–262 (1971).

DeClercq, E., DeSomer, P.: Production of interferon in rabbit cell cultures by mouse L-cell-bound poly I·C. J. Gen. Virol. **16**, 435–439 (1972).

DeClercq, E., DeSomer, P.: Mechanism of the antiviral activity resulting from sequential administration of complementary homopolyribonucleotide to cell cultures. J. Virol. **9**, 721–724 (1972).

DeClercq, E., DeSomer, P.: Protection of rabbits against local vaccinia virus infection by Brucella abortis and polyacrylic acid in the absence of systemic interferon production. Infect. Immun. **8**, 669–673 (1973).

DeClercq, E., Eckstein, F., Merigan, T. C.: Structural requirements for synthetic polyanions to act as interferon inducers. Ann. N.Y. Acad. Sci. **173**, 444 (1970).

DeClercq, E., Edy, V. G., Torrence, P. F., Waters, J. A., Witkop, B.: Antiviral activity of poly (7-deazainosinic acid) derived complexes in vitro and in vivo. Mol. Pharmacol. **12**, 1045–1051 (1976).

DeClercq, E., Georgiades, J., Edy, V. G., Sobis, H.: Effect of human and mouse interferon and of poly rI·poly rC on growth of human fibrosarcoma and melanoma tumors in nude mice. Europ. J. Cancer **14**, 1273–1282 (1978).

DeClercq, E., Huang, G. F., Bhooshan, B., Ledley, G., Torrence, P. F.: Interferon induction by mismatched analogues of polyinosinic acid-polycytidylic acid [(Ix, U)n·(C)n]. Nucl. Acid. Res. **7**, 2003–2074 (1979).

DeClercq, E., Janik, B., Sommer, R. G.: Effect of ionenes on interferon induction by poly I·C. Antimicrob. Agents Chemother. **11**, 756–759 (1977).

DeClercq, E., Merigan, T. C.: Stimulation or inhibition of interferon production depending on time of cycloheximide administration. Virology **42**, 799–802 (1970).

DeClercq, E., Stewart II, W. E.: Het natuurlyk verloop van een acute virusinfective. Tijdschr. Voor Geneeskunde **15**, 10–29 (1973 b).

DeClercq, E., Stollar, B. D., Hobbs, J., Fukui, T., Kakiuch, N., Ikehara, M.: Interferon induction by two 2'-modified double-helical RNAs. Eur. J. Biochem. **107**, 279 (1980).

DeClercq, E., Stollar, B. D., Thang, M. N.: Interferon inducing activity of polyinosinic acid. J. Gen. Virol. **40**, 203 (1978).

DeClercq, E., Torrence, P. F., Fukui, T., Ikehara, M.: Role of purine N-3 in the biologic activities of poly(A) and poly(I). Nucleic Acids Res. **3**, 1591–1601 (1976).

DeClercq, E., Torrence, P. F., Stollar, B. D., Hobbs, J.: Interferon-induction by a 2'-modified double-helical RNA, poly(2'-azido-2'-deoxyinosinic acid)·polycytidylic acid. Europ. J. Biochem. **88**, 341–344 (1978).

Degre, M.: Influence of polyinosinic: polycytidylic acid on the circulating white blood cells in mice. Proc. Soc. Exp. Biol. Med. **142**, 1087–1090 (1973).

Degre, M.: Influence of exogenous interferon on the peripheral white blood cell count in mice. Int. J. Cancer. **14**, 699–703 (1974).

Degre, M.: Effect of human leukocyte interferon on the permeability of the cytoplasma membrane of cultured cells. Acta Pathol. Microbiol. Scand. **B 86**, 303–308 (1978).

Degre, M.: Cholera toxin inhibits antiviral and growth inhibitory activities of human interferon. Proc. Soc. Exp. Biol. Med. **157**, 253–255 (1978).

Degre, M., Elgjo, K.: Methylcholanthrene-induced mouse skin carcinogenesis modified by treatment with polyinosinic: polycytidylic acid (poly I·C). Acta. Path. Microbiol. Scand. **A 79**, 687–688 (1971).

Degre, M., Elgjo, K.: Influence of synthetic polynucleotides and interferon on in vitro growth of cells derived from a mouse sarcoma. Acta. Pathol. Microbiol. Scand. **248**, 61–65 (1974).

Degre, M., Hovig, T.: Functional and ultrastructural studies on the effects of human interferon on cell membranes of in vitro cultured cells. Acta. Path. Microbiol. Scand. **B 84**, 347–349 (1976).

Degre, M., Midtvedt, T.: Effect of standard bacterial vaccine on influenza virus infection and interferon production in germfree mice. Acta. Pathol. Microbiol. Scand. **B 81**, 782–786 (1973).

Degre, M., Rollag, H.: Influence of interferon on the in vivo phagocytic activity of reticuloendothelial cells. J. Reticuloend. Soc. **25**, 489–494 (1979).

Degre, M., Rollag, H.: Pathogenesis of Sendai Virus infection in mice. On the possible role of interferon on the development of disease. Acta Pathol. Microbiol. Scand. **B 88**, 177–182 (1980).

Deinhardt, F., Henle, G.: Interference between polyoma and vesicular stomatitis viruses in tissue culture. J. Immunol. **84**, 608–614 (1960).

DeLaPena, N. C., Bal, E., Puricelli, L., Diaz, A., DeLustig, E. S.: Interferon in the replication of herpes simplex virus in normal and pathological nerve cells. IARC Sci. Publ. **24**, 1055–1066 (1978).

DeLaPena, N. C., Diaz, A., Damel, A., Bal, E., Puricelli, L., Ejden, J., DeLustig, E. S.: Combined therapy of human interferon (HI) and secretory immunoglobulin (S-IgA) in treatment of human herpetic keratitis. Biomedicine **28**, 104 (1978).

DeLey, M., Billiau, A., DeSomer, P.: A semi-continuous system for the production of human interferon in lymphoblastoid cell cultures. J. Gen. Virol. **40**, 455–460 (1978).

DeLey, M., Billiau, A., DeSomer, P.: Interferon-induced synthesis of a 63,000 dalton protein in mouse cells. Biochem. Biophys. Res. Comm. **89**, 701–705 (1979).

DeMaeyer, E.: Interferon twenty years later. Bull. Inst. Pasteur **76**, 303–323 (1978).

DeMaeyer, E.: L'interferon. Nouvelle Presse Medicale **8**, 2871–2872 (1979).

DeMaeyer, E., DeMaeyer-Guignard, J.: Interferons and the immune system, in: Immune System (Doria, G., Eshkol, A., eds.), Vol. 27, pp. 213–226 (1978).

DeMaeyer, E., DeMaeyer-Guignad, J.: Interferons. Comp. Virol. **15**, 205–284 (1979).

DeMaeyer, E., Enders, J. F.: Youth characteristics, interferon production and peocopue formation with different lines of Edmonston measles virus. Arch. ges. Virusforsch. **16**, 151–160 (1965).

DeMaeyer, E., Hoyer, M. C., DeMaeyer-Guignard, J., Bailey, D. W.: Effect of mouse genotype of interferon production. III. Expression of IF-1 by peritoneal macrophages *in vitro*. Immunogenetics **8**, 257–264 (1979).

DeMaeyer-Guignard, J.: La structure de la motiere de l'interferon. La Recherche **2**, 915–922 (1971).

DeMaeyer-Guignard, J., Cachard, A., DeMaeyer, E.: Electrophoretically pure mouse interferon has priming but no blocking activity in poly(I·C)-induced cells. Virology **102**, 222–227 (1980).

DeMaeyer-Guignard, J., Tovey, M. G., Gresser, I., DeMaeyer, E.: Purification of mouse interferon by sequential affinity chromatography on poly(U)- and antibody-agarose columns. Nature **271**, 622–625 (1978).

Demidov, W.: Experience with using interferon in the treatment of patients with chronic tonsillitis. Zh. Ushn. Nos. Gorl. Bolezn. **32**, 86–87 (1972).

Demin, A. A., Vorobieva, N. N., Galenok, V. A.: Leukocytic interferon in systemic lupus erythematosus. Sov. Med. **35**, 43–47 (1972).

DePoux, R.: Fixed rabies virus and interferon. C. R. Acad. Sci. (Paris) **260**, 354–356 (1965).

Derynck, R., Content, J., DeClercq, E., Volckaert, G., Tavernier, J., Devos, R., Fiers, W.: Isolation and structure of a human fibroblast interferon gene. Nature **285**, 542–546 (1980).

DeSomer, P., Declercq, E., Billiau, A., Schonne, E., Clausen, M.: Antiviral activity of polyacrylic and polymethacrylic acids. II. Mode of action in vivo. J. Virol. **2**, 886–890 (1968c).

Desrosiers, R. C., Lengyel, P.: Impairment of reovirus mRNA 'cap' methylation in interferon-treated mouse L929 cells. Biochim. Biophys. Acta **562**, 471–480 (1979).

Dianzani, F.: Viral interference and interferon. Ric. Clin. Lab. **5**, 196–213 (1975).

Dianzani, F., Forni, G., Negroponzi, A., Pugliese, A., Cavallo, G.: Decreased interferon response to poly I·C in rabbits immunized against the inducer. Proc. Soc. Exp. Biol. Med. **139**, 93–95 (1972).

Dianzani, F., Gullino, P., Baron, S.: Rapid activation of the interferon system in vivo. Infect. Immun. **20**, 55 (1970).

Dianzani, F., Monahan, T. M., Scupham, A., Zucca, M.: Enzymatic induction of interferon production by galactose oxidase treatment of human lymphoid cells. Infect. Immun. **26**, 879–882 (1979).

Dianzani, F., Salter, L., Fleischmann, W. R., Zucca, M.: Immune interferon activates cells more slowly than does virus-induced interferon. Proc. Soc. Exp. Biol. Med. **159**, 94–97 (1978).

Diaz, A., Dela Pena, N. C., Bal, E., Ejden, J., DeLustig, E. S.: Combined therapy with immunoglobulin A and human interferon in the rabbit herpetic keratitis. Medicina **38**, 40–44 (1978).

Diener, E.: The 2nd International lymphokine workshop. Cell Immunol. **48**, 427–432 (1979).

430 Appendix

DiStefano, A. D., Buzbar, A. U.: Viral-induced remission in chronic lymphocytic leukemia? Arch. Intern. Med. **139**, 946 (1979).

Djeu, J. Y., Heinbaugh, J. A., Holden, H. T., Herberman, R. B.: Augmentation of mouse natural killer cell activity by interferon and interferon inducers. J. Immunol. **122**, 175–181 (1979 a).

Djeu, J. Y., Heinbaugh, J. A., Holden, H. T., Herberman, R. B.: Role macrophages in the augmentation of mouse natural killer cell activity by poly I·C and interferon. J. Immunol. **11**, 182–185 (1979 b).

Djeu, J. Y., Huang, K. Y., Herberman, R. B.: Augmentation of natural killer activity and induction of interferon by tumor cells in vivo. J. Exp. Med. **151**, 781–789 (1980).

Dodge, W. H., Moscovici, C.: Effect of poly I·C on transformation by Rous Sarcoma virus. Proc. Soc. Exp. Biol. Med. **139**, 1407–1410.

Dolei, A., Colleta, G., Capobianchi, M. R., Rossi, G. B., Vecchio, G.: Interferon effects on Friend leukemia cells. I. Expression of virus and erythroid markers in untreated and DMSO-treated cells. J. Gen. Viurol. **46**, 227–236 (1980).

Dolen, J. G., Carter, W. A., Horoszewicz, J., Vladutiu, A. O., Leibowitz, A., Noland, J. P.: Fibroblast interferon treatment of a patient with chronic active hepatitis increased number of circulating T-lymphocytes and elimination of rosette-inhibitory factor. Amer. J. Med. **67**, 127–131 (1979).

Dolin, R., Baron, S.: Absence of detectable interferon in jejunal biopsies, jejunal aspirates, and sera in experimentally induced viral gastroenteritis in man. Proc. Soc. Exp. Biol. Med. **150**, 377–380 (1975).

Doller, E., Aucker, J., Weissbach, A.: Persistence of herpes simplex virus type 1 in rat neurotumor cells. J. Virol. **29**, 43–50 (1979).

Doshi, H. V., Shah, S. S.: Indian J. Med. Sci. **26**, 759–769 (1972).

Dossenbach, P., Koblet, H., Wyler, R.: Inductive and noninductive effect of interferon containing preparations. Pathol. Microbiol. (Basel) **41**, 141–142 (1974).

Dossenbach, P., Koblet, H., Wyler, R.: Actinomycin-resistant antiviral activity associated with preparations containing chicken interferon. Experientia **32**, 1514–1517 (1976).

Dougherty, J. P., Samanta, H., Farrell, P. J., Lengyel, P.: Interferon double-stranded RNA and RNA degradation. Isolation of homogeneous ppA (2'p5'A)n-1 synthetase from Ehrlich ascites tumor cells. J. Biol. Chem. **255**, 3813–3817 (1980).

Douglas, R. G., Waldman, R. H., Betts, R. F., Ganguly, R.: Lack of effect of an interferon inducer NN-dihexadecyl-m-xylylenediamine on rhinovirus challenge in humans. Antimicrob. Agents Chemother. **15**, 269–272 (1979).

Dowjat, K., Plachcinska, J., Zakazewski, K.: Interferon production and sensitivity in passaged human embryonic fibroblasts. Arch. Immunol. Ther. Exp. (Warsz.) **22**, 725–733 (1974).

Drasner, K., Epstein, C. J., Epstein, L. B.: The antiproliferative effects of interferon on murine embryonic cells. Proc. Soc. Exp. Biol. Med. **160**, 46–50 (1979).

Drobot'ko, L. N., Kuznetsov, V. P., Stulnevz, T. A., Murashova, N. S., Strelkova, L. N.: Treatment of acute herpetic stomatitis in children with interferon ointment. Stomatologia **53**, 53–55 (1974).

Droller, M. J., Borg, H., Perlman, P.: In vitro enhancement of natural and antibody-dependent lymphocytic mediated cytotoxicity against tumor target cells by interferon. Cell Immunol. **47**, 248–260 (1979).

Dubinin, N. P., Zasukhina, G. D., Matusevich, L. L.: Viruses and interferon as possible regulators of repair activity in cells of higher organisms. Dokl. Acad. Naŭk SSSR **212**, 481–482 (1973).

Dunnick, J. K., Galasso, G. J.: Clinical trials with exogenous interferon: summary of a meeting. J. Infect. Dis. **139**, 109–123 (1979).

Ebbesen, P., Olsson, L., Rudkobing, O., Haah, R. S., Kristensen, G.: Correlation in vivo cancer, net outer charge, in vitro migration, interferon activity, in vitro growth rates and chalone-like activity to transformation/reversion in cloned Moloney and Kirsten sarcoma virus-transformed mouse 3T3 cells. Cancer Res. **37**, 4285–4290 (1977).

Edelishtein, E., Shcherbakova, E. G., Rastunova, G. A., Furer, N. M.: Endogenous interferon in the bodies of children with aseptic meningitis caused by parotitis virus. Antibiotiki **19**, 171–175 (1974).

Editorial: A twist on the tale of interferon. Sci. Res. **38** (1967).

Editorial: Interferon therapy in chronic hepatitis B. Lancet **ii**, 1122 (1976).

Edy, V. G., Billiau, A., DeSomer, P.: Non-appearance of injected fibroblast interferon in circulation. Lancet **i**, 451–452 (1978).

Einhorn, S.: Interferon and spontaneous cytotoxicity in man. IV. Evidence for interferon as the factor in human interferon preparations causing enhancement of spontaneous cytotoxicity. J. Clin. Lab. Immunol. **3**, 35–38 (1980).

Einhorn, S., Blomgren, H., Cantell, K., Strander, H.: Effect of prolonged *in vivo* administration of leukocyte interferon on the mitogen responsiveness of human lymphocytes. Acta Med. Scand. **206**, 345–350 (1979).

Einhorn, S., Blomgren, H., Strander, H.: Interferon and spontaneous cytotoxicity in man. I. Enhancement of spontaneous cytotoxicity of peripheral lymphocytes by human leukocyte interferon. Int. J. Cancer **22**, 405–412 (1978a).

Einhorn, S., Blomgren, H., Strander, H.: Interferon and spontaneous cytotoxicity in man. II. Acta Med. Scand. **204**, 477–484 (1978b).

Einhorn, S., Blomgren, H., Strander, H.: Interferon and spontaneous cytotoxicity in man. III. Effect of interferon on lymphocytes and target cells *in vitro*. Cancer Letters **7**, 1–7 (1979).

Eksteen, P. A., Huismans, H.: Interferon induction by bluetongue virus and bluetongue virus RNA. Onderstepoort. J. Vet. Res. **39**, 125 (1972).

Elfenbein, D. S., Murphy, P. A., Chesney, P. J., Seto, D.S.Y., Carner, D. H.: Assessment of the interferon-like activity in preparations of leukocyte pyrogen. J. Gen. Virol. **42**, 185–188 (1979).

Emelianov, B. A., Novokhatsky, A. S.: Reproduction and the interferon-inducing capacity of togaviruses. Vopr. Virusol. **2**, 216 (1977). (In Russian.)

Emelianov, B. A., Uryvaev, L. V.: The mechanism of interferon induction and its effect in tissue culture Arbovirus infections. Vopr. Virusol. **16**, 333–339 (1971). (In Russian.)

Emeny, J. M., Morgan, M. J.: Regulation of the interferon system: evidence that vero cells have a genetic defect in interferon production. J. Gen. Virol. **43**, 247–252 (1979a).

Emeny, J. M., Morgan, M. J.: Susceptibility of various cells treated with interferon to the toxic effect of poly I·poly C treatment. J. Gen. Virol. **43**, 253–255 (1979b).

Emödi, G., Just, M., Grob, P.: Circulating interferon after transfer-factor therapy. Lancet **ii**, 1382 (1973).

Eppstein, D. A., Peterson, T. C., Samuel, C.: Mechanism of interferon action: synthesis and activity of the interferon mediated lowmolecular-weight oligonucleotide from murine and human cells. Virology **98**, 9–13 (1979).

Eppstein, D. A., Samuel, C. E.: Mechanism of interferon action. Properties of an interferon-mediated ribonucleolytic activity from mouse L929 cells. Virology **89**, 240–246 (1978).

Eppstein, D. A., Torrence, P. F., Friedman, R. M.: Double-stranded RNA inhibits a phosphoprotein phosphatase present in interferon treated cells. Proc. Nat. Acad. Sci. USA **77**, 107–111 (1980).

Epstein, L. B.: The comparative biology of immune and classical interferons, in: Biology of the Lymphokines (Cohen, S., Pick, E., Oppenheim, J. J., eds.), pp. 443–514. New York: Academic Press (1979).

Epstein, L. B., Epstein, C. J.: T-lymphocyte function and sensitivity to interferon in trisomy 21. Cellular Immunol. **51**, 303–318 (1980).

Epstein, L. B., Lee, S. H. S., Epstein, C. J.: Enhanced sensitivity of trisomy 21 monocytes to the maturation inhibiting effect of interferon. Cellular Immunol. **50**, 191–199 (1980).

Erickson, J. S., Dalton, B. J., Paucker, K.: Biological properties of human interferon fractions obtained by blue sepharose chromatography. Arch. Virol. **63**, 253–262 (1980).

Erickson, J. S., Paucker, K.: Purification of acid ethanol-extracted human lymphoid interferons by blue Sepharose chromatography. Anal. Biochem. **98**, 214–220 (1979).

Erickson, J. S., Paucker, K.: Molecular species of interferon induced in mouse L cells by Newcastle disease virus and polyrI·polyrC. J. Gen. Virol. **43**, 521–530 (1979a).

Ermolieva, Z. V., Blinova, M. I., Furer, N. M., Ritova, V. V., Kucherenko, L. P.: Children with leukocyte interferon and a stimulator interferon formation (UF virus). Vopr. Virusol. **16**, 442–446 (1972). (In Russian.)

Ershov, F. I.: Mechanism of interferon action. USP Sovrem Biol. **77**, 369–381 (1974).

Ershov, F. I., Novokhatskyi, A. S., Tazulakhova, E. B.: Comparative analysis of interferon inductor action *in vitro* and *in vivo*. Antibiotiki **23**, 557 (1974).

Ershov, F. I., Sokolova, T. M., Tazulakhova, E. B., Kadyrova, A. A., Kisling, U.: Comparative analysis of interferon and antiviral protein mRNAs. Acta Virol. **23**, 32–39 (1979).

Ershov, F. I., Tazulakhova, E. B., Sokolova, T. M., Kadrova, A. A., Novokhatsky, A. S.: Isolation of interferon mRNA and its integration into the genome of a heterologous host. Probl. Virol. **6**, 707 (1976).

Eyckmans, L., Billiau, A., DeSomer, P.: Antibacterial effect of an interferon inducing polycarboxylate. Mechanism of action. Biomedicine **19**, 187–192 (1973).

Fadeeva, L. L., Balezina, T. I., Korneeva, L. E., Korabelnikova, N. I., Tumanova, V. A.: Interferon induction by plant viruses. Antibiotiki **17**, 513–517 (1972).

Fahlbusch, T. B., Zschiesche, W., Schumann, I., Tonew, E.: Induction of lymphokines. Arch. Immunol. Therap. Exper. **25**, 701–706 (1977).

Falcoff, E.: Connaissances actuelles sur les interferons. Pathologie-Biologie **14**, 754–761 (1966).

Falcoff, E., Falcoff, R., Cherby, J., Florent, J., Lunel, J., Ninet, L., Deratuld, Y., Tissier, R., Villemin, B., Werner, G. M.: Doublestranded ribonucleic acid from Mengo virus: production, characterization, and interferon-inducing and antiviral activities in comparison with polyriboinosinic-polyribocytidylic acid. Antimicrob. Agents Chemotherap. **3**, 590–595 (1973).

Falcoff, R.: Translation inhibition factor induced by interferon. In Vitro Monograph **3**, 65 (1974).

Falcoff, R., Falcoff, E., Sanceau, J., Lewis, J. A.: Influence of preincubation on the development of inhibition of protein synthesis in extracts from interferon-treated mouse L-cells. Action on tRNA. Virology **86**, 507–511 (1978).

Falcoff, R., Lebleu, B., Sanceau, J., Falcoff, E., Dirheimer, G., Ebel, J. P.: Study on the interferon-induced translation inhibition of synthetic polynucleotides, in: In Vitro Transcription and Translation of Viral Genomes (Haenvi, A–L., Beaud, G., eds.), p. 363. INSERM. (1975).

Falcoff, R., Sanceau, J.: Mengovirus-induced inhibition of cell protein synthesis and subsequent recovery of cellular activity in interferon-pretreated cells. Virology **98**, 433–438 (1979).

Fan, H., MacIsaac, P.: Virus-specific RNA synthesis in interferon-treated mouse cells productively infected with moloney murine leukemia virus. J. Virol. **27**, 449–452 (1970).

Fanta, D., Soltiziszotz, J.: Interferon and interferon stimulation. Hautarzt **25**, 313–318 (1974).

Fantes, K. H.: Further purification of chick interferon. Nature **207**, 1298–1299 (1965).

Farrar, J. J., Simon, P. L., Farrar, W. L., Koopman, W. J., Follerbonar, J.: Role of mitogenic factor, lymphocyte activating factor and immune interferon in the induction of humoral and cell-mediated immunity. Ann. N.Y. Acad. Sci. **332**, 303–315 (1979).

Farrell, P. J., Broeze, R. J., Lengyel, P.: Accumulation of an mRNA and protein in interferon-treated Ehrlich ascites tumor cells. Nature **279**, 523–525 (1979).

Farrell, P. J., Sen, G. C., Dubois, M. F., Ratner, L., Slattery, E., Lengyel, P.: Interferon action: two distinct pathways for inhibition of protein synthesis by double-stranded RNA. Proc. Nat. Acad. Sci. U.S.A. **75**, 5893–5897 (1978).

Fauconnier, B.: Large-scale production of human interferon from human spleens. J. Interferon Res. **1**, 15–18 (1980).

Fauconnier, B., Ruffault, A.: Human spleen: a new and potent source of human interferon. C. R. Acad Sci. D **290**, 421–422 (1980).

Fayet, M. T., Branche, R., Falcoff, E., Cherby, J., DeRatuld, Y., Werner, G. H.: Study of two double-stranded ribonucleic acids of viral origin: interferon inducing and antiviral activities. Prog. Immunobiol. Standard. **5**, 267 (1972).

Fedorova, Y. B., Neklyudova, L. I.: Distribution of exogenous interferon in experimental animals after intratracheal administration. Vopr. Virusol. **4**, 416–418 (1975). (In Russian.)

Feinerman, B.: Tumor immunology and interferon. Southern Med. J. **71**, 1409–1411 (1978).

Feldmane, G., Loza, V., Duks, A., Yesyacova, I., Vinkele, R., Buicke, A., Meldrajs, J., Erele,

I.: Nucleic acid as interferon inducer. Its antiviral and antitumor activity. Arch. Immunol. Therap. Exper. **25**, 693–700 (1977).

Fellous, M., Kamoun, M., Gresser, I., Bono, R.: Enhanced expression of HLA antigens and beta-2-microglobulin on interferon treated human lymphoid cells. Europ. J. Immunol. **9**, 446–449 (1979).

Fenie, P., Postic, B.: Protection of rabbits against experimental rabies by poly I·poly C. Nature **226**, 171–172 (1970).

Fennestad, K. L., Haahr, S., Bruun, L.: Pleural effusion disease in rabbits. Interferon in body fluids and tissues after experimental infection. Acta. Pathol. Microbiol. Scand. **B 87**, 311–316 (1979).

Ferreira, P. C. P., Peixoto, M. L. P., Silva, M. A. V., Golgher, R. R.: Assay of human interferon in Vero cells by several methods. J. Clin. Microbiol. **9**, 471–475 (1979).

Field, A. K., Tytell, A. A., Lampson, G. P., Hilleman, M. R.: Antigenicity of double-stranded ribonucleic acid including poly I·C. Proc. Soc. Exp. Biol. Med. **139**, 1113–1116 (1972).

Filipic, S., Schauer, P., Likar, M.: Similarities of cellular receptors for interferon and cortisol. Arch. Immunol. Therap. Exper. **25**, 613–616 (1977).

Finkelstein, M. S.: Development of tissue viral resistance in chickens following administration of interferon inducers. J. Immunol. **108**, 1506–1516 (1972).

Finlay, G. J., Booth, R. J., Marbrook, J.: Interferon-induced antibody suppression-selective effect on high density, late responding precursor cells. Europ. J. Immunol. **7**, 123–127 (1977).

Finter, N. B.: Interferons: therapeutic prospects. Mod. Trends Med. Virol. **2**, 262–283 (1970).

Finter, N. B., Brigden, D.: Large scale production of human interferons and their possible uses in medicine. Trends Biochem. Sci. **3**, 76 (1977).

Fitzpatrick, F. A., Stringfellow, D. A.: Prostaglandin D₂ formation by malignant melanoma cells correlates inversely with cellular metastatic potential. Proc. Nat. Acad. Sci. U.S.A. **76**, 1765–1769 (1979a).

Fitzpatrick, F. A., Stringfellow, D. A.: Viruses stimulate prostaglandin formation through interferon induction. Personal Communication (1979b).

Fitzpatrick, F. A., Stringfellow, D. A.: Virus and interferon effects on cellular prostaglandin biosynthesis. J. Immunol. **125**, 431–435 (1980).

Fiume, L., Mattioli, A., Busi, C., Sinibadldi, P., Campadelli-Fiume, G.: An endogenous inhibitor of fibroblast proliferation hinders SV40 replication. Naturwissen. **66**, 265–266 (1979).

Fleischman, W. R., Georgiades, J. A., Osborne, L. C., Dianzani, F., Johnson, H. M.: Induction of an inhibitor of interferon action in a mouse lymphokine preparation. Infect. Immun. **26**, 949–951 (1979).

Fleischmann, W. R., Georgiades, J. A., Osborne, L. C., Johnson, H. M.: Potentiation of interferon activity by mixed preparations of fibroblast and immune interferon. Infect. Immun. **26**, 248–252 (1979).

Fleischmann, W. R., Simon, E. H.: Effect of interferon on virus production from isolated single cells. J. Gen. Virol. **20**, 127–137 (1973).

Flikke, M., Kjeldsberg, E., Lahelle, O.: Interference with cell viability and poliovirus multiplication by polyinosinic-polycytidylic acid. J. Gen. Virol. **9**, 111–117 (1970).

Fomina, A. N., Nosik, N. N., Bukata, L. A., Dauydova, A. A., Barinski, N. F., Doscochil, Y., Ershov, F. I.: Effect of natural interferon inductor (RFf2) on formation of vaccinal immunity to normal encephalitis. Antibiotiki **24**, 67–70 (1979).

Fomina, A. N., Shubladze, A. K., Etkind, R. S., Bektemirov, T. A.: Interferon production *in vitro* by leukocytes in response to arbovirus infection. Vopr. Virusol. **3**, 302 (1975). (In Russian.)

Forestier, F., Geniteau, M., Quero, A. M., Cotte, J., German, A.: Role of macrophages in interferon production in mice. Ann. Immunol. Inst. Pasteur **C130**, 581–586 (1979).

Forman, M. S., Adams, E. W., Vanderpool, E. A., Turner, W.: Induction of acid-stable canine interferon in vivo and in vitro. Amer. J. Vet. Res. **40**, 1440–1442 (1979).

Fournier, F., Chany, C., Rousset, S.: Protentialisation de l'action antivirale de l'interferon par l'actinomycine D. C. R. Acad. Sci. (Paris) **271**, 549–551 (1970).

Fowler, A. K., Reed, C. D., Giron, D. J.: Identification of an interferon in murine placentas. Nature **286**, 266–267 (1980).

Freed, B. M., Patrovic, L., Nadon, N., Hauser, L., Graziade, W. D.: Role of cytotoxicity and antiviral state in the regulation of interferon synthesis. Microbiologica **2**, 75–88 (1979).

Frey, T. K., Jones, E. V., Cardamone, J. J., Youngner, J. S.: Induction of interferon in L cells by defective-interfering particles of vesicular stomatitis virus: lack of correlation with content of [+] snapback RNA. Virology **99**, 95–102 (1979).

Friedman, R. M.: Interferon research in the red queen's kingdom. Arch. Pathol. **98**, 73–75 (1974).

Friedman, R. M.: Guest Editorial: Interferon and Cancer. J. Natl. Cancer Inst. **60**, 1191 (1978).

Friedman, R. M.: Interferon action and the cell surface. Pharm. Therapeut. **2**, 425 (1978).

Friedman, R. M.: Induction and production of interferon. Methods in Enzymology **58**, 292–295 (1979).

Friedman, R. M., Barth, R. F., Stern, R.: Anomalous effects of heterologous normal serum on interferon production in mice. Nature New Biol. **230**, 17–18 (1971).

Friedman, R. M., Levy, M. B., Carter, W. B.: Replication of Semliki forest virus: three forms of viral RNA produced during infection. Proc. Natl. Acad. Sci. **56**, 440–446 (1966).

Friedman, R. M., and Rabson, A. S., Kirkham, W. R.: Variation in interferon production by polyoma virus strains of differing oncogenicity. Proc. Soc. Exp. Biol. Med. **112**, 347–349 (1963).

Friedman, R. M., Sonnabend, J. A., McDevitt, M.: Interferon inhibition of cytoplasmic DNA accumulation in vaccinia virus infection. A radioautographic study. Proc. Soc. Exp. Biol. Med. **119**, 551–553 (1965).

Friedman, W. H., Gresser, I., Bandu, M. T., Aguet, M., Neauport-Sautes, C.: Interferon enhances the expression of Fcj receptors. J. Immunol. **124**, 2436–2440 (1980).

Fruitstone, M. J., Shands, J. W., jr., Gifford, G. E.: Biological effects of poly rI·rC and endotoxin in mice infected with mycobacterium BCG: interferon induction and toxicity. Proc. Soc. Exp. Biol. Med. **139**, 1104–1108 (1972).

Fuchsberger, N., Borecky, L.: Decrease of sensitivity to cellgrowth-inhibitory effect of interferon in human embryo cells after infection with SV40. Acta Virol. **23**, 344–347 (1979 a).

Fuchsberger, N., Borecky, L.: Production of human leukocyte interferon for clinical use under immunoelectrophoretic control. Acta Biol. Med. Germ. **38**, 794–800 (1979 b).

Fuchsberger, N., Borecky, L., Hajnicka, V.: Effect of prolonged interferon treatment on L mouse fibroblast cells. Acta Virol. **18**, 85–87 (1974).

Fuchsberger, N., Borecky, L., Hajnicka, V., Styk, B.: Some biological activities of rabbit anti-interferon serum. Arch. Immuhol. Therap. Exper. **25**, 715–718 (1977).

Fujisawa, J., Iwakura, Y., Kawade, Y.: Nonglycosylated mouse L cell interferon produced by the action of tunicamycin. J. Biol. Chem. **253**, 8677–8679 (1978).

Fujita, T., Saito, S., Kohno, S.: Priming increases the amount of interferon mRNA in poly rI·poly rC treated L cells. J. Gen. Virol. **45**, 301–308 (1979).

Fuller, F. J., Marcus, P. I.: Interferon induction by viruses. IV. Sindbis virus: early passage defective-interfering particles induce interferon. J. Gen. Virol. **48**, 63–74 (1980).

Fulton, R. W., Root, S. K.: Antiviral activity in interferon-treated bovine tracheal organ cultures. Infect. Immun. **21**, 672–675 (1978).

Fung, K. P., Ng, M. H.: Heterocomplexes of human interferon and immunoglobulins: formation and properties. Arch. Virol. **57**, 133–137 (1978).

Furusawa, E., Ramanathan, S., Furusawa, S., Cutting, W.: Antiviral activity of tobacco leaf on encephalomyocarditis (EMC) virus infection. Proc. Soc. Exp. Biol. Med. **138**, 790–795 (1971).

Furusawa, E., Ramanathan, S., Furusawa, S., Woo, Y. K., Cutting, W.: Antiviral activity of higher plants and propiomin on lymphocytic choriomeningitis infection. Proc. Soc. Exp. Biol. Med. **125**, 234–239 (1967).

Furusawa, E., Ramanathan, S., Suzuki, N., Tani, S., Furusawa, S.: Antiviral activity of tobacco smoke condensate on encephalomyocarditis infection in mice. Antimicrob. Agents Chemotherap. **3**, 484 (1973).

Fuse, A., Kuwata, T.: Inhibition of DNA synthesis and alteration of cyclic adenosine 3′5′-monophosphate levels in RSa cells by human leukocyte interferon. J. Natl. Cancer Inst. **60**, 1227–1230 (1978).

Fuse, A., Kuwata, T.: Effect of cholera toxin on the antiviral and anticellular activities of human leukocyte interferon. Infect. Immun. **26**, 235–238 (1979).

Gailonskaia, I. N., Kopelev, M. F., Busuek, G. P., Kuznetsov, V. P., Lozinskaia, T. M.: The clinical course of influenza in patients treated with interferon and symptomatic agents. Klin. Med. (Mosk.) 51, 117–120 (1973).

Gaines, K. C., Sorrell, M. F.: Host resistance in liver disease its evaluation and therapeutic modification. Med. Clin. North Amer. 63, 495–505 (1979).

Gajdosova, E., Doskocil, J., Mayer, V.: Dependence of antiviral activity on molecular weight in an interferon stimulator of the natural double-stranded RNA type. Acta Virol. 17, 196 (1973).

Gajdosova, E., Mayer, V., Doskocil, J.: Viral infection and resistance in immunosuppressed host. IV. Abolition of potentiated togovirus A infection by a resistance inducer of the dsRNA type. Failure of an exogenous interferon. Acta Virol. 17, 327–336 (1973).

Galabov, A. S.: Antiviral effect of simultaneously applied viral, bacterial and synthetic inducers of interferon upon experimental infection in mice. C. R. Acad. Sci. Bulgare 27, 287 (1974).

Galabov, A. S., Eskenazy, M., Konstantinov, G., Mastikova, M.: Effect of solubilization of Salmonella-minnesota glycolipid on its interferon-inducing activity. Experientia 35, 598–599 (1979).

Galabov, A. S., Petrunova, S. S., Galabov, S. M.: Interferon-inducing capacity of detoxicated endotoxin of Serratia marcescens in mouse peritoneal cells, in: Interferon and Interferon Inducers (Fouder, I., Talas, M., eds.), pp. 32–45. Budapest (1976).

Galabov, A. S., Savov, Z. A.: Influence of incubation temperature on interferon mechanism in cells of Testuda graeca kidney. Zentralbl. Bakteriol. 225, 1–6 (1973).

Gardner, L. J., Vilček, J.: Initial interaction of human fibroblast and leukocyte interferons with FS-4 fibroblasts. J. Gen. Virol. 44, 161–168 (1979).

Garry, R. F., Waite, M. R. F.: Na$^+$ and K$^+$ concentrations and the regulations of the interferon system in chick cells. Virology 96, 121–128 (1979).

Gasner, D.: Interferon and beyond. OMNI 1, 54 (1979).

Gatmaitan, B. G., Legaspi, B. C., Levy, H. B., Lerner, A. M.: Modified poly I·poly C complex: induction of serum interferon, fever, and hypotension in rabbits. Antimicrob. Agents Chemother. 17, 49–54 (1979).

Gauntt, C. J., Lockart, R. Z.: Inhibition of Mengo virus by interferon. J. Bacteriol. 91, 176–182 (1966).

Gazit, A., Eylan, E.: Stimulated production of interferon by a low molecular weight factor from chicken egg fluids. Israel J. Med. Sci. 14, 1063–1068 (1978).

Geber, W. F., Lefkowitz, S. S., Hung, C. Y.: Effect of ascorbic acid, sodium salicylate, and caffeine on the serum interferon level in response to viral infection. Pharmacol. 13, 228 (1975a).

Gelb, J., Eidson, C. S., Fletcher, O. J., Kleven, S. H.: Studies on interferon induction by infectious bursal disease virus (IBDV). II. Interferon production in white leghorn chickens infected with attenuated or pathogenic isolates of IBDV. Avian Dis. 23, 634–645 (1979).

Gelb, J., Eidson, C. S., Kleven, S. H.: Studies on interferon induction by infectious bursal disease virus (IBDV). I. Interferon production in chicken embryo cell cultures infected with IBDV. Avian Dis. 23, 485–492 (1979a).

Gelb, J., Eidson, C. S., Kleven, S. H.: Interferon production in embryonated chicken eggs following inoculation with infectious bursal disease virus. Avian Dis. 23, 434–439 (1979b).

Georgiades, J. A., Langford, M. L., Stanton, G. J., Johnson, H. M.: Purification and potentiation of human immune interferon activity. IRCS Med. SCI.-Biochem. 7, 559 (1979).

Georgiades, J. A., Osborne, L. C., Moulton, R. G., Johnson, H. M.: Separation of immune interferon and MIF. Proc. Soc. Exp. Biol. Med. 161, 167–169 (1979).

Gericke, D., Kornhuber, B. C., Chandra, P.: Immunosupressive activity of a heat-stable factor associated with interferon. Naturwissenschaften 60, 482–483 (1973).

Gevaudan, P., Charrel, J., Pieroni, G., Gevaudan, M. J.: Nouveau variant froid de coxsackievirus B5. III. Pouvoir protecteur et aptitude à induire de l'interferon. C. R. Soc. Biol. 164, 1805 (1970).

Gevaudan, P., Charrel, J., Pieroni, G., Gevaudan, M. J.: New cold coxsackie virus B5 variant. II. Evolution of interferon quantities in young mice as a function of time. C. R. Soc. Biol. (Paris) 165, 939–943 (1971).

Ghaffar, A., Cullen, R. T.: In vitro antitumor effect of lymphoid cells from Corynebacterium *parvum*-treated mice: effect of route of *C. parvum* administration. J. Natl. Cancer Inst. **58**, 777 (1977).

Giard, D. J., Loeb, D. H., Thilly, W. G., Wang, D. I. C., Levine, D. W.: Human interferon production with diploid fibroblast cells grown on microcarriers. Biotech. Bioeng. **21**, 433–442 (1979).

Gidlund, M., Ojo, E. A., Orn, A., Wigzell, H., Murgita, R. A.: Severe suppression of the B-cell system has no impact on the maturation of natural killer cells in mice. Scand. J. Immunol. **9**, 167–173 (1979).

Gidlund, M., Orn, A., Wigzell, H., Senik, A., Gresser, I.: Enhanced NK cell activity in mice injected with interferon and interferon inducers. Nature **273**, 759–760 (1978).

Gifford, G. E.: Inhibitory effect of mononucleotide on virus plaque formation. Proc. Soc. Exp. Biol. Med. **119**, 9–12 (1965).

Gifford, G. E.: Interferon and the immune system, in: Clin. Concepts Immunol. (Waldmna, R., ed.), p. 218. Baltimore: Williams and Wilkins (1979).

Gifford, G. E., Ghosh, S. N.: Effect of interferon on vaccinia virus yield and plaque formation. Proc. Soc. Exp. Biol. Med. **120**, 308–310 (1965).

Gifford, G. E., Koch, A. L.: Interferon dose response curve and its possible significance. J. Theoret. Biol. **22**, 271–283 (1969).

Giron, D. J., Liu, R. Y., Hemphill, F. E., Pindak, F. F., Schmidt, J. P.: Role of interferon in the antiviral state elicited by selected interferon inducers. Proc. Soc. Exp. Biol. Med. **163**, 146–148 (1980).

Giron, D. J., Schmidt, J. P., Pindak, F. F.: Induction of viral resistance by poly I·C in cells which apparently produce no interferon. Proc. Soc. Exp. Biol. Med. **141**, 47–50 (1972 a).

Glasgow, L. A.: Interferon: A review. J. Pediat. **67**, 104–121 (1965 b).

Glasgow, L. A., Crane, J. L., jr., Kern, E. R.: Antitumor activity of interferon against murine osteogenic sarcoma cells *in vitro*. J. Natl. Cancer Inst. **60**, 659–663 (1978).

Glasgow, L. A., Crane, J. L., jr., Kern, E. R., Youngner, J. S.: Antitumor activity of interferon against murine osteogenic sarcoma *in vitro* and *in vivo*. Cancer Treat. Res. **62**, 1881–1885 (1978).

Glasgow, L. A., Fischbach, J., Bryant, S. M., Kern, E. R.: Immunomodulation of host resistance to experimental viral infections in mice. Effects of *Corynbacterium acnes*, *C. parvum* and *bacille-calmette-guerin*. J. Infect. Dis. **135**, 763–770 (1977).

Glasky, A. J., Simon, L., Holper, J. C.: Interferon: selectivity and specificity of action in cell-free systems. Science **144**, 1581–1583 (1964).

Glaz, E. T.: Effect of low molecular weight interferon inducers on *Trypanasoma equiperdum* infection of mice. Ann. Trop. Med. Parasitol. **73**, 83–84 (1979).

Gmyria, A. I., Bobrova, I. I., Antonova, A. I.: Use of phonophoresis combined with drug-ultrasonic therapy of various eye diseases. Opthalmol. Zh. **34**, 77–79 (1979).

Gobert, J. G., German, A., Poindron, P., Savel, J.: Interferon and protection of mice against experimental infestation transmitted by the blood forms of plasmadium berghei injected in massive doses. I. methods of protection with a viral inducer of interferon. Ann. Pharm. Fr. **29**, 521–528 (1972).

Gobert, J. G., Poindron, P., German, A., Savel, J.: Studies on the mechanism of action of viral inducer of interferon in the protection of mice against massive infestation by endoerythrocytic forms of plasmodium berghei. C. R. Acad. Sci. (Paris) **274**, 1226–1229 (1972).

Goldblatt, D., McManus, N. H., Epstein, L. B.: A micromethod for preparation of human macrophage cultures for the study of macrophage interactions in immune biosynthesis of interferon and blastogenesis. Immunopharmacol. **1**, 13–20 (1978).

Goldfine, I. D., Smith, G. J., Wong, K. Y., Jones, A. L.: Cellular uptake and nuclear binding of insulin in human cultured lymphocytes: evidence for potential intracellular sites of insulin action. Proc. Natl. Acad. Sci. U.S.A. **74**, 1368–1372 (1977).

Goldstein, L. D., Georgiades, J. A., Langford, M. P., Stanton, G. J., Johnson, H. M.: Human immune interferon-isoelectrofocusing analysis. IRCS Med. Sci. **7**, 560 (1979).

Golosova, T. V., Kuznetsov, V. P., Murasheva, N. S., Ivanova, N. P., Bolkhovitinova, L. A.: Interferon ointment in the complex treatment of burns. Vestn. Kir. **133**, 61–64 (1974).

Golubska, B., Szalaty, M.: Influence of immunosuppressive drugs on replication of Col MM virus and production of interferon *in vivo.* Arch. Immunol. Ther. Exp. (Warsz.) 22, 445–456 (1974).

Goore, M. Y., Dickson, J. H., Lipkin, S.: Human leukocyte interferon produced by use of an antibody-free human serum fraction. Appl. Microbiol. 25, 325–326 (1973).

Goorha, R. M., Gifford, G. E.: Comparison of interferon induction by active and inactive Semliki forest virus. J. Gen. Virol. 10, 117–124 (1971).

Gopalakrishnian, K.: Interferon. Indian J. Cancer 12, 30–38 (1975).

Gordon, G. D., Uhlendorf, C. P., Baer, P. N., Baron, S.: Studies on herpes simplex virus and interferon in human gingival cell cultures. J. Periodontol. 46, 86–89 (1975).

Gordon, I., Stevenson, D.: Kinetics of decay in the expression of interferon-dependent messenger RNAs responsible for resistance to virus. Proc. Nat. Acad. Sci. 77, 452–456 (1980).

Gorshunova, L. B., Bektemirov, T. A., Koshtoian, S. E.: Interferon production and non-specific protective reactions in the CNS of animals vaccinated with live measles vaccine. Vopr. Virusol. 16, 735–739 (1971). (In Russian.)

Gorshunova, L. B., Khasenova, Z. K.: On persistence of vaccinia virus and interferon production in organs of vaccinated white mice. Vopr. Virusol. 5, 523–525 (1979). (In Russian.)

Gough, R. E., Allan, W. H., Knight, D. J., Leiper, J. W. G.: The potentiating effect of an interferon inducer (BRL-5907) on oil based inactivated Newcastle disease virus. Res. Vet. Sci. 17, 280–284 (1974).

Gough, R. E., Allan, W. H., Knight, D. J., Leiper, J. W. G.: Further studies on the adjuvant effect of an interferon inducer (BRL-5907) on Newcastle disease and avian influenza inactivated vaccines. Res. Vet. Sci. 19, 185–188 (1975).

Grandien, M.: Evaluation of tests for rabies antibody and analysis of serum responses after administration of 3 different types of rabies vaccines. J. Clin. Microb. 5, 263–268 (1977).

Granov, L. G., Demodov, V. V., Kuznetson, V. P.: Treatment of persistently unhealing wounds and trophic ulcers with interferon ointment. Vestn. Khir. 108, 69–71 (1972).

Graves, H. E., Meager, A.: Interferon production by human-mouse hybrid cells: dominant mouse control of superinduction and priming. J. Gen. Virol. 47, 489–496 (1980).

Green, J. A., Stanton, G. J., Goode, J., Baron, S.: Vesicular stomatitis virus plaque production in monolayer cultures with liquid overlay medium: description and adaptation to a one-day, human interferon plaque reduction assay. J. Clin. Microb. 4, 479–481 (1976).

Greenberg, S. B., Harmon, M. W., Johnson, P. E., Cough, R. B.: Antiviral activity of intranasally applied human leukocyte interferon. Antimicrob. Agents Chemother. 14, 596–604 (1978).

Greene, J. J., Alderfer, J. L., Tazawa, I., Tazawa, S., Tso, P. O. P., O'Malley, J. A., Carter, W.: Interferon induction and its dependence on the primary and secondary structure of poly rI·poly rC. Biochem. 17, 4214–4220 (1978).

Greene, J. J., Dieffenbauch, C. W., Yang, L. C., T'so, P. O. P.: species-specific posttranscriptional regulation of interferon synthesis. Biochemistry 19, 2485–2490 (1980).

Gresser, I., Bourali-Maury, C.: Antitumor effect of interferon in lymphocyte- and macrophage-depressed mice. Proc. Soc. Exp. Biol. Med. 144, 896–900 (1973).

Gresser, I., DeMaeyer-Guignard, J., Tovey, M. G., DeMaeyer, E.: Electrophoretically pure mouse interferon exerts multiple biologic effects. Proc. Nat. Acad. Sci. U.S.A. 76, 5308–5312 (1979).

Gresser, I., Grogan, E. A.: Inhibition of arboviruses by a constituent of a staphylococcus. Proc. Soc. Exp. Biol. Med. 119, 1176–1181 (1965).

Gresser, I., Maury, C., Kress, C., Blangy, D., Maunoury, M.-T.: Role of interferon in the pathogenesis of virus diseases in mice as demonstrated by the use of anti-interferon serum. VI. Polyoma virus infection. Int. J. Cancer. 24, 178–183 (1979).

Gresser, I., Morel, L., Chatelet, F., Maury, C., Tovey, M., Bandu, M. T., Buywid, J., Delauchs, M.: Delay in growth and the development of nephritis in rats treated with interferon preparations in neonatal period. Amer. J. Pathol. 95, 329–346 (1979).

Gresser, I., Morel-Maroger, L., Verroust, P., Riviere, Y., Guillon, J. C.: Role of interferon in pathogenesis of virus diseases in mice as demonstrated by use of anti-interferon serum. VI. Anti-interferon globulin inhibits development of glomerulonephritis in mice infected at birth with lymphocytic choriomeningitis virus. Proc. Natl. Acad. Sci. U.S.A. 75, 3413–3417 (1978).

Gresser, I., Tovey, M. G.: Antitumor effects of interferon. Biochim. Biophys. Acta 516, 231–250 (1978).

Gresser, I., Tovey, M. G., Maury, C., Bandu, M. T.: Role of interferon in the pathogenesis of herpes simplex virus. IARC Sci. Publ. 24, 1049–1054 (1978).

Grill, L. K., Sun, J. D., Kandel, J.: Effects of dsRNA on protein synthesis in an in vitro wheat germ embryo system. Biochem. Biophys. Res. Comm. 73, 149–156 (1976).

Grob, P. M., Chadha, K. C.: Separation of human leukocyte interferon components by concanavalin A-agarose affinity chromatography and their characterization. Biochem. 18, 5782–5786 (1979).

Groelke, J. W., Camyre, K. P., Mayer, G. D.: Enhancement of interferon production in vitro: a property of tilorone-poly rI·rc/DEAE-dextran. Proc. Soc. Exp. Biol. Med. 148, 1044–1048 (1975).

Grollman, E. F., Lee, G., Ramos, S., Lazo, P. S., Kaback, H. R., Friedman, R. M., Kohn, L. D.: Relationships of the structure and function of the interferon receptors and establishment of the antiviral state. Cancer Res. 38, 4172–4185 (1978).

Gross, H. J., Stephens, E., Jungwirth, C., Winkler, I., Heller, G., Bermauer, H. P., Vienhauser, G., Bodo, G., Boehringer, E., Ostertag, W., Dube, S. K.: In vitro transcription and translation of viral genomes. INSERM, p. 373 (1975).

Grossberg, S. E.: Interferon as a metabolic agent of host resistance. Transplant. Bull. 30, 100–101 (1962).

Grossberg, S. E., Hook, E. W., Wagner, R. R.: Hemorrhagic encephalopathy in chicken embryos infected with influenza virus. III. Viral interference at a distant site induced by prior allantoic infection. J. Immunol. 88, 1–8 (1962).

Grossberg, S. E., Jameson, P., Sedmak, J. J.: Interferon bioassay methods and the development of standard procedures: a critique and analysis of current observations. In Vitro Monographs 3, 26–34 (1974).

Guigues, M., Leng, M.: Antibodies to poly I·poly C. Purification and interaction with polynucleotides. Europ. J. Biochem. 69, 615 (1976).

Guillon, J. C., Gresser, I.: Role of interferon in the pathogenesis of an experimental herpes virus infection in mice. Ann. Inst. Pasteur A 129, 207 (1978).

Gunby, P.: Looking for biological response modifiers. Arch. Intern. Med. 139, 957 (1979).

Gupta, S. L.: Specific phosphorylation in interferon-treated uninfected and virus-infected mouse L929 cells: enhancement by doublestranded RNA. J. Virol. 29, 301–311 (1979).

Gupta, S. L., Rubin, B. Y., Holmes, S. L.: Interferon action-induction of specific proteins in mouse and human cells by homologous interferons. Proc. Natl. Acad. Sci. U.S.A. 76, 4817–4821 (1979).

Gurari-Rotman, D., Revel, M., Tartakovsky, B., Segal, S., Hahn, T., Handzel, S., Levin, S.: Lymphoblastogenesis in Down's syndrome and its inhibition by human interferon. FEBS Letters 94, 187–190 (1978).

Haahr, S.: The occurrence of interferon in the cerebrospinal fluid in patients with bacterial meningitis. Acta Path. Microbiol. Scand. 73, 264–274 (1968).

Hadhazy, G., Horvath, E., Gergely, L.: Simultaneous inhibitory action on virus multiplication of interferon and some natural micropolysaccharides (heparin, hyaluronic acid). Acta Microbiol. Acad. Sci., Hung. 13, 193–196 (1966).

Hafkin, B., Pollard, R. B., Tiku, M. L., Robinson, W. S., Merigan, T. C.: Effect of interferon and adenine arabinoside treatment of hepatitis B virus infection on cellular immune responses. Antimicrob. Agents Chemother. 16, 781–787 (1979).

Haghihara, B., Kobayashi, S., Kishida, T., Nagano, Y., Kojima, Y.: Effect du facteur inhibiteur du virus sur la phosphorylation oxydative dans la cellule de tetrahymena geleii. C. R. Soc. Biol. 159, 264 (1965).

Hahn, T., Levin, S., Handzel, Z. T.: Production of immune and viral interferon by lymphocytes of newborn infants. Isreal J. Med. Sci. 16, 33–36 (1980).

Hahn, T., Levin, S., Handzel, Z. T., Ashkenazi, A. Chemke, J., Shterk, V.: An apparently immunoregulatory effect of human leukocyte interferon on the blastogenic response in Down's syndrome. Israel J. Med. Sci. 15, 775–777 (1979).

Hahon, N.: Counteraction of poly (4-vinylpyridine-N-oxides) on the depression of viral interferon induction by coal dust. Infect. Immun. **13**, 1334–1337 (1976).

Hahon, N., Booth, J. A.: Hemadsorption cell-counting assay of interferon. Arch. ges. Virusforsch. **44**, 160–163 (1974).

Hahon, N., Booth, J. A., Eckert, H. L.: Interferon assessment by the immunofluorescent, immunoperoxidase and hemadsorption cell-counting techniques. Arch. Virol. **48**, 239–249 (1975).

Hahon, N., Booth, J. A., Stewart, J. D.: Aflatoxin inhibition of viral interferon induction. Antimicrob. Agents Chemother. **16**, 277–282 (1979).

Hajnicka, V., Borecky, L.: Antiviral and anticellular effects of interferon on the mouse embryonic cells transformed by viruses and/or chemical carcinogens. Acta Biol. Med. Germ. **38**, 821–827 (1979).

Hajnicka, V., Fuchsberger, N., Borecky, L.: Purification of mouse interferon on specifically purified immunoadsorbent. Arch. Immunol. Therap. Exp. **25**, 619 (1977).

Halbach, M., Koschel, K., Jungwirth. C.: Interferon enhances the fragility of lysosomes in L-929 mouse fibroblasts. J. Gen. Virol. **39**, 387–390 (1978).

Haliotis, T., Roder, J., Klein, M., Ortaldo, J., Fauci, A. S., Herberman, R. B.: *Chediak-Higashi* gene in humans. I. Impairment of natural-killer function. J. Exp. Med. **151**, 1039–1048 (1980).

Hall, C. B., Douglas, R. G., Simons, R. L., Geiman, J. M.: Interferon production in children with respiratory syncytial, influenza and parainfluenza virus infections. J. Pediatrics **93**, 28–30 (1978).

Haller, O., Arnheiter, H., Gresser, I., Lindenmann, J.: Genetically determined, interferon-dependent resistance to influenza virus in mice. J. Exp. Med. **149**, 601–612 (1979).

Haller, O., Arnheiter, H., Lindenmann, J., Gresser, I.: Host gene influences sensitivity to interferon action selectively for influenza virus. Nature **283**, 660–661 (1980).

Hallum, J. V., Thacore, H. R., Youngner, J. S.: Effect of exogenous interferon on L cells persistently infected with Newcastle disease virus. Infect. Immun. **5**, 145–146 (1972).

Hamburg, S. I., Cassell, G. H., Rabinovitch, M.: Relationship between enhanced macrophage phagocytic activity and the induction of interferon by Newcastle disease virus in mice. J. Immunol. **124**, 1360–1365 (1980).

Hamburg, S. I., Manejias, R. E., Rabinovitch, M.: Macrophage activation: increased ingestion of IgG-coated erythrocytes after administration of interferon inducers to mice. J. Exp. Med. **147**, 593–598 (1978).

Hanley, D. F., Wiranowska-Stewart, M., Stewart II, W. E.: Pharmacology of interferons. I. Pharmacologic distinctions between human leukocyte and fibroblast interferons. Int. J. Immunopharmac. **1**, 219–226 (1979).

Hare, J. D., Morgan, H. R.: Polyoma virus and L cell relationship. II. A curable carrier system not dependent on interferon. J. Natl. Cancer Inst. **33**, 765–775 (1964).

Harmon, M. W., Greenberg, S. B., Johnson, P. E.: Rapid onset of the interferon-induced antiviral state in human nasal epithelial and foreskin fibroblast cells. Proc. Soc. Exp. Biol. Med. **164**, 146–148 (1980).

Harrington, D. G., Crabbs, C. L., Hilmas, D. E., Brown, J. R., Higbee, G. A., Cole, F. E., Levy, H. B.: Adjuvant effects of low doses of a nuclease-resistant derivative of poly I·poly C on antibody responses of monkeys to inactivated Venezuelan equine encephalitis virus vaccine. Infect. Immun. **24**, 160–166 (1979).

Harte, D. E.: Natural defense-interferon. OMNI **2**, 12 (1979).

Hashimoto, H., Shibukawa, N., Kojima, Y.: The mode of production of endotoxin-induced interferon in rabbit tissue cells. I. Development of priming by pretreatment with interferon. Microbiol. Immunol. **22**, 673–681 (1978).

Hashimoto, H., Shibukawa, N., Kojima, Y.: The mode of production of endotoxin-induced interferon in rabbit lymphoid cell cultures. II. Priming effect of interferon on apparently noninducible cells. Microbiol. Immunol. **23**, 1033–1037 (1979).

Havell, E. A.: Isolation of a subspecies of murine interferon antigenically related to human leukocyte interferon. Virology **92**, 324–330 (1979).

Havell, E. A., Hayes, T. G., Vilček, J.: Synthesis of two distinct interferons by human fibroblasts. Virology **89**, 330–333 (1978).

Havemann, K.: Interferon and so-called interferon inducers. Wien. klin. Wschr. **85**, 461–466 (1973).

Hayashi, M., Sharpless, N. S., Logrippo, G. A.: Comparative study between immunoglobulin status and interferon response in health and disease. J. Reticuloendothel. Soc. **3**, 107 (1966).

Hayes, T. G., Yip, Y. K., Vilček, J.: Le interferon production by human fibroblasts. Virol. **98**, 351–363 (1979).

Hayflick, L.: The choice of a cell substrate for preparation of human interferon. In Vitro Monograph **3**, 4–11 (1974).

Heath, R. B.: The pathogenesis of respiratory viral infection. Postgrad. Med. J. **55**, 122–127 (1979).

Heidel, G.: Artificial polynucleotides as inducers of interferon. Z. Gesamte Hyg. **20**, 116 (1974).

Heine, J. W., Adler, W. H.: Kinetics of interferon production by mouse lymphocytes and its modulating effect on virus plaqueforming cell assay as a quantitative method to determine activated lymphocytes. J. Immunol. **117**, 1045–1052 (1976).

Heine, J. W., Mikulski, A. J., Sulkowski, E., Carter, W. A.: Stabilization of human fibroblast interferon purified on concanavalin A-agarose. Arch. Virol. **57**, 185–190 (1979).

Hellmann, W., Kohlhage, H.: Isoelectric behaviour of different rabbit interferons induced by Newcastle disease virus. Z. Naturforsch. **27**, 1411–1414 (1972 a).

Hellmann, W., Kohlhage, H.: Gel chromatography of virusinduced interferon from exudate granulocytes. Archiv ges. Virusforsch. **40**, 128–131 (1973 c).

Hellstrom, I.: Sensitivity of mouse tumor cells to the antiviral action of interferon. J. Natl. Cancer Inst. **33**, 209–123 (1964).

Henderson, D. R., Joklik, W. K.: The mechanism of interferon induction by UV-irradiated reovirus. Virology **91**, 320–328 (1978).

Henle, W.: Interference and interferon in persistent viral infections of cell cultures. J. Immunol. **91**, 145–151 (1963).

Henle, G., Hinze, H. C., Henle, W.: Persistent infection of L cells with polyoma virus: Periodic destruction and repopulation of the cultures. J. Natl. Cancer Inst. **31**, 125–141 (1963).

Henry, C. J., Slifkin, M., Graver, R. C.: Inhibition of adenovirus type II by human and monkey interferon. Proc. Soc. Exp. Biol. Med. **137**, 1431–1436 (1971).

Herberman, R. B., Djeu, J. Y., Ortaldo, J. R., Holden, H. T., West, W. H., Bonnard, G. D.: Role of interferon in augmentation of natural and antibody-dependent cell-mediated cytotoxicity. Cancer Treat. Res. **62**, 1893–1898 (1978).

Herberman, R. B., Ortaldo, J. R., Bonnard, G. D.: Augmentation by interferon of human natural and antibody-dependent cell-mediated cytotoxicity. Nature **277**, 221–223 (1979).

Heremans, H., Billiau, A., Columbatti, A., Hilgers, J., DeSomer, P.: Interferon treatment of NZB mice: Accelerated progression of autoimmune disease. Infect. Immun. **21**, 925–928 (1978).

Heremans, H., Deley, M., Vockaert-Vervliet, G., Billiau, A.: Interferon production and virus replication in lymphoblastoid cells infected with different viruses. Arch. Virol. **63**, 317–321 (1980).

Hernandez-Asensio, M., Hooks, J. J., Ida, S., Siraganian, R. P., Notkins, A. L. Interferon-induced enhancement of IgE-mediated histamine release form human basophils requires RNA synthesis. J. Immunol. **122**, 1601–1603 (1979).

Heron, I., Berg, K.: Human leukocyte interferon: analysis of effect on MLC and effector cell generation. Scand. J. Immunol. **9**, 517–526 (1979).

Heron, I., Hokland, M., Berg, K.: Enhanced expression of beta-2-microglobulin and HLA antigens on human lymphoid cells by interferon. Proc. Soc. Natl. Acad. Sci. U.S.A. **75**, 6215–6219 (1978).

Heron, I., Hokland, M., Moller-Larsen, A., Berg, K.: The effect of interferon on lymphocyte mediated effector cell functions: selective enhancement of natural killer cells. Cellular Immunol. **42**, 183–187 (1979).

Herr, H. W., Kemeny, N., Yagoda, A., Whitmore, W. F.: Poly I. C. immunotherapy in patients with papillomas on superficial carcinomas of the bladder. Natl. Cancer Inst. Monogr. **49**, 325 (1978).

Higashihara, M., Koyama, H., Igarashi, Y.: Induction of interferon in mice by strains of different virulence of Rift Valley fever virus. Kitasato Arch. Exp. Med. **45**, 33–43 (1972).

Hilfenhaus, J.: Propagation of Semliki forest virus in various human lymphoblastoid cell lines. J. Gen. Virol. **33**, 539–542 (1976).

Hilfenhaus, J.: The impossibility of defining unequivocally the antiviral activity of human fibroblast interferon in terms of a human leukocyte interferon standard. J. Biol. Stand. **6**, 159 (1978).

Hilfenhaus, J., Hinz, J., Mauler, R.: Induction of interferon by formaldehyde inactivated influenza viruses in the mouse. Z. Immun. Forsch. **146**, 377–388 (1974).

Hilfenhaus, J., Mauler, R.: Requirement of cellular RNA-synthesis for the inhibition of Semliki Forest virus by poly(rI)·poly(rC). Z. Naturforsch. **27**, 320 (1972).

Hill, N. O.: Production of interferon for clinical trials. Cancer **29**, 53 (1979).

Hill, N. O., Loeb, L., Pardue, A.: Leukocyte interferon production and its effectiveness in acute lymphatic leukemia. J. Clin. Hematol. Oncol. **8**, 66 (1978).

Hilleman, M. R.: Immunologic, chemotherapeutic and interferon approaches to control of viral disease. Am. J. Med. **38**, 751–766 (1965).

Hilleman, M. R.: Advances in control of viral infections by nonspecific measures and by vaccines with special reference to live mumps and rubella virus vaccines. Clin. Pharmacol. Therapeutic. **7**, 752–762 (1966).

Hiller, G., Jungwirth, C., Bodo, G., Schultze, B.: Biological activity of poly rI·poly rC: Effect on poxvirus-specific functions. Virology **52**, 22–28 (1973).

Hiller, G., Viehhauser, G., Winkler, I., Pohl, D., Jungwirth, C.: In vitro translation of natural mRNAs in a cell-free system containing components from interferon-treated chicken fibroblast and factor preparations from mouse ascites cells or rabbit reticulocytes. Z. Naturforsch. **30**, 398–405 (1975).

Hiller, G., Winkler, I., Viehhauser, G., Jungwirth, C., Bodo, G., Dube, S., Ostertag, W.: Failure of globin mRNA to stimulate globin synthesis in cell-free extracts of interferon-treated globin-synthesizing mouse erythroleukemic cells. Virology **69**, 360–368 (1976).

Hillian, F. M., Bishop, J., Lee, S. H. S., Rozee, K. R.: The characteristics of enhanced DNA synthesis in L cell treated with interferon and arginine-deprived. Exper. Cell. Res. **110**, 283–288 (1977).

Hirsch, M. S.: Interferon – Its hour come at last? N. Engl. J. Med. **298**, 1022 (1978).

Hirt, H. M., Becker, H., Kirchner, H.: Induction of interferon production in mouse spleen cell cultures by *Corynebacterium parvum*. Cell. Immunol. **38**, 168–172 (1978).

Hirt, H. M., Kochen, M., Kirchner, H.: Interferon production in murine spleen cell cultures stimulated by Corynebacterium parvum, in: The Macrophage and Cancer (James, K., McBride, B., Stuart, A., eds.), p. 60. University of Edinburgh, Dept. of Surgery Medical School (1977).

Hitchcock, G., Tyrrell, D. A. J.: Some virus isolation from common colds. II. Virus interference in tissue cultures. Lancet **i**, 237–239 (1960).

Ho, M.: Kinetics considerations of the inhibitory action of an interferon produced in chick cultures infected with Sindbis virus. Virology **17**, 262–275 (1962a).

Ho, M.: Effect of an interferon on synthesis of viral RNA and plaque formation. Proc. Soc. Exp. Biol. Med. **112**, 511–515 (1963).

Ho, M.: The promise of interferon. Med. Times **100**, 150–159 (1972).

Ho, M.: Interferon and hepatitis B virus. N. Engl. J. Med. **295**, 562 (1976).

Ho, M.: Interferon and its therapeutic potential. Med. J. Australia **2**, 11–12 (1979).

Ho, M., Breinig, M. K., Maehara, N.: Cellular basis of interferon formation and hyporeactivity after exposure to bacterial lipopolysaccharide. J. Infect. Dis. **133**, A30–A38 (1976).

Hof, M.: Interferon sensitivity of various strains of influenza A2 viruses. Zentralbl. Bakteriol. Orig. A **222**, 415–427 (1972).

Hofmann, H.: Interferon production in infections with influenza A2 Hong Kong virus. Wien. klin. Wschr. **85**, 90 (1973).

Hofmann, H., Radda, A., Pretzmann, G.: Interferon production by two species of mice after infection with tick-borne encephalitis virus. Archiv ges. Virusforsch. **34**, 385–387 (1971).

Holmes, H. C., Darbyshire, J. H.: Induction of chicken interferon by avian infectious bronchitis virus. Res. Vet. Sci. **25**, 178–181 (1978).

Holstein, B. D., Kohan, S. S., DeLaPena, N. C., Pirosky, R. R.: Interferon as viral inhibitor induced by heterologous DNA. Acta Virol. **15**, 381–386 (1971).

Holstein, B. D., Lustig, E. D., Teyssie, A. R.: Circulating interferon in chickens inoculated with Rous viruses: action corticoids. Medicina (Buenos Aires) 34, 219–222 (1974).

Hooks, J. J., Moutsopoulos, H. M., Geis, S. A., Stahl, N. I., Decker, J. L., Notkins, A. L.: Immune interferon in the circulation of patients with autoimmune disease. N. Engl. J. Med. 301, 5–9 (1979).

Hopps, H. E.: Potential safety requirements for human interferon. In Vitro Monograph 3, 63–64 (1974).

Horak, I., Hilfenhaus, J., Siegert, W., Jungwirth, C., Bodo, G., Palese, P.: Interferon action: effect on the formation of poxvirus specific polysomes and viral RNA. Zeitschr. Naturforsch. 256, 1164–1170 (1970).

Horoszewicz, J. S., Leong, S. S., Carter, W. A.: Noncycling tumor cells are sensitive targets for the antiproliferative activity of human interferon. Science 206, 1091–1093 (1979).

Horoszewicz, J. S., Leong, S. S., Ito, M., Buffett, R. F., Karakousis, C., Holyoke, E., Job, J. L., Dolen, J., Carter, W. A.: Human fibroblast interferon in human neoplasia: clinical and laboratory study. Cancer Treatment Res. 62, 203 (1978).

Hortobagyi, G. N., Guttermann, J. U., Blumenschein, G. R., Buzbar, A. V., Richman, S. P., et al.: Immunotherapy of human breast cancer, in: Immunotherapy of Human Cancer, pp. 321–345. New York: Raven Press (1978).

Houghton, M., Eaton, M. A. W., Stewart, A. G., Smith, J. C., Doel, S. M., Catlin, G. H., Lewis, H. M., Patel, T. P., Emtage, J. S., Carey, N. H., Porter, A. G.: The complete amino acid sequence of human fibroblast interferon as deduced using synthetic oligodeoxyribonucleotide primers of reverse transcriptase. Nucl. Acids Res. 8, 2885–2894 (1980).

Houghton, M., Stewart, A. G., Doel, S. M., Entage, J. S., Eaton, M. A. W., Smith, J. C., Patel, T. P., Lewis, H. M., Porter, A. G., Birch, J. R., Cartwright, T., Carey, N. H.: The amino-terminal sequence of human fibroblast interferon deduced from reverse transcripts obtained using synthetic oligonucleotide primers. Nucl. Acids Res. 8, 1913–1932 (1980).

Houston, W. E., Crabbs, C. L., Stephen, E. L., Levy, H. B.: Modified polyriboinosinic · polyribocytidylic acid, an immunological adjuvant. Infect. Immun. 14, 318–320 (1976).

Hovanessian, A. G.: Intracellular events in interferon-treated cells. Differentiation 15, 139–152 (1979).

Hovanessian, A. G., Kerr, I. M.: The (2'-5')oligoadenylate (pppA2'-5'A2'-5'A) synthetase and protein kinase(s) from interferon treated cells. Europ. J. Biochem. 93, 518–526 (1979).

Hovanessian, A. G., Wood, J., Meurs, E., Montagnier, L.: Increased nuclease activity in cells treated with pppA2'p5'A2'A. Proc. Natl. Acad. Sci. U.S.A. 76, 3261–3265 (1979).

Hren-Vencelj, H., Schauer, P.: A contribution to understanding the mechanism of interferon activity. I. Induction of the antiviral state. Zdrav. Vestn. 43, 599–603 (1974).

Huang, A. S., Wagner, R. R.: Inhibition of cellular RNA synthesis by nonreplicating vesicular stomatitis virus. Proc. Natl. Acad. Sci. U.S.A. 54, 1579–1584 (1965).

Huddlestone, J. R., Merigan, T. C., Oldstone, B. A.: Induction and kinetics of natural killer cells in humans following interferon therapy. Nature 282, 417–419 (1979).

Huffman, J. H., Anderson, M. A., Allen, L. B., Sidwell, R. W.: Lack of suppression of resistance factors to influenza infections in mice pretreated with virazole. J. Antimicrob. Chemother. 3, 79–85 (1977).

Huffman, J. H., Sidwell, R. W., Khare, G. P., Witkowski, J., Allen, L. B., Robis, R. K.: In vitro effect of 1-D-ribo-furanosyl-1,2,4-triazole-3-carboxamide (virazole, 1 CN 1229) on deoxyribonucleic acid and ribonucleic acid viruses. Antimicrob. Agents Chemother. 3, 235 (1973).

Hugh, R., Huang, K., Elliott, T. B.: Enhancement of bacterial infections in mice by Newcastle disease virus. Infect. Immun. 3, 488–493 (1971).

Hughes, T. K., Blalock, J. E., Baron, S.: Various heterologous cells exhibit interferon induced transfer of viral resistance. Arch. Virol. 58, 77–80 (1978).

Hunkapiller, M. W., Hood, L. E.: New protein sequenator with increased sensitivity. Science 207, 523–525 (1980).

Hunt, J. M., Marcus, P. I.: Mechanism of Sindbis virus-induced intrinsic interference with vesicular stomatitis virus replication. J. Virol. 14, 99–109 (1974).

Hunt, T.: Interferon, dsRNA and the pleiotypic effector. Nature **273**, 97 (1978).

Huziak, T., Petrak, M., Brudnjak, Z.: Persistent ulcerative vaccinia treated with human leukocyte interferon. Lijec. Vjes. **95**, 640–642 (1973).

Idestrom, K., Cantell, K., Killander, D., Nilsson, K., Strander, H., Willems, J.: Interferon therapy in multiple myeloma. Acta Med. Scand. **205**, 149–154 (1979).

Igoshin, I., Kuznetsov, V. P., Kharitonov, V. A.: Treatment of psoriasis with human leukocyte interferon and interferon combined with deoxyribonuclease and cytostatics (preliminary report). Vestn. Dermatol. Venerol. **46**, 10–13 (1972).

Ikic, D., Pistotnik, M., Grgievic, D., Soos, E., Jusic, D.: The use of human leukocytic interferon in patients with trophic ulcer. Proc. Symp. Clin. Use of interferon; Yugoslav. Acad. Sci. and Arts, pp. 219–222 (1975).

Ikic, D., Smerdel, S., Soos, E., Jusic, D.: Immunological protection and therapy of human genital herpes. Radova. Immunol. Zavoda **13**, 1113 (1971).

Ikic, D., Smerdel, S., Soos, E., Jusic, D., Orescanin, M.: The therapy of some skin virus diseases of the genital region with human leucocytic interferon. Proc. Symp. Field Trials of Vaccines. Yugoslav. Acad. Sci. and Arts, Zagreb, pp. 193–197 (1973).

Ikic, D., Soos, E., Smerdel, S., Jusic, D.: Experience with clinical use of human leukocyte interferon. Radovi Immunol. Zavada **18**, 47 (1975).

Ikic, D., Soos, E., Smerdel, S., Jusic, D., Cupak, K., Trajer, S.: Edipemic keratoconjunctivitis treated with human leukocytic interferon. Proc. Symp. Field Trials of Vaccines. Yugoslav. Acad. Sci. and Arts, Zagreb, pp. 199–204 (1973).

Imanishi, J., Pak, C. B., Kishida, T.: Effect of interferon on the enhancement of the reduction of nitroblue tetrazolium (NBT). C. R. Soc. Biol. **173**, 1004 (1979).

Ingimarsson, S., Cantell, K., Strander, H.: Side effects of long-term treatment with human leukocyte interferon. J. Infect. Dis. **140**, 560–566 (1979).

Inglot, A. D.: A rich source of replicative ribonucleic acid of Sindbis virus – a potent interferon inducer. Archiv. Immunol. Therap. Exper. **18**, 401–408 (1970).

Inglot, A. D.: Antiviral drugs in human therapy. Acta Microb. **5**, 183–186 (1973).

Inglot, A. D., Albin, M., Chudzio, T.: Persistent infection of mouse cells with Sindbis virus: role of virulence of strains, auto-interfering particles, and interferon. J. Gen. Virol. **20**, 105–110 (1973).

Inglot, A. D., Chudzio, T., Albin, M.: Role of incomplete virus and interferon in persistent infection of mouse cells with Sindbis virus. Acta Microbiol. Pol. **5**, 181–182 (1973).

Inglot, A. D., Godzinska, H., Chudzio, T.: Use of polyethylene glysol-treated calf serum for cell cultures in virus and interferon studies. Acta Virol. **19**, 250 (1975).

Inglot, A. D., Inglot, O., Kisielow, B.: Antiserum to type I mouse interferon neutralizes endotoxin-induced interferon in mice. Acta Virol. **23**, 350 (1979).

Inglot, A. D., Inglot, O., Zoltowska, A., Oleszak, E.: Effect of anti-mouse type I interferon globulin on the evaluation of moloney sarcoma virus-induced disease in mice. Int. J. Cancer **24**, 445–449 (1979).

Inglot, A. D., Kisielow, B., Inglot, O.: Biological properties of mouse interferon bound to a high molecular weight carrier, blue dextran 2000. Arch. Virol. **60**, 43–50 (1979).

Inglot, A. D., Lobodzinska, M., Biernacka, I., Niedzwiedzka, E.: Changes in the production of interferon in the process of adaptation of influenza type A2 virus to the mouse lung. Arch. Immunol. Ther. Exp. **14**, 333 (1966).

Inglot, A. D., Niedzwiedzka, E.: Observation on the production of interferon by polyoma virus. Arch. Immunol. Ther. Exp. **13**, 506 (1965).

Inglot, A. D., Oleszak, E., Kisielow, B.: Antagonism in action between mouse or human interferon and platelet growth factor. Arch. Virol. **63**, 291–296 (1980).

International Colloquium on Interferon and Interferon inducers. Catholic University of Leuven, Belgium, September 13–16 (1971).

Isaacs, A.: Metabolic effects of interferon on chick fibroblast. Virology **10**, 144–146 (1960).

Isaacs, A.: Studies on interferon. Austral. J. Exp. Biol. Med. Sci. **43**, 405–412 (1965).

Isaacs, A., Burke, D. C.: Interferon: A possible check to virus infections. New Scientist (1958).

Ito, F., and Aoki, H., Kimura, Y., Takano, M., Maeno, K., Shimokata, K.: Enumeration of immune interferon-producing cells induced by allogeneic stimulation. Infect. Immun. **28**, 542–545 (1980).

Ito, Y., Nishiyama, Y., Shimokata, K., Kimura, Y., Nagata, I., Kunii, A.: Interferon production in L cells persistently infected with hemagglutinating virus of Japan (HVJ). Virology **71**, 463–466 (1976 c).

Ito, Y., Nishiyama, Y., Shimokata, K., Takeyama, H., Kunii, A.: Immune interferon produced in vitro as a quantitative indicator of cell-mediated immunity. Microbiol. Immunol. **23**, 1169–1177 (1979).

Ito, Y., Nishiyama, Y., Shimokata, K., Nagata, I., Kunii, A.: Interferon susceptibility of various cell lines persistenly infected with hemagglutinating virus of Japan. J. Gen. Virol. **43**, 103–110 (1979).

Ito, Y., Nishiyama, Y., Shimokata, K., Nagata, I., Kunii, A.: Temperature sensitivity of interferon susceptibility in L cells persistently infected with hemagglutinating virus of Japan (HVJ). Virology **89**, 342–346 (1978).

Ito, Y., Nishiyama, Y., Shimokata, K., Nagata, I., Takeyama, H., Kunii, A.: The mechanism of interferon induction in mouse spleen cells stimulated with HVJ. Virology **88**, 128–132 (1978).

Ito, Y., Nishiyama, Y., Shimokata, K., Takeyama, H., Kunii, A.: Suppression of interferon production in mouse spleen cells by cytochalasin D. J. Gen. Virol. **41**, 129–134 (1978).

Ito, Y., Nishiyama, Y., Shimokata, K., Takeyama, H., Kunii, A.: Active component of HVJ (Sendai virus) for interferon induction in mice. Nature **274**, 801 (1978).

Itoh, K., Inoue, M., Kataoka, S., Kumagai, K.: Differential effect of interferon on expression of IgG- and IgM-Fc receptors on human lymphocyte. J. Immunol. **124**, 2589–2600 (1980).

Iwakura, Y., Yonehara, S., Kawade, Y.: Purifcation of mouse L cell interferon. Essentially pure preparations with associated cell growth inhibitory activity. J. Biol. Chem. **253**, 5074–5078 (1978).

Iwakura, Y., Yonehara, S., Kawade, Y.: Presence of a common structure in the two molecular species of mouse L cell interferon. Biochem. Biophys. Res. Commun. **84**, 557–563 (1978).

Iwasaki, T., Nozima, T.: Defense mechanisms against primary influenza virus infection in mice. I. Roles of interferon and neutralizing antibodies and thymus dependence of interferon and antibody production. J. Immunol. **118**, 256–260 (1977).

Izbicky, A., Drevo, M., Domorazkova, E., Slonim, D.: Negative sero conversion and circulating interferon in children vaccinated with live measles vaccine. J. Hyg. Epidemiol. Microbiol. **21**, 191 (1977).

Jacobs, J. P.: Serially propagated human diploid cells: a synopsis of the present position concerning their use for producing viral vaccines and interferon. Devl. Biol. Stand. **42**, 13–18 (1979).

Jacquet, M., Caput, D., Falcoff, E., Falcoff, R., Gros, F.: The use of a complementary DNA probe to detect accumulation of mengo RNA in infected cells pretreated with interferon. Biochim. **59**, 189–195 (1977).

Jahiel, R. I., Vilček, J., Nussenzweig, R., Vanderberg, J.: Interferon inducers protect mice against *Plasmodium berghei* malaria. Science **161**, 802–803 (1968).

Jameson, P., Greiff, D., Grossberg, S. E.: Thermal stability of freeze-dried mammalian interferons. Analysis of freeze-drying conditions and accelerated storage tests for murine interferon. Cryobiol. **16**, 301–314 (1979).

Jameson, P., Grossberg, S. E.: Production of interferon by human tumor cell lines. Arch. Virol. **62**, 209–220 (1979).

Janik, B., DeClercq, E., Sommer, R. G.: Interferon inducing activity of (A)n·(U)n complexes of varying chain length. Biochim. Biophys. Acta **517**, 265–268 (1978).

Jaouni, K. C.: Entamoeba histolytica: genetic control of susceptibility in chicken eggs. Exp. Parasitol. **47**, 54–64 (1979).

Jarvis, A. P., Ozer, H. L., Colby, C.: A murine cell possessing a dominant mutation affecting the regulation of interferon production: characterization by interspecific hybrids. Somatic Cell Genet. **4**, 677–698 (1978).

Jarvis, A. P., White, C., Ball, A., Gupta, S. L., Ratner, L., Sen, G. C., Colby, C.: Interferon-associated, dsRNA-dependent enzyme activities in mutant 3T6 cell engaged in the semiconstitutive synthesis of interferon. Cell **14**, 879–884 (1978).

Jasmin, C.: What purpose does interferon serve? Presse Med. **79**, 1373–1375 (1971).

Jennings, R.: Interferon induction by influenza type C. J. Hyg. (Camb.) **70**, 13–21 (1972).

Jensen, K. E., Neal, A. L., A. L., Owens, R. E., Warren, J.: Interferon responses of chick embryo fibroblasts to nucleic acids and related compounds. Nature **200**, 433–434 (1963).

Joffe, B. K. E., Puricelli, L., deLustig, E. S.: Mouse interferon action on a murine neuroblastoma in vitro. Cell Mol. Biol. **24**, 257–264 (1979).

Johnson, H. M.: Cyclic AMP regulation of mitogen-induced interferon production and mitogen suppression of immune response. Nature **265**, 154–155 (1977).

Johnson, H. M.: Differentiation of the immunosuppressive and antiviral effects of interferon. Cell. Immunol. **36**, 220 (1979).

Johnson, H. M.: Similarities in the supression of the immune response by interferon and by a thiol-oxidizing agent. Proc. Soc. Exp. Biol. Med. **164**, 380–385 (1980).

Johnson, H. M., Baron, S.: Interferon: effects on the immune response and the mechanism of activation of the cellular response. CRC Crit. Rev. Biochem. **4**, 203–227 (1976 a).

Johnson, H. M., Ohtsuki, K.: Suppression of in vitro antibody response by ribosome-associated factor(s) from interferon-treated cells. Cell. Immunol. **44**, 125–130 (1979).

Johnson, P. E., Greenberg, S. B., Harmon, M. W., Alford, B. R., Couch, R. B.: Recovery of applied human leukocyte interferon from the nasal mucosa of chimpanzees and humans. J. Clin. Microbiol. **4**, 106–108 (1976).

Johnson, T., Rasmussen, A. F.: Emotional stress and susceptibility to poliomyelitis virus infection in mice. Archiv ges. Virusforsch. **17**, 392–397 (1965).

Johnston, M. D., Christofinis, G., Ball, G. D., Fantes, K., Finter, N. B.: A culture system for producing large amounts of human lymphoblastoid interferon. Dev. Biol. Stand. **42**, 189–192 (1979).

Johnston, M. I., Stollar, B. D.: Antigenic structure of dsRNA analogues having varying activity in interferon induction. Biochem. **17**, 1959 (1978).

Johnstone, D. E., Douglas, R. G., jr., Simon R.: Attempted induction of interferon by bacterial vaccines in allergic and nonallergic humans. Ann. Allergy **32**, 40 (1974).

Joncas, J. H., Robillard, L. R., Boudreault, A., Leyritz, M., Miclaughilin, B. Y. M.: Interferon in serum and cerebrospinal fluid in subacute sclerosing panencephalitis. Can. Med. Ass. J. **115**, 299 (1976).

Jordan, G. W., Merigan, T. C.: Quantitative aspects of interferon-induced plaque reduction: effects of cell age and dose of challenge virus. Proc. Soc. Exp. Biol. Med. **145**, 1037–1047 (1974).

Juhlin, L., Cantell, K.: Interferon response of lymphocytes and resistance to infections. Lancet **8065**, 667–668 (1978).

Jullien, P., DeMaeyer-Guignard, J.: Toxic effect of polyriboinosinic-polyribocytidylic acid on mouse hemopoietic stem cells. Int. J. Cancer **7**, 468–475 (1971).

Jungwirth, C., Bodo, G.: Bestimmung des Molekulargewichtes von Interferon durch Gelfitration. Biochem. Ztschr. **339**, 382–389 (1964).

Kading, V. H., Blalock, J. E., Gifford, G. E.: Effect of serum on the antiviral and anticellular activities of mouse interferon. Arch. Virol. **56**, 231–237 (1978).

Kadish, A. S., Tansey, F. A., Yu, G. S. M., Doyle, A. T., Bloom, B. R.: Interferon as a mediator of human lymphocyte suppression. J. Exp. Med. **151**, 637–650 (1980).

Kaempfer, R., Israeli, R., Rosen, H., Knoller, S.: Reversal of the interferon-induced block of protein synthesis by purified preparations of eucaryotic initiation factor 2. Virology **99**, 170–173 (1979).

Kajander, A., et al.: Interferon treatment of rheumatoid arthritis. Lancet **8123**, 984 (1979).

Kalmakoff, J., Austin, F. Y.: Failure of interferon production following large doses of dsRNA. Proc. Univ. Otago Med. Sch. **50**, 56 (1972).

Kalmakoff, J., Williams, B. R., Austin, F. J.: Antiviral response in insects? J. Invert. Pathol. **29**, 44–49 (1977).

Kamalian, L. A., Engoian, M. N., Vartevanian, Z.: Production of leukocyte interferon in irradiated and intact dogs. Vopr. Virusol. **16**, 552–555 (1971). (In Russian.)

Kanady, M. Y., Smith, W. R.: Variations in the interferogenic responses of two strains of mice. Proc. Soc. Exp. Biol. Med. **141**, 794 (1972).

Kaplan, M. M., Wecker, E., Forsek, Z., Koprowski, H.: An indicator plaque-forming system for demonstration of interference by noncytocidal strains of rabies virus. Nature 186, 821–822 (1960).

Kara, J.: Inhibitory effect of chick interferon and inducers (I·C) on transformation with Rous sarcoma virus. Folia Biol. 19, 194–202 (1973).

Karakuyumchian, M. K., Bektemirova, M. S., Polkovnikova, V. I. A.: Determination of the degree of antirabies immunity in mice with different capabilities for interferon formation. Vopr. Virusol. 18, 275–277 (1973). (In Russian.)

Karpetsky, T. P., Winchurch, R. A., Burman, C. J., Fantes, K. H.: Ribonuclease activity of preparations of human lymphoblastoid interferon. J. Gen. Virol. 44, 241–244 (1979).

Kascskak, R. J., Lyons, M. J.: Attempts to demonstrate the interferon defense mechanism in cultured mosquito cells. Archiv ges. Virusforsch. 45, 149–154 (1974).

Kasparov, A. A., Zeitlenok, N. A., Zaitseva, N. S., Fadeeva, L. L., Vilner, L. M.: Experimental bases of therapeutic-prophylatic use of interferon induced-interferonogene in viral infections of the eye. Ophthalmol. Zh. 27, 49–55 (1972).

Kato, N., Nakashima, I., Ohta, M., Naito, S.: Interferon and cytotoxic factor (cytotoxin) released in blood of mice infected with Mycobacterium bovis BCG. II. Influence of time after BCG on production of interferon or cytotoxin by capsular polysaccharide of Klebsiella pneumoniae or by bacterial lipopolysaccharide and on the hyperreactivity to their lethal effects. Microbiol. Immunol. 23, 395–402 (1979).

Kato, N., Nakashma, I., Ohta, M., Naito, S., Kojima, T.: Interferon and cytotoxic factor (cytotoxin) released in blood of mice infected with Mycobacterium bovis BCG. I. Enhanced production of interferon and appearance of cytotoxin stimulated by capsular polysaccharide of Klebsiella pneumoniae or bacterial lipopolysaccharide. Microbiol. Immunol. 23, 383–394 (1979).

Katz, E., Margalith, E., Winer, B.: The effect of Tilorone hydrochloride on the growth of several animal viruses in tissue cultures. J. Gen. Virol. 31, 125–130 (1976).

Katz, E., Margalith, E., Winer, B.: Inhibition of herpesvirus DNA and protein synthesis by tilorone-HCl. Antimicrob. Agents Chemother. 9, 189–195 (1977).

Kaufman, H. E.: Treatment of herpes keratitis with human leukocyte interferon. Marefuah. 85, 467–468 (1973).

Kaufman, H. E., Ellison, E. D., Centifanto, Y. M.: Difference in interferon response and protection from ocular virus infection in rabbits and monkeys. Am. J. Ophtholmol. 74, 89–92 (1972).

Kaufman, H. E., Sugar, J., Varnell, E. D.: Effect of exogenous interferon on herpetic keratitis in rabbits and monkeys. Invest. Ophthalmol. 12, 378–380 (1973).

Kawakita, M., Cabrer, B., Taira, H., Rebello, M., Slattery, E., Weideli, H., Lengyel, P.: Purification of interferon from mouse Ehrlich ascites tumor cells. J. Biol. Chem. 253, 598–602 (1978).

Kaznacheev, V. P., Vorobieva, A. M., Kononova, V. K., Riazanov, V. N.: Study of leukocytic interferon in rheumatism. Pediatria 52, 30–32 (1973).

Kern, E. R., Olsen, G. A., Overall, J. C., Glasgow, L. A.: Treatment of murine cytomegalovirus infection with exogenous interferon, polyinosinic-polycytidylic acid, and polyinosinic-polycytidylic acid-poly L lysine complex. Antimicrob. Agents and Chemother. 13, 344–348 (1978).

Khadzhibaeva, G. S., Pogodina, V. V., Latypova, R. V., Vilner, L. M.: Interferonogenic activity of gossipol, a low molecular substance. Antibiotiki 23, 365 (1978).

Khaitovich, A. G., Lvosky, P., E. A., Kiselev, P. N.: Radioprotective action of exogenous interferon. Radiobiologia 14, 356–358 (1974).

Khan, A., Hill, N. O.,: Interferon treatment of immunosuppressed patients. Ann. Allergy 44, 289 (1980).

Khesin, Y. E., Aliabieva, T. N., Malinovskaia, V. V., Kuznetsou, V. P., Gerasimov, A. M.: Ribonuclease activity in preparations of human leukocyte interferon. Biull. Eksp. Biol. Med. 82, 805–807 (1976).

Khesin, Y. E., Gulevich, N. E., Amenenkova, A. N., Sonove, N. S., Pokidysheva, L., Norovlansky, A. N.: Association of the feature of human cell culture chromosome set with production of antiviral effect of interferon. Vopr. Virusol. 4, 358–362 (1973). (In Russian.)

Khesin, Y. A. E., Voronina, F. V., Amchenkova, A. M.: Morphological and histochemical studies on cultures of mosue peritoneol leucocytes during interferon formation. Acta Virol. 14, 445–452 (1970).

Khesin, Y. A. E., Voronina, F. V., Marchenko, V. I., Rusanove, N. A., Balandin, I. G.: Morphological, cytochemical and biochemical changes in peritoneal macrophages (normal, activated and tolerant) in process of interferon formation. Vopr. Virusol. 18, 302–308 (1973).

Kilbourne, E. D., Smart, K. M., Pokorny, B. A.: Inhibition by cortisone of the synthesis and action of interferon. Nature 190, 650–651 (1961).

Kilham, L., Bucker, C. E., Fern, V. H., Baron, S.: Production of interferon during rat virus infection. Proc. Soc. Exp. Biol. Med. 129, 274–276 (1968).

Killander, D., Lindahl, P., Lundin, L., Leary, P., Gresser, I.: Relationship between the enhanced expression of histocompatibility antigens on interferon-treated 1210 cells and their position in the cell cycle. 1976.

Kimball, P. C., Duesberg, P. H.: Virus interference by cellular double-stranded ribonucleic acid. J. Virol. 7, 697–706 (1971).

Khoobyarian, N., Fischinger, J. Y.: Role of heated adenovirus 2 in viral interference. Proc. Soc. Exp. Biol. Med. 120, 533–538 (1965).

Kimchi, A., Shulman, L., Schmidt, A., Chernajovsky, Y., Fradin, A., Revel, M.: Kinetics of the induction of 3 translation-regulatory enzymes by interferon. Proc. Nat. Acad. Sci. U.S.A. 76, 3208–3212 (1979).

Kimchi, A., Shure, H., Revel, M.: Regulation of lymphocyte mitogenesis by 2'5'-oligoisoadenylate. Nature 282, 849–851 (1979).

Kimchi, A., Zilberstein, A., Schmidt, A., Shulman, L., Revel, M.: The interferon-induced protein kinase PK-i from mouse L cells. J. Biol. Chem. 254, 9846–9853 (1979).

Kimura, Y.: Inhibition of interferon action by chinoform. Med. Microbiol. Immunol. 167, 189–196 (1979).

Kingham, J. G., Ganguly, N. K., Shaari, Z. D., Mendelson, R., McGuire, M. J., Holgate, S. J., Cartwright, T., Scott, G. M., Richards, B. M., Wright, R.: Treatment of HBsAg-positive chronic active hepatitis with human fibroblast interferon. Gut 19, 91–94 (1978).

Kingman, S. M., Samuel, C. E.: Mechanism of interferon action: interferon-mediated inhibition of Simian virus-40 early RNA accumulation. Virology 101, 458–465 (1980).

Kingman, S. M., Smith, M. D., Samuel, C. E.: Mechanism of interferon action: Simian virus 40-specific early polypeptides synthesized in untreated and interferon treated monkey kidney cells. Proc. Nat. Acad. Sci. U.S.A. 77, 2419–2423 (1980).

Kinoshita, R., Miura, K., Suzuki, S., Uchino, H.: Lack of correlation between interferon production of mononuclear cells and virus replication in chronic hepatitis B virus infection. J. Clin. Microb. 10, 923 (1979).

Kirchner, H., Fenkl, H., Zawatzky, R., Engler, H., Becker, H.: Dissociation between interferon production induced by phytohemagglutinin and concanavalin A in spleen cell cultures of nude mice. Eur. J. Immunol. 10, 224 (1980).

Kirchner, H., Peter, H. H., Hirt, H. M., Zawatzky, R., Dawggee, H., Bradstreet, P.: Studies of the produce cell of interferon in human lymphocyte cultures. Zeit. Immun. Immunobiol. 156, 65–75 (1979).

Kirchner, H., Zawatzky, R., Engler, H., Schirrmacher, V., Becker, H., Wussow, P. V.: Production of interferon in the murine mixed lymphocyte culture. 2. Interferon production is a T-cell dependent function, independent of proliferation. Europ. J. Immunol. 9, 824–826 (1979).

Kirchner, H., Zawatzky, R., Hirt, H. M.: In vitro production of immune interferon by spleen cells of mice immunized with Herpes simplex virus. Cell Immunol. 40, 204–210 (1978).

Kirchner, H., Zawatzky, R., Schirrmacher, V.: Interferon production in murine mixed lymphocyte culture. I. Interferon production caused by differences in the H-2K and H-2D region but not by I-Region or M-locus. Europ. J. Immunol. 9, 97–99 (1979).

Kishida, T.: In: Interferon. Effect of interferon on inclusion formation by Shope fibroma virus (Nagano, Y., Levy, H. B., eds.). Tokyo: I. Shein, Ltd. (1970).

Kishida, T., Arakawa, J., Suzuki, K.: Effet du facteur inhibiteur sur l'infection virale d'animaux hétérologues. Acad. Sci. 158, 1774 (1964).

Kishida, T., Kato, S., Nagano, Y.: Effet du facteur inhibiteur du virus sur le fibrome de shope. C. R. Acad. Sci. **159**, 782 (1965).

Kishida, T., Kawamata, J., Miyamato, H., Kato, S.: Effet du facteur inhibiteur du virus sur l'inclusion intracellulaire produite par le virus de fibrome de Shope. Acad. Sci. **160**, 1765 (1966).

Kishida, T., Morikawa, K., Ito, M., Yokota, Y.: Influence of interferon of the inhibition by macrophages of the in vitro multiplication of murine malignant cells (FM3A). C.R. Soc. Biol. (Paris) **167**, 1503–1505 (1973).

Kisielow, B., Inglot, A. D., Chudzio, T.: Biological activity of sera obtained by hyperimmunizing rabbits with interferon from mouse L cells. Biological activity of anti-interferon sera. Arch. Immunol. Ther. Exp. **27**, 37–44 (1979).

Kjeldsberg, E., Flikke, M.: Antiviral activity of polyinosinic polycytidylic acid in the absence of cell-controlled RNA synthesis. J. Gen. Virol. **10**, 147–154 (1971).

Klein, F., Ricketts, R. T., Jones, W. I., DeArmon, I. A., Temple, M. J., Zoon, K. C., Bridgen, P. J.: Large-scale production and concentration of human lymphoid interferon. Antimicrobial Agents Chemother. **15**, 420–435 (1979).

Klein, G., Vilček, J.: Attempts to induce interferon production by IdUrd induction of EBV superinfection in human lymphoma lines and their hybrids. J. Gen. Virol. **46**, 111–118 (1979).

Kliachko, V. R., Fedorova, I. U. A., Bektemirov, T. A.: Leukocyte interferon in primary hypothyroidism. Pold. Eudokrinal. (Mosk.) **17**, 29–32 (1971).

Knight, E., jr.: Preparation of ^{125}Iodine-labelled human fibroblast interferon. J. Gen. Virol. **40**, 681 (1978a).

Knight, E., jr.: Purification of interferons. Pharm. Therapeutics **2**, 439 (1978b).

Knight, E., jr., Hunkapiller, M. W., Korant, B. D., Hardy, R. W., Hood, L. E.: Human fibroblast interferon: amino acid analysis and amino terminal amino acid sequence. Science **207**, 525–527 (1980).

Knight, E., jr., Korant, B.: Fibroblast interferon induces synthesis of 4 proteins in human fibroblast cells. Proc. Natl. Acad. Sci. U.S.A. **76**, 1824–1827 (1979).

Kobayashi, S.: Interferon: from fundamental research to applications. Gendai Kagaku **35**, 10–16 (1974).

Kobayashi, S.: Titration of interferon using a new type VSV (New Jersey serotype). Virus (Tokyo) **214**, 1–7 (1974).

Kobayashi, S., Kojima, Y., Nagano, Y., Hagihara, B.: Mode d'action du facteur inhibiteur du virus plans l'inhibition de la phosphorylation oxyalative. C.R. Soc. Biol. **159**, 261 (1965).

Koblet, M., Kohler, U., Wyler, R.: Optimization of the interferon assay using inhibition of Semliki forest virus-ribonucleic acid synthesis. Appl. Microbiol. **24**, 323–327 (1972).

Koblet, M., Wyler, R., Kohler, U.: Kinetics of interferon action. Experientia **34**, 1164 (1978).

Koblet, H., Wyler, R., Kohler, U.: Increase of interferon antiviral activity by exogenous cyclic adenosine-3'5' monophosphate. Experientia **35**, 575–576 (1979a).

Koblet, H., Wyler, R., Kohler, U.: Altered or increased transfer RNA methylation in the course of interferon action on cells in culture. Experientia **35**, 576–577 (1979b).

Kobus, M., Sawicki, W., Korbecki, M.: Effect of poly I:C on cell proliferation *in vivo*. Arch. Immunol. Therap. Exp. **25**, 673–678 (1977).

Kociskova, D., Borecky, L., Oravec, C.: The effect of interferon induction on complement level in rat. Acta Biol. Med. Germ. **38**, 837–841 (1979).

Koenig, E. L.: Interferon: A review. Delaware Med. Found. **42**, 4–8 (1970).

Kohase, M., Vilček, J.: Studies on the enhancement of interferon production in human diploid (FS-4) cells by ultraviolet. Jap. J. Med. Sci. Biol. **31**, 17–26 (1978).

Kohase, M., Vilček, J.: Interferon induction with NDV in FS4 cells: effect of DRB. Arch. Virol. **62**, 263–272 (1979a).

Kohase, M., Vilček, J.: Interferon induction with NDV in FS4 cells: effect of priming with interferon and of virus inactivating treatments. Jap. J. Med. Sci. Biol. **32**, 281–294 (1979b).

Kohlhage, H.: Interferon and its clinical use. Med. Klin. **70**, 1319–1325 (1975).

Kohn, A.: The mode of action of interferon. Harefuah **84**, 667–678 (1973).

Kohn, A.: Early interactions of viruses with cellular membranes. Adv. Virus Res. **24**, 223–276 (1979).

Kohn, L. D., Lee, G., Grollman, E. F., Ledley, F. D., Mullin, B. R., Friedman, R. M., Meldolesi, M. F., Aloj, S. M.: Membrane glycolipids and their relationship to structure and function of cell surface receptors for glycoprotein hormones, bacterial toxins and interferon, in: Cell Surface Carbohydrate Chemistry (Harmon, R. E., ed.), p. 103. New York: Academic Press (1978).

Kohno, S., Shirasawa, N., Yukiko, U., Matsuno, T., Kohase, M.: Binding of polyriboinosinic acid-polyribocytidylic acid with cultured cells. Arch. Virol. 49, 229–232 (1975).

Kolaczkowska, M. K.: Properties of interferon from mouse brains. Arch. Immunol. Ther. Exp. (Warsz.) 21, 453–459 (1973).

Kolaczkowska, M. K.: Purification and physicochemical properties of interferons. Postepy. Hyg. Med. Dosw. 28, 229–242 (1974).

Kolaczkowska, M. K., Sypula, A., Zielinska-Jenczylik, J.: Proteins in mouse embryonic cell (MEC) culture fluids following interferon induction. Arch. Immunol. Ther. Exp. (Warsz.) 23, 233–239 (1975).

Koltai, M., Meces, E.: Inhibition of the acute inflammatory response by interferon inducers. Nature 242, 525–527 (1973).

Kono, S., Koase, M., Sakata, H., Shimizu, Y.: Variable interferon productivity of vero cells. Archiv ges. Virusforsch. 37, 141–143 (1972).

Korbecki, M., Luczak, M., Kobus, M.: Effect of poly I·C on parainfluenza 3 virus multiplication in wish cells. Acta. Virol. 15, 175 (1971).

Korsantiya, B. M., Bakhutashvili, V. I.: Transmission of endogenic interferon to the progeny during pregnancy and lactation. Vopr. Virusol. 18, 479–484 (1973). (In Russian.)

Korsantiya, B., Bakhatashvili, V. I., Smorodintsev, A. A.: Endogenous interferon transmission via milk: protection of suckling white mice against lethal influenza infection. Acta Virol. 18, 217–221 (1974).

Kortsaris, A., Taylor-Papadimitriou, J., Georgatsos, J. G.: Interferon inhibition of protein synthesis by isolated mitochondia. Biochem. Biophys. Res. Commun. 68, 1317–1321 (1976).

Kosower, N. S., Kosower, E. M.: Interferon- an altered initiation factor (a hypothesis for its formation and action. J. Mol. Med. 1, 11 (1975).

Kotai, A., Mecs, I., Granti, T.: Increase of interferon induction by basically modified polypeptides. Acta. Pharm. Hung. 46, 145–148 (1976).

Kovalyova, T. P., Selivanov, A. A., Krylou, V. A., Yurlova, T. I., Smorodinstev, A. A.: Anti-interfering and anti-interferon-inducing properties of adenoviral soluble antigens. Acta Virol. 17, 170 (1973).

Kovanen, J., Haltia, M., Cantell, K.: Failure of interferon to modify Creutzfeldt-Jakob disease. Brit. Med. J. 280, 902 (1980).

Kowal, K. J., Youngner, J. S.: Induction of interferon by temperature sensitive mutants of Newcastle disease virus. Virology 90, 90–102 (1978).

Kozlova, Vi., Kuznetsev, V. P., Pukhner, A. F.: The therapeutic efficacy of human leukocyte interferon in the treatment of viral diseases of genitalia. Akush. Ginerol. (Mosk.) 48, 40–41 (1972).

Kreuz, L. E., Levy, A. H.: Density homgeniety and estimated molecular weight of interferon. Nature 200, 883–884 (1963).

Krieg, C. J., Ostertag, W., Clauss, U., Pragnell, I., Swetly, P., Roesler, G., Weimann, B. J.: Increase in intracisternal A-type particles in Friend cells during inhibition of Friend virus release by interferon or azidothymidine. Exp. Cell Res. 116, 21–30 (1978).

Krim, M.: Toward tumor therapy with interferons: I. Interferons: production and properties. Blood 55, 711–721 (1980).

Krim, M.: Towards tumor therapy with interferons: II. Interferons in vivo effects. Blood 55, 875–884 (1980).

Krishnan, I., Baglioni, C.: 2'5'-oligo(A) polymerase activity in serum of mice infected with EMC virus or treated with interferon. Nature 285, 485–487 (1980).

Krispin, T. I., Kolisov, V. D., Balandin, I. G.: Investigation of the initial stages of interaction of mouse interferon with L929 cells. Vopr. Virusol. 5, 510–514 (1979).

Kroath, H., Gross, H. J., Jungwirth, C., Bodo, G.: RNA methylalion in vaccinia virus-infected chick embryo fibroblasts treated with homologous interferon. Nucleic Acids Res. 5, 2441–2444 (1978).

Kroath, H., Janda, H. G., Hiller, G., Kuhn, E., Jungwirth, C., Gross, H. J., Bodo, G.: Methylation of vaccinia virus specific on RNA in the interferon-treated chick cell. Virology **92**, 572–577 (1979).

Kronenberg, L. H.: Interferon production by individual cells in culture. Virology **76**, 634–642 (1977).

Kuan, Fu, C.: Application of the interference phenomenon in tissue culture for the detection of Jap. B. Enceph. virus. Acta Virol. **3**, 82–88 (1959).

Kucera, L. S., Edwards. I.: Herpes simplex virus type 2 functions expressed during stimulation of human cell DNA synthesis. J. Virol. **29**, 83–90 (1979).

Kulberg, A. I. A., Priimiagi, L. S., Bartova, L. M., Shmeleva, N. E., Fadeeva, L. L.: Biull. Eksp. Biol. Med. **73**, 63–66 (1972).

Kumar, V., Gen-Ezra, J., Bennett, M., Sonnenfeld, G.: Natural killer cells in mice treated with Strontium-89; normal target-cell binding cell numbers but inability to kill even after interferon administration. J. Immunol. **123**, 1832–1838 (1979).

Kunze, M.: Production of interferon in the white mouse by dimethyl sulfoxide. Ann. N.Y. Acad. Sci. **243**, 308 (1975).

Kurimura, T., Hirano, A.: Depression of multinucleation by interferon in Simean Virus 40-transformed cells treated with cytochalasin B. GANN Jap. J. Cancer Res. **67**, 751 (1976).

Kuruts, V. M.: Use of interferon in the complex treatment of young children with cytomegalic inclusion disease. Pediatr. Akush. Ginekol. **71**, 23–24 (1971).

Kuwata, T., Fuse, A., Morinaga, N.: Effects of oubain on the anticellular and antiviral activities of human and mouse interferon. J. Gen. Virol. **34**, 537–540 (1977 a).

Kuwata, T., Fuse, A., Suzuki, N., Morinaga, N.: Comparison of the suppression of cell and virus growth in transformed human cells by leukocyte and fibroblast interferon. J. Gen. Virol. **43**, 435–441 (1979).

Kuwata, T., Handa, S., Fuse, A., Morinaga, N.: Effect of glycolipids detectable in transformed human cell on interferon activities. Biochem. Biophys. Res. Commun. **85**, 77–84 (1978).

Kuznekov, V. P.: Human leukocytic interferon. Cas. Lek. Cesk. **111**, 430–433 (1972).

Lab, M., Koehren, F., Krin, M. A.: Inhibition de la production et de l'action antivirale de l'interferon de poulet par le virus 3 de la grenouille. C. R. Acad. Sci. (Paris) **271**, 1227–1230 (1974).

Labzo, S. S., Novokhatsky, A. S., Kabirov, S. K., Knyazeva, V. F.: Stimulation of interferon production by natural and synthetic inducers in human tonsillar cell cultures. Vopr. Virusol. **1**, 81–84 (1980). (In Russian.)

Lackovic, V., Borecky, L.: Patterns of interferon induction in leukocytes. Acta Microbiol. Polonica **22**, 148–151 (1973).

Lackovic, V., Borecky, L.: Production of antiviral and migration inhibitory activity in the peritoneum of mice after inoculation with allegeneic Ehrlich ascites tumor cells. Acta Biol. Med. Germ. **38**, 781–789 (1979).

Lackovic, V., Borecky, L., Kresakovr, J.: Effect of impulsin treatment on interferon production and antiviral resistance of mice. Arch. Immunol. Therap. Exper. **25**, 655–662 (1977).

Lackovic, V., Borecky, L., Youngner, J. S.: Enhancement of interferon production by lowered temperature and/or cycloheximide in endotoxin-stimulated mouse leucocytes. Acta Virol. **16**, 217–225 (1972).

Lackovic, V., Borecky, L., Zschiesche, W., Fahlbusch, B., Schumann, I.: Production of interferon and other lymphokines during murine tumour growth. 2. Induction of an interferon by Ehrlich ascites cells in outbred mice. Acta Virol. **24**, 45–54 (1980).

Lackovic, V., Kontsek, P., Svobodova, J., Borecky, L.: Long-term culture of guinea-pig tongue cells-suitable interferon system. Acta Virol. **23**, 162–164 (1979).

Lacour, F., Delage, G., Spira, A., Nahon-Merlin, E., Lacour, J., Michelson, A. M., Bayst, S.: Randomized trial with poly A-poly U as adjuvant therapy complementing surgery in patients with breast cancer: in vitro study of cellular immunity. Recent Results Cancer Res. **68**, 129–138 (1978).

Lampson, G. P., Nemes, M. M., Field, A. K., Tytell, A. A., Hilleman, M. F.: The effect of altering the size of poly C on the toxicity and antigenicity of poly I.C. Proc. Soc. Exp. Biol. Med. **141**, 1068–1071 (1972).

Lampson, G. P., Tytell, A. A., Field, A. K., Nemes, M. M., Hilleman, M. F.: Influence of polyamines on induction of interferon and resistance to viruses by synthetic polynucleotides. Proc. Soc. Exp. Biol. Med. 132, 212–218 (1969).

Lampson, G. P., Tytell, A. A., Nemes, M. M., Hilleman, M. R.: Characterization of chick embryo interferon induced by DNA virus. Proc. Soc. Exp. Biol. Med. 118, 441–448 (1965).

Lancz, G. J., Johnson, T. C.: Biochemical events during interferon synthesis in L-cells infected with Newcastle disease virus. Proc. Soc. Exp. Biol. Med. 136, 1078–1081 (1971).

Landolfo, S., Marcucci, F., Giovarelli, M., Forni, G.: Does macrophage production of interferon after alloantigens stimulation depend on factors from activated T lymphocytes. Transplantation 29, 87–89 (1980).

Landolfo, S., Marcucci, F., Giovarelli, M., Viano, I., Forni, G.: Lymphokine production in mouse mixed lymphocyte reaction (MLR). II. Tentative mapping of murine alloantigens activating MIF and interferon release and their relationship to proliferation. Immunogenetics 9, 245–254 (1979).

Langford, M. P., Georgiades, J. A., Stanton, G. J., Dianzani, F., Johnson, H. M.: Large-scale production and physicochemical characterization of human immune interferon. Infect. Immun. 26, 36 (1979).

Larin, N. M.: Interferon. IInd Intl. Symp. Chemother. 2, 9–18 (1963).

Larke, R. P. B.: The effects of therapeutic measures in diseases caused by viruses. Canad. Med. Assoc. J. 95, 961–969 (1966a).

Larke, R. P. B.: Interferon: a changing picture. Canad. Med. Assoc. J. 94, 23–31 (1966b).

Larsson, I., Landstrom, L.-E., Larner, E., Lundgren, E., Miorner, H., and Strannegard, O.: Interferon production in glia and glioma cell lines. Infect. Immun. 22, 786–803 (1978).

Larsson, I., Lundgren, E., Nilsson, K., Strannegard, O.: A human neoplastic hematopoietic cell line producing a fibroblast type of interferon. Den. Biol. Stand. 42, 193–197 (1979).

Lawton, J. W. M., Shortridge, K. F., Wong, R. L. C., Ng, M. H.: Interferon synthesis by human colostral leucocytes. Arch. Dis. Childhood 54, 127–130 (1979).

Lazar, R., Breinig, M. K., Armstrong, J. A., Ho, M.: Response of cloned progeny of clinical isolates of herpes simplex virus to human leukocyte interferon. Infect. Immun. 28, 708–712 (1980).

Lebedev, D. D.: Information of interferon, interferonogens, and their importance in pediatric practice. Pediatriia 1, 76–78 (1974).

Lebleu, B., Hubert, E., Content, J., DeWit, L., Braude, I. A., Declercq, E.: Translation of mouse interferon in Xenopus laevis oocytes and in rabbit reticulocyte lysates. Biochem. Biophys. Res. Commun. 82, 665 (1978).

Lebleu, B., Sen, G. C., Brown, G. E., Shaila, S., Lengyel, P.: Studies on mechanism of action of interferon. 2. Increased endonuclease activity in extracts from interferon-treated Ehrlich ascites tumour cells-dependence on ATP and dsRNA. Arch. Int. Physiol. Biochim. 85, 179 (1977).

Lebleu, B., Sen, G. C., Gupta, S. L., Galster, R., Brown, G. E., Rebello, M. A., Lengyel, P.: In vitro transcription and translation of viral genomes. INSERM Meeting, p. 379 (1975).

Lebon, P., Commoy-Chevalier, M., J., Robert-Galliot, B., Morin, A., Chany, C.: Type I interferon induced by culturing human leukocytes with cells infected with herpesvirus and treated by glutaraldehyde. C. R. Acad. Sci. D 290, 37–40 (1980).

Lebon, P., Moreau, M. C.: Inhibition of interferon activity by ouabain. C. R. Acad. Sci. D 276, 3061–3064 (1973).

Lebon, P., Ponsot, G., Aicardi, J., Goutieres, F., Arthuis, M.: Early intrathecal synthesis of interferon in herpes encephalitis. Biomed. Exp. 31, 267–270 (1980).

Lee, S. H. S., Epstein, L. B.: Reversible inhibition by interferon of the maturation of human peripheral blood monocytes to macrophages. Cell. Immunol. 50, 177–190 (1980).

Lee, S. H. S., Ozere, R. L.: Production of interferon by human mononuclear leucocytes. Proc. Soc. Exp. Biol. Med. 118, 190–195 (1965).

Lee, S. H. S., Rozee, K. R.: Variation of interferon production during the cell cycle. Appl. Microbiol. 20, 11–15 (1970).

Lemon, S. M., Bancroft, W. H.: Lack of specific effect of adenine arabinoside, human interferon and ribavirin on in vitro production of hepatitis B surface antigen. J. Infect. Dis. 140, 798–801 (1979).

Leong, J. C., Kane, J. P., Oleszko, O., Levy, J. A.: Antigenspecific non-immunoglobulin factor that neutralizes xenotropic virus is associated with mouse serum lipoproteins. Proc. Natl. Acad. Sci. U.S.A. **74**, 276–280 (1977).

Leontieva, N. A., Fomina, A. N., Idrisova, Z. Y., Shubladze, A. K., Galegov, G. A.: Combined use of interferon and various strylquinolines in cell cultures and experimental arbovirus infections. Vopr. Virusol. **17**, 482–485 (1972). (In Russian.)

Levin, M. J., Rinaldo, C. R., Leary, P. L., Zaia, J. A., Hirsch, M. S.: Immune response to herpes antigens in adults with acute cytomegalovirus mononucleosis. J. Infect. Dis. **140**, 851–857 (1979).

Levin, S., Schlesinger, M., Handzel, Z., Hahn, T., Altman, Y., Czernobilsky, B., Boss, J.: Thymic deficiency in Down's syndrome. Pediatrics **63**, 80–87 (1979).

Levine, A. S., Levy, H. B.: Phase I–II trials of poly I·C stabilized with poly L-lysine. Cancer Treat. Res. **62**, 1907–1912 (1978).

Levine, A. S., Sivulich, M., Wiernik, P. H., Levy, H. B.: Initial clinical trials in cancer patients of poly ICLC, a highly effective interferon inducer. Cancer. Res. **39**, 1645–1650 (1979).

Levine, S., Magee, W. E., Miller, O. V., Hamilton, R. D.: Interferon as a tool for separating viral from host-cell functions. Symp. in Interferon, Lyon, France, pp. 126–135 (1969).

Levy, H. B.: Polymers as interferon-inducers, in: Polymeric Drugs (Donaruma, L. G., Vogl, O., eds.). New York: Academic Press (1978).

Levy, H. B., Lvovsky, E.: Topical treatment of vaccinia virus infection with an interferon-inducer in rabbits. J. Infect. Dis. **137**, 78–81 (1978).

Levy, M. H., Wheelock, E. F.: The role of macrophages in suppression of established Friend virus leukemia. J. Reticulo. Soc. **20**, 243–254 (1976).

Lewis, J. A., Falcoff, E., Falcoff, R.: Dual action of doublestranded RNA in inhibiting protein synthesis in extracts of interferon-treated mouse L-cells. Translation is impaired at level of initiation and by mRNA degradation. Europ. J. Biochem. **86**, 497–500 (1978).

Leyritz, M., Joncas, J. H.: Interaction of hydrocortisone, interferon and Epstein-Barr virus in lymphoid cells. Europ. J. Cancer **14**, 1377–1382 (1978).

Libikova, H., Rajcani, J.: Experimental mixed infection with two tick-borne viruses and interferon-mediated interference. Acta Virol. **19**, 1–8 (1975).

Libikova, H., Stancek, D., Wiedermann, V., Hasto, J., Breier, S.: Psychopharmaca and electroconvulsive therapy in correlation to viral antibodies and interferon. Experimental and clinical study. Arch. Immunol. Therap. Exper. **25**, 641 (1977).

Lin, L. S., Abreu, S. L.: Production, purification and characterization of rat interferon. Arch. Virol. **62**, 221–227 (1979).

Lindenbaum, A., Rosenthal, M. W.: Removal of polymeric plutonium from mouse liver by interferon inducing compounds. Radiat. Res. **62**, 575 (1975).

Lindenmann, J.: Interferon, future applications. Deut. Med. Wschr. **103**, 1317 (1978).

Link, F., Blaskovic, D., Raus, J.: Interferon formation during virus adaption. Acta Virol. **8**, 561 (1964).

Lipinsky, M., Virelizier, J. L., Tursz, T., Griscelli, C.: Natural killer and killer cell activities in patients with primary immunodeficiencies or defects in immune interferon production. Eur. J. Immunol. **10**, 246–249 (1980).

Lipp, M., Brandner, G.: Inhibition of herpes simplex virus type I specific translation in cells treated with poly rI.poly rC. J. Gen. Virol. **47**, 97–112 (1980).

Liu, J. L.: Protective effect of interferon on mice experimentally injected with Japanese encephalitis virus. Chin. J. Microbiol. **5**, 1–9 (1972).

Liu, J. L., Peng, S. Y.: Purification and characterization of mouse serum interferon. Chin. J. Microbiol. **8**, 111–119 (1975).

Liu, C. P., Slate, D. L., Gravel, R., Ruddle, F. H.: Biological detection of specific mRNA molecules by microinjection. Proc. Natl. Acad. Sci. U.S.A. **76**, 4503–4506 (1979).

Livovski, I., Kiselev, P., Tendler, E., Tokarevich, N., Turbina, I.: Formation of interferon in cultures of bone marrow and peripheral blood cells in lymphogranulomatosis. Vopr. Onkol. **20**, 84–85 (1974).

Livovski, I., Shimanovsk, I., Kiselev, P., Livshits, R., Panomareva, T.: Role of lymphoid bone marrow hematopoietic tissues in interferon formation in the irradiated organism. Vopr. Virusol. **5**, 564–568 (1974). (In Russian.)

Lo, G., Treagan, L.: Selective decrease in interferon production in immunotolerant mice. Infect. Immun. **9**, 192–194 (1974).

Lobodzinska, M., Albin, M.: Rat interferon. VI. Heterologous interferon in the treatment of viral infection. Arch. Immunol. Ther. Exp. **27**, 247–252 (1979).

Lockart, R. Z., jr.: Interference and interferon with respect to herpesviruses, in: The Herpesviruses (Kaplan, A. S., ed.), pp. 261–270. Academic Press (1975).

Lockart, R. Z., jr., Sreevalsan, T.: The effect of interferon on the synthesis of viral nucleic acid, in: Viruses Nucleic Acids and Cancer, pp. 448–461 (1963).

Lodenmann, E., Diederich, J., Sattler, V., Wacker, A.: Induction of interferon in L cells by Poly I.C. in the presence of cationic compounds. Archiv ges. Virusforsch. **40**, 87–92 (1973).

Lombardi, P. S., Cole, B. C.: Induction of a pH-stable interferon in sheep lymphocytes by Mycoplasmatales virus MuL2. Infect. Immun. **20**, 209–212.

Lomniczi, B.: Studies on interferon production and interferon sensitivity of different strains of Newcastle diseases virus. J. Gen. Virol. **21**, 305–313 (1973).

Lomniczi, B.: Interferon induction by different strains of infectious bronchitis virus. Acta Vet. Acad. Sci. Hung. **24**, 199–204 (1974b).

Lomniczi, B.: The role of interferon in interference and autointerference elicited by Newcastle Disease virus. Acta Microbiol. **22**, 137 (1975).

Long, W. F.: Effect of metabolic inhibitors on viral and polynucleotide induction of chick cell interferon. Microbios **4**, 253–259 (1971).

Lotem, J., Sachs, L.: Genetic dissociation of different cellular effects of interferon on myeloid leukemic cells. Int. J. Cancer **22**, 214–218 (1976).

Louis, J. A., Lambert, P. H. Kobayakawa, T., Izui, S.: Relevance of polyclonal antibody formation to the development of autoimmunity. Adv. Exp. Biol. Med. **114**, 667–671 (1979).

Louisot, P., Vallier, P., Morelis, P.: Induction d'une activité antivirale contre myxovirus influenza A par un acide ribonucléique d'espèce hétérologue. C. R. Soc. Biol. **161**, 2551 (1967).

Lowell, A.: Editorial: Interferon, 1973. South. Med. J. **67**, 1–3 (1974).

Lubiniecki, A. S., Armstrong, J. A., Ho, M.: Eastern equine encephalitis virus. Quantitative study of the effects of interferon on virus replication. Archiv ges. Virusforsch. **45**, 52–64 (1974a).

Lubiniecki, A. S., Armstrong, J. A., Ho, M.: The pattern of virus-specific peptide synthesis in rabbit cells infected with Eastern equine encephalitis virus and its response to interferon. Proc. Soc. Exp. Biol. Med. **145**, 1014–1017 (1974b).

Lubiniecki, A. S., Blattner, W. A., Cruttenden, V., Gunnell, M., Tarr, G. C., Fraumeni, J. F., jr.: T-antigen expression in human skin fibroblasts is not regulated by an endogenous interferon response to SV40 infection. Arch. Virol. **57**, 349 (1978).

Lubiniecki, A. S., Jones, V., Eatherly, C.: Cytogenetic analysis of the sensitivity to anti-viral and anti-cell growth activities of human fibroblast interferon in aneuploid human tumor cell lines. Arch. Virol. **60**, 341–346 (1979).

Luby, J. P.: Sensitivities of neurotropic arboviruses to human interferon. J. Infect. Dis. **132**, 361 (1975).

Luby, J. P.: Antivirals with clinical potential. Adv. Intern. Med. **24**, 229–254 (1979).

Lucas, C. J., Ubels-Postma, J. Galama, J. M. D., Rezee, A.: Studies on the mechanism of measles virus-induced suppression of lymphocyte functions in vitro. Cell. Immunol. **37**, 448 (1978).

Ludwig, H.: Absent serum interferon in chronic lymphatic leukemia. N. Eng. J. Med. **301**, 1007 (1979).

Luftig, R. B., Conscience, J.-F., Skoultchi, A., McMillan, P., Revel, M., Ruddle, F. H.: Effect of interferon on DMSO-stimulated friend erythro-leukemic cells: ultrastructural and biochemical study. J. Virol. **23**, 799–810 (1977).

Lumb, M., Macey, P. E., Spyvee, J., Whitmarsh, J. H., Wright, R. D.: Isolation of vivomycin and borrelidin, two antibiotics with anti-viral activity from a species of streptomyces. Nature **206**, 263–265 (1965).

Lundgren, E., Larsson, I. Miorner, H., Strannegard, O.: Effects of leukocyte and fibroblast interferon on events in the fibroblast cell cycle. J. Gen. Virol. **42**, 589–596 (1979).

Lunger, P. D., Clark, H. F.: Reptilia-related viruses. Adv. Virus Res. **23**, 159–204 (1978).

MacCallum, F. O.: The problems of viral chemotherapy. Ann. Appl. Biol. **81**, 441 (1975).

MacDonald, R. D., Kennedy, J. C.: Infectious pancreatic necrosis virus persistently infects chinook salmon embryo cells independent of interferon. Virology **95**, 260–264 (1979).

Machida, H., Kuninaka, A., Yoshino, H.: Interferon production and resistance to viral infection by poly I.C in chick embryo cells. I. Effect of growth medium. Japan. J. Microbiol. **18**, 427–432 (1974).

Machida, H., Kuninaka, A., Yoshino, H.: Interferon production and resistance to viral infection induced by poly I.poly C in chick embryo cells. II. Lack of enhancement by DEAE-dextran. Japan. J. Microbiol. **19**, 65–68 (1975).

Machida, H., Kuninaka, A., Yoshino, H.: Relationship between the molecular size of poly I.poly C and its biological activity. Japan. J. Microbiol. **20**, 71–76 (1976).

Machida, H., Kuninaka, A., Yoshino, H.: Effect of nucleosides on interferon production and development of antiviral state induced by poly I.poly C. Microbiol. Immunol. **23**, 643–650 (1979).

Machida, H., Kuninaka, A., Yoshino, H., Yamada, K., Okumura, H.: Interferon production in human diploid cell strains derived from embryonic lungs. Microbiol. Immunol. **24**, 31–37 (1980).

Mackanzie, A. M.: Variations in interferon production by lymphocytes from patients with chronic lymphatic leukemia. J. Clin. Pathol. **25**, 768–771 (1972).

MacLeod, A. R.: Therapy with interferon. N. Eng. J. Med. **301**, 106 (1979).

Madiarova, R. S., Nikolaeva, N., Morogova, V. M., Gilidina, S. S.: The effect of splenectomy and anti-lymphocyte serum on interferon and antibody formation. Vopr. Virusol. **18**, 68–73 (1973). (In Russian.)

Magee, W. E.: Potentiation of interferon production and stimulation of lymphocytes by polyribonucleotide entrapped in liposomes, in: Liposomes and their uses in biology and medicine (Papahadjopoulos, D., ed.). Ann. N. Y. Acad. Sci. **207**, 308 (1976).

Magee, W. E., Levine, S.: The effects of interferon on vaccinia virus infection in tissue culture. Ann. Acad. Sci. **173**, 362–378 (1970).

Maheshwari, R. K., Demsey, A. E., Mohanty, S. B., Friedman, R. M.: Interferon-treated cells release vesicular stomatitis virus particles lacking glycoprotein spikes: correlation with biochemical data. Proc. Natl. Acad. Sci. U.S.A. **77**, 2284–2287 (1980).

Maheshwari, R. K., Friedman, R. M.: Production of VSV with low infectivity by interferon-treated cells. J. Gen. Virol. **44**, 261–264 (1979).

Maheshwari, R. K., Friedman, R. M.: Effect of interferon treatment on vesicular stomatitis virus (VSV): release of unusual particles with low infectivity. Virology **101**, 399–407 (1980).

Maheshwari, R. K., Jay, F. T., Friedman, R. M.: Selective inhibition of glycoprotein and membrane protein of vesicular stomatitis virus from interferon-treated cells. Science **207**, 504–541 (1980).

Malinovskaya, V. V., Khesin, Ya. E., Pokidysheva, L. N.: Influence of sera of different origins on interferon production and the activity of lysomal apparatus of cells of the abdominal exudate of newborn mice. Vopr. Virusol. **3**, 346 (1978). (In Russian.)

Mallucci, L., Taylor-Papadimitriou, J.: Inhibition by interferon of polyoma virus-induced cell DNA synthesis in mouse peritoneal macrophages. J. Gen. Virol. **21**, 391–388 (1973).

Mamontova, T. V., Mentkevich, L. M., Orlova, T. G.: Antiviral activity of mouse interferons induced by bacterial and animal cell mRNA – interferon translation. Vopr. Virusol. **1**, 63–66 (1980). (In Russian.)

Mamontova, T. V., Orlova, T. G.: Effect of Ca ions on the efficiency of translation by bacteria of interferon messenger RNA. Acta Virol. **23**, 271 (1979).

Manejias, R. E., Hamburg, S. I., Rabinovitch, M.: Serum interferon and phagocytic activity of macrophages in recombinant inbred mice inoculated with Newcastle Disease Virus. Cell. Immunol. **38**, 209–212 (1978).

Mantei, N., Schwarzstein, M., Streuli, M., Panem, S., Nagata, S., Weissmann, C.: The nucleotide sequence of a cloned human leukocyte interferon cDNA. Gene **10**, 1–10 (1980).

Manthey, K. F., Hilfenhaus, J., Karges, H. E.: Human interferon as therapeutic agent. Behring Inst. Mitteilung **54**, 81 (1976).

Manzella, J. P., Roberts, N. J.: Human macrophage and lymphocyte responses to mitogen stimulation after exposure to influenza viruses ascorbic acid and hyperthermia. J. Immunol. **123**, 1940–1944 (1979).

Marchenko, V. I., Pokidyshzva, L.: The interaction of interferon antibodies and leukocyte in experiments *in vitro*. Vopr. Virusol. **16**, 456–459 (1971). (In Russian.)

Marchenko, V. I., Pokidysheva, L. N., Orlova, T. G.: Cryomethod for interferon concentration. Vopr. Virusol. **5**, 568 (1975). (In Russian.)

Marchenko, V. I., Pokidysheve, L. N., Malinovskaya, V. V., Alyabieva, T. I., Khesin, Y. E.: Differences in the antiviral and antiongenic effect of interferons produced in peritoneal cells of mice and in Krebs – 2 ascitic carcinoma cells. Vopr. Virusol. **3**, 344 (1977). (In Russian.)

Marchenko, V. I., Zubanova, N. A., Dyuisalieve, R. G., Voronina, F. V., Delimbetova, G. A., Bocharov, A. F.: Investigation of association between manifestations of hyporeactivity (tolerance) in interferon induction and the presence of virus in cells of a tolerant animal. Probl. Virol. **2**, 206 (1977). (In Russian.)

Marcus, P. I., Fuller, F. J.: Interferon induction by viruses. II Sindbis virus: induction requires one-quarter of the genome-genes G and A. J. Gen. Virol. **44**, 169–178 (1979).

Marcus, P. I., Sekellick, M. J.: Interferon Action: III The rate of primary transcription f vesicular stomatitis virus is inhibited by interferon action. J. Gen. Virol. **38**, 391–396 (1978).

Marcus, P. I., Sekellick, M. J.: Interferon induction by viruses. III. Vesicualr stomatitis virus: interferon-inducing particle activity requires partial transcription of gene N. J. Gen. Virol. **47**, 89–96 (1980).

Marecki, N. M., Bradley, S. G.: Enhanced toxicity for mice of combinations of bacterial endotoxin with antitumor drugs. Antimicrob. Agents Chemother. **3**, 599 (1973).

Markovits, P., Coppey, J.: Studies on interferon induction by the Avian adenovirus CELO in chicken cells. J. Gen. Virol. **17**, 157–160 (1972).

Maroun, L. E.: Interferon-mediated effect on ribosomal RNA metabolism. Biochem. Biophys. Acta **517**, 109–114 (1978).

Maroun, L. E.: Interferon effect on ribosomal ribonucleic acid related to chromosome 21 ploidy. Biochem. J. **179**, 221–225 (1979).

Marquard, M.: Polyriboinosinic-Polyriboytidylic acid prevents chemically induced malignant transformation *in vitro*. Nature New Biol. **246**, 228–229 (1973).

Martin, B. A. B., Kroath, H., Jungwirth, C., Hofschneider, P. H., Bodo, G., Wengler, G.: Action of interferon on aged chick embryo cells. Contrast of *in vivo* and *in vitro* studies. Exp. Cell Biol. **48**, 31–44 (1980).

Martin, E. M., Birasall, N. J., Brown, R. E., Kerr, I. M.: Enzymic synthesis, characterization and nuclear-magnetic-resonance spectra of 2-5A and related obligonucleotides: comparison with chemically synthesised material. Eur. J. Biochem. **95**, 295–307 (1979).

Martynova, T. I., Kuznetsov, V. P., Korneva, T. K., Pestovskaia, G. N., Markova, E. V.: Interferon treatment of perineal wounds. Khirurgiia (Mosk.) **10**, 110–113 (1974).

Marx, J. L.: Interferon (I): On the threshold of clinical application. Science **204**, 1183 (1979).

Marx, J. L.: Interferon (II): learning about how it works. Science **204**, 1293–1294 (1979).

Masucci, M. G., Masucci, G., Klein, E., Berthold, W.: Target selectivity of interferon-induced human killer lymphocytes related to their Fc-receptor expression. Proc. Natl. Acad. Sci. U.S.A. **77**, 3620–3624 (1980).

Masucci, M. G., Szigeti, R., Klein, E., Klein, G., Gruest, J., Montagnier, L., Taira, H., Hall, A., Nagata, S., Weissmann, C.: Effect of human leukocyte interferon-alpha1 polypeptide produced by *E. coli* on cell growth and on some immunological functions of blood lymphocytes. (1980, in press.)

Matsubara, S., Suzuki, F., Ishida, N.: The induction of interferon by levamisole in mice. Cellular Immunol. **43**, 214–218 (1979a).

Matsubara, S., Suzuki, F., Ishida, N.: Induction of immune interferon in mice treated with a bacterial immunopotentiator. Cancer Immunol. Immunother. **6**, 41–46 (1979b).

Matsubara, S., Suzuki, M., Ishida, N.: Impaired induction of type II interferon in tumor-bearing mice. Cancer Res. **40**, 873–876 (1980).

Matusbara, S., Suzuki, M., Nakamura, M., Edo, K., Ishida, N.: Isolation of an inhibitor of type II interferon induction from tumor ascites fluids. Cancer Res. **40**, 2534–2538 (1980).

Matsuno, T., Shirasawa, N.: Interferon suppresses steroidinducible glutamine synthetase biosynthesis in embryonic chick neutral retina. Biochem. Biophys. Acta **538**, 188–194 (1978).

Matsuno, T., Shirasawa, N., Kohno, S.: Reversible inhibition of interferon-induced antiviral state by deoxyadenosine. Acta Virol. **20**, 466 (1976 a).

Matsuyama, M.: Cell interaction with poly I.poly C and interferon induction in chick and mouse cells. J. Gen. Virol. **24**, 503–514 (1974).

Matsuyama, M.: Action of interferon on cell membrane of mouse lymphocytes inhibition of ligand-induced redistribution of surface receptors. Exp. Cell. Res. **124**, 253–260 (1979).

Matsuyama, M., Kawade, Y.: Cell growth inhibitory activity of electrophoretic fractions of L-cell interferon preparation. Acta Virol. **18**, 383–390 (1974).

Matsuyama, M., Kawade, Y., Fukada, T.: RNA-induced interference with animal virus infection dependence on cellular metabolic activity. Jap. J. Microbiol. **14**, 303–309 (1970).

Matthews, N.: Tumour-necrosis factor from the rabbit 3. Relationship to interferons. Brit. J. Cancer **40**, 534–539 (1979).

Matthews, T. H. J., Lawrence, M. K.: Serum interferon assay as a possible test for virus infection of man. Arch. Virol. **59**, 35–38 (1979).

Matthews, T. H. J., Nair, C. D. G., Lawrence, M. K., Tyrrell, D. A. J.: Antiviral activity in milk of possible clinical importance. Lancet **8000**, 1387 (1976).

May, D. C., Stanton, G. J.: The inhibitory effect of high concentrations of human and chicken sera on the activity of interferon. Tex. Rep. Biol. Med. **32**, 876 (1974).

Mayer, G. D.: Structural and biological relationships of low molecular weight interferon inducers. Pharmacol. Ther. **8**, 173–192 (1980).

Mayer, V., Mitrova, E., Gajdoskova, E., Doskocil, J.: Viral infection and resistance in immunosuppressed host. V. conversion of enhanced fatal tick-bourne encephalitis to a nonlethal form by a resistance stimulator of the double-stranded RNA type. Acta Virol. **18**, 31–40 (1974).

McGhee, J. R., Michalek, S. M., Moore, R. N., Mergenhagen, S. E., Rosenstreich, D. L.: Genetic control of in vivo sensitivity to lipopolysaccharide: evidence for codominant inheritance. J. Immunol. **122**, 2052–2058 (1979).

McIntosh, K.: Interferon in nasal secretions from infants with viral respiratory tract infections. J. Pediat. **93**, 33 (1978).

McLaren, C., Potter, C. W.: The relationship between interferon and virus virulence in influenza virus infections of the mouse. J. Med. Microbiol. **6**, 21–32 (1973).

McPherson, T. A., Tan, Y. H.: Phase I pharmacotoxicology study of human fibroblast interferon in human cancer. J. Natl. Cancer Inst. **65**, 75–80 (1980).

Meager, A., Graves, H. E., Bradshaw, T. K.: Stimulation of interferon yields from cultured human cells by calcium salts. Fed. Europ. Biochem. Soc. **87**, 303–307 (1978).

Meager, A., Graves, H. E., Bucke, D. C., Swallow, D. M.: Involvement of a gene on chromosome 9 in human fibroblast interferon production. Nature **280**, 493–495 (1979).

Meager, A., Graves, H. E., Shuttleworth, J., Zucker, N.: Interferon production: variation in yields from human cell lines. Infect. Immun. **25**, 658–671 (1979).

Meager, A., Graves, H. E., Walker, J. R., Burke, D. C., Swallow, D. M., Westerveld, A.: Somatic cell genetics of human interferon production in human-rodent cell hybrids. J. Gen. Virol. **45**, 309–322 (1979).

Mecs, I.: The kinetics of formation and sensitivity to interferon of viral intermediates appearing in chick cells infected with Semliki Forest virus. Acta Virol. **17**, 177–188 (1973).

Melinichenko, E. M., Shcmerbakova, E. G.: The detection of interferon in the saliva of children with acute herpetic stomatitis. Stomatologiia (Mosk.) **50**, 51–54 (1971).

Mellstedt, H., Bjorkholm, M., Johansson, B., Ahre, A., Holm, G., Strander, H.: Interferon therapy in myelomatosis. Lancet **8144**, 245–247 (1979).

Melnick, J. L.: Viral vaccines: new problems and prospects. Hosp. Pract. **13**, 104–112 (1978).

Mendelson, J., Dick, V.: Production of interferon by murine peritoneal leukocytes: enhancement by mineral oil. J. Infect. Dis. **123**, 351–355 (1971).

Mendelson, J., Dick, V.: Enhancement of interferon production of murine peritoneal leukocytes by mineral oil: the effect of experimental EMC infection in mice. Can. J. Microbiol. **19**, 544–546 (1973).

Mendlowski, B., Field, A. K., Tytell, A. A., Hilleman, M. R.: Safety assessment of poly I·C in NZB, NZW mice. Proc. Soc. Exp. Biol. Med. **148**, 476 (1975).

Menezes, J., Bourkas, A. E.: Interferon-sensitive expression of membrane-bound IgM on a human lymphoid B-cell line persistently infected with herpes simplex virus. Biomed. Exp. 31, 2–3 (1979).

Mentkevich, L. M., Shcheglovitova, O. N.: Formation of serum and bone marrow (in vitro) interferon in immune mice. Vopr. Virusol. 17, 735–736 (1972). (In Russian.)

Mentkevich, L. M., Shcheglovitova, O. N.: Species specificity of interferon induced by influenza virus and poly I·C in a xenogenic chimera. Radiobiologiia 15, 630–632 (1975). (In Russian.)

Mentkevich, L. M., Shcheglovitova, O. N., Chakhava, O. B., Shustrova, M. M.: Formation of serum and tissue interferon induced by NDV in germfree guinea-pigs. Vopr. Virusol. 18, 374–375 (1973). (In Russian.)

Mentkevich, L. M., Shcheglovitova, O. N., Gulianskii, L. N., Shevelev, N. L.: Suppression of interferon synthesis during the ,,GVH" reaction in F1 (CBAXC57B1/6) mice. Bull. Eksp. Biol. Med. 82, 1098–1100 (1976).

Mentkevich, L. M., Zhdanova, L. V.: Homologous interference of Newcastle disease virus in conditions of suppression of interferon formation. Vopr. Virusol. 17, 292–294 (1972). (In Russian.)

Merigan, T. C.: Interferons of mice and men. N. Engl. J. Med. 276, 913–920 (1967).

Merigan, T. C.: Interferon: its inducers and some aspects of host resistance in malignancy. Cancer Chemother. Res. 58, 571–578 (1974 a).

Merigan, T. C.: Interferon inducers revisited. New Engl. J. Med. 246, 95–96 (1974 b).

Merigan, T. C.: Clinical testing of human interferon in infectious diseases. In Vitro 3, 49–56 (1974 c).

Merigan, T. C.: Book Review: Interferon and its clinical potential by D. A. J. Tyrrell. Nature 266, 479 (1977).

Merigan, T. C.: Human interferon as a therapeutic agent. N. Engl. J. Med. 300, 42 (1979).

Merigan, T. C., et. al.: Interferon in chronic hepatitis B infection. Lancet 8165, 422 (1980 a).

Merigan, T. C.: Clinical virology, interferon and infectious diseases in the People's Republic of China in 1979. J. Infect. Dis. 141, 265 (1980 b).

Merigan, T. C., Gregory, D. E., Petralli, J. K.: Physical properties of human interferon prepared in vitro and in vivo. Virology 29, 515–522 (1966).

Merigan, T. C., Rand, K. H., Pollard, R. B., Abdallah, P. S., Jordan, G. W., Fried, R. P.: Interferon for the treatment of herpes zoster in patients with cancer. N. Engl. J. Med. 298, 981 (1978).

Merigan, T. C., Sikora, K., Breeden, J. H., Levy, R., Rosenberg, S. A.: Preliminary observations on the effect of human leukocyte interferon in non-Hodgkin's lymphoma. N. Engl. J. Med. 299, 1449–1453 (1978).

Metz, D. H.: Interferon deglycosylated. Nature 261, 192 (1976 a).

Metz, D. H.: Interferon translated. Nature 259, 362 (1976 b).

Mezencio, J., Peixoto, M. C. P., Ferreira, P. C. P., Golgher, R. R.: Induction of interferon by group C arboviruses. Arch. Virol. 58, 355 (1978).

Mezentseva, L. M.: Activation of lymphoid elements by interferon in the ,,graft vs host" reaction. Microbiol. 38, 778–779 (1976).

Michaels, B. S., Waddell, G. M., Zinner, D. D., Sigel, M. M.: Viral inhibitory activity of polyvinylpyrrolidone. Nature 212, 101–102 (1966).

Mifune, K., Desmyter, J., Rawls, W. E.: Effect of exogenous interferon on Rubella virus production in carrier cultures of cells defective in interferon production. Infect. Immun. 2, 132–138 (1970).

Mikmailova, E. V., Kliachko, V. R., Fedorova, I., Bektemirov, T. A.: Leukocyte interferon in patients with diabetic obesity. Prob. Endocrinol. (Mosk.) 18, 13–16 (1972).

Mikulski, A. J., Heine, J. W., Le, H. V., Sulkowski, E.: Large scale purification of human fibroblast interferon. Prep. Biochem. 10, 102–120 (1980).

Miles, D. L., Miles, D. W., Eyring, H.: Interferon induction conformational hypothesis. Proc. Nat. Acad. Sci. U.S.A. 76, 1018–1021 (1979).

Minagawa, T., Ho, M.: Hyporeactivity factor produced after induction of immune interferon in mice sensitized with BCG. Infect. Immun. 22, 371–375 (1978).

Minato, N., Reid, L., Cantor, H., Lengyel, P., Bloom, B. R.: Mode of regulation of natural killer cell activity by interferon. J. Exp. Med. 152, 124–137 (1980).

Minks, M. A., Benvin, S., Baglioni, C.: Mechanism of pppA (2'p5'A) 2'p5'AOH synthesis in extracts of interferon-treated cells. J. Biol. Chem. **255**, 5031–5035 (1980).

Minks, M. A., Benvin, S., Maroney, P. A., Baglioni, C.: Metabolic stability of 2'5'oligo(A) and activity of 2'5' oligo(A)-dependent endonuclease in extracts of interferon-treated and control HeLa cells. Nucl. Acids Res. **6**, 767–780 (1979a).

Minks, M. A., Benvin, S., Maroney, P. A., Baglioni, C.: Synthesis of 2'-5'olgio(A) in extracts of interferon-treated HeLa cells. J. Biol. Chem. **254**, 5088–5064 (1979b).

Minks, M. A., West, D. K., Benvin, S., Baglioni, C.: Structural requirements of dsRNA for activation of 2–5A polymerase and protein kinase of interferon-treated HeLa cells. J. Biol. Chem. **254**, 10180–10183 (1979).

Miorner, H., Landstrom, E., Larner, E., Larsson, I., Lundgren, E. A., Strannegard, O.: Regulation of mitogen-induced lymphocyte DNA synthesis by human interferon of different origins. Cell. Immunol. **35**, 15–24 (1978).

Mitrov, A. E., Mayer, V.: Morphological changes in the spleen induced by an interferon stimulator in the immunosuppressed host. Folia Morfol. (Praha) **20**, 94–96 (1972).

Mitrov, A. E., Mayer, V.: Viral infection and resistance in immunosuppressed host. II stimulatory effect and morphology following a single injection of an interferon inducer of the double-stranded RNA type. Acta Virol. **17**, 18–28 (1973).

Mitsuhashi, S., Saito, K., Kurashige, S., Yamaguchi, N.: Ribonucleic acid in the immune response. Molec. Cell. Biochem. **20**, 131 (1978).

Mizrahi, A., O'Malley, J. A., Carter, W. A., Takatsuki, A., Tamura, G., Sulkowski, E.: Glycosylation of interferons. Effects of tunicamycin on human immune interferon. J. Biol. Chem. **253**, 7612–7615 (1978).

Mizunoe, K., Hiraki, M., Nagano, Y., Maehara, N.: Suppression of intracellular multiplication of Mycobacterium tuberculosis by interferon. Japan. J. Microbiol. **19**, 235–236 (1975).

Mogensen, K. E., Cantell, K.: Non-specific adsorption of interferon to immobilized serum immunoglobulin. J. Gen. Virol. **45**, 171–176 (1979).

Mogensen, K. E., Tovey, M. G., Pirt, S. J., Mathison, G. E.: Induction of mouse interferon in a chemically defined system. J. Gen. Virol. **16**, 111–114 (1972).

Moller-Larsen, A.: Cell-mediated cytotoxicity during vaccinia virus revaccination in man: influence of antibodies and interferon. Scand. J. Immunol. **10**, 543–548 (1979).

Moore, M., Potter, M. R.: Enhancement of human natural cell-mediated cytotoxicity by interferon. Brit. J. Cancer **41**, 378 (1980).

Moore, M., White, W. J., Potter, M. R.: Modulation of target cell susceptibility to human natural killer cells by interferon. Intern. J. Cancer **25**, 565–572 (1980).

Morahan, P. S., Grossberg, S. E.: Age-related cellular resistance of chicken embryo to viral infections. I. Interferon and natural resistance to myxoviruses and VSV. J. Infect. Dis. **121**, 615–623 (1970).

Morahan, P. S., Grossberg, S. E.: Age-related cellular resistance of the chicken embryo to viral infections. II. Inducible resistance produced by influenza virus and *E. coli.* J. Infect. Dis. **121**, 624–634 (1970).

Morahan, P. S., Grossberg, S. E.: Age-related cellular resistance of the chicken embryo to viral infections. III *E. coli* resistance-inducing protein. Proc. Soc. Exp. Biol. Med. **134**, 342–347 (1978).

Morahan, P. S., McCord, R. S.: Resistance to herpes simplex type 2 virus induced by an immunopotentiator (pyran) in immunosuppressed mice. J. Immunol. **115**, 311 (1975).

Mordhorst, C. H., Reinicke, V.: Tric (trachoma-inclusion conjunctivitis) agents and interferon. Acta Path. Microbiol. Scand. **65**, 545–553 (1965).

Morel-Morager, I., Sloper, J. C., Vinter, J., Woodrow, D., Gresser, I.: An ultrastructural study of the development of nephritis in mice treated with interferon in the neonatal period. Lab. Invest. **39**, 513–522 (1978).

Moreno, J. A., Baughcum, S. D., Levy, H. B., Baer, G. M.: Further studies on rabies post-exposure prophylaxis in mice: comparison of vaccine with interferon and vaccine. J. Gen. Virol. **42**, 219–222 (1979).

Morris, A. G., Barrett, A. D., Bird, R. M., Burke, D. C.: The effect of malignant transformation on the sensitivity of murine fibroblasts to the antiviral effect of interferon. FEMS Microbiol. Lett. **6**, 139–142 (1979).

Morris, A. G., Burke, D. C.: An interferon-sensitive early step in the establishment of infection of murine cells by murine sarcoma/leukemia virus. J. Gen. Virol. **43**, 173–182 (1979).

Morris, A. G., Clegg, C.: The effect of mouse interferon on the transformation of NIH/3T3 mouse cells by murine sarcoma virus. Virology **88**, 400–404 (1978).

Morser, J., Burke, D.: Interferon and double-stranded RNA. Nature **277**, 435 (1979).

Morser, J., Flint, J., Meager, A., Graves, H., Baker, P. N., Colman, A., Burke, D. C.: Characterization of interferon messenger RNA from human lymphoblastoid cells. J. Gen. Virol. **44**, 231–234 (1979).

Morser, J., Kabayo, J. P., Hutchinson, D. W.: Differences in sialic acid content of human interferons. J. Gen. Virol. **41**, 175–178 (1978).

Morser, J., Meager, A., Coleman, A.: Enhancement of interferon in RNA levels in butyric acid-treated Namalva cells. FEBS Letter **112**, 203–206 (1980).

Morton, J. I., Brown, M., Siegel, B. V.: Influence of cytoxan and poly I:C on early antinuclear antibody responses in New Zealand black mice. Proc. Soc. Exp. Biol. Med. **139**, 1417–1419 (1972).

Moschini, G. B.: Experimental vaccinial kerato-conjunctivitis. Effect of an interferon inducer (poly I·C). Arch. Ophthalmol. **87**, 211–215 (1972).

Moshkin, S. A., Smorodintsev, A. A., Rudenko, V. I.: Luminescent microscopy analysis of the antitoxic effect of interferon upon intravenous inoculation of massive doses of influenza virus. Vopr. Virusol. **4**, 423–427 (1970). (In Russian.)

Mozes, L. W., Defendi, V.: Effect of interferon on the early functions of simian virus-40. Virology **85**, 315 (1978).

Mozes, L. W., Defendi, V.: The differential effect of interferon on T antigen production in Simian virus-40 infected or transformed cells. Virology **93**, 558–568 (1979).

Munk, K., Frick, T.: Effect of poly IC-induced interferon on herpes virus hominis infection *in vitro* and *in vivo*. Z. Naturforsch. B **27**, 220–222 (1972).

Murphy, P. A., Chesney, P. J., Seto, D. S. Y., Carver, D. H.: Assessment of interferon-like activity in preparations of leukocyte pyrogen. J. Gen. Virol. **42**, 185–188 (1979).

Murphy, Y. K. S., Anders, H. P.: Interferons. Angew. Chem. Internat. Edit. **9**, 480–488 (1970).

Muyembe, J. J., Billiau, A., DeSomer, P.: Mechanism of resistance to virus challenge in mice infected with *Brucella abortus*. Archiv ges. Virusforsch. **38**, 290–296 (1971).

Nagano, Y., Kimura, Y., Takano, S.: Hyper-reactivity and hyporeactivity in mice on the induction of virus-inhibiting factor on interferon. C. R. Soc. Biol. **172**, 809 (1978).

Nagano, Y., Kojima, Y., Oda, M., Kim, T., Shiraska, M., Haneishi, T.: Inactivation du facteur inhibiteur du virus par 1 anti-serum. C. R. Soc. Biol. **159**, 280 (1965).

Nagano, Y., Kojima, Y., Shirasaka, M., Haneishi, T.: Propriétés chimiques du facteur inhibiteur du virus. Jap. J. Exp. Med. **35**, 133–140 (1965).

Nagano, Y., Komatsu, H.: Effect of activation of reticuloendothelial system on formation of interferon. Japan. J. Microbiol. **19**, 228–231 (1975).

Nagano, Y., Komatsu, H.: Influence of urethane on the granulopoetic activity of the reticuloendothelial system and the production of interferon. C. R. Soc. Biol. **172**, 1099–1106 (1978).

Nagano, Y., Lee, T.: Different types of virus inhibiting factor of interferon produced by different organs. C. R. Soc. Biol. **172**, 805 (1978).

Nagano, Y., Maehara, N.: Molecular weight species of virusinhibiting factor or interferon produced in the rabbit. Jap. J. Microbiol. **16**, 433–435 (1972).

Nagano, Y., Maehara, N.: Role of spleen cells in formation of virus-inhibiting factor or interferon. Japan. J. Microbiol. **19**, 232–234 (1975).

Nagano, Y., Maehara, N.: Virus-inhibitory factor or interferon activity on heterologous animal cells. Japan. J. Microbiol. **19**, 447–448 (1976).

Nagano, Y., Saito, H.: Effect of virus inhibiting factor or interferon on the division and diffusion and differentiation of murine leukemia cells. C. R. Soc. Biol. **173**, 967–972 (1979 a).

Nagano, Y., Saito, H.: Effect of interferon on the in vitro multiplication of mouse tumor cells. C. R. Soc. Biol. **173**, 20–25 (1979 b).

Nagano, Y., Saito, H., Kurashima, S., Kumazawa, Y.: Role of host cells in suppression of the *in vivo* multiplication of Ehrlichs ascites cancer cells by interferon. C. R. Soc. Biol. **173**, 960–966 (1979).

Nagata, S., Mantei, N., Weissmann, C.: Not less than eight distinct chromosomal genes for human interferon: Structure of the gene for interferon alpha-1 (1980, in press).

Nagata, S., Taira, H., Hall, A., Johnsrud, L., Streuli, M., Escodi, J., Boll, W., Cantell, K., Weissmann, C.: Synthesis of *E. coli* of a polypeptide with human leukocyte interferon activity. Nature **284**, 316–320 (1980).

Nahon-Merlin, E., Lacour, F., Friend, C., Revoltella, R.: Protective effect of immunization with nonviral antigens against friend leukemia virus in mice. Proc. Nat. Acad. Sci. U.S.A. **76**, 2018–2021 (1979).

Nain, M., Kohlhage, H.: Effects of splenectomy on production of poly I:C induced serum interferon in rabbits. Arch. Virol. **51**, 151 (1976).

Naora, H.: Some aspects of double-stranded hairpin structures in heterogeneous nuclear RNA. Int. Rev. Cytol. **56**, 255–313 (1979).

Naysmith, J. D., Sharpe, T. J., Plantdrose, D. N.: The anti-virus activity of double-stranded RNA in the presence of antibody to double-stranded RNA. Europ. J. Immunol. **4**, 629–632 (1974).

Neighbour, P. A., Bloom, B. R.: Absence of virus-induced lymphocyte suppression and interferon production in multiple sclerosis. Proc. Natl. Acad. Sci. U.S.A. **76**, 476–480 (1979).

Nekliudova, L. I., Bektemirov, T. A.: Interferon formation in persons vaccinated with genetically heterogenous strains of Hong Kong influenza. Vopr. Virusol. **16**, 689–692 (1971). (In Russian.)

Nekliudova, L. I., Fedorova, I. U. B.: Use of leukocytic interferon for treatment of influenza. Klin. Med. (Mosk.) **52**, 119–122 (1974).

Neta, R., Salvin, S. B.: In vivo release of lymphokines in different strains of mice. Cell Immunol. **51**, 173–178 (1980).

Neumann, C., Sorg, C.: Immune interferon. 1. Production by lymphokine-activated murine macrophages. Europ. J. Immunol. **7**, 719–725 (1977).

Neumann, C., Sorg, C.: Immune interferon. 2. Different cellular site for production of Murine Macrophage Migration Inhibitory Factor and Interferon. Europ. J. Immun. **8**, 582 (1978).

Neumann, C., Sorg, C.: Different cellular sites for the production of murine macrophage migration inhibitory factory and immune interferon. Adv. Exp. Med. Biol. **114**, 479–483 (1979).

Neumann-Haefelin, D.: Abwehr und Bekämpfung von Virusinfektionen durch Interferon. Deutsche Med. Wschr. **102**, 766 (1977).

Newmark, P.: New routes to polypeptide hormones. Nature **280**, 637–638 (1979).

Nichols, W. W., Bradt, C., Paucker, K., Kjellen, L., Farrell, E.: Inhibition of virus-induced chromosome damage by interferon. Mutat. Res. **16**, 340–344 (1972).

Nicholson, K. G., Cole, P. J., Turner, G. S., Harrison, P.: Immune responses of humans to a human diploid cell strain of rabies virus vaccine: lymphocyte transformation, production of virus-neutralizing antibody and induction of interferon. J. Infect. Dis. **140**, 176–182 (1979).

Nicholson, K. G., Kuwert, E. K., Werner, J., Harrison, P.: Interferon response to human diploid cell strain rabies vaccines in man. Arch. Virol. **61**, 35–40 (1979).

Nikoskii, I. S., Novolotskii, Y. L., Krivokhatskaya, L. A., Chernenko, O. D.: Effect of thymus extract and of late thymectomy on interferon production. Bull. Exp. Biol. Med. **84**, 1439–1443 (1977).

Nilsen, T. W., Baglioni, C.: Mechanism for discrimination between viral and host messenger RNA in interferon-treated cells. Proc. Natl. Acad. Sci. U.S.A. **76**, 2600–2604 (1979).

Nilsen, T. W., Wood, D. L., Baglioni, C.: Virus-specific effects of interferon in embryonal carcinoma cells. Nature **286**, 178–179 (1980).

Nishiyama, Y., Ito, Y., Shimokata, K., Kimura, Y.: The induction of interferon by vesicular stomatitis virus in mouse L cells. Microbiol. Immunol. **23**, 233–247 (1979).

Nolewajka, E., Mikozajski, K., Kapp-Burzynska, Z., Trzeciak, J., Wrona, M.: Induction and properties of guinea pig serum. Arch. Immunol. Therap. Exper. **25**, 623 (1977).

Norby, E.: Interferon – its function and significance. Lakartidningen **69**, 988–998 (1972).

Norris, D., Loh, P. C.: Coxsackievirus myocarditis: prophylaxis and therapy with an interferon stimulator. Proc. Soc. Exp. Biol. Med. **142**, 133 (1973).

Novokhatsky, A. S.: Role of double-stranded RNA in the process of viral induction of interferon formation. Vopr. Virusol. **4**, 49–492 (1974). (In Russian.)

Novokhatsky, A. S., Berezina, L. K.: Multiplication of arboviruses in mosquito cells treated with interferon inducer. Vopr. Virusol. **3**, 357 (1975). (In Russian.)

Novokhatsky, A. S., Berezina, L. K., Kadyrova, A. A., Lvov, D. K., Ershov, F. I.: The interferon inducing activity of Okholsky virus. Vopr. Virusol. **3**, 328 (1976). (In Russian.)

Novokhatsky, A. S., Cherkashina, N. P., Ershov, F. I.: A rapid method for determination of antiviral activity of interferon inducers in experimental infection. Vopr. Virusol. **3**, 303–306 (1979). (In Russian.)

Novokhatsky, A. S., Ershov, F. I.: Inhibition of multiplication of RNA-containing viruses in tissue culture on combined use of interferon production inducter and ribonuclease. Antibiotiki **7**, 629 (1973).

Novokhatsky, A. S., Ershov, F. I.: The dynamics of development of cell resistance to viruses induced by synthetic polynucleotides. Acta Virol. **20**, 23 (1976).

Novokhatsky, A. S., Ershov, F. I., Timkovsky, A. L., Bressler, S. E., Kogan, E. N., Tikhomirova-Sidorova, N. S.: Double-stranded complex of polyguanylic and polycytidylic acids and its antiviral activity in tissue culture. Acta Virol. **19**, 121–129 (1975).

Novokhatsky, A. S., Labzo, S. S., Tsareva, A. A.: Antiviral activity of interferon and its inductors in lymphoblastoid and somatic human cells. Antibiotiki **24**, 294–299 (1979).

Nozakirenard, J.: Induction of interferon by *Bacillus-subtilis*. Ann. Microbiol. **A129**, 525 (1978).

Oaten, S. W., Webb, H. E., Bowen, E. T.: Enhanced resistance of mice to infection with langut (TP21) virus following pre-treatment with Sindbis or Semliki Forest virus. J. Gen. Virol. **33**, 381–388 (1976).

Obrosova-Serova, N. P., Fedorova, G. I., Glukhov, P. I., Shalinov, M. I., Litvinov, V. G.: Effectiveness of midantan and interferon inducers as means of non-specific prevention of influenza. Antibiotiki **17**, 734–738 (1972).

Ochoa, S., DeHaro, C.: Regulation of protein synthesis in eukaryotes. Ann. Rev. Biochem. **48**, 549–580 (1979).

Oddo, F. G., Sinatra, A.: Produzione di un fattore interferonesimile in colture di cellule heLa infettale con virus morbilloso. Inst. Microbiol. Palermo, p. 38 (1963).

Oddo, F. G., Sinatra, A., Tomasino, R. M., Chiarini, A.: An interferon-like inhibitor as a possible factor in the selection of measles virus variants. Archiv ges. Virusforsch. **16**, 148–150 (1965).

Ognianov, D., Fernandez, A.: Isolation and properties of interferon from chicken embryo and mouse strains infected with eastern encephalomvalitis virus (EEE). Zentralbl. Veterinaermed. **B 19**, 94–98 (1972).

Ogurtsov, R. P., Zheleznikova, G. F.: The influence of exogenous interferon on the transplantation reactions in mice. Immunobiol. **3**, 45–49 (1978).

Oh, J. O.: Role of immunity in the pathogenesis of herpes simplex uveritis, in: Immunology and Immunopathology of the Eye (Silverstein, A. M., O'Conner, G. R., eds.), pp. 248–255. New York: Masson.

Ohmori, K., Kawata, M., Okumura, K., Kuwata, T., Tada, T.: Natural killing of human fibroblast cell lines differing in interferon sensitivity. Immunol. Letters **1**, 57–60 (1979).

Ohtsuki, K., Baron, S.: Regulation of interferon-impaired initiation factor activity *in vitro* by cAMP and dsRNA. Proc. Soc. Exp. Biol. Med. **159**, 453–455 (1979).

Ohtsuki, K., Baron, S.: An interferon-induced ribosome-associated protein kinase which reduces the activity of initiation factor. J. Biochem. **85**, 1495–1502 (1979).

Ohtsuki, K., Dianzani, F., Baron, S.: Decreased initiation factor activity in mouse L cells treated with interferon. Nature **269**, 536 (1977).

Ohtsuki, K., Maeda, J., Yamamoto, H., Tsubokura, M.: Studies on avian infectious bronchitis virus (IBV). III. Interferon induction by and sensitivity to interferon of IBV. Arch. Virol. **60**, 249–256 (1979).

Oishi, K., Imanishi, J., Kishida, T.: Bactericidal effect of mouse macrophage treated with interferon. C.R. Soc. Biol. **173**, 1000–1003 (1979).

Okamura, H., Berthold, W., Hool, L., Hunkapiller, M., Inove, M., Smith-Johannsen, H., Tan, Y. H.: Human fibroblastoid interferon: immunosorbent column chromatography and N. terminal amino acid sequence. Biochem. (1980, in press).

Okazaki, H.: Purification and properties of an inhibitory factor of virus infection. Jap. J. Exp. Med. **37**, 159–168 (1967).

Olden, K., Yamada, K. M.: Direct detection of antigens in SDS-PAGels. Anal. Biochem. **78**, 483 (1977).

Olsen, G. A., Kern, E. R., Overall, J. C., jr., Glasgow, L. A.: Effect of treatment with exogenous interferon, polyriboinosinic-polyribocytidylic acid or polyriboinosinic-polyribocytidylic acid-poly-L-lysine comples on herpesvirus kominis infection in mice. J. Infect. Dis. **137**, 428–432 (1970).

O'Malley, J. A., Carter, W. A.: Human interferons: characterization of the major molecular components. J. Reticuloendothel. Soc. **23**, 299 (1978).

O'Malley, J. A., Leong, S. S., Horoszewicz, J. S., Carter, W. A.: Polyinosinic acid-polycytidylic acid and its mismatched analogues: differential effects on human cells function. Molec. Pharmacol. **15**, 165–173 (1979).

Orinda, D., Drahovsky, D., Wacker, A.: Induction of interferon by poly I·C in synchronized mouse L cells. Naturwissenschaften **59**, 519–520 (1972).

Orinda, D. A. O., Gericke, D., Chandra, P.: Antitumour activity of poly I·C in combination with some biologically active compounds. Z. Krebsforsch. **78**, 219–224 (1972).

Orlova, T. G., Georgadze, I. I., Kognovitskaya, A. I., Karmanov, P.: Characteristics of messenger RNA for interferon and interferon-inducing RNA isolated from Newcastle disease virus-infected cells. Vopr. Virusol. **4**, 412 (1975). (In Russian.)

Orlova, T. G., Golovanova, T. A., Shcheglovitova, O., Mysyakin, E. B., Bokhonko, A., Kaulen, D. R.: Comparative studies on the anticellular and antiviral effects of interferon and hemopoetic stem cell inhibition factor. Acta Virol. **23**, 177–182 (1979).

Orlova, T. G., Kognovitskaya, A. I., Mamontova, T. V., Mentkevich, L. M., Soloviev, V. D.: Translation of messenger RNA for interferon by bacterial cells and properties of interferon obtained. Acta Biol. Med. Germ. **38**, 759–763 (1979).

Orlova, T. G., Yeryomkina, E. I.: Interferonogenicity and other properties of partially inactivated influenza virus. Acta Virol. **15**, 126–132 (1971).

Orlova, T. G., Zhdanova, L. V., Mentkevich, L. M., Shcheglovitova, O. N., Soloviev, V. D.: Interferon-producing activity of bone marrow cells treated with mRNA for interferon when transplanted to irradiated mice. Vopr. Virusol. **5**, 541–543 (1979). (In Russian.)

Ortaldo, J. R., McCoy, J. L.: Protective effects of interferon in mice previously exposed to lethal irradiation. Rad. Res. **81**, 262–266 (1980).

Ortega, J., Ma, A., Shore, N. A., Dukes, P. P., Merigan, T. C.: Suppressive effect of interferon on erythroid cell proliferation. Exp. Hematol. **7**, 145–150 (1979).

Osborne, L. C., Georgiades, J. A., Johnson, H. M.: Large-scale production and partial purification of mouse immune interferon. Infect. Immun. **23**, 80–86 (1979).

Osborne, L. C., Georgiades, J. A., Johnson, H. M.: Antibody to mouse immune interferon. IRCS Med. Sci.: Biochem. **8**, 212 (1980).

Osterberg, S.: Interferon, a substance which does what you want it to do. Lakartidningen **72**, 473–474 (1975).

Osterman, L. A.: Participation of tRNA in regulation of protein biosynthesis at the translation level in eukaryotes. Biochemie **61**, 323–342 (1979).

Ostrovski, I., N. N., Vengerov, I. I., Lazukina, L. N., Koiudenko, L. G., Alekseeva, A. K.: Application of an interferonogen-oral live influenza vaccine A213 for treating influenza. Zh. Mikrobiol. Epidemiol. Immunol. **10**, 54–56 (1974).

Ovsyannikova, N. V., Karmysheva, V. Y.: Effect of exogenous interferon on virus-specified immune cytolysis. Vopr. Virusol. **1**, 72–75 (1980). (In Russian.)

Palmblad, J., Cantell, K., Holm, G., Borberg, R., Strander, H., Sunblad, L.: Acute energy deprivation in man: effect on serum immunoglobulins antibody response, complement factors 3 and 4 acute phase reactants and interferon-production capacity of blood lymphocytes. Clin. Exp. Immunol. **30**, 50–55 (1977).

Palmbald, J., Cantell, K., Strander, H., Freoberg, J., Karlsson, C. G., Levi, L., Granstrom, M., Unger, P.: Stressor exposure and immunological response in man: Interferon-producing capacity and phagocytosis. J. Psychosom. Res. **20**, 193–199 (1976).

Paucker, K.: Interferon. Clin. Pediat. **3**, 671–678 (1964).

Paucker, K.: Antigenic properties of human interferons. Tex. Rep. Biol. Med. **35**, 23–28 (1977).

Paucker, K., Dalton, B. J., Torma, E. T.: Antigenic properties and heterospecific activities of human leukocyte interferon species. Conference on Production of Human Interferon and Investigation of its Clinical Use. W. Alton Jones Cell Science Center. Tissue Culture Assoc. Inc., May 19–20 (1977).

Pazin, G. J., Armstrong, J. A., Lam, M. T., Tarr, G. C., Jannetta, P. J., Ho, M.: Prevention of reactivated herpes simplex infection by human leukocyte interferon. N. Eng. J. Med. **301**, 225–229 (1979).

Perez-Bercoff, R., Carrara, C., Dolei, A., Rita, G.: Herpes virus and double-stranded RNA. Experientia **29**, 1171 (1973).

Perez-Bercoff, R., Cioe, L., Degener, A. M., Meo, P., Rita, G.: Infectivity of mengovirus replicative form. IV. Intracellular conversion into replicative intermediate. Virology **96**, 307–310 (1979).

Peries, J. R., Canivet, M., Boiron, M.: Studies of interferon and murine sarcoma virus group. Bibl. Haematol. **39**, 331–334 (1973).

Peries, J. R., Canivet, M., Godard, C., Sall, E. M., Tavitian, A.: Inhibition of interferon action by toyocamycin. J. Gen. Virol. **23**, 347–350 (1974).

Peries, J. R., Canivet, M., Olivie, M., Salle, M., Boiron, M.: Decrease of sensitivity to interferon in cells infected with murine leukemia-sarcoma viruses. J. Natl. Cancer Inst. **51**, 455–463 (1973).

Peries, J. R., Canivet, M., Olivie, M., Tavitian, A.: Effect of selective inhibitor of ribosomal RNA synthesis on the antiviral action of interferon. C. R. Acad. Sci. **278**, 2079–2082 (1974).

Peries, J., Canivet, M., Rhodes-Feuillette, A., Todaro, G. J.: Effect of interferon on chronic infecton of human cells by xenotropic type-C viruses. Int. J. Cancer **23**, 798–802 (1979).

Peterhans, E., Charrey, J., Richoz, Y., Wyler, R.: Production of large quantities of interferon with calf testicular cells and leucocytes. Res. Vet. Sci. **20**, 99 (1979).

Peterhans, E., Wyler, R.: Interferon. Schweiz. Arch. Tierheilkd. **118**, 133–139 (1976).

Petric, H., Prevec, L.: Vesicular stomatitis virus – a new interfering particle – intracellular structures and virus-specific RNA. Virology **41**, 615–630 (1970).

Petricciani, J. C.: Bacteriophages and interferon. In vitro Monographs **3**, 24 (1974).

Petrivic, I., Soldo, I., Soos, E., Smerdel, S., Jusic, D., Kunsten, D.: Use of human leukocytic interferon in the therapy and prevention of postvaccinal complications following mass vaccination against smallpox. Lijec. Vjesn. **96**, 349–354 (1974).

Petukhova, M. B., Blinova, E. N., Karmysheva, V. Y., Ershov, F. I.: Immunofluorescent analysis of regularities of human interferon biosynthesis. Vopr. Virusol. **4**, 450 (1978). (In Russian.)

Pfeffer, L. M., Murphy, J. S., Tamm, I.: Interferon effects on the growth and division of human fibroblasts. Exp. Cell. Res. **121**, 111–120 (1979).

Pfeffer, L. M., Wang, E., Tamm, I.: Interferon effects on microfilament organization, cellular fibronectin distribution and cell motility in human fibroblasts. J. Cell Biol. **85**, 9–17 (1980).

Phillipson, L., Dinter, Z.: The role of interferon in persistent infection with foot and mouth disease virus. J. Gen. Microbiol. **32**, 277–285 (1963).

Pieroni, R. E., Bundeally, A. E., Levine, L.: The effect of actinomycin D on the lethality of poly I·C. J. Immunol. **106**, 1128–1129 (1971).

Pilich, D. J. F., Planterose, D. N.: Effects on friend disease of double-stranded RNA of fungal origin. J. Gen. Virol. **10**, 155–166 (1971).

Pitha, P. M., Fernie, B., Maldarelli, F., Hattman, T., Wivel, N. A.: Effect of interferon on mouse leukemia virus (MuLV). V. Abnormal proteins in virions of Rauscher MuLV produced in the presence of interferon. J. Gen. Virol. **46**, 97–110 (1980).

Pitha, P. M., Fernie, B., Maldarelli, F., Wivel, N. A.: The errors in assembly of MuLV in interferon-treated cells. J. Supramolec. Struct. **12**, 35–46 (1979).

Pitha, P. M., Rowe, W. P.: Effect of interferon on exogenous, endogenous, and chronic murine leukemia virus, in: Prog. Cancer Res. Ther. (Chirigos, M. A., ed.), Vol. 2, p. 361. New York: Raven Press (1977).

Pitha, P. M., Rowe, W. P., and Oxman, M. N.: Effect of interferon on exogenous, endogenous, and chronic murine leukemia virus infection. Virology **70**, 324–337 (1976).

Pitha, P. M., Staal, S. P.: Effect of interferon on murine leukemia virus infection. III. Effect of interferon on MSV-induced transformation. Virology **90**, 151–155 (1978).

Pitha, P. M., Wivel, N. A., Fernie, B. F., Harper, H. P.: Effect of interferon on murine leukemia virus infection. IV. Formation of noninfectious virus in chronically-infected cells. J. Gen. Virol. **42**, 462–480 (1979).

Poindron, P., Coupin, G., Illinger, D., Richards, M.: Action mechanism and therapeutic value of interferon. Lyon Pharm. **27**, 121–133 (1976).

Poindron, P., Gobert, J. G., Savel, J., German, A.: Interferon and protection of the mouse against experimental infestation transmited by the erythrocytic forms of plasmodium berghei injected in massive doses. II. Effects of several immunosuppressive agents on protection patterns by a viral interferon inducer. Ann. Pharm. Fr. **31**, 81–90 (1973).

Pokidysheva, L. N., Marchenko, V. I., Kuznetsov, V. P.: Study of methods of stimulating interferon formation. Vopr. Virusol. **19**, 280–283 (1974). (In Russian.)

Pokidysheva, L. N., Marchenko, V. I., et al.: Differences in properties of interferons produced by blood leukocytes of normal subjects, patients with cancer and leukemia. Vopr. Virusol. **5**, 532–534 (1979). (In Russian.)

Pokidysheva, L. N., Voronina, F. V., Khesin, I. E., Marchenko, V. I.: Stimulation of the inhibiting effect of interferon on the growth of ascitic carcinoma in relation to host responsiveness and cells. Vopr. Virusol. **5**, 591–596 (1976). (In Russian.)

Pokrovski, V. I., Ostrovski, N. N., Kashin, A. M., Nekliudova, L. I., Kuznetsov, V. P.: Effect of intrapulmonary administration of leukocytic interferon on the course of viro-bacterial pneumonia in patients with influenza. Klin. Med. **54**, 61–64 (1976).

Pollard, R. B., Merigan, T. C.: Experience with clinical applications of interferon and interferon inducers. Pharma. Therap. **2**, 783 (1978).

Ponomareva, T. I., Borovkova, N. M., Vikmnovich, E. M., Dreizin, R. S.: Interferongenetic activity and sensitivity of rhinoviruses to interferon. Vopr. Virusol. **18**, 239–240 (1973). (In Russian.)

Popescu, C., Pencea, J., Coiculescu, C., Hoisie, S., Ficiu, H.: The induction of interferon-like agents in the serum and spleen of mice treated with two polymicrobial products. Arch. Roum. Pathol. Exp. Microbiol. **34**, 285–294 (1975).

Porterfield, J. S., Burke, D. C., Allison, A. C.: An estimate of the molecular weight of interferon as measured by its rate of diffusion through agar. Virology **12**, 197–203 (1960).

Postic, B., Singh, B., Squeglia, N. L., Guevarra, L. O.: Inactivation of clinical isolates of herpevirus hopvirus, types I and II, by chemical contraceptives. Sex. Trans. Dis. **5**, 22–24 (1978).

Pottathil, R., Chandrabose, K. A., Cuatrecasas, P., Lang, D. J.: Establishment of the interferon-mediated anitiviral state: role of fatty acid cycloxygenase. Proc. Natl. Acad. Sci. U.S.A. **77** (1980, in press).

Potter, J. E., Banatvala, J. E., Best, J. M.: Interferon studies with Jap. and U.S. rubella virus strains. Brit. Med. J. **1**, 197–199 (1973).

Povolotsky, Y. L., Krivokhatskaya, L. D.: Effect of dibazol and ascorbic acid on antiviral activity of human interferon in cell cultures. Antibiotiki **24**, 291–293 (1979).

Pribyl, D., Treagan, L.: A comparison of the effect of metal carcinogens, chromium, cadmium and nickel on the interferon system. Acta Virol. **21**, 507 (1977).

Price, W. H., Thind, I. S., O'Leary, W., El Dadam, A. H.: A protective mechanism induced by live group B arboviruses against heterologous group B arboviruses independent of serum neutralizing antibodies or interferon. Amer. J. Epidemiol. **86**, 11–17 (1967).

Priestman, T. J.: Initial evaluation of human lymphoblastoid interferon in patients with advanced malignant disease. Lancet **ii**, 113–117 (1980).

Priimagi, L., Iyks, S., Kulberg, A.: Heterologous gamma globulin as interferon inducer: differences in the properties of aggregated and aggregate-free gamma globulin preparations. Arch. Virol. **49**, 89 (1975) [also in: Radiography **41**, 89 (1975)].

Priimyagi, L. S., Iyks, S. R., Kulberg, A.: Production of interferon and of virus-neutralizing antibodies in adult mice infected with enteroviruses in the neonatal period. Bull. Exp. Biol. Med. **85**, 334 (1978).

Pudov, V. I.: Effect of interferon on metastasis of brown-pearce carcinoma. Bull. Exp. Biol. Med. **72**, 91–92 (1971 b).

Puesteri, A. M., Ewalt, L. C., Lodmell, D. A.: Non-specific inhibition of encephalomyocarditis virus replication by a type II interferon released from unstimulated cells of M. tuberculosis sensitized mice. J. Immunol. **124**, 1277 (1980).

Pugliese, A.: Interferon and experimental neoplasms. G. Batteriol. Virol. Immunol. **67**, 300–307.

Pugliese, A.: Interaction of poly I·C with membranes of cells stimulated to produce interferon and of cells not so stimulated. G. Batteriol. Virol. Immunol. **67**, 231–237 (1974b).

Pugliese, A., Cavallo, G.: Effect of synthetic polyribonucleotides on the growth of transplantable tumors in Balb c/mice. Experientia **35**, 536–538 (1979).

Pugliese, A., Tovo, P. A.: Potentiation of poly I.C-induced interferon production in mice using a calf thymus extract (TP-1). Thymus **1**, 305–310 (1980).

Pullman, A.: Blockade of virus synthesis. Nucleic acid induced interferon inhibitor. Ther. GGW **110**, 7241 (1971).

Pumper, R. W., Molander, L.: Interferon production by mammalian cells grown in a serum-free medium. In vitro Monographs **15**, 388 (1979).

Purcell, R. H.: The viral hepatitides. Hosp. Pract. **13**, 51–63 (1978).

Pusztai, R., Szabo, E.: Sensitivity of formation of adenovirus specific tumour antigen to leukocyte interferon. Acta Virol. **2**, 325–328 (1978).

Pusztai, R., Szabo, E., Beladi, I.: T antigen synthesis and resistance to interferon in human adenovirus type 12 infected chick cells. Acta Virol. **21**, 449–455 (1977).

Pyhala, L.: Neutralizing antibodies to human leukocyte, lymphoblastoid and fibroblast interferons elicited by immunization with human leukocyte interferon. Acta Pathol. Microbiol. Scand. C **86**, 291–298 (1978).

Quinnan, G. V., Manishewitz, J. E.: The role of natural killer cells and antibody-dependent cell-mediated cytotoxicity during murine cytomegalo-virus infection. J. Exp. Med. **150**, 1549–1554 (1979).

Rada, B.: The influence of cell-free extracts from Ehrlich ascitic carcinoma and Rous sarcoma on the action of antiviral inhibitors. Acta Virol. **16**, 498 (1972).

Rainte-Audinene, A. B., Klenova, A. N., Palaikene, Z. I.: Results of treatment of acute respiratory viral infections of children with exogenous leukocytic interferon. Pediatriia **7**, 45–49 (1976).

Raj, N. B. K., Fernie, B. F., Pitha, P. M.: Correlation between the induction of mouse interferon and the amount of its mRNA. Eur. J. Biochem. **98**, 215–221 (1979).

Raj, N. B. K., Pitha, P. M.: Biosynthesis of human interferon by translation of its messenger RNA in a wheat germ cell-free system. Abst. Ann. Meet. Am. Soc. Microbiol., p. 253 (1976).

Ramoni, C., Rossi, G. B., Grappelli, C.: Expresson of viral and/or hemoglobin antigens in Friend virus erthyroleukemic cells treated with dimethyl sulfoxide and/or interferon. Bibl. Haematol. **43**, 445–447 (1975).

Ramseur, J. M., and Friedman, R. M.: Prolonged infection of interferon-treated cells by vesicular stomatitis virus: possible role of temperature-sensitive mutants and interferon. J. Gen. Virol. **37**, 523–534 (1977).

Rapp, F., Butel, J. S., Feldman, L. A., Kitahara, T., Melnick, J. I.: Differential effects of inhibitors on the steps leading to the formation of SV40 tumor and virus antigens. J. Exp. Med. **121**, 935–944 (1965).

Rapp, F., Nishiyama, Y.: Inhibition of herpes simplex virus type II induced biochemical transformation by interferon. J. Virol. **33**, 543–546 (1980).

Rasmussen, L. E., Armstrong, J. A., Ho, M.: Interference mediated by a variant of Sindbis virus. I. Isolation of an avirulent variant and in vivo interference. J. Infect. Dis. **128**, 156 (1973).

Rathova, V., Kociskova, D., Borecky, L.: Activation of the complement system by interferon inducers. Acta Virol. **16**, 508 (1972).

Rathova, V., Kociskova, D., Borecky, L.: Levels of complement during interferon induction. Arch. Immunol. Therap. Exp. **25**, 707–714 (1977).

Rathova, V., Kociskova, D., Krizanova, O., Borecky, L.: Consumption of complement in chelated and nonchelated guinea pig serum after challenge with some viral and nonviral interferon inducers. Acta Virol. **20**, 86 (1976).

Ratner, L., Nordlund, J. J., Lengyel, P.: Interferon as an inhibitor of cell growth: studies with mouse melanoma cells. Proc. Soc. Exp. Biol. Med. **163**, 267–270 (1980).

Ratner, L., Wiegand, R. C., Farrell, P. J., Sen, G. C., Cabrer, B., Lengyel, P.: Interferon, double-stranded RNA and DNA degradation. Fractionation of the endonuclease INT system into two macromolecular components: role of a small molecule in nuclease activation. Biochem. Biophys. Res. Comm. **81**, 947–952 (1978).

Raveche, E. S., Tjio, J. H., Steinberg, A. D.: Genetic studies in NZB mice. III. Induced antinucleic acid antibody production. J. Immunol. **122**, 1454–1460 (1979).

Raychaudhuri, A., Megel, H.: The effect of tilorone on immunoglobulin-bearing lymphocytes (B cells) in peripheral blood and spleens of mice. J. Reticuloendothel. Soc. **20**, 127 (1976).

Rech, J., Brunel, C., Jeanteur, P.: Hn RNP from HeLa cells contain a ribonuclease active on double-stranded RNA. Biochem. Biophys. Res. Commun. **88**, 422–427 (1979).

Regelson, W.: Clinical immunoadjuvant studies with tilorone, DEAE-fluorene and *Corynebacterium parvum* and some observations on the role of host resistance and herpes-like lesions in tumor growth. Ann. N. Y. Acad. Sci. **277**, 269–281 (1976).

Regnard, J., Bricout, F.: Viruses and interferon. Can. Med. **13**, 1049–1055 (1972).

Reizin, F. N., Roikhel, V. M.: Effect of colchicine on virus-induced interferonogenesis in chick embryo cells. Lint. Tsitolog. **20**, 87 (1978).

Reizin, F. N., Roikhel, V. M., Chumako, M. P.: The influence of substances changing the intracellular concentration of cyclic adenosine 3'–5'-monophosphate on interferon synthesis in chick embryo cell culture. Arch. Virol. **49**, 307 (1975a).

Reizin, F. N., Roikhel, V. M., Chumako, M. P.: Effect of substances modifying the intracellular cyclic AMP level on interferon formation in chick embryos of different ages. Bull. Exp. Biol. Med. **79**, 647.

Reizin, F. N., Zeitlenok, N. A.: Physiology of interferonogenesis. III. Effect of DL-ornithine on interferonogenesis in chick embryo fibroblast. Acta Virol. **17**, 11–17 (1973).

Reizin, F. N., Zeitlenok, N. A., Chumakov, M. P.: Amino acids and membrane transport in the interferonogenesis system. USP Sov. Biol. **78**, 254–272 (1974).

Remington, J. S., Hackman, R.: Changes in mouse serum proteins during acute and chronic infection with an intracellular parasite (Toxoplasma gondii). J. Immunol. **95**, 1023–1033 (1966).

Renis, H. E.: Effect of poly I·C on experimental respiratory infection in hamsters. Appl. Microbiol. **20**, 821–824 (1970).

Renton, K. W., Keyler, D. E., Mannering, G. J.: Suppression of the inductive effects of phenobarbital and 3-methylcholanthrene on ascorbic acid synthesis and hepatic cytochrome P-450-linked monooxygenase systems by the interferon inducers poly I·C and tilorone. Biochem. Biophys. Res. Commun. **88**, 1017–1023 (1979).

Renton, K. W., Mannering, G. J.: Depression of hepatic cytochrome-P-450-dependent mono-oxygenase systems with administered interferon inducing agents. Biochem. Biophys. Res. Comm. **73**, 343–348 (1976).

Reuss, K., Scheit, K. H., Saiko, O.: Induction of interferon by polyribonucleotides containing thiopyrimidines. Nucl. Acid Res. **3**, 2861 (1976).

Revel, M.: Effect of thermostable mutation in leu-tRNA synthetase on the antiviral state induced by interferon. IRCS Med. Sci. **3**, 609 (1975).

Revel, M., Content, J., Zilberstein, A., Lebleu, B., Falcoff, E., Falcoff, R.: Mechanism of interferon-induced block in messenger RNA translation, in: Perspectives in Virology (Pollard, M., ed.), Vol. 9, p. 233. New York: Academic Press.

Revel, M., Content, J., Zilberstein, A., Nudel, U., Berissi, H., Dudock, B.: Control of mRNA translation by specified tRNAs in extracts from interferon treated mouse cells. Coll. INSERM **47**, 397–406 (1975).

Reznik, V. I., Shangina, D. A., Zdanovskaya, N. I.: Use of leukocyte interferon in foci of acute respiratory diseases. Vopr. Virusol. **6**, 732–733. (In Russian.)

Rhoads, A. R., West, W. L., Morris, M. P.: Interferon induction and suppression of solid tumor growth in rats with tilorone hydrochloride. Res. Commun. Chem. Path. Pharmacol. **6**, 741 (1973).

Rhodes-Feuillette, A., Canivet, M., Andrieu, J. M., Peries, J.: Effect of levamisole on interferon production by PHA-stimulated human leukocyte cultures. Biomed. Express **31**, 170–172 (1979).

Rhodes-Feuillette, A., Cavalieri, F., Canivet, M., Peries, J.: Effect of interferon on chronic infection of human cells by a xenotropic type D virus (Mason-Pfizer virus). C. R. Acad. Sci. D **288**, 1239–1242 (1979).

Ribalko, S. L.: Experimental endogenic interferon induction by prodigiosan. Microbiol. Zh. **34**, 55 (1972).

Riccardi, C., Santoni, A., Barlozzari, T., Fuccetti, P., Herberman, R. B.: In vivo natural reactivity of mice against tumor cells. Int. J. Cancer **25**, 475–486 (1980).

Richman, D. D., Wong, K. T., Robinson, W. S., Merigan, T. C.: Effect of interferon on the replication of Sendai virus. J. Gen. Virol. **9**, 141–150 (1970).

Richmond, J. Y., Campbell, C. H.: Foot-and-mouth disease virus: protection induced in infected mice by two orally-administered interferon inducers. Archiv ges. Virusforsch. **42**, 102 (1973).

Richmond, J. Y., Polatnick, J., Knudsen, R. C.: Microassay for interferon using [3H]-uridine, microculture plates and multiple automated sample harvester. Appl. Environ. Microbiol. **39**, 823–827 (1980).

Riedel, B., Brown, D. T.: Novel antiviral activity found in the media of Sindbis virus persistently infected mosquito (Aedes albopictus) cell cultures. J. Virol. **29**, 51–60 (1979).

Riesenfeld, I., Tufveson, G., Alm, G. V.: Lymphoma development from transplanted murine leukemia virus infected organ cultured thymuses inhibitory effect of *in vitro* interferon treatment. Int. J. Cancer **25**, 529–534 (1980).

Rissanen, A., Palo, J., Myllyla, G., Cantell, K.: Interferon therapy for ALS. Ann. Neurol. **7**, 392 (1980).

Robert, D., Quillon, J. P., Ivanoff, B., Beaudry, Y., Fontages, R., Normierg, G., Pinel, A. M., Dussoord, D., Hunterland, L.: Role of interferon in mice protection against influenza A virus by bacterial ribosomes together with membrane glycoprotein of K pneumoniae as adjuvant. Infect. Immun. **26**, 515–527 (1979).

Roberts, N. J., Diamond, M. E., Douglas, R. G., Simons, R. L., Steigbigel, R. T.: Mitogen responses and interferon production after exposure of human macrophages to infectious and inactivated influenza viruses. J. Med. Virol. **5**, 17–24 (1980).

Roberts, N. J., Douglas, R. G., Simons, R. M., Diamond, M. E.: Virus-induced interferon production by human macrophages. J. Immunol. **123**, 365–369 (1979).

Robinson, R. A., DeVita, V. I., Levy, H. B., Baron, S., Hubbard, S. P., Levine, A. S.: A phase I–II trial of multiple-dose poly I·poly C in patients with leukemia or solid tumors. J. Natl. Cancer Inst. **57**, 599–602 (1976).

Roboz, J. P., Holland, J. F., Bekesi, J. G.: Effectiveness of exogenous mouse interferon in AKR leukemia. Prog. Cancer Res. Ther. 2 (Chirigos, M. A., ed.), p. 369. New York: Raven Press (1977).

Rocklin, R. E.: Mediators of cellular immunity their nature and assay. J. Invest. Dermatol. **67**, 372–380 (1976).

Roder, J. C.: The beige mutation in the mouse. I. A stem cell predetermined impairment in natural killer cell function. J. Immunol. **123**, 2168–2173 (1979).

Roder, J. C., Duwe, A.: The beige mutation in the mouse selectively impairs natural killer cell function. Nature **278**, 451–453 (1979).

Rodgers, R., Merigan, T. C.: Interferon and its inducers: antiviral and other effects. CRC Crit. Rev. Clin. Lab. Sci. **3**, 131–162 (1972).

Rodhe, G., Schurian, E., Meyer, G.: Influence of whole body irradiation with 60CO on poly I·C. induced interferon in mice. Zentralb. Bakteriol. **23**, 535–540 (1975).

Rosenfelt, F.: Interferon therapy in myelomatosis. Lancet **i**, 674 (1979).

Rosenquist, B. D.: Induction and biological significance of interferon with particular reference to cattle. J. Amer. Vet. Med. Assoc. **163**, 821 (1973).

Rossi, C. R., Kiesel, G. K.: Factors affecting the production of bovine type I interferon on bovine embryonic living cells by polyI–polyC. Amer. J. Vet. Res. **41**, 557–560 (1980).

Rossi, C. R., Kiesel, G. K., Hoff, E. J.: Factors affecting the assay of bovine type I interferon on bovine embryonic cells. Amer. J. Vet. Res. **41**, 552–556 (1980).

Rossi, G. B.: Globulin gene expression in dimethyl-sulfoxide-stimulated friend leukemia cells: influence of interferon. Bull. Mol. Biol. Med. **3**, 338–341 (1978).

Rossi, G. B., Dolei, A., Cioe, L., Affabris, E., Belardelli, F., Gambari, R., Fantoni, A.: Expression of erythroid-markers in differentiating friend-leukemia cells: influence of interferon, in: Oncogenic Viruses and Host Cell Genes (Ikawa, Y., Odaka, T., ed.), p. 377. Academic Press (1979).

Rosztoczy, I.: Kinetic and metabolic studies on the priming effect of interferon in L cells. Arch. Immunol. Therap. Exper. **25**, 631 (1977 b).

Rosztoczy, I.: Attempt to transfer priming by cocultivation of L cells and chick embryo fibroblasts. Acta Virol. **23**, 437–438 (1980).

Rotem, Z., Charlwood, P. A.: Molecular weights of interferons from different animal species. Nature **198**, 1066 (1963).

Rouse, B. T., Babiuk, L. A.: Mechanisms of recovery from herpesvirus infections-a-review. Can. J. Comp. Med. **42**, 414–427 (1978).

Rouse, B. T., Wardley, R. C., Babiuk, L. A., Mukkur, T. K. S.: The role of neutrophils in antiviral defense-in vitro studies on the mechanism of antiviral inhibition. J. Immunol. **118**, 1957 (1977).

Rubin, B. Y., Gupta, S. L.: Interferon-induced proteins in human fibroblasts and development of the antiviral state. J. Virol. **34**, 446–454 (1980).

Rubinstein, M., Rubinstein, S., Familletti, P., Gross, M. S., Waldman, A., Pestka, S.: Human leukocyte interferon purified to homogeneity. Science **202**, 1289–1290 (1978).

Rubinstein, M., Rubinstein, S., Familletti, P. C., Miller, R. S., Waldman, A. A., Pestka, S.: Human leukocyte interferon: production purification to homogeneity, and initial characterization. Proc. Natl. Acad. Sci. U.S.A. **76**, 640–644 (1979).

Rudenko, V. I., Smorodintsev, A. A., Aksenov, O. A., Lyabina, L. M.: On the nature of interferon producing cells. Vopr. Virusol. **4**, 52–56 (1970). (In Russian.)

Rudneva, I. A., Korabelnikova, N. I., Germanov, A. B., Sokolov, M. I., Fadeeva, L. L.: Study of interferonogenic activity of herpes simplex virus. Arch. ges. Virusforsch. **37**, 1–5 (1972).

Ruiz-Gomez, J., Avitia-Gonzalez, R.: Inhibition by interferon of chromosome damage by Sendai virus. Rev. Lat. Amer. Microbiol. **16**, 89–93 (1974).

Runti, C.: Antiviral chemotherapeutics XII. Interferon and interferon inducers. Farmaco Sci. **29**, 3–26 (1974).

Rustigian, R., Winston, S. H., Darlington, R. W.: Variable infection of Vero cells and homologous-interferance after co-cultivation with HeLa cells with persistent defective infection by measles virus. Infect. Immun. **23**, 775–786 (1979).

Ryd, W., Hagmar, B., Lundgren, E., Strannegard, O.: Discrepant effects of interferon on murine syngeneic ascites tumors and their solid metastasizing counterparts. Int. J. Cancer **23**, 397–401 (1979).

Rytel, M. W.: Induction of interferon in man by vaccines. Proc. Soc. Exp. Biol. Med. **149**, 266 (1975 b).

Rytel, M. W., Balay, J.: Impaired production of interferon in lymphocytes from immuno-suppressed patients. J. Infect. Dis. **127**, 445–449 (1973).

Sabioncello, A., Rabatic, S., Dekaris, D., Jusic, D., Soos, E., Ikic, D.: Detection of lymphokine activity in human leukocyte interferon preparations. Periodicum Biologorum **78**, 25 (1976).

Saito, N., Matsuno, T., Sudo, T., Furuya, E., Kohno, S.: Priming activity of mouse interferon: effect on interferon messenger RNA synthesis. Arch. Virol. **52**, 159 (1976).

Sakaguchi, A. Y., Stevenson, D., Gordon, I.: Inhibition of interferon production and antiviral action in mouse cells by 4,5'8-trimethylpsoralen activated with near ultraviolet light. Arch. Virol. **63**, 69–74 (1980).

Sakseka, E., Timonen, T., Cantell, K.: Human natural killer cell activity is augmented via recruitment of "pre-NK" cells. Scand. J. Immunol. **10**, 257–266 (1979).

Salaman, J. R., Miller, J. J.: Nonspecific chemical immunosuppression. Transplant. Proc. **11**, 845–850 (1979).

Salit, M. G., Ogburn, C. A.: Human leukocyte interferon: separation of biologically different species by modification of carbohydrate moieties. Arch. Virol. **63**, 133–142 (1980).

Salzberg, S., Heller, A., Aboud, M., Gurari-Rotman, D., Revel, M.: Effect of interferon on human cells releasing oncornaviruses: an assay for human interferon. Virology **93**, 209–214 (1979).

Samuel, C. E.: Mechanism of interferon action: phosphorylation of protein synthesis initiation factor eIF-2 in interferon-treated human cells by a ribosome-associated kinase possessing site specificity similar to hemin-regulated rabbit reticulocyte kinase. Proc. Natl. Acad. Sci. U.S.A. **76**, 600–604 (1979a).

Samuel, C. E.: Mechanism of interferon action. Kinetics of interferon action in mouse L929 cells: phosphorylation of protein synthesis initiation factor eIF-2 and ribosome-associated protein P1. Virology **93**, 281–285 (1979b).

Santoli, D., Trinchieri, G., Koprowski, H.: Cell mediated cytotoxicity against virus-infected target cells in humans. II. Interferon induction and activation of natural killer cells. J. Immunol. **121**, 532–537 (1978).

Sapozhnikov, I. V., Kornilova, N. I. A.: A study of the interferon forming function of mouse leukocytes following inoculation with Bordetella pertussis. Vopr. Virusol. **18**, 64–67 (1973).

Sato, T., Fuse, A., Kuwata, T.: Enhancement by interferon of natural cytotoxic activities of lymphocytes from human cord blood and peripheral blood of aged persons. Cell Immunol. **45**, 458–463 (1979).

Sato, T., Tomita, Y., Kuwata, T.: Inhibition by interferon of Sendai virus cytolysis. Infect. Immun. **28**, 6–10 (1980).

Sauvager, F., Fabiani, G., Fauconnier, B.: Production of interferon after infection by various doses of Plasmodium berghei in mice. Ann. Microbiol. **A130**, 373–388 (1979).

Sauvager, F., Fauconnier, B.: Protective effect of endogenous interferon in mouse malaria as demonstrated by use of anti-interferon globulins. Biomed. Express. **29**, 184–186 (1978).

Sawada, T., Fujita, T., Kusunoki, T., Imanishi, J., Kishida, T.: Preliminary report on the clinical use of human leukocyte interferon in neuroblastoma. Cancer Treat. Rep. **63**, 2111–2114 (1979).

Sawicki, L., Chowchuvech, E., Weissenbacher, M., Baron, S., Galin, M.: Pathogenic studies of herpes simplex virus infection of the rabbit eye. Proc. Soc. Exp. Biol. Med. **144**, 705 (1973).

Schafer, M. P., Chirigos, M. A., Papas, T. S.: Inhibition of Rauscher leukemia virus and avian myeloblastosis virus DNA polymerases by tilorone (NSC-143969) and its analogs. Cancer Chemother. Res. **58**, 821–827 (1974).

Schat, K. A., Gonzalez, J., Solorzano, A.: Interferon production by strains of herpesvirus associated with Marek's disease. Avian Dis. **18**, 531 (1974).

Schauer, P., Hren-Vencelj, H.: Contribution to the mechanism of interferon action. II. Influence of the interferon treatment on polysomal sedimentation in vaccinia infected cells. Zdrav. Vestn. **44**, 147–150 (1975a).

Schauer, P., Hren-Vencelj, H.: Contribution to understanding the mechanism of interferon activity. III. Electrophoretic separation of interferon-induced material. Zdrav. Vestn. **44**, 213–217 (1975b).

Scheiffahrt, F.: Interferon production. Dtsch. Med. Wschr. **96**, 1814 (1971).

Schellekens, H., DeWilde, G. A., Weimar, W.: Production and initial characterization of rat interferon. J. Gen. Virol. **46**, 243–248 (1980).

Schelleken, H., Weimar, W., Cantell, K., Stitz, L.: Antiviral effect of interferon *in vivo* may be mediated by the host. Nature **278**, 742 (1979).

Scherbakova, E. G., Eidelshtein, S. I., Furer, N. M.: Pharmacological study of human leucocytic interferon. Antibiotici **18**, 256–259 (1973).

Scherrer, R., Bic, E., Cohen, J.: Infectious pancreatic necrosis virus: a study of its replication and of its effect on interferon production in different cells and at different temperatures. Ann. Microbiol. **125**, 455 (1974).

Schlesinger, C., Ohlbaum, A., Grex, L., Stekel, A.: Decreased interferon production by leukocytes in marasmus. Amer. J. Clin. Nutrit. **29**, 758 (1976).

Schmidt, A., Chernajovsky, Y., Shulman, L., Federman, P., Berissi, H., Revel, M.: Interferon-induced phosphodiesterase degrading (2'–5') A and the C. C. A terminus transfer RNA. Proc. Natl. Acad. Sci. U. S. A. **76**, 4788–4792 (1979).

Schmidt, A., Zilberstein, A., Shulman, L., Federman, P., Berissi, H., Revel, M.: Interferon action: isolation of nucelase F, a translation inhibitor activated by interferon-induced (2'–5')oligo-isoadenylate. FEBS Letters **95**, 257–265 (1978).

Schramm-Thiel, N., Freiskorn, R., Kettner, M., May, G., Wacker, A.: Macromolecular virostatic substances and their interferon inducing activity. Arzneim. Forsch. **21**, 1382–1392 (1971).

Schroder, E. W., Chou, I. N., Jaken, S., Black, P.: Interferon inhibits the release of plasminogen activator from SV3T3 cells. Nature **276**, 828–829 (1978).

Schultz, R. M., Chirigos, M. A.: Similarities among factors that render macrophages tumoricidal in lymphokine and interferon preparations. Cancer Res. **38**, 1003 (1978).

Schultz, R. M., Chirigos, M. A.: Selective neutralization by antiinterferon globulin of macrophage activation by L-cell interferon, Brucella abortus ether extract, Salmonella typhimum lipopolysaccharide, and polyanions. Cell. Immunol. **48**, 52–58 (1979).

Schultz, R. M., Chirigos, M. A., Heine, U. I.: Functional and morphologic characteristics of interferon-treated macrophages. Cell. Immunol. **35**, 84–91 (1978).

Schultz, R. M., Pavlidis, N. A., Stoychkov, J. N., Chirigos, M. A.: Prevention of macrophage tumoricidal activity by agents known to increase cellular cylic AMP. Cell Immunol. **42**, 71–78 (1979).

Schultz, R. M., Pavlidis, N. A., Stylos, W. A., Chirigos, M. A.: Cytotoxic activity of interferon-treated macrophages studied by various inhibitors. Cancer Treat. Res. **62**, 1889–1892 (1978).

Schultz, R. M., Stoychkov, J. N., Pavlipis, N., Chirigos, M. A., Olkowski, Z. L.: Role of E-type prostaglandins in the regulation of interferon-treated macrophage cytotoxic activity. J. Reticuloendo. Soc. **26**, 93 (1979).

Schwartz, J.: Interferon sales $2 Billion-plus? Nature **285**, 4 (1980).

Scott, G. M., Cartwright, T., LeDu, G., Dicker, D.: Effect of human fibroblast interferon on vaccination in volunteers. J. Biological Standardization **6**, 73 (1977).

Scott, G. M., Csonka, G. W.: Effect of injections of small doses of human fibroblast interferon into genital warts-pilot study. Brit. J. Vener. Dis. **55**, 442–445 (1979).

Scott, G. M., Reed, S., Cartwright, T., Tyrrell, D.: Failure of human fibroblast interferon to protect against rhinovirus infection. Arch. Virol. (1980, in press).

Scott, G. M., Tyrrell, D. A. J.: Interferon: therapeutic fact or fiction for the 80's? Brit. Med. J. **280**, 1558–1562 (1980).

Seaman, W. E., Merigan, T. C., Talal, N.: Natural killing in estrogen-treated mice responds poorly to polyI·polyC despite normal stimulation of circulating interferon. J. Immunol. **123**, 2903 (1979).

Secher, D. S., Burke, D. C.: A monoclonal antibody for large-scale purification of human leukocyte interferon. Nature **285**, 446–449 (1980).

Sehgal, P. B., Gupta, S. L.: Regulation of the stability of polyI·polyC induced human fibroblast interferon messenger RNA. Proc. Natl. Acad. Sci. U.S.A. **77**, 3489–3493 (1980).

Sehgal, P. B., D. S., Lyles, Tamm, I.: Superinduction of human fibroblast interferon production: Further evidence for increased stability of interferon mRNA. Virology **89**, 186–190 (1978).

Sehgal, P. B., Sagar, A. D.: Heterogeneity of poly(I)·poly(C) induced human fibroblast interferon mRNA species. Nature (1980, in press).

Sehgal, P. B., Soreq, H., Tamm, I.: Does 3'-terminal poly(A) stabilize human fibroblast interferon messenger RNA in oocytes of xenopus laevis? Proc. Nat. Acad. Sci. U. S. A. **75**, 5030–5033 (1978).

Sehgal, P. B., Tamm, I.: Two mechanisms contribute to the superinduction of poly(I)·poly(C)-induced human fibroblast interferon production. Virology **92**, 240–244 (1979).

Sehgal, P. B., Tamm, I.: The transcription for poly(I)·poly(C)-induced human fibroblast interferon mRNA. Virology **102**, 245–250 (1980).

Sekellick, M. J., Marcus, P. I.: Persistent infection. 1. Interferon-inducing defective-interfering particles as mediators of cell sparing: Possible role in persistent infection by vesicular stomatitis virus. Virology **85**, 175–180 (1978).

Sekellick, M. J., Marcus, P. I.: Persistent infection. II. Interferon inducing temperature-sensitive mutants as mediators of cell sparing. Virology **95**, 36–47 (1979).

Sela, B. A., Gurari-Rotman, D.: Interferon abrogates the arrest of DNA synthesis in heterologous thymocytes treated with lectins. Biochem. Biophys. Res. Commun. **84**, 550–556 (1978).

Selgrade, M. J., Osborn, J. E.: Divergence of mouse brain interferon responses following virulent or avirulent NDV inoculation. Proc. Soc. Exp. Biol. Med. **143**, 12–18 (1973).

Sellers, R. F.: Multiplication, interferon production and sensitivity of virulent and attenuated strains of the virus of foot-and-mouth disease. Nature **198**, 1228–1229 (1963).

Sellers, R. F.,, Bennett, J. M., Mowat, G. N., Snowdown, W. A.: Some factors affecting interferon production by foot-and-mouth disease virus in bovine tissue cultures. Arch. ges. Virusforsch. **23**, 1–11 (1968).

Sellers, R. F., Mowat, G. N.: Interference between modified and virulent strains of foot-and-mouth disease virus. Arch. ges. Virusforsch. **23**, 20–26 (1968).

Sen, G. C., Hidehara, T., Lengyel, P.: Interferon, doublestranded RNA and protein phosphorylation. Characteristics of double-stranded RNA-activated protein kinase system partially purified from interferon-treated Ehrlich ascites tumor cells. J. of Biol. Chem. **253**, 5915–5920 (1978).

Sen, G. C., Sarkar, N. H.: Effects of interferon on the production of murine mammary tumor virus by mammary tumor cells in culture. Virology **102**, 431–443 (1980).

Sena, J. D., Rio, G. J.: Partial purification and characterization of RTG-2 fish cell interferon. Infect. Immun. **11**, 815 (1975).

Senik, A., Gresser, I., Maury, C., Gidlund, M., Orn, A., Wigzell, H.: Enhancement of mouse NK cells by interferon. Transplant. Proc. **11**, 993–996 (1979).

Senik, A., Gresser, I., Maury, C., Gidlund, M., Orn, A., Wigzell, H.: Enhancement by interferon of natural killer cell activity in mice. Cell. Immunol. **44**, 186–200 (1979).

Senik, A., Kolb, J. B., Orn, A., Gidlund, M.: Study of the mechanism for in vitro activation of mouse NK cells by interferon. Scand. J. Immunol. **12**, 51–60 (1980).

Senussi, O. A., Cartwright, T., Thompson, P.: Resolution of human fibroblast interferon into two distinct classes by thiol exhange chromatography. Arch. Virol. **62**, 323–332 (1979).

Sergiescu, D., Cerutti, I., Efthmiou, E., Kahan, A., Chany, C.: Adverse effects of interferon treatment on the life span of NZB mice. Biomed. Exp. **31**, 48 (1979).

Serkedzhieva, I.: Double-interferon induction in cell cultures. Acta Microbiol. Bulg. **1**, 82–89 (1978).

Sethi, K. K., Brandis, H.: Interferon enhances T cell mediated cytotoxicity of H-2 compatible target cells infected with UV-inactivated Herpes simplex virus. Arch. Virol. **57**, 177–183 (1978).

Seto, D. S., Brown, D. G., Gerring, J. P., Levy, D. A.: The effect of cell density on the production of interferon. Proc. Soc. Exp. Biol. Med. **145**, 434–437 (1974).

Seto, D. S., Carver, D. W.: Circulating interferon in sudden infant death syndrome. Proc. Soc. Exp. Biol. Med. **157**, 378 (1968).

Shcheglovitova, O. N., Ershov, F. I., Mentkevich, L. M.: Comparative studies of interferon production in mice with graft versus host (1978).

Shcherbakov, I. M.: Use of interferons and interferonogens in dermatology. Vestn. Dermatol. Venerol. **47**, 8–13 (1973).

Shcherbakova, E. G., Rastunova, G. A., Furer, N. M.: Use of the method of double induction for intensifying the process of interferon biosynthesis. Antibiotiki **19**, 539–542 (1971).

Sherbakova, E. G., Furer, N. M., Rastunova, G. A., Lituinov, A. N., Zhigachev, V. E.: Study of the antiviral action of a new boromolecular weight interferon inducer. Antibiotiki **21**, 838–842 (1976).

Shimizu, F., Satoh, J., Tada, M., Kumagai, K.: Suppression of in vitro growth of virulent and a virulent herpes simplex viruses by cell-mediated immune mechanisms, antibody and interferon. Infect. Immun. **22**, 752–757 (1978).

Shimizu, N., Sokawa, Y.: 2'5'-oligoadenylate synthetase activity in lymphocytes from normal mouse. J. Biol. Chem. **254**, 12034–12037 (1979).

Shingu, H., Sugiyama, M., Watanabe, M., Nakajima, T.: Effects of ozone and photochemical oxidants on interferon production by rabbit alveolar macrophages. Bull. Environ. Contam. Toxicol. **24**, 433–438 (1980).

Shinkai, K., Nishimura, T.: Efficient filtration of interferon through membrane filters. Jap. J. Microbiol. **20**, 251 (1976).

Shirasawa, N., Matsuno, T.: Suppression of the accumulation of steroid-inducible glutamine synthetase mRNA on embryonic chick retinal polysomes by interferon preparation. Biochim. Biophys. Acta **552**, 271–280 (1979).

Shitikova, G. S., Boldasov, V. K.: The interfering and interferon-inducing activity of attenuated and original parainfluenza virus strains. Prob. Virol. **4**, 445 (1977).

Shoham, J., Eshel, I., Aboud, M., Salzberg, S.: Thymic hormonal activity on human peripheral blood lymphocytes in vitro. II. Enhancement of the production of immune interferon by activated cells. J. Immunol. **125**, 54 (1980).

Shope, R. E.: An antiviral substance from Pencillum funiculosum. VI. Prevention of the establishment of passive immunity to Semliki Forest virus infection in mice by Melanine. J. Exp. Med. **124**, 15–32 (1966).

Shortridge, K. F.: Colostrum as a source of togavirus inhibitors. Arch. Dis. Child. **52**, 164 (1977).

Shpak, T. N.: Experimental basis for use of phonophoresis of interferon in herpetic keratitis. Ofthalmol. Zh. **34**, 82–84 (1979).

Shu, H. L.: Interfering and interferon-inducing capacity of NDV. I. Quantitative analysis and physicochemical characteristics. Arch. ges. Virusforsch. **46**, 179 (1974).

Shu, H. L.: Interfering and interferon-inducing capacity of NDV. II. Relationship between pyrogenic interfering and interferon-inducing activities. Arch. ges. Virusforsch. **46**, 191 (1974).

Shulitsev, G. P., Bertemirov, T. A., Dibizheva, G. V., Burtsev, V. I.: Interferon formation in chronic pyelonephritis patients. Klin. Med. **50**, 6265 (1972).

Sidwell, R. W., Huffman, J. M.: Use of disposable micro tissue culture plates for antiviral and interferon induction studies. Appl. Microbiol. **22**, 797–801 (1971).

Siegel, B. V.: Enhancement of interferon production by poly rI·poly rC in mouse cell cultures. Nature **254**, 531 (1975).

Silva, A., Bonavida, B., Targan, S.: Mode of action of interferon-mediated modulation of natural killer cytotoxic activity: recruitment of pre-NK cells and enhanced kinetics of lysis. J. Immunol. **125**, 479–484 (1980).

Simili, M., DeFerra, F., Baglioni, C.: Inhibition of RNA and protein synthesis in interferon-treated HeLa cells infected with vesicular stomatitis virus. J. Gen. Virol. **47**, 373–384 (1980).

Simon, P. L., Farrar, J. J., Kind, P. D.: Biochemical relationship between mouse immune interferon and a killer cell helper factor. J. Immunol. **122**, 127–132 (1979).

Sinatra, A.: Effect of actinomycin D on viral multiplication and on interferon production in cell cultures infected with 2 variants of measles virus. Boll. Ist. Sieroter. **50**, 453–461 (1971).

Singer, S. H., Ford, M.: The influence of mycoplasma infection on the induction of the antiviral state by polyinosinic-polycytidilic acid. Proc. Soc. Exp. Biol. Med. **139**, 1413 (1972).

Sinyachenko, O. V.: Bases and prospects for using interferon in treating patients with systemic lupus erythematosus. Ter. Arkh. **47**, 434–438 (1975).

Skurkovich, S. V., et al.: Interferon-containing plasma: preparation for treatment of viral infections. Biomed. Exp. **29**, 227 (1978).

Skurkovich, S. V., Klinova, E. G., Eremkina, E. I., Levina, N. V.: Immunosuppressive effect of an anti-interferon serum. Nature **247**, 551–552 (1974).

Skurkovich, S. V., Olshansky, A. Y., Klinova, E. G., Eremkina, E. I.: Preparation of nonspecific immunoglobulin against human leukocyte interferon. Bull. Exp. Biol. Med. **86**, 1473–1476 (1978).

Skurkovich, S. V., Olshansky, A. J., Samoilova, R. S., Eremkina, E. I.: Quantitative determination of human leukocyte interferon by microfluorometric immunoassay with FITC-labelled anti-interferon immunoglobulin. J. Immunol. Meth. **19**, 119 (1978).

Skurkovich, S. V., Sabashvili, M. K.: The obtainment of donor plasma containing interferon for clinical parenteral use. Probl. Germatol. Pereliv. Krov. **16**, 11–44 (1971).

Skurkovich, S. V., Skorikova, A. S., Eremkina, E. I.: Enhancement by interferon of lymphocyte cytotoxicity in normal individuals to cells of man lymphoblastoid lines. J. Immunol. **121**, 1173 (1978).

Skwarek, J.: Effects of some plant preparations on the influenza virus propogation. II. Induction of interferon. Acta. Pol. Pharm. **36**, 715–720 (1979).

Slate, D. L., Ruddle, F. H.: Antibodies to chromosome 21 coded cell surface components can block response to human interferon. Cyto. Cell Genet. **22**, 265–269 (1978).

Slate, D. L., Ruddle, F. H.: Sensitivity of human-mouse somatic cell hybrids to human interferon. Cyto. Cell Genet. **22**, 270–274 (1978).

Slate, D. L., Ruddle, F. H.: Fibroblast interferon in man is coded by two loci on separate chromosomes. Cell **16**, 171–180 (1979).

Slate, D. L., Ruddle, F. H.: Genetics of the interferon system. Pharmacol. Therap. **4**, 221–230 (1979).

Slattery, E., Gosh, N., Samanta, H., Lengyel, P.: Interferon, dsRNA and RNA degration-activation of an endonuclease by (2'-5') A. Proc. Nat. Acad. Sci. U. S. A. **76**, 4778–4782 (1979).

Slattery, E., Taira, H., Broeze, R., Lengyel, P.: Mouse interferons: production by Ehrlich ascites tumor cells infected with Newcastle disease virus and its enhancement of theophylline. J. Gen. Virol. **49**, 91–96 (1980).

Slavina, E. G., Karmanova, N. V., Leipunskaya, L., Zinzar, S. N., Reinhoper, J., Svet-Moldavsky, G. J.: Rapidly acquired cytotoxity of lymphoid cells from mice inoculated with allogeneic spleen cells. J. Nat. Can. Inst. **57**, 1233–1236 (1976).

Smirnova, T. D., Kagan, G.: Effect of mycoplasma-viral infection of a primary culture of chick embryo cells on interferon production induced by langat virus. Zh. Mikrobiol. Epidemiol. Immunobiol. **48**, 54–58 (1971).

Smith, H.: Interferon therapy in myelomatosis. Lancet in: 1248–1249 (1979).

Smith, K. A., Cornwell, G. G., McIntyre, O. R.: The effect of polyI:C and interferon on lymphocyte DNA synthesis, in: Lymphocyte Recognition and efector mechanisms (Lindahl-Kiessling, K., Osoba, D., eds.), p. 101. Academic Press (1974).

Sodja, I.: Interferon production by rabies virus strains isolated from wild rodents. Acta Virol. **19**, 84 (1975).

Sokawa, Y., Ando, T., Ishihara, Y.: Induction of 2'5-oligoadenylate synthetase and interferon in mouse trigeminal ganglia infected with herpes simplex virus. Infect. Immun. **28**, 719–723 (1980).

Sokolova, T. M., Kisling, U.: Molecular fundamentals of interferon synthesis and action. Antibiotik. **23**, 1112 (1978).

Soloviev, V. D., Baktemirov, T. A., Feddorova, I. U. B., Marova, E. I., Kliachko, V. P.: Determination of interferon formation by blood leukocytes in patients with endocrine diseases. Probl. Endokrinol. (Mosk.) **20**, 21 (1974).

Soloviev, V. D., Bektemirov, T. A., Moisiadi, S. A.: Interferon and antibody in rabbits during experimental herpetic keratitis. Vopr. Virusol. **19**, 323–325 (1974a). (In Russian.)

Soloviev, V. D., Bektemirov, T. A., Moisiadi, S. A.: Relation between interferon production and susceptibility to herpetic keratitis in rabbits. Vopr. Virusol. **19**, 325–327 (1974b). (In Russian.)

Soloviev, V. D., Gutman, RN. R., Manakhova, L. S.: The interferon inducing capacity of influenza B virus strains and their sensitivity to exogenous interferon. Vopr. Virusol. **3**, 312 (1976). (In Russian.)

Soloviev, V. D., Kitsak, V. Y., Bektemirov, T. A., Bocharov, A. F., Moisiadi, S. A., Delimbetova, G. A., Chuev, Y. V.: The influence of exogenous interferon on the course of latent oncornavirus infection of J-96 cells. Vopr. Virusol. **2**, 196 (1977). (In Russian.)

Soloviev, V. D., Malinovskaia, V., Khesinia, E., Pokidysheva, L. N., Marchenko, V. I.: The acid phosphatase activity and capacity for interferon production of peritoneal exudate cells from mice of different ages. Vopr. Virusol. **18**, 533–538 (1973). (In Russian.)

Soloviev, V. D., Mentkevich, L. M., Shheglovitova, O. N., Orlova, T. G.: Bone marrow interferon of mice. Bull. Exp. Biol. Med. **73**, 74–77 (1972).

Soloviev, V. D., Mentkevich, L. M., Orlova, T. G., Shcheglovitova, O. N., Osidze, N. G., Gunenkov, V. V.: Bone-marrow interferon. Bull. Exp. Biol. Med. **80**, 786 (1975).

Soloviev, V. D., Nekliudova, L. I., Bektemirova, T. A., Fedorova, I. U. B.: Interferon formation in Hong-Kong influenza. Vopr. Virusol. **16**, 548–552 (1971). (In Russian.)

Soloviev, V. D., Orlova, T. G., Mentkevich, L. M., Shcheglovitova, O. N., Kuznetsov, V. P.: Human bone marrow interferon. Vopr. Virusol. **2**, 173 (1976). (In Russian.)

Soloviev, V. D., Sorokin, A. M.: Comparative effect of actinomycin D. imuran, hydrocortisone on interferon and antibody formation in mice. Bull. Exp. Biol. Med. **81**, 65 (1976).

Soloviev, V. D., Sorokin, A. M., Gutman, N. R.: Effect of immunodepression on virus multiplication and interferon and antibody formation in animals. Bull. Exp. Biol. Med. **80**, 1456 (1976).

Sonnenfeld, G., Harned, C. L., Thaniyavarn, S., Huff, T., Mandel, A. D., Nerland, D. E.: Type II interferon induction and passive transfer depress the murine cytochrome P-450 drug metabolism system. Antimicrob. Agents Chemother. **17**, 969–972 (1980).

Sonnenfeld, G., Mandel, A. D., Merigan, T. C.: Time and dosage dependence of immunoenhancement by murine type II interferon preparations. Cell. Immunol. **40**, 285–293 (1978).

Sonnenfeld, G., Mandel, A. D., Merigan, T. C.: In vitro production and cellular origin of murine type II interferon. Immunol. **36**, 883–390 (1979).

Sonnenfeld, G., Merigan, T. C.: The role of interferon in viral infections. Springer Seminars Immunopath. **2**, 311–338 (1979 a).

Sonnenfeld, G., Merigan, T. C.: A regulatory role for interferon in immunity. Ann. N. Y. Acad. Sci. **332**, 345–355 (1979 b).

Sonnenfeld, G., Salvin, B., Youngner, J. S.: Cellular source of interferons in the circulation of mice with delayed hypersensitivity. Infect. Immun. **18**, 283–290 (1977).

Sorokin, A. M.: Action of x-rays and imuran on the formation of interferon and antibodies. Vopr. Virusol. **18**, 443–446 (1973). (In Russian.)

Sreevalsan, T., Lockart, R. Z., jr.: Inhibition by puromycin of the initiation of synthesis of infectious RNA and virus by chicken cells infected with WEE virus. Virology **24**, 91–94 (1964).

Sreevalsan, T., Taylor-Papadimitriou, J., Rozengurt, E.: Selective inhibition by interferon of serum-stimulated biochemical events in 3T3 cells. Biochem. Biophys. Res. Commun. **87**, 679–685 (1979).

Stahlman, S. A., Sakguchi, A. Y., Hiti, A.: Interferon production and activity in mouse neuroblastoma cells. Arch. Virol. **57**, 91 (1971).

Stancek, D.: Interferon production by and recovery of persistently infected L cells after treatment with immune serum. Acta Virol. **9**, 275–278 (1965).

Stancek, D., Taborsky, I.: In vitro studies on mouse interferons induced with phage doublestranded RNA synthetic double-stranded polynucleotides and viral inducers. Med. Microbiol. Immunol. **160**, 65–70 (1974).

Stanton, G. J., Johnson, H. M., Baron, S.: Role of interferon in virus infections and antibody formation, in: Pathobiology Annual (Ioachim, H. L., ed.), Vol. 8 (1979).

Stanton, G. J., Langford, M. P., Baron, S.: Effect of interferon, elevated temperature, and cell type on replication of acute hemorrhagic conjunctivitis viruses. Infect. Immun. **18**, 370–376 (1977).

Stanwick, T. L., Hallum, J. V.: Role of interferon in 6 cells lines persistently infected with rubella virus. Infect. Immun. **10**, 810–815 (1974).

Stark, G. R., Dower, W. J., Schimke, R. T., Brown, R. E., Kerr, I. M.: 2–5A synthetase: assay, distribution, and variation with growth or hormone status. Nature **278**, 471–473 (1979).

Starr, S. E., Tolpin, M. D., Friedman, H. M., Paucker, K., Plotkin, S. A.: Impaired cellular immunity to cytomegalovirus in congenitally infected children and their mothers. J. Infect. Dis. **140**, 500–505 (1979).

Stebbing, N.: Interferon and inducers *in vivo*. Nature **279**, 581 (1979).

Stebbing, N.: Protection of mice against infection with wild-type Mengo virus and interferon-sensitive mutant (IS-1) by polynucleotides and interferons. J. Gen. Virol. **44**, 255–260 (1979).

Stebbing, N., Dawson, K. M.: The formation of complexes between polynucleotides, carboxymethylcellulose and polylysine which are antiviral in mice without inducing interferon. Molec. Pharmacol. **16**, 313–323 (1979).

Stebbing, N., Dawson, K. M., Lindley, I. J. D.: Requirement for macrophages for interferon to be effective against encephalomyocarditis virus infection in mice. Infect. Immun. **19**, 5–11 (1978).

Stebbing, N., Grantham, C. A.: Antiviral activity against EMC virus and SFV and acute toxicity of poly I·poly C administered sequentially to mice. Arch. Virol. **51**, 199–215 (1976).

Stebbing, N., Grantham, C. A., Carey, N. H.: Antiviral activity of single-stranded homopolynucleotides against encephalomyocarditis virus and Semliki forest virus in adult mice without interferon induction. J. Gen. Virol. **30**, 21 (1976).

Stebbing, N., Grantham, C. A., Kaminski, F. K.: Investigation of the antiviral mechanism of poly I and poly C against EMC virus infection in mice in absence of interferon induction. J. Gen. Virol. **32**, 25–30 (1976).

Stefanos, S., Catinot, L., Wietzerbin, J., Falcoff, E.: Production of antibodies against mouse immune T (Type II) interferon and their neutralizing properties. J. Gen. Virol. **50**, 225–229 (1980).

Steinberg, A. D., Baron, S., Uhlendorf, C., Talal, N.: Depression of the interferon response to polyinosinic-polycytidylic acid by specific antibody. Proc. Soc. Exp. Biol. Med. 137, 558–561 (1971).

Stephen, E. L., Hilmas, D. E., Levy, H. B., Spertzel, R. O.: Protective and toxic effects of a nuclease-resistant derivative of poly I·C on Venezuelan equine encephalomyelitis virus in rhesus monkeys. J. Infect. Dis. 139, 267–272 (1979).

Stewart II., W. E.: Antiviral and other activities of pure interferons and interferoids. Proceedings of the IVth Intl. Cong. Virology, Den Haag, Netherlands (1978).

Stewart II, W. E.: Varied biologic effects of interferon, in: Interferon – 1979 (Gresser, I., ed.), pp. 29–51. London: Academic Press.

Stewart II, W. E.: Purification and properties of interferon proteins, in: Microbiology – 1980. ASM Publ. (1980, in press).

Stewart II, W. E., Blalock, J. E., Burke, D. C., Chany, C., Dunnick, J. K., Falcoff, E., Friedman, R. M., Galasso, G. J., Joklik, W. K., Vilcek, J. T., Youngner, J. S., Zoon, K. C.: Interferon Nomenclature. Nature 286, 110 (1980).

Stewart II, W. E., Havell, E. A.: Characterization of a subspecies of mouse interferon cross-reactive on human cells and antigenically related to human leukocyte interferon. Virology 101, 315–318 (1980).

Stewart II, W. E., LeGoff, S., Wiranowska-Stewart, M.: Characterization of two distinct molecular populations of type I mouse interferons. J. Gen. Virol. 37, 277–284 (1977).

Stewart II, W. E., Lin, L. S.: Antiviral activities of interferons. Pharm. Therap. 6, 443–512 (1979).

Stewart II, W. E., Sarkar, F. H., Taira, H., Hall, A., Nagata, S., Weissmann, C.: Comparisons of some biological and physiocochemical properties of human leukocyte interferons produced by human leukocytes and by E. coli. Gene 11, 181–186 (1980).

Stewart II, W. E., Wiranowska-Stewart, M., Koistinen, V., Cantell, K.: Effect of glycosylation inhibitors on the production and properties of human leukocyte interferon. Virology 97, 473–476 (1979).

Stinebring, W. R.: Interferon. Ann. N. Y. Acad. Sci. 284, 666 (1977).

Stitz, L., Schellekens, H.: Influence of input multiplicity of infection on the antiviral activity of interferon. J. Gen. Virol. 46, 205–210 (1980).

Stohlmon, S. A., Sakaguchi, A. Y., Hiti, A.: Interferon production and activity in mouse neuroblastoma cells. Arch. Virol. 57, 91–96 (1978).

Stohlmon, S. A., Sakagushi, A. Y., Weiner, L. P.: Rescue of a positive stranded RNA virus from antigen negative neuroblastoma cells. Life Sci. 24, 1029–1035 (1979).

Strander, H., Adamson, U., Aparisi, T., Brostrom, L. A., Cantell, K., Einhorn, S., Hall, K., Ingimarsson, S., Nilsonne, U., Soderberg, G.: Adjuvant interferon treatment of human osteosarcoma. Recent Results Cancer Res. 68, 40–44 (1978).

Strannegard, O., Larsson, I., Lundgren, E., Miorner, H., Persson, H.: Modulation of immune responses in newborn and adult mice by interferon. Infect. Immun. 20, 334–338 (1978).

Strauchen, J. A., Young, N. A., Friedman, R. M.: Interferon-mediated inhibition of mouse mammary tumor virus expression in cultured cells. Virology 82, 232–236 (1977).

Streuli, M., Nagata, S., Weissmann, C.: Not less than three different species of type alpha (leukocyte) interferon in man: nucleotide sequence of the cDNA for interferon alpha2 (1980, in press).

Stringfellow, D. A.: Prostaglandin restoration of the interferon response of hyporeactive animals. Science 201, 376 (1979).

Stringfellow, D. A.: Antiviral and interferon-inducing properties of interferon inducers administered with prostaglandins. Antimicrob. Agents Chemother. 17, 455–460 (1980).

Stringfellow, D. A., Weed, S. D.: Interferon induction by and toxicity of polyI·polyC., mismatched analogs and polyI·polyC L-lysine with carboxymethycellulose. Antimicrob. Agents Chemother. 17, 988–992 (1980).

Stringfellow, D. A., Weed, S. D., Underwood, G. E.: Antiviral and interferon inducing properties of 1,5-diamino anthraquinones. Antimicrob. Agents Chemother. 15, 111–119 (1979).

Strutsovskaia, A. L., Ulanovskaia, T. I., Furer, N. M., Ermolieva, Z. V.: Experience with using leukocytic interferon with methacil in influenza in children. Antibiotiki 20, 170–173 (1975).

Suarez, M. G., Chany, C., Cassingena, R., Vignal, M., Lemaitre, J.: Localization of chromosome coding for simian interferon synthesis. C. R. Acad. Sci. (Paris) D 274, 3632–3634 (1972).

Suenaga, T., Okuyama, T., Yashida, I., Azuma, M.: Effect of mycobacterium tuberculosis BCG on the resistance of mice to ectromelia virus infection: Participation of interferon in enhanced resistance. Infect. Immun. **20**, 312 (1978).

Sugiyama, M., Epstein, L. B.: Effect of Corynebacterium parvum on human T-lymphocyte interferon production and T-lymphocyte proliferation in vitro. Cancer Res. **38**, 4467–4473 (1978).

Sugiyama, M., Shingu, H., Shibata, T., Kausumoto, S., Nakajima, T.: The effect of ozone and photo-chemical oxidants on the interferon production of tonsillar lymphocyte. Acta Oto-Laryng. **87**, 567–575 (1979).

Sundmacher, R., Cantell, K., Houg, P., Neumann-Haefelin, D.: Role of debridement and interferon in treatment of dendritic keratitis. Ophthalmologie **207**, 77–80 (1978).

Sundmacher, R., Cantell, K., Skoda, R., Hallermann, C., Neumann-Haefelin, D.: Human leukocyte and fibroblast interferon in a combination therapy of dendritic keratitis. Albrecht von Graefes Arch. Ophthalmol. **208**, 229–234 (1978).

Suzuki, F., Suzuki, C., Shimura, E., Maeda, H., Fujii, T., Ishida, N.: Antiviral and interferon inducing activities of a new peptidomannon KS-2 extracted from culture mycelia of Lentinus edodes. J. Antibiot. **32**, 1336–1345 (1979).

Svec, J., Svec, P.: On the mechanism of interferon induction by polynucleotides. Suppressive effect of poly(rI)poly(rC) on the liberation of histamine by polycations. Arch. ges. Virusforsch. **44**, 307–312 (1974).

Sypula, A., Zielinska-Jenczylik, J.: Production of interferon in human diploid cell cultures. II. Effect of various factors on interferon production in human diploid cell cultures. Arch. Immunol. Therap. Exp. **27**, 561–570 (1979).

Sypula, A., Zielinska-Jenczylik, J., Maresz-Babcyszyn, J.: Effect of bacteriocins on interferon production. Arch. Immunol. Therap. Exp. **25,** 651 (1977).

Sypula, A., Zielinska-Jenczylik, J., Tomaszewska, Z., Skurska, Z.: Comparative studies on chikken and mouse interferons induced with NDV. Arch. Immunol. Therap. Exp. **21**, 219–226 (1973).

Syulowa, A., Zielinska-Jenczylik, J., Skurska, L.: Inhibition of cowpox virus infection in mice by interferon therapy. Arch. Immunol. Therap. Exp. **20**, 837–840 (1972).

Taborsky, I.: Effect of cychoheximide on *in vitro* formation of rabbit granulocyte pyrogen induced with influenza A/PR8 virus or endotoxin. Acta Virol. **16**, 376–381 (1972).

Taborsky, I.: Heterogeneity of rabbit serum interferon induced by poly I·C. Arch. ges. Virusforsch. **44**, 51–57 (1974a).

Taborsky, I.: Electrofocusing of interferons induced by poly I·C in the serum and peritoneal exudate granulocytes of rabbits. Arch. ges. Virusforsch. **44**, 58–61 (1974 b).

Taborsky, I., Dolnik, V.: Physico-chemical properties of interferon produced by a mixed leukocyte suspension. Acta Virol. **21**, 359 (1977a).

Taborsky, I., Dolnik, V.: Ability of polymorphonuclear blood cells to produce interferon after induction with phage double-stranded RNA. Acta Virol. **21**, 499–502 (1977).

Taborsky, I., Doskocil, J., Stancek, D.: Purification of mouse interferon induced by isotopically labelled double-stranded F2 phage RNA. J. Hyg. Epidem. Microbiol. Immunol. **21**, 261 (1977).

Taborsky, I., Doskocil, J., Zajicova, V.: Pyrogenic activity of dsRNA from E. coli F2 phage. Acta Virol. **18**, 106–112 (1974).

Tagliabue, A., Mantovani, A., Kilgallen, M., Herberman, R. B., McCoy, J. L.: Natural cytotoxicity of mouse monocytes and macrophages. J. Immunol. **122**, 1263–1270 (1979).

Taira, H., Broeze, R. J., Jayaram, B. M., Lengyel, P., Hunkapiller, M. W., Hood, L. E.: Mouse interferons: amino terminal amino acid sequences of various species. Science **207**, 528–530 (1980).

Taira, H., Broeze, R. J., Slattery, E., Lengyel, P.: Large-scale production of mouse interferon from monolayers of Ehrlich ascites tumor cells. J. Gen. Virol. **49**, 231–234 (1980).

Takehara, M., Kuida, K., Mori, K.: Antiviral activity of virus-like particles from Lentinus edodes. Arch. Virol. **59**, 269–274 (1979).

Takeyama, H., Kawashima, K., Kobayashi, M., Yamada, K., Ito, Y.: Antitumor effect of interferon preparation on murine transplantable tumors. GANN **69**, 641–648 (1978).

Takeyama, H., Kawashima, K., Yamada, K., Ito, Y.: Properties of interferon-induced by purified protein derivative of tuberculin in mice sensitized with BCG or cell-wall skeleton of BCG. GANN 70, 421–428 (1979).

Talas, M., Glaz, T.: Type I interferon-induced in mice by infection with *Trypanosoma equiperdum*. J. Infect. Dis. 139, 595–598 (1979).

Talas, M., Novokhatsky, A. S., Batkai, L.: Induction of interferon and radioprotective activity of poly G-polyC in mice. Acta Microb. Acad. Sci. Hung. 26, 213–216 (1979).

Talas, M., Szolgay, E.: Radioprotective activity of interferon inducers. Arch. Virol. 56, 309–315 (1978).

Tamm, I., Sehgal, P. B.: New evidence for regulated transcription of hnRNA and for regulated translation of interferon mRNA in human cells, in: Specific Eukaryotic Genes (Engberg, J., et al., eds.), pp. 424–441. Copenhagen: Munksgaard (1978).

Tamm, I., Sehgal, P. B.: Interferons. Amer. J. Med. 66, 3–5 (1979).

Tan, Y. H., Barakat, F., Berthold, W., Smith-Johannsen, H., Tan, C.: The isolation and amino acid/sugar composition of human fibroblastoid interferon. J. Biol. Chem. 254, 8067–8073 (1979).

Tan, Y. H., Smith-Johannsen, H., Okamura, H.: Isolation of human fibroblastoid interferon for structure and function analyses. Ann. N. Y. Acad. Sci. (1980, in press).

Tanamoto, K., Abe, C., Homma, J. Y., Kojima, Y.: Regions of the lipopolysaccharide of Pseudomonas aeruginosa essential for antitumor and interferon inducing activities. Europ. J. Biochem. 97, 623 (1979).

Tanamoto, K., Abe, C., Homma, Y., Kuretani, K., Hoshi, A., Kojima, Y.: A compound possessing antitumor and interferon inducing activities derived from common antigen (OEP) Pseudomonas aeruginosa. J. Biochem. 83, 711–718 (1978).

Taniguchi, T., Mantei, N., Schwarzstein, M., Nagata, S., Muramatsu, M., Weissmann, C.: Human leukocyte and fibroblast interferons are structurally related. Nature 285, 547–549 (1980).

Taniguchi, T., Ohno, S., Fujiikuriyama, Y., Muramatsu, M.: The nucleotide sequence of human fibroblast interferon cDNA. Gene 10, 11–16 (1980).

Taniguchi, T., Sakai, M., FujllKuriyama, T., Muramatsu, M., Kobayashi, S., Sudo, T.: Construction and identification of a bacterial plasmid containing the human fibroblast interferon gene sequence. Proc. Jap. Acad. B. 55, 464–469 (1979).

Targan, S., Dorey, F.: Interferon activation of pre-spontaneous killer (Pre-SK) cells and alteration in kinetics of both Pre-SK and active SK cells. J. Immunol. 124, 2156–2160 (1980).

Tarodi, B., Metz, D. H., Douglas, A., Russell, W. C.: A study of events in chick cells infected with human adenovirus type 5 and their relationship to the induction of interferon. J. Gen. Virol. 36, 425–436 (1977).

Tarr, G. C., Armstrong, J. A., Ho, M.: Production of interferon and serum hyporeactivity factor in mice infected with murine cytomegalovirus. Infect. Immun. 19, 903 (1975).

Taylor-Papadimitriou, J., Stoker, M. G., Riddle, P.: Further manifestations of abortive transformation of BHK 21 cells by polyoma virus. Int. J. Cancer 7, 269–276 (1977).

Tazulakhova, E. B., Ershov, F. I.: Mechanisms of action of interferon. Antibiotiki 17, 940–945 (1972).

Tazulakhova, E. B., Ershov, F. I.: Protein repressor of interferon. Vopr. Virusol. 6, 703–706 (1978). (In Russian.)

Tazulakhova, E. B., Novokhatsky, A. S., Ershov, F. I.: Interferon induction by, and antiviral effect of poly I.C in experimental viral infection. Acta Virol. 17, 487–492 (1973).

Tazulakhova, E. B., Zaitseva, O. V., Ershov, F. I.: Biological characteristics of interferon production repressor. Antibiotiki 75, 145 (1980).

Tennant, R. W., Schluter, B., Myer, F. E., Otten, J. A., Yang, W. K.: Genetic evidence for a product of the Fv-1 locus that transfers resistance to mouse leukemia virus. J. Virol. 20, 589–596 (1976).

ter Meulen, V.: Present state of antiviral therapy. Monschr. Kinderheilkd. 127, 367–371 (1979).

ter Meulen, V., Katz, M., Kackell, Y. M., Barbant-Brodano, G., Koprowski, H., Lennette, E. H.: Subacute sclerosing panencephalitis: In vitro characterization of viruses isolated from brain cells in culture. J. Infect. Dis. 126, 11–23 (1972).

ter Meulen, V., Martin, S. J.: Genesis and maintenance of a persistent infection by canine distemper virus. J. Gen. Virol. 32, 431–440 (1976).

Ternovyi, M. K.: Effect of interferonogenic complex on thymidine 3H-labelling of DNA, RNA and proteins of marrow cells after total x-irradiation of mice. Ukr. Biokhim. Zh. 50, 98–101 (1978). (In Russian.)

Tevethia, S. S., Greenfield, R. S., Rieder, V., Tevethia, M. J.: Biology of Simian virus 40 transplantation antigen. IV. Inhibition by human interferon of expression of SV40 TrAg in SV40 infected monkey cells. Virology 95, 587–592 (1979).

Teyssie, A. R., Holstein, B. A., Pirosky, R. R., Kohan, S. S.: Interferon induced by tumoral DNA in a homologous system. Acta Virol. 17, 151–154 (1973).

Teyssie, A., Knecher, L., DeHolstein, B.: Interferon in vitro infections with Junin virus. Medicina 37, 53 (1977).

Thacore, H. R.: Rescue of vesicular stomatitis virus from homologous and heterologous interferon-induced resistance in human cell cultures by poxvirus. Infect. Immun. 14, 311–314 (1976).

Thacore, H. R.: Effect of interferon in transcription and translation of vesicular stomatitis virus in human and simian cell cultures. J. Gen. Virol. 41, 421–426 (1978).

Thacore, H. R., Youngner, J. S.: Cells persistently infected with Newcastle disease virus. II. Ribonucleic acid and protein synthesis in cells infected with mutants isolated from persistently infected L cells. J. Virol. 6, 42–48 (1970).

Thang, M. N., Thang, D., Chelbialix, M. K., Robertgalliot, B., Commoychevalier, M. J., Chany, C.: Human leukocyte interferon relationship between molecular structure and species specificity. Proc. Nat. Acad. Sci. 76, 3717–3721 (1979).

Theil, K. W., Mohanty, S. B., Hetrick, F. M.: Effect of poly I:C on infectious bovine rhinotracheitis virus infection in calves. Proc. Soc. Exp. Biol. Med. 137, 1176–1179 (1971).

Thilly, W. G., Levine, D. W.: Microcarrier culture; a homogeneous environment for studies of cellular biochemistry. Methods Enzymol. 58, 184–194 (1979).

Thind, I. S., Price, W. H.: A new specific humoral viral resistance factor serum protective factor some biologic and physical properties. J. Immunol. 106, 1559–1565 (1971).

Thomopoulos, S. P., Kosmakos, F. C., Pastan, I., Lovelace, E.: Cyclic AMP increases the concentration of insulin receptors in cultured fibroblast and lymphocytes. Biochem. Biophys. Res. Comm. 75, 246 (1977).

Thormar, H., Wisniewski, H. M., Lin, F. H.: Sera and cerebrospinal fluids from normal uninfected sheep containing a visna virus inhibiting factor. Nature 279, 245–246 (1979).

Thygeson, P., Ostler, H. B.: Zoster and herpes simplex virus uveitis: a comparison, in: Immunology and Immunopathology of the Eye (Silverstein, A. M., O'Connor, G. R., eds.), pp. 230–240. New York: Masson (1979).

Toba, M., Suzuki, H., Sekine, N.: Absence of interferon production in a newly established human cell line. Intervirology 11, 221–226 (1979).

Tokmadze, T. L., Lezhava, Z. M. M., Georgadze, I. I., Korsantiia, B. M.: Mechanism of the production of interferon in the lymphoid formations of the throat. Vest. Otorinolaringol. 6, 18–23 (1975).

Tomida, M., Takenaga, K., Yamamoto, Y., Hozumi, M.: Enhancement by dsRNA of production of cultured mouse peritoneal macrophages of differentiation-stimulating factors for mouse myeloid leukemic cells Biochem. J. Molecular Aspects 176, 665–669 (1978).

Tomita, Y., Kuwata, T.: Suppression of murine leukemia virus production by ouabain and interferon in mouse cells. J. Gen. Virol. 38, 223–230 (1978).

Tomita, Y., Kuwata, T.: Suppressive effects of interferon on syncytuim formation by RD-114 virus in human transformed cells. J. Gen. Virol. 43, 111–118 (1979).

Toneva, V.: Swine cell systems as interferon producers. IV. Comparative studies on the correlation between virulence of different Newcastle disease virus strains and their potency as interferon inducers. Arch. Immunol. Therap. Exp. 25, 679–682 (1977).

Tongaonkar, S. S., Ghosh, S. N.: Interferon induction by arboviruses. Indian J. Med. Res. 69, 865–873 (1979).

Torosov, T. M., Gaeva, L. L., Kurbatova, G. E.: The effect of methacil and nerobol on the formatin of interferon and specific antibodies in rabbits vaccinated with vaccinia. Vopr. Virusol. 17, 1460–1463 (1972). (In Russian.)

Torrence, P. F., Declercq, E., Waters, J. A., Witkop, B.: A potent interferon inducer derived from poly (7-deazaino sinic acid). Biochem. 13, 440 (1974).

Torrence, P. F., Friedman, R. M.: Are dsRNA-directed inhibition of protein synthesis in interferon-treated cells and interferon induction related phenomena? J. Biol. Chem. **254**, 1259–1267 (1979).

Torrence, P. F., Kovidov, S., Witkop, B.: Dependence of interferon induction on nucleic acid conformation. Proc. Natl. Acad. Sci. U.S.A. **73**, 3785–3789 (1976).

Toth, F., Talas, M.: Effect of the interferon inducer tilorone in inbred CBA mice. Acta Microb. Acad. Sci. Hung. **23**, 325 (1976).

Tovey, M. G., Brouty-Boye, D.: The use of the chemostat to study the relationship between cell growth rate, viability and the effect of interferon on L1210 cells. Exp. Cell Res. **118**, 383 (1979).

Tovey, M. G., Lenoir, G., Begon-Lours, J., Tapiero, H., Rochette-Egly, C.: The effects of mitogens on the expression of Epstein-Barr virus antigen in human lymphoid cell lines. J. Immunol. **123**, 138–142 (1979).

Tovey, M. G., Mathison, G. E., Pirt, S. J.: The production of interferon by chemostat cultures of mouse LS-cells grown in chemically-defined protein free medium. J. Gen. Virol. **20**, 29–35 (1973).

Tovey, M. G., Rochetteegly, C., Castagna, M.: Effect of interferon on concentrations of cyclic nucleotides in cultured cells. Proc. Nat. Acad. Sci. **76**, 3890–3893 (1979).

Toy, S. T., Gifford, G. E.: Interferon production with different multiplicities of Semliki Forest virus. Proc. Soc. Exp. Biol. Med. **126**, 787–780 (1967).

Trapman, J.: A systematic study of interferon production by mouse L929 cells induced by polyI·polyC and DEAE-dextran. FEBS Lett. **98**, 107–110 (1979).

Trapman, J.: Distinct antigenic character of two components of polyI·polyC-induced mouse L cell interferon. FEBS Lett. **109**, 137–140 (1980).

Traugh, J. A., Sharp, S. B.: Protein modification enzymes associated with the protein synthesizing complex from rabbit reticulocytes. Protein kinase, phosphoprotein phosphatase and acetyltransferase. J. Biol. chem. **252**, 3738 (1977).

Treagan, L., Furst, A.: Inhibition of interferon synthesis in mammalian cell cultures after nickel treatment. Res. Commun. Chem. Pathol. Pharmacol. **1**, 395–402 (1970).

Treagan, L., Jayne, A., Prato, C.: Variable response of normal and transformed mouse cells to interferon inducers. Acta Virol. **20**, 83 (1976).

Treuner, J., Dannecker, G., Niethammer, D.: Effect of interferon on the cell growth under experimental and clinical conditions. Eur. J. Pediat. **133**, 185 (1980).

Treuner, J., Niethammer, D., Dannecker, G., Hagmann, R., Neef, V., Hofschneider, P. H. Successful treatment of nasopharyngeal carcinoma with interferon. Lancet **i**, 817–818 (1980).

Trinchieri, G., Perussia, B., Santoli, D., Cerottini, J. C.: Human natural killer cells. Transplant. Proc. **11**, 807–810 (1979).

Trinchieri, G., Santoli, D.: Antiviral activity induced by culturing lymphocytes with tumor-derived or virus transformed cells. Enhancement of human natural killer cell activity by interferon and antagonistic inhibition of susceptibility of target cells to lysis. J. Exp. Med. **147**, 1314–1320 (1978).

Trinchieri, G., Santoli, D., Dee, R. R., Knowles, B. B.: Antiviral activity induced by culturing lymphocytes with tumor-derived or virus transformed cells. Identification of the antiviral activity as interferon and characterization of the human effector lymphocyte subpopulation. J. Exp. Med. **147**, 1299 (1978).

Trinchieri, G., Santoli, D., Koprowski, H.: Spontaneous cell-mediated cytotoxicity in humans: Role of interferon and immunoglobulins. J. Immunol. **120**, 1849 (1978).

Trofatter, K. F., jr., Daniels, C. A.: Effects of prostaglandins and cyclic AMP modulators on herpes simplex virus growth and interferon response in human cells. Infect. Immun. **27**, 158–167 (1980).

Trousdale, M. D., Paque, R. E., Nealon, T., Gauntt, C. J.: Assessment of coxsackievirus B3 ts mutants for induction of myocarditis in a murine model. Infect. Immun. **23**, 486–495 (1979).

Trubina, L. M., Yakovenko, Z. F., Itkis, S. N., Zakharchenko, E. M.: Interferon production induced by various viruses in cultures of leukocytes from children vaccinated against measles. Acta Virol. **16**, 446 (1972).

Trueblood, M. S., Manjara, J.: Response of bovine viruses to interferon. Cornell Vet. **62**, 3–12 (1972).

Tsai, S. C., Appel, M. J.: Interferon induction in dogs. Amer. J. Vet. Res. **40**, 356–361 (1979).

Tsiang, H., Atanasiu, P.: Immunosuppression and role of interferon in hamsters infected with rabies virus. C. R. Acad. Sci. **D276**, 1085–1088 (1973).

Turgunbaev, O. T.: Use of interferon for prevention of acute respiratory viral diseases in children's collectives (literature survey). Zdravookhr. Kirg. **5**, 57–59 (1975).

Turkin, D.: The interferon-newest weapon in the fight against viral diseases. Amer. Pharmacy **20**, 33–35 (1980).

Turner, E. V., Sonnenfeld, G.: Interferon induction by the immunomodulating polyanion lambda corrageénan. Infect. Immun. **25**, 467–469 (1979).

Turner, G. S.: Rabies vaccines and interferon. J. Hyg. **70**, 445–453 (1972).

Tyring, S., Klager, K., Luk, A., Messiha, F., Lefkowitz, S.: Ethanol, disulfiram, and pyrazole: effects on interferon production in mice. Immunopharm. **2**, 63–72 (1979).

Tyrrell, A. A., Field, A. K.: Interferons and host resistance with particular emphasis on induction by complexed polynucleotides. CRC Crit. Rev. Biochem. **1**, 1–32 (1972).

Tyurina, G. P.: Activity of pig embryo kidney culture in interferon production. Vopr. Virusol. **2**, 216 (1976). (In Russian.)

Uhlendorf, G., Gordon, P., Baron, S., Baer, N.: Studies of Herpes Simplex virus and interferon in human gingival cell cultures. J. Periodont. **46**, 86 (1975).

Umenai, T., Suzuki, F., Ishida, N.: Effect of an interferon inducer 9-methylstreptimidone on *Candida albicans* infection in mice. Antimicrob. Agents Chemother. **13**, 939 (1978).

Umino, Y., Kono, S., Saito, S.: UV-irradiation of interferon-treated chick embryo cells enhances Sindbis virus growth. Arch. Virol. **52**, 351 (1976).

Underwood, P. A.: Herpes simplex infection of HEP-2 and L-929 cells. Microbios. **5**, 167–176 (1972).

Urbaniak, S. J., et al.: Neutropenia and thrombocytopenia after repeated courses of leukocyte interferon. Lancet **i**, 553–554 (1978).

Ustacelebi, S., Williams, J. F.: Temperature-sensitive mutants of adenovirus defective in interferon induction at non-permissive temperature. Nature **235**, 52–53 (1972a).

Ustacelebi, S., Williams, J. F.: Depression of interferon production in chick embryo cells by rifampicin. J. Gen. Virol. **15**, 139–148 (1972b).

Vaisrub, S.: Hepatitis B-pathways to prevention and therapy. J. A. M. Med. Assoc. **236**, 2321 (1976).

Valle, M., Cantell, K.: The ability of Sendai virus to overcome cellular resistance to vesicular stomatitis virus. Ann Med. Exp. Fenn. **43**, 57–60 (1965).

Vandenbussche, P., Content, J., Lebleu, B., Werenne, J.: Comparison of interferon action in interferon resistance and sensitive L1210 cells. J. Gen. Virol. **41**, 161–166 (1978).

Vanky, F. T., Argov, S. A., Einhorn, S. A., Klein, E.: Role of alloantigens in natural killing. Allogeneic but not autologous tumor biopsy cells are sensitive for interferon-induced cytotoxicity. J. Exp. Med. **151**, 1151–1165 (1980).

Van't Hull, E., Schellekens, H., Lowenberg, B., de Vries, M. J.: Influence of interferon preparation on the proliferative capacity of human and mouse bone marrow cell in vitro. Cancer Res. **38**, 911 (1977).

Vaquero, C. M., Clemens, M. J.: Inhibition of protein synthesis and activation of nuclease in rabbit reticulocyte lysates by the unusual oligonucleotide ppp As 'p5'A2'p5'A. Eur. J. Biochem. **98**, 245–252 (1979).

Veckenstedt, A., Witkowski, W., Hoffmann, S.: Comparison of antiviral properties in mice of bis-pyrrolidinoacetamido fluorenone and tilorone. Acta Virol. **23**, 153–158 (1979).

Vengris, V. E., Mare, C. J.: Swine interferon. I. Induction in procine cells with viral and synthetic inducers. Can. J. Comp. Med. **36**, 282–287 (1972a).

Vengris, V. E., Mare, C. J.: Swine interferon. II. Induction in pigs. Can. J. Comp. Med. **36**, 288–293 (1972b).

Vengris, V. E., Mare, C. J.: Lead poisoning in chickens and the effect of lead on interferon and antibody production. Can. J. Comp. Med. **38**, 328–335 (1974).

Veomett, M. J., Veomett, G. E.: Species specificity of interferon action: maintenance and establishment of the antiviral state in the presence of a heterospecific nucleus. J. Virol. 31, 785–794 (1979).

Veomett, M. J., Veomett, G. E.: Characteristics of the interferon system of an embryonal carcinomal cell are recessive in intraspecific somatic cell hybrids. Somatic Cell Genet. 6, 325–332 (1980).

Verma, D. S., Spitzer, G., Gutterman, J. V., Zander, A. R., McCredie, K. B., Dicke, K. A.: Human leukocyte interferon preparation blocks granulopoietic differentiation. Blood 54, 1423–1427 (1979).

Vethamany, V. G., Lee, S. H. S., Blair, D. M., Rozeee, K. R.: Scanning electron microscopy of L929 cells exposed to interferon and reovirus. Acta Virol. 21, 456–462 (1977).

Vieuchange, J., Fayaz, A., de Lalun, E.: Interférence entre le virus de la maladie de Newcastle et la virus de la rage expérimentale. C. R. Acad Sci. (Paris) D 271, 734 (1970).

Vignaux, F., Gresser, I.: Enhanced expression of histocompatibility antigens on interferon-treated mouse embryonic fibroblasts. Proc. Soc. Exp. Biol. Med. 157, 456 (1977).

Vilček, J., Freer, J. H.: Inhibition of Sindbis virus plaque formation by extracts of Escherichia coli. J. Bacter. 92, 1716–1722 (1966).

Vilček, J., Havell, E. A., Gradoville, M. L., Mika-Johnson, M. S., Douglas, W. H. J.: Selection of new human foreskin fibroblast cell strains for interferon production, in: Human interferon (Stinebring, W. R., ed.), pp. 101–118. Plenum Publ. (1978).

Vilček, J., Sulea, I. T., Zerebeckyj, I. L., Yip, Y. K.: Pharmacokinetic properties of human fibroblast and leukocyte interferon in rabbits. J. Clin. Microbiol. 11, 102–105 (1980).

Vilner, L. M., Brodskaya, L. M., Chumakov, M. P., Rodin, I. M.: Interferon-inducing activity of a double-stranded complex of polyguanilate-polycytidilate (poly-G)(poly-C) in mice and its effectiveness in experimental tick-borne encephalitis. Vopr. Virusol. 5, 545 (1972). (In Russian.)

Vilner, L. M., Finogenova, E. V., Tikhomirova-Sidorova, N. S., Rodin, I. M., Krophachev, Y. A., Kogan, E. M., Trukhmanova, L. B.: The influence of interferon inducers on formation of specific resistance to tick-borne encephalitis. Vopr. Virusol. 9, 70–75 (1976). (In Russian.)

Vilner, L. M., Kogan, E. M., Timkovsky, A. L., Tyufanov, A. V., Finogenova, E. V., Platonova, G. A.: Effects of various polyribonucleotides interferonogens on acute and latent viral infections in mice. Vopr. Virusol. 1, 67–71 (1980). (In Russian.)

Virelizier, J. L.: Effects of immunosuppressive agents on leucocyte interferon production in normal or thymus-deprived mice. Transplantation 27, 353–354 (1979).

Virelizier, J. L., Chan, E. L., Allison, A. C.: Immunosuppressive effects of lymphocyte (type II) and leucocyte (type I) interferons on primary antibody responses in vivo and in vitro. Clin. Exp. Immunol. 30, 299–305 (1977).

Virelizier, J. L., Gresser, I.: Roles of interferon in the pathogenesis of viral diseases of mice as demonstrated by the use of antiinterferon serum. V. Protective role in mouse hepatitis virus type 3 infection of susceptible and resistant strains of mice. J. Immunol. 120, 1616 (1978).

Virelizier, J. L., Guygrand, D.: Immune interferon secretion as as expresion of immunological memory to transplantation antigens – in vivo generation of long-lived recirculating memory cells. Eur. J. Immunol. 10, 375–378 (1980).

Virelizier, J. L., Lipinsky, M., Tursz, J., Griscelli, C.: Defects of immune interferon secretion and natural killer activity in patients with immunological disorders. Lancet 8144, 696 (1979).

Vladutiu, A. O.: Immune mechanisms and the action of interferon in chronic hepatitis B virus infection. Immunol. Commun. 7, 371 (1978).

Vodopija, A.: Clinical use of interferon. Lijec. Vjesn. 96, 375–377 (1974).

Vogel, S. N., Moore, R. N., Sipe, J. D., Rosenstreich, D. L.: BCG-induced enhancement of endotoxin sensitivity in C3H/HeJ mice. I. In vivo studies. J. Immunol. 124, 204–209 (1980).

Vogt, H. H.: New results in interferon research. Naturwiss. Rundsch. 29, 84–96 (1976).

Volckaert-Vervliet, G., Heremans, H., DeLey, M., Billiau, A.: Interferon induction and action in human lymphoblastoid cells infected with measles virus. J. Gen. Virol. 41, 459–466 (1978).

Von Sprockhoff, H., Rohde, G., Meyer, G.: Demonstration of antigen and interferon in rabbits infected with Borna virus. Zentralb. Bakt. Orig. A 232, 549–553 (1975).

Vorotyntseva, N. V., Baramykova, G. P., Kuznetsov, V. P., Lozovskaia, L. S., Nefedova, L. A.:
    Use of human leukocytic interferon for the prevention and treatment of respiratory viral dis-
    eases in children under hospital conditions. Pediatriia 1, 37–42 (1975).

Wade, N.: Interferon victory claimed and disclaimed. Science 207, 745 (1980).

Wagner, R. R.: Interferon control of viral infection. Assoc. Amer. Physicians 76, 92 (1963a).

Wagner, R. R.: Cellular resistance to viral infection with particular reference to endogenous inter-
    feron. Bact. Rev. 27, 72–86 (1963b).

Wagner, R. R.: Interferon. A review and analysis of recent observations. Am. J. Med. 38,
    726–737 (1965).

Waldman, R. H., Ganguly, R.: Effect of CP-20, an interferon inducer on upper respiratory tract
    infections due to Rhinovirus type 21 in volunteers. J. Infect. Dis. 138, 531–535 (1978).

Walker, S. E.: Accelerated mortality in young NZB/NZW mice treated with interferon inducer
    tilorone HCL. Clin. Immunol. Immunopathol. 8, 204 (1977).

Wallach, D., Revel, M.: Hormonal protection of interferon-treated cells against double-stranded
    RNA induced cytolysis. FEBS Lett. 101, 364–368 (1979).

Wardley, R. C., Babiuk, L. A., Rouse, B. T.: Polymorph-mediated antibody dependent cyto-
    toxicity: modulation of activity by drugs and immune interferon. Can. J. Microbiol. 22,
    1222 (1976).

Ware, C. F., Granger, G. A.: A physicochemical and immunologic comparison of the cell growth
    inhibitory activity of human lymphotoxins and interferons in vitro. J. Immunol. 122, 1763
    (1979).

Warhmofsky, F.: You can kill your own viruses. True, the man's magazine (1966).

Waschke, K., Waschke, S., Hoffman, S., Witkowski, W.: Interferon induction by double-
    stranded-like complexes of vinyl copolymers with polynucleotides. Arch. Immunol. Therap.
    Exp. 25, 627 (1977).

Watanabe, M., Sato, M.: Production of interferon induced by hyaluronic acid from Rous sarcoma.
    Cancer 29, 511–523 (1972).

Watanabe, Y., Sokawa, Y.: Effect of interferon on the cell cycle of BALB/c 3T3 cells. J. Gen.
    Virol. 41, 411–416 (1978).

Watson, K.: Immunology: damage from immune response. Nurs. Mirror 148, 40–41 (1979).

Webb, D., Braun, W., Plescia, O. J.: Antitumor effects of polynucleotides and theophylline.
    Cancer Res. 32, 1814 (1972).

Webb, H. E., Wetherley-Mein, G., Smith, C. E. G., McMahon, D.: Leukemia and neoplastic
    processes treated with Langat and Kyasanur Forest disease viruses: a clinical and laboratory
    study of 28 patients. Brit. Med. J. 1, 258–266 (1966).

Weimar, W., et al.: Fibroblast interferon in HBs-Ag positive chronic active hepatitis. Lancet ii,
    1270 (1977).

Weimar, W., Heijtink, R. A., Schalm, S. W., Schellekens, H.: Differential effects of fibroblast
    and leukocyte interferon in HBs-Ag positive chronic active hepatitis. Europ. J. Clin. Invest.
    9, 151–154 (1979).

Weimar, W., Heijtink, R. A., TenKate, F. J. P., Schalm, S. W., Masurel, N., Schellekens, H.,
    Cantell, K.: Double-blind study of leucocyte interferon administered in chronic HBs positive
    hepatitis. Lancet i, 336 (1980).

Weimar, W., Lameijer, L. D. F., Edy, V. G., Schellekens, H.: Prophylactic use of interferon in
    renal allograft recipients. Transplant. Proc. 11, 69–70 (1979).

Weimar, W., Schellekens, H.: Is it true what they say about interferon? N. Eng. J. Med. 300, 923
    (1979).

Weimar, W., Schellekens, H.: Interferon therapy for chronic hepatitis B. Lancet i, 590 (1980).

Weimar, W., Schellekens, H., Lameijer, L. D. F., Masurel, N., Edy, V. G., Billiau, A., De-
    Somer, P.: Double-blind study of interferon administration in renal transplant recipients.
    Europ. J. of Clin. Invest. (1979).

Weimar, W., Stitz, L., Billiau, A., Cantell, K., Schellekens, H.: Prevention of vaccinia lesions in
    Rhesus monkeys by human leukocyte and fibroblast interferon. J. Gen. Virol. 48, 25–30
    (1980).

Weinmann, E., Majer, M., Hilfenhaus, J.: Intramuscular and/or intralumbar postexposure treatment of rabies virus infected monkeys with human interferon. Infect. Immun. **24**, 24–31 (1979).

Weinstein, Y., Brodeur, B. R., Melmon, K. L., Merigan, T. C.: Interferon inhibition of lymphocyte mitogenesis. Immunology **33**, 313 (1977).

Weintraub, M., Sheagren, J. N.: Interferon in malaria. Ann. Intern. Med. **13**, 1045–1046 (1970).

Weissenbach, J., Zeevi, M., Landau, T., Revel, M.: Identification of the translation products of human fibroblast interferon mRNA in reticulocyte lysates. Eur. J. Biochem. **98**, 1–8 (1979).

Weissenbacher, M., Chowchuvech, E., Schmunis, G., Sawicki, L., Galin, M. A.: Sensitivity of human conjunctival tissue cultures to adenovirus 8, herpes simplex and vaccinia viruses. Induction of resistance by an interferon inducer. Proc. Soc. Exp. Biol. Med. **142**, 997 (1973).

Welsh, R. M., Hallenbeck, L. A.: Effect of virus infections on target cell susceptibility to natural killer cell-mediated lysis. J. Immunol. **124**, 2491–2497 (1980).

Werenne, J., Revel, M.: Triggering of protein phosphorylation in human cell system by interferon and double-stranded RNA. Arch. Int. Physiol. Biochem. **86**, 471 (1978).

West, D. K., Baglioni, C.: Induction by interferon in HeLa cells of a protein kinase activiated by dsRNA. Europ. J. Biochem. **101**, 461–468 (1979).

Westhues, M., Mayr, A.: Human interferon inducer therapy in clinical use. Arch. Oto. Rhino. Laryngol. **210**, 257 (1975).

Wheelock, E. F.: Inhibition of virus induced leukemia in mice by a non-tumor virus. Natl. Cancer Inst. Monograph **22**, 73–76 (1965).

Whitley, R. J., Arvin, A., Merigan, T., Galasso, G., Dunnick, J.: Distribution of adenine arabinoside and interferon. J. Amer. Med. Ass. **242**, 1259 (1979).

Wieranga, W., Skulnick, H. I., Stringfellow, D. A., Weed, S. D., Renis, H. E., Eidson, E. E.: 5-substituted 2-amino-6-phenyl-4(5H)-pyrimidinones, antiviral and interferon-inducing agents. J. Medicinal Chem. **23**, 237–239 (1980).

Wietzerbin, J., Stefanos, S., Falcoff, R., Lucero, M., Catinot, L., Falcoff, E.: Immune interferon-induced by phytohemagglutinin in nude mouse spleen cells. Infect. Immun. **21**, 966 (1978).

Wietzerbin, J., Stefanos, S., Lucero, M., Falcoff, E., O'Malley, J. A., Sulkowski, E.: Physicochemical characterization and partial purification of mouse immune interferon. J. Gen. Virol. **44**, 773–783 (1979).

Wietzerbin, J., Stefanos, S., Lucero, M., Falcoff, E., Thang, D. C., Thang, M. N.: Presence of a polynucleotide binding site on murine immune interferon (T-type). Biochem. Biophys. Res. Commun. **85**, 480–489 (1978).

Wildstein, A., Stevens, L., Applebaum, H., McCabe, R. E., Hashim, G.: Prolongation of allografts in animals with a new agent tilorone. Proc. Clin. Diai. Transplant Forum **5**, 47–50 (1975).

Williams, B. R. G., Golgher, R. R., Brown, R. E., Gilbert, C. S., Kerr, I. M.: Natural occurrence of 2–5 A in interferon-treated EMC virus-infected L cells. Nature **282**, 582 (1979).

Williams, B. R. G., Kalmakoff, J.: Detection of dsRNA in Semliki forest virus infected cells by an indirect solid phase radioimmunoassay: an assay for interferon. Intervirology **8**, 110 (1977).

Williams, B. R. G., Kerr, I. M.: Inhibition of protein synthesis by 2'–5'-linked adenine oligonucleotides in intact cells. Nature **276**, 88–90 (1978).

Williams, B. R. G., Kerr, I. M.: The 2-5A (pppA2'p5'A2'p5'A) system in interferon-treated and control cells. Trends Biochem. Sci. **5**, 138–139 (1980).

Williams, B. R. G., Kerr, I. M., Gilbert, C. S., White, C. N., Ball, L. A.: Synthesis and breakdown of ppp A2'p5'A2'p5'A and transient inhibition of protein synthesis in extracts from interferon treated and control cells. Europ. J. Biochem. **92**, 455–470 (1978).

Williams, R., Eddleston, A. L.: Chronic active hepatitis: immunopathogenesis and immunotherapy. Isr. J. Med. Sci. **15**, 261–275 (1979).

Winston, S. H., Rustigian, R.: Enhancement and suppression by actinomycin D of a Vero cell nontransmissible measles infection. Infect. Immun. **24**, 967–970 (1979).

Wiranowska-Stewart, M., Lin, L. S., Braude, I. A., Stewart II, W. E.: Production, partial purification and characterization of human and murine interferons-type II. Molecular Immunol. **17**, 625–634 (1979).

Wiranowska-Stewart, M., Lin, L. S., Braude, I. A., Stewart II, W. E.: Comparisons of the physicochemical and biological properties of human, murine and bovine interferons, types I and II, in: Biochemical Characterization of Lymphokines (deWeck, A., ed.), pp. 331–338. New York: Academic Press (1980).

Wirth, J. J., Levy, M. H., Wheelock, E. F.: Use of silica to identify host mechanism involved in suppression of established Friend virus leukemia. J. Immunol. 117, 2124–2130 (1976).

Wohlenberg, C., Openshaw, H., Notkins, A. L.: In vitro system for studying the efficacy of antiviral agents in preventing the reactivation of latent herpes simplex virus. Antimicrob. Agents Chemother. 15, 625–627 (1979).

Wolinsky, J. S., Dau, P. C., Buimovici-Klein, E., Melnick, J., Berg, B. O., Lang, P. B., Cooper, L. Z.: Progressive rubella panencephalitis: immunovirological studies and results of isoprinosine therapy. Clin. Exp. Immunol. 35, 397–404 (1979).

Wong, K. T., Robinson, W. S., Merigan, T. C.: Inhibition of rubella virus – specific RNA synthesis by interferon. Proc. Soc. Exp. Biol. Med. 136, 615–618 (1971).

Wood, J. N.: Lack of detectable nuclease activity in highly purified preparations of murine fibroblast interferon. Molec. Biol. Rep. 5, 253–256 (1979).

Wood, J. N., Hovanessian, A. G.: Interferon enhances 2–5'A synthetase in embryonal carcinoma cells. Nature 282, 74–76 (1979).

Worthington, M.: Interferon system in mice infected with the scrapie agent. Infect. Immun. 6, 643–645 (1972).

Worthington, M., Baron, S.: Effect of polyriboinosinic·polyribocytidylic acid and antibody on infection of immunosuppressed mice with vaccinia virus. J. Infect. Dis. 128, 308 (1973).

Wu, J. M., Cheung, C. P., Bruzel, A. R., Suhadolnik, R. J.: The reversal of inhibition of protein synthesis by dsRNA in lysed rabbit reticulocytes with fructose 6-phosphate. Biochem. Biophys. Res. Commun. 86, 648–653 (1979).

Yabrov, A. A.: Nonantiviral protective action of interferon and the problem of nonspecific resistance of the cell. Adv. Mod. Biol. (Mosc.) 74, 97–120 (1972).

Yabrov, A. A.: Interferon and cell-mediated immunity. Med. Hypotheses 5, 769–798 (1979).

Yagi, M. J., King, N. W., Bekesi, J. G.: Alterations of a mouse mammary tumor virus glycoprotein with interferon treatment. J. Virol. 34, 225–233 (1980).

Yakobson, E., Revel, M., Gurari-Rotman, D.: Monkey interferon: activity on human cells and chromatographic properties. Arch. Virol. 59, 251–256 (1979).

Yamamoto, Y.: Two molecular species of mouse L-cell interferon differing in lectin binding. J. Gen. Virol. 42, 533–540 (1979).

Yamamoto, Y., Kawade, Y.: Antigenicity of mouse interferons: distinct antigenicity of the two L cell interferon species. Virology 103, 80–88 (1980).

Yamamoto, Y., Tomida, M., Hozumi, M.: Stimulation of differentiation of mouse myeloid leukemic cells and induction of interferon in the cells by double-stranded polyribonucleotides. Cancer Res. 39, 4170–4174 (1979).

Yamamura, Y., Y., Cochran, K. W.: Effect of diethylpyrocarbonate on the antiviral and interferon-inducing activities of viral and non-viral agents. Antimicrob. Agents Chemother. 9, 675 (1976).

Yamamura, Y., Kato, H., Hanazawa, S., Yamaguchi, Y.: Induction of interferon in mice injected with heat-killed corynebacterium-anaerobium. Jap. J. Exp. Med. 48, 69 (1978).

Yang, S. C., Hsia, S.: Interferon production of human leukemic cells and in vitro assay. J. Formosan Med. Assoc. 72, 612–618 (1973).

Yaron, M., Yaron, I., Wiletzki, C., Zor, U.: Interferon in synovial fibroblast culture. Arthrit. Rheum. 21, 694 (1978).

Yasuhiko, I., Nagata, I., Kunii, A.: Mechanism of endotoxin-type interferon production in mice. Virology 52, 439 (1973).

Yau, P. M. P., Godefroy-Colburn, T., Birge, C. H., Ramabhadran, T. V., Thach, R. E.: Specificity of interferon action in protein synthesis. J. Virol. 27, 648 (1978).

Yonehara, S., Iwakura, Y., Kawade, Y.: Rapid purification of mouse L-cell interferon labeled with radioactive amino acid by immune precipitation. Virology 100, 125–129 (1980).

Yoshida, I., Azuma, M., Suenaga, T., Mizuno, F.: Regulation of interferon production by dibutyryl cyclic GMP in serum-free human diploid cell cultures. J. Gen. Virol. 39, 303 (1978).

Young, C. W.: Interferon. CA, A Cancer J. for Clinicians 22, 27–29 (1972).

Youngner, J. S., Salvin, S. B.: Type I and II interferons and migration inhibitory factor: production in mycobacterium bovis BCG-infected mice desensitized with old tuberculin or lipopolysaccharide. Infect. Immun. **19**, 912 (1974).

Zagorodnaia, I. S., Rybalko, S. L.: Interferon formation in influenza. Vrach. Delo **7**, 135–137 (1973).

Zaitseva, O. V., Tazulakhova, E. B., Ershov, F. I.: Isolation and characterization of informative RNA of interferon production repressor. Antibiotiki **25**, 215–217 (1980).

Zaratskii, I. Z., Petukhova, M. B., Ershov, F. I.: An isoelectric focusing study of chick and mouse interferons. Bull. Exp. Biol. Med. **86**, 1040–1042 (1978).

Zarling, J. M., Eskra, L., Borden, E. C., Horoszowicz, J., Carter, W. A.: Activation of human natural killer cells cytotoxic for human leukemia cells by purified interferon. J. Immunol. **123**, 63–70 (1979).

Zarling, J. M., Soaman, J., Eskra, L., Borden, E., Horoszowicz, J. S., Carter, W. A.: Enhancement of T cell cytotoxic responses by purified human fibroblast interferon. J. Immunol. **121**, 2002–2004 (1978).

Zasukhina, G. D., Barkova, E. P., Shvetsova, T. P., Andronova, A. V., Bektemirov, T. A., Andzhaparide, O. G.: Effect of the interferon in vitro on development of chromosomal aberrations and mytotic activity of human diploid cells after the action of 4-nitroguinolin-1-oxide. Vopr. Virusol. **5**, 544–546 (1979). (In Russian.)

Zawatzky, R., Hilfenhaus, J., Kirchner, H.: Resistance of nude mice to Herpes simplex virus and correlation with *in vitro* production of interferon. Cell. Immunol. **47**, 424–428 (1979).

Zee, Y. C., Osebold, J. W., Dotson, W. M.: Antibody responses and interferon titers in the respiratory tracts of mice after aerosolized exposure to influenza virus. Infect. Immun. **25**, 202–212 (1979).

Zeitlenok, N. A., Konosh, O. V., Kasparov, A. A., Fadeeva, L. L.: Determination of the interferon level in the blood, conjunctival washings and urine of patients with herpetic keratoiridocyclitis treated with interferonogen. Antibiotiki **19**, 759–762 (1974).

Zielinska-Jenczylik, J., Rzucidlo, Z., Sypula, A., Blach-Olszen, H., Kidankiewicz, T.: Production of interferon in human diploid cell cultures. Arch. Immunol. Ther. Exp. (Warsz.) **24**, 769–775 (1976).

Zilberstein, A., Content, J., Lebleu, B., Berissi, M., Shulman, L. M., Revel, M.: Mechanism of the interferon-induced block of mRNA translation in mouse L cells and its reversal by t-RNA. Isr. J. Med. Sci. **11**, 1211 (1975).

Zilberstein, A., Kimchi, A., Schmidt, A., Revel, M.: Isolation of 2 interferon-induced translational inhibitors: protein kinase and an oligo-isoadenylate synthetase. Proc. Natl. Acad. Sci. U.S.A. **75**, 4734–4738 (1978).

Zoon, K. C., Bridgen, P. J., Smith, M. E.: Production of human lymphoblastoid interferon by Namalva cells cultured in serum-free media. J. Gen. Virol. **44**, 227–230 (1979).

Zoon, K. C., Buckler, C. E., Bridgen, P. J., Gurari-Rotman, D.: Production of human lymphoblastoid interferon by Namalva cells. J. Clin. Microbiol. **7**, 44–51 (1978).

Zoon, K. C., Smith, M. E., Bridgen, P. J., ZurNedden, D., Anfinsen, C. B.: Purification and partial characterization of human lymphoblastoid interferon. Proc. Natl. Acad. Sci. U.S.A. **76**, 5601–5605 (1979).

Zoon, K. C., Smith, M. E., Bridgen, P. J., Anfinsen, C. B., Hunkapiller, M. W., Hood, L. E.: Amino-terminal sequence of the major component of human lymphoblastoid interferon. Science **207**, 527–528 (1980).

Zozikov, W., Mietens, C.: Multiplication of virulent and attenuated poliovirus strains during inhibition of interferon synthesis by actinomycin D. Immun. Infekt. **2**, 83–84 (1974).

Zschiesche, W., Fahlbusch, B., Schumann, I., Lackovic, V., Borecky, L.: Production of interferon and other lymphokines during murine tumor growth. I. Lymphokines in cell-free fluid or rat ascites hepatoma. Acta Virol. **23**, 37–44 (1980).

Zschiesche, W., Slavina, E., Leipunskaya, I.: The interferonogenic agent tilorone as a modulator of GvH reaction in mice. Arch. Immun. Therap. Exp. **25**, 725–730 (1977).

Zuckerman, A. J.: Recent advances in viral hepatitis types A and B. Isr. J. Med. Sci. **15**, 231–239 (1979).

Subject Index

By Robert Zolnerzak, Brooklyn, New York

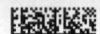